The New American Heart Association Cookbook

9TH EDITION

9TH EDITION

The New American Heart Association Cookbook

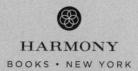

HARMONY

BOOKS · NEW YORK

Copyright © 2019 by American Heart Association

All rights reserved.

Previous editions published in the United States in 1973, 1975, 1979, 1984, 1991, 1998, 2004, 2010, and 2017.

Published in the United States by Harmony Books, an imprint of Random House, a division of Penguin Random House LLC, New York. harmonybooks.com

Harmony Books is a registered trademark, and the Circle colophon is a trademark of Penguin Random House LLC.

Your contributions to the American Heart Association support research that helps make publications like this possible. For more information, call 1-800-AHA-USA1 (1-800-242-8721) or contact us online at www.heart.org.

Library of Congress Cataloging-in-Publication Data has been applied for.

ISBN 978-0-553-44720-0

Ebook ISBN 978-0-553-44719-4

Printed in the United States of America

Cover design by Jennifer Carrow
Front cover photographs: Broiled Salmon over Garden-Fresh Corn and Bell Peppers (page 149) and Poached Eggs with Pesto Bulgur (page 309). Spine photograph: Gazpacho (page 49). Back cover photographs: Ginger-Berry Wonton Baskets (page 500) and Chili Meatballs (page 283). Cover photographs by Ben Fink.

10 9 8 7 6 5 4 3

First Paperback Edition

Contents

Acknowledgments

American Heart Association Consumer Publications

MANAGING EDITOR
Deborah A. Renza

ASSISTANT MANAGING EDITOR
Roberta Westcott Sullivan

Recipe Developers for This and Previous Editions

Ellen C. Boeke

Janice Cole

Claire Criscuolo

Sarah Fritschner

FRP

Nancy S. Hughes

Ruth Mossok Johnston

Jackie Mills, M.S., R.D.

Carol Ritchie

Julie Shapiro, R.D., L.D.

Francine Wolfe Schwartz

Marjorie Steenson

Linda Foley Woodrum

NUTRITION ANALYST
Tammi Hancock, R.D.

Healthy Eating, Healthy Heart

In this new edition of the American Heart Association's cornerstone cookbook, you'll find more than 800 recipes, with heart-healthy dishes covering every meal of the day, including breakfasts, snacks, beverages, and desserts, designed to satisfy every craving. More than 100 of the recipes are new and 250 of them are refreshed from the association's previous cookbooks, which means they've been updated for the way we cook and eat today, whether it's new ingredients, spices, or herbs or a different cooking technique. In the headnotes throughout, you'll find suggestions for complementary recipes to help you easily plan a meal. In some cases, we've suggest pairing entrées with side dishes or desserts that bake at the same temperature in the oven or that both use the grill so that putting together a meal can be convenient and time-saving. Also new to this edition is a special chapter with more than 20 delicious slow-cooker recipes, including Italian Wedding Soup (page 109), Chicken Sofrito (page 113), and Smoky Pulled Pork with Barbecue Sauce (page 122).

As you plan your meals at home—and when you make food choices away from home—what matters most is to establish a well-balanced diet. To do this, keep the following basics in mind, and then eating well can be as easy as 1-2-3.

1. Include a wide variety of nutritious foods from all the food groups.
2. Limit foods that include nutrients that are detrimental to good health.
3. Choose the right foods in the right portions.

Here's what to include in your diet:

- Fruits and vegetables
- Whole grains
- Fat-free, 1%, and low-fat dairy products
- Oily fish
- Skinless poultry
- Lean cuts of meat
- Healthy fats and oils
- Legumes, nuts, and seeds

FRUITS AND VEGETABLES

Whether they are fresh, frozen, or canned, vegetables and fruits are beneficial sources of potassium, magnesium, and fiber. If buying canned, choose the no-salt-added and no-sugar-added varieties.

To increase fruits and vegetables in your diet, try these three steps:

1. Make fruits and vegetables your go-to snack and dessert choices. Enjoy Luscious Berry Dip (page 16), Crunchy Parmesan-Garlic Snap Peas (page 27), Apple Pie Pops (page 504), Peach-Plum Crumble (page 491), or Spiced Skillet Bananas (page 503).

2. Choose entrées that include fruits and/or vegetables, such as Grilled Pineapple-Lime Salmon (page 150), Cider-Glazed Turkey Tenderloin with Harvest Vegetables (page 233), Jamaican Jerk Pork and Vegetables with Mango-Coconut Rice (page 294), or Pasta Primavera (page 345) to get in more servings of these food groups each day.

3. Vary your choices by color; fill your grocery cart with a rainbow of fruits and vegetables to get the widest variety of vitamins and minerals.

WHOLE GRAINS

Grains are a major source of energy and fiber. Any food made of wheat, rice, oats, corn, or another cereal is a grain product. There are two main types of grains: whole and refined. A whole grain is a healthier choice than a refined grain because a whole grain contains the bran, germ, and endosperm—where many of the grain's nutrients are stored.

To increase whole grains in your diet, try these three steps:

1. Eat whole-grain products for at least half of the grains you eat. For example, replace the white bread with whole wheat on a turkey sandwich and choose whole-grain pasta for a spaghetti and meatball dinner.

2. Get your day started out with a healthy breakfast including a whole-grain cold cereal, oatmeal, or whole-wheat toast. Try Cocoa-Banana Oatmeal (page 472), Apple-Berry Couscous (page 471), or Raisin Bran Bread (page 451).

3. Choose side dishes that include a whole grain such as brown rice, quinoa, buckwheat, wild rice, barley, bulgur, farro, couscous, grits, and corn. Give these a try: Bulgur Pilaf with Lemon and Spinach (page 416), Toasted Farro with Caramelized Carrots and Sweet Potatoes (page 420), or Couscous with Dates and Walnuts (page 417).

FAT-FREE, 1%, AND LOW-FAT DAIRY PRODUCTS

Dairy foods are an important part of a healthy diet, providing calcium, protein, potassium, and vitamin D in fortified products. You can easily avoid the high levels of saturated fat found in whole milk and whole-milk products by choosing fat-free and low-fat dairy counterparts.

To healthfully include dairy in your diet, try these three steps:

1. If you drink whole milk, gradually transition to 2% fat, then 1%, and finally fat-free, which has the fewest calories and the least unhealthy fats. To get started and let your taste buds adjust, pour half of a glass of whole milk and then fill the other half with a reduced-fat version.

2. Enjoy fat-free and low-fat plain yogurt for breakfast or an afternoon snack just by itself or in a smoothie or parfait. Be sure to get creative with adding chopped unsalted nuts and a variety of fruits—and even vegetables! Try Carrot Cake Smoothie (page 30) and Blackberry-Pomegranate Yogurt Parfaits (page 479) as delicious examples.
3. Read Nutrition Facts panels on dairy products. If you compare a cup of whole milk to a cup of fat-free milk, for example, you'll see that by choosing the fat-free version, you'll save about 65 calories and 4.5 grams of saturated fat. Also, be mindful of the amount of sodium in cheese and added sugars in yogurt. Often these nutrients are higher in low-fat cheeses and yogurts than in their full-fat versions, so compare products and make healthy choices.

OILY FISH

Fish is a good source of protein, magnesium, and omega-3 fatty acids. Omega-3s have positive cardiovascular benefits so they're important to include in your diet.

To healthfully include fish in your diet, try these three steps:

1. Include fish rich in omega-3s, such as salmon, lake trout, herring, sardines, mackerel, and albacore tuna. Prepare Salmon Cakes with Creole Aïoli (page 151), Trout with Fresh Tomatoes and Capers (page 163), Sautéed Lemon-Garlic Sardines and Fennel with Fettuccine (page 152), or Tuna-Artichoke Casserole with Basil and Dill (page 167).

2. Eat fish that's been prepared with a healthy cooking technique, such as baked, poached, grilled, or broiled, rather than battered and fried. Choose Baked Trout with Tartar Sauce (page 162), Fish in Crazy Water (page 134), Grilled Tuna with Smoky-Sweet Fruit Salsa (page 164), or Ginger Broiled Fish (page 133).
3. When buying the frozen or canned varieties, be sure to read the Nutrition Facts panel and choose lower sodium options.

SKINLESS POULTRY

Lean skinless poultry is a source of essential protein, which helps you feel full and satisfied until your next meal.

To healthfully include poultry in your diet, try these three steps:

1. Read the front packaging labels and choose poultry that hasn't been injected with broth, salt, or seasonings.
2. Trim away any visible fat before cooking.
3. Remove the skin before eating.

LEAN CUTS OF MEAT

Meat can be part of a heart-healthy diet if eaten in moderation.

To healthfully include meat in your diet, try these three steps:

1. Trim away any visible fat before cooking.
2. Choose lean and extra-lean meats such as sirloin, top sirloin, round steak, and eye-of-round, extra-lean ground beef, flank steak, pork loin chops, pork tenderloin, and the lowest sodium available center-cut ham.

Buy "choice" or "select" grades of beef rather than "prime."

3. Limit processed meats such as bacon, hot dogs, bologna, salami, and sausage; they contain sodium, nitrates, and other food additives.

HEALTHY FATS AND OILS

Fats are divided into two types: saturated ("bad") and unsaturated ("good"). The good fats, polyunsaturated and monounsaturated, are found in healthy unsaturated vegetable oils, nuts, and oily fish.

To healthfully include oils and fats in your diet, try these three steps:

1. Cook with liquid nontropical vegetable oil including canola, corn, olive, safflower, sesame, soybean, and sunflower.

2. Choose trans-fat-free soft margarines and trans-fat-free stick margarines.

3. Read ingredient labels and choose products whose first ingredient is unsaturated liquid vegetable oil rather than hydrogenated or partially hydrogenated oil.

LEGUMES, NUTS, AND SEEDS

Legumes, nuts, and seeds are beneficial sources of energy, magnesium, protein, and fiber. They are excellent alternatives to animal sources of protein that contain saturated fat.

To healthfully include legumes, nuts, and seeds in your diet, try these three steps:

1. Eat small portions of nuts and seeds since they are high in calories.

2. Choose unsalted varieties of nuts and seeds including almonds, pecans, walnuts, peanuts, pistachios, hazelnuts, pumpkin seeds, sunflower

seeds, and peanut butter (low sodium) and enjoy them as is or in side dishes, breads, and desserts. Try Pecan Broccoli (page 376), Zucchini Bread with Pistachios (page 458), or Dark Chocolate Walnut Cookies (page 487).

3. Include dried and no-salt-added canned legumes such as green peas, black-eyed peas, chickpeas, split peas, kidney beans, navy beans, black beans, and lentils not only in vegetarian main meals but also in snacks, such as Edamame Guacamole (page 15) and Pizza-Flavored Roasted Chickpeas (page 28), and soups, such as Lentil Chili Soup (page 61) and Tuscan Kale and Cannellini Bean Soup (page 59).

Here's what to limit in your diet:

- Saturated fat
- Trans fat
- Sodium
- Added sugars

SATURATED FAT AND TRANS FAT

There are two kinds of "bad" fats that are harmful to heart health: saturated fat and trans fat. Saturated fats are found in animal products and some tropical oils; trans fats are found primarily in commercial products created in an industrial process that adds hydrogen to liquid vegetable oils to make them more solid. Saturated and trans fats raise blood cholesterol. High levels of blood cholesterol is a risk factor for heart disease and stroke.

To reduce saturated and trans fats in your diet, try these three steps:

1. Fats and oils high in saturated fat tend to become hard at room

temperature, including butter, some stick margarines, and shortening; replace these with healthier unsaturated choices (see page 4).

2. Read the Nutrition Facts panel on packaged or commercially processed products such as fried foods and baked goods. Since products can be listed as "0 grams of *trans* fats" if they contain 0 grams to less than 0.5 grams of *trans* fat per serving, also read ingredients lists and look for "partially hydrogenated oils" to spot a product that contains *trans* fats.

3. Limit full-fat dairy products as well as fatty cuts of meats.

SODIUM

Most of the sodium—75 percent—that we consume comes from salt added to packaged and processed foods and restaurant foods. The top six types of food that contribute the most sodium in our diets include bread/rolls, cured meats/cold cuts, pizza, burritos/tacos, soups, and sandwiches. Eating too much sodium can raise your high blood pressure, which is a risk factor for heart disease and stroke.

To reduce the sodium in your diet, try these three steps:

1. Compare the Nutrition Facts label on foods when you grocery shop and choose no-salt-added or lowest-sodium products.

2. Eat more home-cooked meals so you can better control the sodium in your foods.

3. When dining out, review online menus and nutritional information ahead of time to make smart choices.

ADDED SUGARS

Sugars in foods can be naturally occurring or added. Naturally occurring sugars are found *naturally* in foods such as fruit (fructose) and milk (lactose). Added sugars are those put in foods during preparation or processing, or added at the table. Added sugars contribute zero nutrients but many additional calories that can lead to overweight or even obesity, which are both risk factors for heart disease and stroke.

To reduce the added sugars in your diet, try these three steps:

1. Replace beverages and foods that contain high levels of added sugars including regular soft drinks, fruit drinks, sports drinks, candy, baked goods, and ice cream with sparkling water, unsweetened tea, sugar-free beverages, and 100% fruit juice, as well as fresh and dried fruits.

2. Read ingredients lists on food packages and look for words such as *syrup, molasses, honey, cane juice, corn sweetener,* or *fruit juice concentrate,* which all are forms of added sugar, and limit these foods. Keep in mind that the closer these words are to the beginning of the ingredients list, the more sugar is in the product.

3. Read the Nutrition Facts panel on products and look for Added Sugars. For products that don't have the new labeling, it may be helpful to calculate the calories per serving from *total* sugars (added sugars and naturally occurring sugars). To do this, you can multiply the grams of sugar by 4 (there are 4 calories per 1 gram of sugar). For example, a product containing 15 grams of

sugar has 60 calories from sugar per serving.

PORTION CONTROL

As part of an overall healthy eating plan, it's important to know not only what to eat but also how much to eat. Recognizing and eating reasonable serving sizes is a key element in maintaining a weight that's healthy for you. Visualizing healthy servings of foods is a good way to do this. A healthy portion of an entrée is 3 ounces of cooked meat, poultry, or fish, which is about equal to the size of a deck of playing cards. A portion-controlled side dish is usually a 1/2 cup serving; picture this as about the size of a baseball.

By keeping a few simple guiding principles in mind along with a variety of delicious recipes on hand, you'll enjoy a lifetime of healthy eating. Combine smart eating with a few healthy lifestyle recommendations and you'll be well equipped to live a heart-healthy life.

Healthy Lifestyle, Healthy Heart

Although some risk factors for heart disease and stroke, such as increasing age, family history, and ethnicity, can't be changed, many of the most damaging risk factors are things you can control as part of a healthy lifestyle.

MAINTAIN A HEALTHY WEIGHT

Being overweight or obese increases your likelihood of developing heart disease and stroke even if you have no other risk factors. If you consistently take in more calories than you burn through physical activity, you will gradually gain weight. To best manage your weight, eat the right amount of calories for you and participate in regular physical activity. Talk to your healthcare provider who will determine what a healthy weight is for you.

EXERCISE REGULARLY

The American Heart Association suggests at least 150 minutes of moderately intense physical activity per week or 75 minutes of vigorous physical activity per week (or a combination of both) and moderate-to-high-intensity muscle strengthening activity at least twice per week. Preferably, aerobic activity should be spread throughout the week. Keep in mind that some physical activity is better than none. Examples of moderate activities are walking briskly, general gardening, yoga, and water aerobics; vigorous activities include swimming laps, aerobic dancing, and jogging. Even light intensity activities are better for you than sitting. Any amount of activity results in at least some benefit.

DON'T SMOKE OR BREATH TOBACCO SMOKE

If you smoke, ask your healthcare provider about the best ways to quit. When you stop smoking, your risk for heart disease and stroke drops rapidly.

DRINK ALCOHOL IN MODERATION—OR NOT AT ALL

If you do drink alcohol, do so in moderation. Drinking in moderation means no more than one drink per day for women or two drinks per day for men. One drink is equal to 12 ounces of beer, 5 ounces of wine, or 1 1/2 ounces of 80-proof distilled spirits. If you don't drink, don't start.

SCHEDULE REGULAR MEDICAL CHECKUPS

Make an appointment with your healthcare provider for a heart checkup to find out your numbers for your blood pressure, cholesterol, blood sugar, and weight. Be sure to discuss your personal risk for cardiovascular disease and create an appropriate action plan for you to reduce your risk for heart attack and stroke.

About the Recipes

Each recipe in the book includes a nutrition analysis so you can decide how that dish fits with your dietary needs. These guidelines will give you some details on how the analyses were calculated.

Because of the many variables involved, the nutrient values provided should be considered approximate. When figuring portions, also remember that the serving sizes are approximate.

- Each analysis is for a *single* serving; garnishes or optional ingredients are *not* included unless otherwise noted.
- When ingredient options are listed, the first one is analyzed.
- When a range of amounts is given, the average is analyzed.
- All the recipes are analyzed using unsalted or low-sodium ingredients whenever possible. In some cases, we call for unprocessed foods or no-salt-added and low-sodium products, then add table salt sparingly for flavor. If only a regular commercial product is available, we use the one with the lowest sodium.

- We specify canola, corn, and olive oils in these recipes, but you can also use other heart-healthy unsaturated oils, such as safflower, soybean, and sunflower.
- Values other than fats are rounded to the nearest half gram. Because of rounding, values for saturated, trans, monounsaturated, and polyunsaturated fats may not add up to the amount shown for total fat value.
- For recipes that call for broth, we used our homemade broths (pages 35–37) in the analyses. We encourage you to make your own broth to keep sodium low and flavor high. If you do use store-bought broths, be sure to choose the products lowest in sodium and fat.
- Meats are analyzed as lean, with all visible fat discarded. Values for ground beef are based on lean meat that is 95 percent fat free.
- When meat, poultry, or seafood is marinated and the marinade is

discarded, the analysis includes all the sodium from the marinade but none of the other nutrients from it.

- If alcohol is used in a cooked dish, we estimate that most of the alcohol calories evaporate as the food cooks.
- Because product labeling in the marketplace can vary and change quickly, we use the generic terms "fat-free" and "low-fat" throughout to avoid confusion.
- We use the abbreviations *g* for gram and *mg* for milligram.

Appetizers, Snacks, and Beverages

ARTICHOKE DIP

SERVES 16

Surround a bowl of this dip with unsalted whole-grain crackers or baked chips, or serve with crisp carrot, celery, and jicama sticks.

- 1/2 cup fat-free plain yogurt
- 4 ounces light tub cream cheese, at room temperature
- 2 medium green onions (green part only), thinly sliced
- 1 1/2 teaspoons cream sherry
- 1 teaspoon dried Italian seasoning, crumbled
- 1/8 teaspoon garlic powder
- 1/8 teaspoon salt
- 9 ounces frozen artichoke hearts, thawed, patted dry, and finely chopped

In a medium bowl, stir together all the ingredients except the artichokes.

Stir in the artichokes. Cover and refrigerate for at least 1 hour. Stir just before serving.

PER SERVING

calories 29	sodium 65 mg
total fat 1.0 g	carbohydrates 3 g
saturated fat 0.5 g	fiber 1 g
trans fat 0.0 g	sugars 1 g
polyunsaturated fat 0.0 g	protein 1 g
monounsaturated fat 0.5 g	DIETARY EXCHANGES
cholesterol 5 mg	free

SMOKED SALMON PARTY DIP

SERVES 20

A hollowed-out red cabbage bowl makes a striking container for this dip, especially when you surround it with strips of brilliantly colored bell peppers. What a great way to lure your guests to a heart-healthy dip!

- 1 cup fat-free cottage cheese
- 1 cup fat-free sour cream
- 3 ounces smoked salmon, chopped
- 4 medium green onions, finely chopped
- 2 teaspoons fresh lemon juice
- 1/4 teaspoon garlic powder

In a food processor or blender, process the cottage cheese for 30 seconds, or until smooth. Transfer to a medium bowl.

Stir in the remaining ingredients. Cover and refrigerate until serving time.

PER SERVING

calories 27	sodium 139 mg
total fat 0.0 g	carbohydrates 3 g
saturated fat 0.0 g	fiber 0 g
trans fat 0.0 g	sugars 2 g
polyunsaturated fat 0.0 g	protein 3 g
monounsaturated fat 0.0 g	DIETARY EXCHANGES
cholesterol 4 mg	1/2 lean meat

YELLOW SPLIT PEA DIP

SERVES 4

This mildly flavored dip, commonly known as Greek Fava, is traditional in Santorini, but can be found in other parts of Greece as well. It's best served warm with crusty whole-grain bread, but is also delicious when served at room temperature or even cold.

- 1 cup yellow split peas, sorted for stones and shriveled peas, rinsed, and drained
- 1/2 cup chopped onion
- 2 medium garlic cloves, chopped
- 1/4 cup fresh lemon juice (about 1 large lemon)
- 2 tablespoons olive oil (extra-virgin preferred)
- 3/8 teaspoon salt
- 1 medium lemon, cut into 4 wedges

In a large saucepan, stir together the peas, onion, and garlic. Add enough water to cover by 1 inch. Bring to a boil over high heat. Discard any foam. Reduce the heat and simmer, covered, for 1 1/2 to 2 hours, or until the peas are thick and creamy and the liquid is absorbed. Remove from the heat. Let stand for 10 minutes.

In a food processor or blender, process the pea mixture, lemon juice, oil, and salt for 30 seconds to 1 minute, or until smooth. Serve with the lemon wedges.

Cook's Tip: If you have an immersion blender, you can stir the lemon juice, oil, and salt into the peas and purée in the saucepan.

PER SERVING

calories 241	carbohydrates 33 g
total fat 7.5 g	fiber 13 g
saturated fat 1.0 g	sugars 5 g
trans fat 0.0 g	protein 13 g
polyunsaturated fat 1.0 g	DIETARY EXCHANGES
monounsaturated fat 5.0 g	2 starch, 1 lean meat,
cholesterol 0 mg	1 fat
sodium 226 mg	

ROASTED-PEPPER HUMMUS

SERVES 8

Roasted bell pepper not only boosts the flavor of this creamy chickpea spread but adds vibrant color as well. Serve with Peppercorn-Dill Flatbread *(page 449), heart-healthy crackers, or vegetable dippers, such as broccoli florets, sugar snap peas, or even asparagus spears.*

> 2 tablespoons sesame seeds, dry-roasted
> 1 15.5-ounce can no-salt-added chickpeas, rinsed and drained
> 1/2 cup diced roasted red bell pepper, drained if bottled
> 1/4 cup water
> 2 tablespoons fresh lime juice
> 1 medium garlic clove, minced
> 1/4 teaspoon salt
> 1/8 teaspoon pepper

In a food processor or blender, process the sesame seeds for 30 seconds.

Add the remaining ingredients. Process until smooth. Serve at room temperature or refrigerate in an airtight container to serve chilled.

PER SERVING

calories 69	sodium 94 mg
total fat 1.5 g	carbohydrates 11 g
saturated fat 0.0 g	fiber 3 g
trans fat 0.0 g	sugars 1 g
polyunsaturated fat 0.5 g	protein 3 g
monounsaturated fat 0.5 g	DIETARY EXCHANGES
cholesterol 0 mg	1 starch

CURRY YOGURT DIP

SERVES 8

The curry in this dip jazzes up raw vegetables or apple slices with its notes of cumin, coriander, and turmeric.

> 1 cup fat-free plain Greek yogurt
> 3 tablespoons light mayonnaise
> 2 teaspoons curry powder

In a small bowl, whisk together all the ingredients. Cover and refrigerate until serving time.

PER SERVING

calories 30	sodium 60 mg
total fat 1.5 g	carbohydrates 2 g
saturated fat 0.0 g	fiber 0 g
trans fat 0.0 g	sugars 1 g
polyunsaturated fat 1.0 g	protein 3 g
monounsaturated fat 0.5 g	DIETARY EXCHANGES
cholesterol 2 mg	1/2 lean meat

SPINACH DIP

SERVES 6

Watercress adds a peppery bite and avocado provides a lush richness to this appetizer, a heart healthy take on the cream-heavy, fat-laden traditional version of the dip.

> 10 ounces frozen chopped spinach
> 5 medium green onions, coarsely chopped
> 1/2 cup watercress or baby arugula leaves
> 1/4 cup fresh parsley, stems discarded
> 8 ounces fat-free plain yogurt
> 1 medium avocado, chopped
> 1 1/4 teaspoons salt-free garlic herb seasoning blend
> 1/8 teaspoon pepper
> 1/8 teaspoon salt
> 1/8 teaspoon red hot-pepper sauce, or to taste

Prepare the spinach using the package directions, omitting the salt and margarine. Drain well in a colander. Squeeze dry.

(continued)

In a food processor or blender, process the spinach, green onions, watercress, and parsley until just blended. The mixture should be coarse. Transfer to a colander to drain well.

Process the remaining ingredients until smooth. Transfer to a medium bowl.

Stir the spinach mixture into the yogurt mixture. Cover and refrigerate for at least 1 hour.

Cook's Tip: To keep the avocado chunkier, mash it with a fork instead of processing it. Stir the avocado into the spinach and yogurt mixture.

PER SERVING

calories 93	sodium 120 mg
total fat 5.5 g	carbohydrates 9 g
saturated fat 1.0 g	fiber 4 g
trans fat 0.0 g	sugars 4 g
polyunsaturated fat 0.5 g	protein 5 g
monounsaturated fat 3.5 g	**DIETARY EXCHANGES**
cholesterol 1 mg	1 vegetable, 1 fat

RANCH DIP

SERVES 8

This version of a tried-and-true traditional dip is low in saturated fat and makes a great appetizer or snack when served with a variety of fresh vegetables, such as cucumber rounds, red and yellow bell pepper strips, green beans, and fennel slices. The fresh parsley really perks up the flavor.

    2 ounces light tub cream cheese
    3/4 cup low-fat buttermilk
    2 tablespoons chopped fresh parsley
    1/2 teaspoon garlic powder
    1/2 teaspoon onion powder
    1/4 teaspoon dried oregano, crumbled
    1/8 teaspoon pepper

In a medium bowl, using an electric mixer on medium speed, beat the cream cheese for 1 minute, or until fluffy.

Reduce the speed to medium low and gradually beat in the buttermilk for 1 to 2 minutes, or until smooth.

Add the remaining ingredients. Beat for about 30 seconds, or until combined. Serve immediately or cover and refrigerate for up to four days for a more pronounced flavor.

PER SERVING

calories 27	sodium 57 mg
total fat 1.5 g	carbohydrates 2 g
saturated fat 1.0 g	fiber 0 g
trans fat 0.0 g	sugars 2 g
polyunsaturated fat 0.0 g	protein 1 g
monounsaturated fat 0.5 g	**DIETARY EXCHANGES**
cholesterol 6 mg	free

FIRE-AND-ICE CREAM CHEESE SPREAD

SERVES 6

Easy but elegant, this classic cream cheese spread heats up your palate with crushed red pepper and cools it down with the sweetness of apricots. Serve with pear slices or heart-healthy crackers.

    1/4 cup light tub cream cheese
    1/4 cup fat-free sour cream
    1/4 cup all-fruit apricot spread
    1/4 teaspoon crushed red pepper flakes
    2 tablespoons finely chopped red bell pepper

In a small mixing bowl, using an electric mixer on medium speed, beat the cream cheese and sour cream until well blended.

Line a small bowl with plastic wrap. Spoon the cream cheese mixture into the bowl. Press the mixture lightly to get rid of any air pockets. Smooth the surface with a rubber scraper. Cover and refrigerate for at least 30 minutes to firm slightly.

Meanwhile, in a small saucepan, cook the apricot spread and red pepper flakes over medium heat for 3 minutes, or until the spread just begins to melt, stirring occasionally. Remove from the heat.

Stir in the chopped bell pepper. Let cool to room temperature.

Uncover and invert the cream cheese mixture onto a small serving plate. Top the cream cheese mixture with the apricot spread mixture.

PER SERVING

calories 59
total fat 1.5 g
  saturated fat 1.0 g
  trans fat 0.0 g
  polyunsaturated fat 0.0 g
  monounsaturated fat 0.5 g
cholesterol 8 mg

sodium 51 mg
carbohydrates 9 g
  fiber 0 g
  sugars 7 g
protein 1 g
DIETARY EXCHANGES
  1/2 fruit

EDAMAME GUACAMOLE

SERVES 8

Edamame pairs well with avocado in this modernized twist on a traditional guacamole. Forgo the expected chips and serve it in colorful mini bell peppers for a perfectly pleasing party appetizer.

1 medium ripe avocado, peeled, seeded, and coarsely chopped
1 cup frozen shelled edamame, thawed
1 medium ripe tomato, or 12 to 16 cherry tomatoes, coarsely chopped (about 1 cup)
1 tomatillo, husk discarded, chopped (optional)
2 tablespoons chopped onion
2 tablespoons chopped fresh cilantro
1 tablespoon fresh lime juice
1 large garlic clove, minced
1/2 medium fresh jalapeño, seeds and ribs discarded, chopped (optional; see Cook's Tip on Handling Hot Chiles, page 24)
1/4 teaspoon ground cumin
Pepper to taste (freshly ground preferred)
16 baby bell peppers, assorted colors, halved

In a food processor or blender, process all the ingredients except the bell peppers until creamy. For a chunkier texture, pulse the ingredients until the desired consistency.

Spoon 1 tablespoon guacamole into each bell pepper half.

PER SERVING

calories 79
total fat 4.0 g
  saturated fat 0.5 g
  trans fat 0.0 g
  polyunsaturated fat 1.5 g
  monounsaturated fat 1.5 g
cholesterol 0 mg

sodium 5 mg
carbohydrates 8 g
  fiber 3 g
  sugars 4 g
protein 4 g
DIETARY EXCHANGES
  2 vegetable, 1 fat

LOTS OF LAYERS DIP

SERVES 16

A classic for football parties, this traditionally high-calorie, fat-laden dip goes light with fat-free dairy products and a quick tomato salsa. Heating the chili powder for just a few minutes gives this dip an extra punch of flavor.

1/3 cup chopped avocado
1/4 teaspoon fresh lime juice
1 15.5-ounce can no-salt-added pinto beans or no-salt-added black beans, rinsed and drained
2 tablespoons canned diced green chiles, drained
1/2 teaspoon canola or corn oil
1/4 teaspoon garlic powder
1 14.5-ounce can no-salt-added diced tomatoes, drained
1 teaspoon ground cumin
1 teaspoon cider vinegar
3/4 cup sliced green onions
1 1/2 teaspoons chili powder
3/4 cup fat-free sour cream
1/2 cup shredded fat-free Cheddar cheese
3 tablespoons sliced black olives, chopped

In a small bowl, gently stir together the avocado and lime juice. Set aside.

In an 8-inch square glass baking dish, mash the beans until broken into medium-size pieces. (A potato masher works well for this.) Stir in the chiles, oil, and garlic powder. Spread to cover the bottom of the dish.

(continued)

In a medium bowl, stir together the tomatoes, cumin, and vinegar. Spread over the bean mixture. Sprinkle with the green onions.

In a small nonstick skillet, heat the chili powder over low heat for 5 minutes, or until fragrant, stirring frequently.

Put the sour cream in a small bowl. Stir in the chili powder. Spread over the green onions.

Sprinkle with the Cheddar, then with the olives, and finally with the reserved avocado.

Cook's Tip: For a light lunch, warm the dip and some corn tortillas separately in the microwave, spread the dip over the tortillas, top with the shredded lettuce, and roll up the tortillas jelly-roll style. Enjoy with a cup of soup, such as Roasted Corn Soup (page 40).

PER SERVING

calories 57	sodium 80 mg
total fat 1.0 g	carbohydrates 9 g
saturated fat 0.0 g	fiber 2 g
trans fat 0.0 g	sugars 3 g
polyunsaturated fat 0.0 g	protein 4 g
monounsaturated fat 0.5 g	DIETARY EXCHANGES
cholesterol 3 mg	1/2 starch

LUSCIOUS BERRY DIP

SERVES 8

This rich-tasting fruit and cheese dip is the perfect complement to any of your favorite fruits.

> 1 cup fat-free ricotta cheese
> 3/4 cup halved fresh strawberries, hulled, or 3/4 cup frozen strawberries, thawed
> 1/2 cup fresh raspberries, or 3/4 cup frozen unsweetened raspberries, thawed, undrained
> 1/4 cup fat-free vanilla yogurt
> 1 tablespoon light brown sugar
> 1/2 teaspoon ground cinnamon

In a food processor or blender, process all the ingredients until smooth. Transfer to a small serving bowl. Cover and refrigerate until ready to serve.

Cook's Tip: Frozen raspberries lose quite a bit of volume when they thaw, which is why the recipe calls for a larger amount of frozen raspberries than of fresh.

PER SERVING

calories 45	sodium 66 mg
total fat 0.0 g	carbohydrates 6 g
saturated fat 0.0 g	fiber 1 g
trans fat 0.0 g	sugars 5 g
polyunsaturated fat 0.0 g	protein 5 g
monounsaturated fat 0.0 g	DIETARY EXCHANGES
cholesterol 3 mg	1/2 fruit

MUSHROOM AND NUT PÂTÉ

SERVES 8

This vegetarian version of pâté, the French word for "paste," has an earthy, exotic flavor thanks to the variety of mushrooms included. Serve this on Whole-Wheat French Bread (page 443) or whole-grain crackers. Use any leftovers as a sandwich spread.

> 2 tablespoons light tub margarine
> 1 pound mixed exotic mushrooms, such as brown (cremini), chanterelle, morel, oyster, or shiitake (stems discarded), sliced
> 1 small onion, chopped
> 1 medium garlic clove, minced
> 1 cup walnuts
> 2 tablespoons canola or corn oil
> 1/4 teaspoon dried oregano, crumbled
> 1/4 teaspoon dried thyme, crumbled
> Dash of red hot-pepper sauce
> 2 tablespoons chopped fresh parsley (optional)
> 1 tablespoon sesame seeds, dry-roasted (optional)

In a large skillet, melt the margarine over medium-high heat, swirling to coat the bottom. Cook the mushrooms, onion, and garlic for about 5 minutes, or until the mushrooms and onion are soft and the liquid has evaporated, stirring frequently. Set aside.

In a food processor or blender, coarsely chop the walnuts. Remove 2 tablespoons. Set aside.

Gradually pour in the oil, processing after each addition, until well blended.

Add the mushroom mixture, oregano, thyme, and hot-pepper sauce to the mushroom mixture. Process until well blended. Stir in the reserved walnuts.

Transfer the pâté to a small serving bowl. Sprinkle with the parsley and sesame seeds.

PER SERVING

calories 156	**sodium** 26 mg
total fat 14.5 g	**carbohydrates** 5 g
saturated fat 1.0 g	fiber 2 g
trans fat 0.0 g	sugars 2 g
polyunsaturated fat 8.0 g	**protein** 4 g
monounsaturated fat 4.0 g	**DIETARY EXCHANGES**
cholesterol 0 mg	1 vegetable, 3 fat

EGGPLANT PÂTÉ

SERVES 10

This Mediterranean spread is rich in flavor without putting a squeeze on your wallet. Broiling the eggplant gives it an intense smokiness that adds depth to this dish. Serve with baked whole-wheat pita chips or whole-grain toast wedges.

1 tablespoon olive oil and 1 tablespoon olive oil, divided use
1 large eggplant, halved lengthwise
1 small onion, finely chopped
1 medium garlic clove, minced
1/4 cup finely chopped green bell pepper
1 1/2 tablespoons fresh lemon juice
Pepper to taste (coarsely ground preferred)
1/4 cup chopped fresh parsley (optional)

Preheat the broiler.

Rub 1 tablespoon olive oil on the cut sides of the eggplant. Put the eggplant on a large, sturdy baking sheet with the cut side down. Put the baking sheet on the middle rack of the oven.

Broil the eggplant for 20 to 25 minutes, or until very soft. Remove from the oven and let cool slightly.

Using a large spoon, scoop out the eggplant pulp and transfer it to a medium bowl, discarding the skin. Using a fork, mash the pulp well.

In a small nonstick skillet over medium-high heat, heat the remaining 1 tablespoon oil, swirling to coat the bottom. Cook the onion for 7 to 9 minutes, or until browned, stirring frequently. Stir in the garlic. Cook for 30 seconds, stirring occasionally. Stir the onion mixture, bell pepper, lemon juice, and pepper into the eggplant until well mixed.

Refrigerate, covered, for 2 to 3 hours. Just before serving, sprinkle with the parsley.

PER SERVING

calories 42	**sodium** 2 mg
total fat 3.0 g	**carbohydrates** 4 g
saturated fat 0.5 g	fiber 2 g
trans fat 0.0 g	sugars 2 g
polyunsaturated fat 0.5 g	**protein** 1 g
monounsaturated fat 2.0 g	**DIETARY EXCHANGES**
cholesterol 0 mg	1 vegetable, 1/2 fat

TORTILLA PINWHEELS

SERVES 10

It will be party time when you bring out a plate of this Tex-Mex finger food. Turn up the heat by varying the type of salsa you choose.

4 ounces light tub cream cheese
1/2 15.5-ounce can no-salt-added black beans, rinsed, drained, and mashed
1/2 medium red bell pepper, finely chopped
1/4 cup salsa (lowest sodium available), such as Salsa Cruda (page 437)
1 medium green onion, thinly sliced
1/4 teaspoon ground cumin
1/8 teaspoon salt
5 6-inch corn tortillas

(continued)

Preheat the oven to 350°F.

In a medium bowl, using an electric mixer on medium speed, beat the cream cheese until smooth. Stir in the remaining ingredients except the tortillas.

Wrap the tortillas in aluminum foil. Bake for 5 minutes, or until heated through. Remove from the oven.

Put one tortilla on a cutting board, leaving the others wrapped. Spread 1/4 cup bean mixture over the top of the tortilla. Roll up jelly-roll style and place with the seam side down on the cutting board. Insert four wooden toothpicks about 1 inch apart into the tortilla roll. Using a sharp knife, slice between the toothpicks to make 4 pieces. Leaving the toothpicks in place, arrange the pieces on a serving plate. Repeat with the remaining tortillas and filling.

PER SERVING

calories 69	**sodium** 108 mg
total fat 2.0 g	**carbohydrates** 9 g
saturated fat 1.0 g	fiber 2 g
trans fat 0.0 g	sugars 2 g
polyunsaturated fat 0.0 g	**protein** 3 g
monounsaturated fat 0.5 g	**DIETARY EXCHANGES**
cholesterol 7 mg	1/2 starch, 1/2 fat

PLUM TOMATOES WITH BLUE CHEESE

SERVES 8

Sweet and juicy plum tomatoes are topped with a spicy cheese mixture and green onions in this holiday party appetizer. Allow some time for the flavors to marry.

> 1 1/2 ounces blue cheese
> 1 tablespoon plus 2 teaspoons fat-free milk
> 1/4 teaspoon red hot-pepper sauce
> 12 medium Italian plum (Roma) tomatoes
> 2 tablespoons finely chopped green onions

In a medium mixing bowl, using an electric mixer on low speed, beat the blue cheese, milk, and hot-pepper sauce until completely blended,

scraping the side of the bowl with a rubber scraper. Transfer to a small container. Cover and refrigerate for 30 minutes to 24 hours.

Cut the tomatoes in half lengthwise. Top each half with the blue cheese mixture. Sprinkle with the green onions. Serve immediately or cover and refrigerate for up to 1 hour.

PER SERVING

calories 37	**sodium** 82 mg
total fat 1.5 g	**carbohydrates** 4 g
saturated fat 1.0 g	fiber 1 g
trans fat 0.0 g	sugars 3 g
polyunsaturated fat 0.0 g	**protein** 2 g
monounsaturated fat 0.5 g	**DIETARY EXCHANGES**
cholesterol 4 mg	1 vegetable

PLUM TOMATOES WITH FETA CHEESE

Substitute 2 ounces fat-free feta cheese for the blue cheese. Substitute fat-free plain Greek yogurt for the milk.

PER SERVING

calories 26	**sodium** 117 mg
total fat 0.0 g	**carbohydrates** 4 g
saturated fat 0.0 g	fiber 1 g
trans fat 0.0 g	sugars 3 g
polyunsaturated fat 0.0 g	**protein** 3 g
monounsaturated fat 0.0 g	**DIETARY EXCHANGES**
cholesterol 0 mg	1 vegetable

RED POTATOES WITH FETA CHEESE AND BASIL

Replace the tomatoes with 8 small red potatoes, halved lengthwise. Steam for 10 minutes. Plunge the potatoes into a bowl of ice water for 2 minutes. Drain well. Pat dry. Top each half with the feta mixture in Plum Tomatoes with Feta Cheese above. Sprinkle with 2 tablespoons finely chopped fresh basil or green onions.

PER SERVING

calories 49	**sodium** 123 mg
total fat 0.0 g	**carbohydrates** 10 g
saturated fat 0.0 g	fiber 1 g
trans fat 0.0 g	sugars 1 g
polyunsaturated fat 0.0 g	**protein** 3 g
monounsaturated fat 0.0 g	**DIETARY EXCHANGES**
cholesterol 0 mg	1/2 starch

COCONUT HALIBUT BITES

SERVES 12

Warm, crusted seafood poppers, served with a triple-citrus sweet-and-sour dipping sauce, are a sure way to get the party started.

Cooking spray
1/4 cup egg substitute
1/2 teaspoon dried dillweed, crumbled
1/8 teaspoon pepper
1/4 cup all-purpose flour
1/4 cup sweetened shredded coconut
1 pound halibut fillets, rinsed and patted dry, cut into 24 1-inch cubes

Sauce
1/2 cup sweet orange marmalade
1 teaspoon grated lime zest
1 tablespoon fresh lime juice
1 tablespoon fresh lemon juice

Preheat the oven to 400°F. Lightly spray a baking sheet with cooking spray.

In a small shallow dish, whisk together the egg substitute, dillweed, and pepper. In a separate small shallow dish, stir together the flour and coconut. Set the dishes and baking sheet in a row, assembly-line fashion. Working in batches, put the fish in the egg substitute mixture, turning to coat. Using a slotted spoon, transfer the fish to the flour mixture, turning to coat and gently shaking off any excess. Place the fish on the baking sheet, spacing the cubes slightly apart so they brown evenly.

Bake for 7 to 8 minutes, or until the fish flakes easily when tested with a fork.

Meanwhile, in a small serving bowl, whisk together the sauce ingredients. Serve with the fish.

PER SERVING

calories 87	carbohydrates 12 g
total fat 1.0 g	fiber 0 g
saturated fat 0.5 g	sugars 8 g
trans fat 0.0 g	protein 8 g
polyunsaturated fat 0.0 g	DIETARY EXCHANGES
monounsaturated fat 0.0 g	1 other carbohydrate,
cholesterol 19 mg	1 lean meat
sodium 44 mg	

ORANGE CHICKEN LETTUCE WRAPS

SERVES 8

Crisp lettuce leaves enfold tender cubes of chicken. Bell pepper, broccoli slaw, and water chestnuts give these wraps a triple crunch. Bright with citrus, they're perfect as appetizers, but you could make this recipe as an entrée for four.

2 heads iceberg lettuce
1 teaspoon grated orange zest
1/4 cup fresh orange juice
1/4 cup fat-free, low-sodium chicken broth, such as on page 36
1 tablespoon plain rice vinegar
2 teaspoons soy sauce (lowest sodium available)
1 1/2 teaspoons cornstarch
1/2 teaspoon toasted sesame oil
1 teaspoon canola or corn oil
1 pound boneless, skinless chicken breasts, all visible fat discarded, cut into 1/2-inch cubes
1 medium bell pepper (yellow preferred), diced
1 cup packaged broccoli slaw or 1 cup chopped broccoli florets
1/2 cup sliced canned water chestnuts, drained and chopped
2 medium green onions, thinly sliced

Cut each head of lettuce in half vertically. Discard the cores. Carefully remove 4 outside leaves from each half. Set aside.

In a small bowl, whisk together the orange zest, orange juice, broth, vinegar, soy sauce, cornstarch, and sesame oil. Set aside.

In a large nonstick skillet, heat the canola oil over medium-high heat, swirling to coat the bottom. Cook the chicken for 3 to 4 minutes, or until lightly browned on the outside and no longer pink in the center, stirring constantly.

Stir in the bell pepper. Cook for 1 to 2 minutes, or until tender-crisp, stirring constantly.

(continued)

Stir in the broccoli slaw, water chestnuts, and green onions. Cook for 1 to 2 minutes, or until the broccoli is tender-crisp and the water chestnuts are heated through.

Stir in the reserved orange zest mixture. Reduce the heat and simmer for 2 to 3 minutes, or until the sauce has thickened, stirring occasionally. Transfer to a serving bowl.

Place the bowl of chicken filling in the center of a platter. Arrange the lettuce leaves around the bowl. Let each person spoon some chicken mixture onto the lettuce leaves and gently roll to enclose the filling.

PER SERVING

calories 98	**sodium** 111 mg
total fat 2.5 g	**carbohydrates** 6 g
saturated fat 0.5 g	fiber 2 g
trans fat 0.0 g	sugars 3 g
polyunsaturated fat 0.5 g	**protein** 14 g
monounsaturated fat 1.0 g	**DIETARY EXCHANGES**
cholesterol 36 mg	1 vegetable, 1 lean meat

SKEWERED CHICKEN STRIPS WITH SOY-PEANUT MARINADE

SERVES 16

Make this juicy chicken strip appetizer for your next book club gathering and you won't be putting away any leftovers. Or try this recipe for dinner for four, keeping the chicken breasts whole (not using the skewers) and serving them on a bed of brown rice with a side of steamed snow peas.

Marinade
- 2 tablespoons fresh lime juice
- 1 tablespoon low-sodium peanut butter
- 1 tablespoon soy sauce (lowest sodium available)
- 1 tablespoon plain rice vinegar
- 2 medium garlic cloves, minced
- 1/2 teaspoon ground cumin
- 1/2 teaspoon toasted sesame oil
- 1/4 teaspoon pepper

■ ■ ■

- 4 boneless, skinless chicken breast halves (about 4 ounces each), all visible fat discarded, flattened to 1/4- to 1/2-inch thickness and each cut lengthwise into 8 strips
- Cooking spray

In a large shallow glass dish, whisk together the marinade ingredients. Add the chicken, turning to coat. Cover and refrigerate for 30 minutes to 8 hours, turning occasionally. Discard the marinade.

Soak 32 wooden skewers 4 to 6 inches long in cold water for at least 10 minutes to prevent charring, or use metal skewers.

Lightly spray the grill rack with cooking spray. Preheat the grill on medium high.

Thread one strip of chicken onto each skewer.

Grill for 2 to 3 minutes on each side (6 to 8 minutes on each side for unsliced chicken if making an entrée) or until no longer pink in the center. Serve immediately.

PER SERVING

calories 28	**sodium** 39 mg
total fat 1.0 g	**carbohydrates** 0 g
saturated fat 0.0 g	fiber 0 g
trans fat 0.0 g	sugars 0 g
polyunsaturated fat 0.0 g	**protein** 4 g
monounsaturated fat 0.5 g	**DIETARY EXCHANGES**
cholesterol 11 mg	1/2 lean meat

MEATBALL SLIDERS WITH BEER SAUCE

SERVES 12

You can make the sauce while these easy-to-prepare meatballs bake. These mini sandwiches make a great game-time snack, or pair one with a leafy green salad for a light lunch.

Cooking spray

Meatballs
- 2 slices whole-grain bread (lowest sodium available), cut into cubes
- 4 ounces beer (light or nonalcoholic)

1 pound extra-lean ground beef

1/2 cup shredded low-fat mozzarella cheese

1/2 teaspoon pepper, or to taste

Sauce

1 teaspoon light tub margarine

1/2 cup chopped onion

1 tablespoon all-purpose flour

8 ounces beer (light or nonalcoholic)

2 tablespoons light brown sugar

2 tablespoons cider vinegar

2 tablespoons fat-free, low-sodium beef
broth, such as on page 35

■ ■ ■

12 whole-wheat slider or dinner rolls (lowest
sodium available)

Preheat the broiler. Lightly spray the broiler pan and rack with cooking spray.

In a medium bowl, soak the bread cubes in 4 ounces beer for 2 to 3 minutes.

Add the beef, mozzarella, and pepper. Using your hands or a spoon, combine the ingredients. Shape into twelve 1/2-inch balls (about 1 1/2 teaspoons each). Transfer to the broiler rack.

Broil the meatballs about 4 inches from the heat for 10 to 15 minutes, or until the tops are browned. Turn over the meatballs. Broil for 10 to 15 minutes, or until the meatballs are browned on the outside and no longer pink in the center. Drain on paper towels.

Meanwhile, in a medium skillet, melt the margarine over medium-high heat, swirling to coat the bottom. Cook the onion for 3 minutes, or until soft, stirring frequently.

Stir in the flour. Cook for 1 to 2 minutes, stirring constantly.

Stir in the remaining sauce ingredients. Reduce the heat and simmer for 10 minutes.

Add the meatballs to the sauce, stirring gently to coat. Simmer for 20 minutes, stirring occasionally and turning the meatballs to coat with the sauce.

Just before serving, split open the rolls and toast them. Top the bottoms of the rolls with the meatballs and sauce. Put the tops of the rolls on the sliders.

Cook's Tip: If you can't find whole-wheat, lower-sodium slider or dinner rolls, you can use 4 whole-wheat hot dog buns. Cut the buns crosswise into thirds to create slider rolls.

PER SERVING

calories 188	carbohydrates 24 g
total fat 4.5 g	fiber 3 g
saturated fat 1.5 g	sugars 6 g
trans fat 0.0 g	protein 13 g
polyunsaturated fat 1.0 g	DIETARY EXCHANGES
monounsaturated fat 1.5 g	1 1/2 starch, 1 lean
cholesterol 23 mg	meat
sodium 268 mg	

CRUMB-CRUSTED MUSHROOMS WITH LEMON

SERVES 4

Now you see them, now you don't! Coat whole button mushrooms with yogurt and top with lightly seasoned bread crumbs, bake them for a few minutes, and watch them disappear.

1 1/2 teaspoons light tub margarine

2 slices whole-grain bread (lowest sodium
available), processed into crumbs

4 medium garlic cloves, minced

1 teaspoon dried Italian seasoning, crumbled

1/8 teaspoon salt-free lemon pepper

1 tablespoon grated lemon zest

Cooking spray

8 medium button mushrooms, stems
discarded

1/3 cup fat-free plain yogurt

1/4 teaspoon paprika

1 medium lemon, cut into 4 wedges

In a large nonstick skillet, melt the margarine over medium-high heat, swirling to coat the bottom. Add the bread crumbs, garlic, Italian seasoning, and lemon pepper, stirring to combine. Cook for 6 minutes, or until the mixture is golden brown, stirring frequently. Remove from the heat.

(continued)

Stir in the lemon zest.

Preheat the oven to 450°F. Lightly spray a baking sheet with cooking spray.

In a large bowl, gently stir together the mushrooms and yogurt to coat. Place the mushrooms in a single layer about 1/4 inch apart on the baking sheet. Sprinkle the bread crumb mixture and then the paprika over the mushrooms.

Bake for 5 minutes, or until heated through.

Gently transfer the mushrooms to a serving plate. Sprinkle with any bread crumbs remaining on the baking sheet. Garnish with the lemon wedges.

PER SERVING

calories 69	**sodium** 87 mg
total fat 1.5 g	**carbohydrates** 11 g
saturated fat 0.0 g	fiber 2 g
trans fat 0.0 g	sugars 4 g
polyunsaturated fat 0.5 g	**protein** 5 g
monounsaturated fat 0.5 g	**DIETARY EXCHANGES**
cholesterol 0 mg	1/2 starch

CRUMB-CRUSTED TOMATO SLICES

Lightly spray a 9-inch square baking pan with cooking spray. Substitute 2 large tomatoes (about 8 ounces each) for the mushrooms. Cut the tomatoes into 4 slices each. Place the tomatoes in the pan. Spoon the yogurt over each slice. Top with the crumb topping. Bake at 450°F for 20 minutes, or until soft. Garnish with the lemon wedges.

PER SERVING

calories 77	**sodium** 90 mg
total fat 1.5 g	**carbohydrates** 13 g
saturated fat 0.0 g	fiber 3 g
trans fat 0.0 g	sugars 6 g
polyunsaturated fat 0.5 g	**protein** 4 g
monounsaturated fat 0.5 g	**DIETARY EXCHANGES**
cholesterol 0 mg	1/2 starch, 1 vegetable

MARINATED MUSHROOMS
SERVES 8

This appetizer is fast to prep but needs adequate time for the marinade to infuse the porous mushrooms with its bite from hot chiles and tartness from fresh citrus.

Marinade
    1 medium garlic clove, minced
    2 tablespoons finely chopped green onions
    2 tablespoons finely chopped fresh cilantro
    1/3 cup olive oil (extra-virgin preferred)
    2 teaspoons adobo sauce (from chipotle
        peppers canned in adobo sauce)
    3 small strips lime zest
    1/3 cup fresh lime juice
    2 tablespoons dry white wine (regular or
        nonalcoholic)
    1/4 cup low-fat plain yogurt

■ ■ ■

8 ounces button mushrooms, quartered

In a shallow glass baking dish, whisk together the marinade ingredients. Add the mushrooms, stirring to coat. Refrigerate, covered, for several hours or overnight, stirring occasionally.

Drain the mushrooms, discarding the marinade. Serve cold.

PER SERVING

calories 28	**sodium** 3 mg
total fat 2.5 g	**carbohydrates** 1 g
saturated fat 0.5 g	fiber 0 g
trans fat 0.0 g	sugars 1 g
polyunsaturated fat 0.5 g	**protein** 1 g
monounsaturated fat 1.5 g	**DIETARY EXCHANGES**
cholesterol 0 mg	1/2 fat

STUFFED MUSHROOMS

SERVES 6

Savor these plump mushrooms as an appetizer or jazz up your next spaghetti dinner by serving them over sauce and pasta as you would meatballs.

18 medium button mushrooms (about
    1 pound), stems minced
2 teaspoons olive oil
3 medium garlic cloves, minced
1/4 medium red bell pepper, diced
1/4 medium yellow bell pepper, diced
2 medium green onions, sliced
3/4 cup fresh soft whole-grain bread crumbs
    (lowest sodium available)
1/4 cup egg substitute
2 tablespoons shredded or grated Parmesan
    cheese
1/2 teaspoon dried Italian seasoning,
    crumbled

Preheat the oven to 425°F.

Place the mushroom caps with the smooth side down in a 13 x 9 x 2-inch baking pan. Set aside.

In a medium nonstick skillet, heat the oil over medium heat, swirling to coat the bottom. Cook the mushroom stems and garlic for 5 minutes, stirring occasionally.

Stir in both bell peppers. Cook for 2 to 3 minutes, or until tender.

Stir in the green onions. Cook for 2 minutes. Remove from the heat.

Stir in the remaining ingredients. Spoon the filling into the mushroom caps, packing the mixture lightly.

Bake for 25 minutes, or until heated through.

PER SERVING

calories 67	sodium 92 mg
total fat 2.0 g	**carbohydrates** 7 g
saturated fat 0.5 g	fiber 2 g
trans fat 0.0 g	sugars 1 g
polyunsaturated fat 0.0 g	**protein** 6 g
monounsaturated fat 1.5 g	**DIETARY EXCHANGES**
cholesterol 1 mg	1/2 starch

SWEET-AND-SOUR SPRING ROLLS

SERVES 4

These vegetarian spring rolls make a great starter for an Asian dinner, or serve them as finger food at your next party. Spring roll wrappers can be hard to find, so crisp phyllo dough stands in quite nicely.

1 teaspoon canola or corn oil and 1 teaspoon
    canola or corn oil, divided use
1 1/2 cups shredded cabbage
4 medium garlic cloves, minced
4 medium green onions, chopped
1 8-ounce can bamboo shoots, drained
2 teaspoons soy sauce (lowest sodium
    available)
1/8 teaspoon pepper
3 18 x 14-inch sheets frozen phyllo dough,
    thawed in refrigerator
Cooking spray
1 tablespoon plus 1 teaspoon bottled
    sweet-and-sour sauce (lowest sodium
    available)

In a large nonstick skillet, heat 1 teaspoon oil over medium-high heat for 1 minute, swirling to coat the bottom. Cook the cabbage and garlic for 3 minutes, stirring constantly.

Stir in the green onions and bamboo shoots. Cook for 30 seconds, stirring constantly. Remove from the heat.

Stir in the soy sauce and pepper.

Keeping the unused phyllo covered with a damp cloth or damp paper towels to prevent drying, lightly spray one sheet of dough with cooking spray. Working quickly, cut that sheet into four 9 x 7-inch pieces. Put three of the quarter-sheets under the cloth. On the remaining quarter, put 1 rounded tablespoon cabbage mixture 2 to 3 inches from one short end. Fold that end up to enclose the filling. Fold in the left and right sides. Roll tightly. Transfer with the seam side down to a large plate. Repeat with the remaining phyllo and filling to make an additional 11 spring rolls.

(continued)

Wipe the skillet with paper towels. Heat the remaining 1 teaspoon oil over medium-high heat for 1 minute, swirling to coat the bottom. Cook the spring rolls for 6 minutes, turning occasionally, until they are browned on all sides. Transfer to a serving plate. Brush with the sweet-and-sour sauce.

PER SERVING

calories 105	carbohydrates 18 g
total fat 3.0 g	fiber 2 g
saturated fat 0.0 g	sugars 4 g
trans fat 0.0 g	**protein** 3 g
polyunsaturated fat 1.0 g	**DIETARY EXCHANGES**
monounsaturated fat 1.5 g	1 starch, 1 vegetable,
cholesterol 0 mg	1/2 fat
sodium 145 mg	

JALAPEÑO POPPERS

SERVES 12

Charring fresh jalapeños imparts a smoky flavor and makes the coating adhere better to the surface of these cheese-filled delights.

Cooking spray

12 large fresh jalapeños (about 1 pound), halved lengthwise, seeds and ribs discarded (see Cook's Tip on Handling Hot Chiles in the next column)

8 ounces fat-free block cream cheese, softened

1/2 cup shredded low-fat Cheddar cheese

1 teaspoon ground cumin

1/4 cup all-purpose flour

1/2 cup egg substitute

1/3 cup plain dry bread crumbs (lowest sodium available)

1 teaspoon salt-free all-purpose seasoning blend

Preheat the broiler. Lightly spray a broiler pan and rack and a large baking sheet with cooking spray.

Place the jalapeños with the cut side down on the broiler rack.

Broil about 2 inches from the heat for 3 to 4 minutes, or until slightly charred. Using tongs, turn over the jalapeños. Broil for 2 to 3 minutes, or until tender-crisp. Transfer the broiler pan and rack to a cooling rack.

Preheat the oven to 400°F.

In a small mixing bowl, using an electric mixer on low speed, beat the cream cheese until smooth. Stir in the Cheddar and cumin. Spoon the mixture into the jalapeños.

Put the flour and egg substitute in separate shallow dishes. In a third shallow dish, stir together the bread crumbs and seasoning blend. Put the dishes and baking sheet in a row, assembly-line fashion. Lightly dip each jalapeño in the flour, then in the egg substitute, and finally in the bread crumbs. Place with the stuffed side up on the baking sheet.

Bake for 8 to 10 minutes, or until golden brown and heated through. Transfer the baking sheet to a cooling rack. Let cool for 3 to 4 minutes.

Cook's Tip: You can also grill the jalapeños (whole) before stuffing them. Using the tip of a knife, make a small hole in the stem ends of the jalapeños to keep them from bursting as they cook. Grill over medium-high heat for 4 to 5 minutes, or until the skins are slightly charred, turning after each minute of cooking time. When cool enough to handle, cut the jalapeños in half lengthwise, discarding the stems, seeds, and ribs, and stuff and bake as directed.

Cook's Tip on Handling Hot Chiles: Hot chiles contain oils that can burn your skin, lips, and eyes. Wear disposable gloves or wash your hands thoroughly with warm, soapy water immediately after handling hot chiles. Examples of hot chiles are Anaheim, ancho, bhut jolokia (ghost), cascabel, cayenne, cherry, chipotle, habañero, Hungarian wax, jalapeño, poblano, Scotch bonnet, serrano, and Thai. A rule of thumb is that the smaller the pepper, the hotter it is.

MEXICAN POTATO SKINS

SERVES 4

For after-school snacking or chilling and grilling with friends, these tasty appetizers satisfy the need for something with a hint of heat. Use the reserved potato skins from Baked Potato Soup *(page 63), or you can bake your own (see Cook's Tip below).*

8 potato-skin quarters from Baked Potato
    Soup, or 2 8-ounce baked potato skins
2 tablespoons plus 2 teaspoons fat-free sour
    cream
8 fresh cilantro leaves, finely chopped
1/4 cup salsa (lowest sodium available), such
    as Salsa Cruda (page 437)
1 small fresh jalapeño, seeds and ribs
    discarded, thinly sliced (optional; see
    Cook's Tip on Handling Hot Chiles,
    page 24)

Preheat the oven to 400°F.

Place the potato skins on a baking sheet.

Bake for 8 to 10 minutes, or until hot and crisp. For extra-crisp skins, use a toaster oven (the time is the same as for the oven). Transfer to a plate.

Meanwhile, in a small bowl, stir together the sour cream and cilantro.

Spoon the salsa onto each potato skin. Top with a dollop of the sour cream mixture and the jalapeño slices.

Cook's Tip on Baked Potato Skins: Preheat the oven to 425°F. Bake the potatoes on the oven rack for 1 hour 15 minutes, or until slightly over-done (the skins will be crisp and crackle slightly when you gently squeeze the potatoes using an oven mitt or tongs). Transfer to a cooling rack. Let stand for 15 to 20 minutes, or until cool enough to handle. Halve the potatoes length-wise, then halve crosswise (to make 4 quarters each). Using a spoon, scoop out the flesh, leaving about an 1/8-inch shell.

SPINACH AND CHEESE MINI QUICHES

SERVES 24

From bridal showers to brunch get-togethers, these rich mini quiches are the perfect size for party finger foods. They freeze well, so you can make them in advance.

Cooking spray
16 ounces fat-free cottage cheese
10 ounces frozen chopped spinach, thawed,
    well drained, and squeezed dry
1 cup shredded low-fat Swiss cheese
3/4 cup egg substitute
1/2 cup low-fat all-purpose baking mix
    (lowest sodium available)
2 medium green onions, thinly sliced
2 tablespoons shredded or grated Parmesan
    cheese
2 tablespoons fat-free half-and-half
1 tablespoon chopped fresh dillweed or
    1 teaspoon dried dillweed, crumbled
1 tablespoon olive oil
1/4 teaspoon pepper

Preheat the oven to 350°F. Lightly spray two 24-cup mini muffin pans with cooking spray.

In a large bowl, stir together the remaining in-gredients until the baking mix is just moistened. Don't overmix. Spoon 1 heaping tablespoon bat-ter into each muffin cup.

(continued)

With the pans on separate oven racks, bake for 15 minutes. Switch the pans from top to bottom. Bake for 10 to 15 minutes, or until a wooden toothpick inserted in the center of a quiche comes out clean. Transfer the pans to a cooling rack. Let cool for 5 minutes. Using a thin spatula, loosen the quiches. Transfer to a serving platter.

PER SERVING

calories 44
total fat 1.0 g
  saturated fat 0.5 g
  trans fat 0.0 g
  polyunsaturated fat 0.0 g
  monounsaturated fat 0.5 g
cholesterol 3 mg

sodium 138 mg
carbohydrates 4 g
  fiber 0 g
  sugars 1 g
protein 5 g
DIETARY EXCHANGES
  1 lean meat

ASIAN SNACK MIX

SERVES 16

By varying healthy cereals and nuts, you can create lots of different snack mixtures that are perfect when you're craving crunch. Package 1/2-cup servings in snack-size baggies for a grab-and-go treat.

> 5 cups rice squares cereal
> 2 cups unsalted pretzel sticks, broken in half
> 1/4 cup light tub margarine
> 2 teaspoons soy sauce (lowest sodium available)
> 1 teaspoon ground ginger
> 1 teaspoon garlic powder
> 1/4 to 1/2 teaspoon wasabi powder (optional)
> 1/2 cup almonds

Preheat the oven to 275°F.

In a large bowl, stir together the cereal and pretzel sticks.

In a small saucepan, melt the margarine over low heat. Stir in the remaining ingredients except the almonds. Stir into the cereal mixture.

Stir in the almonds. Transfer the mixture to a shallow roasting pan.

Bake for 1 hour, stirring every 10 minutes. Serve warm or let cool completely and store in an airtight container for up to seven days.

PER SERVING

calories 91
total fat 3.5 g
  saturated fat 0.0 g
  trans fat 0.0 g
  polyunsaturated fat 1.0 g
  monounsaturated fat 2.0 g
cholesterol 0 mg

sodium 120 mg
carbohydrates 13 g
  fiber 1 g
  sugars 1 g
protein 2 g
DIETARY EXCHANGES
  1 starch, 1/2 fat

SOUTHWESTERN SNACK MIX

Substitute puffed corn cereal or corn squares for the rice squares, ground cumin for the ginger, chili powder for the garlic, red hot-pepper sauce for the wasabi powder, and pecans for the almonds.

PER SERVING

calories 91
total fat 4.0 g
  saturated fat 0.0 g
  trans fat 0.0 g
  polyunsaturated fat 1.0 g
  monounsaturated fat 2.0 g
cholesterol 0 mg

sodium 106 mg
carbohydrates 14 g
  fiber 1 g
  sugars 2 g
protein 1 g
DIETARY EXCHANGES
  1 starch, 1/2 fat

INDIAN SNACK MIX

Stir together 2 1/2 cups of rice squares, 2 1/2 cups of corn squares, and the pretzels. Stir the mixture with the melted margarine (don't use the soy sauce). Replace the spices with 1 teaspoon curry powder, 1 teaspoon onion powder, and 1/4 to 1/2 teaspoon cayenne. Stir in the almonds just before baking.

PER SERVING

calories 93
total fat 3.5 g
  saturated fat 0.0 g
  trans fat 0.0 g
  polyunsaturated fat 1.0 g
  monounsaturated fat 2.0 g
cholesterol 0 mg

sodium 102 mg
carbohydrates 14 g
  fiber 1 g
  sugars 1 g
protein 2 g
DIETARY EXCHANGES
  1 starch, 1/2 fat

ORANGE PUMPKIN-SPICED PECANS

SERVES 8

Bake a batch of these pecans spiced with the flavors of fall to nibble or package in decorative tins or jars to give away as gifts.

Cooking spray
1 large egg white, lightly beaten using a fork
1 teaspoon pumpkin pie spice
1 teaspoon grated orange zest
1 teaspoon pure maple syrup
1 teaspoon vanilla extract
2 cups pecan halves
1/3 cup sweetened dried cranberries (optional)

Preheat the oven to 250°F. Line a rimmed baking sheet with aluminum foil. Lightly spray with cooking spray. Set aside.

In a medium bowl, whisk together the egg white, pumpkin pie spice, orange zest, maple syrup, and vanilla. Stir the pecans into the mixture until well coated. Transfer the pecans to the baking sheet, arranging them in a single layer.

Bake for 50 minutes to 1 hour, or until the pecans are crisp, stirring occasionally. Transfer the baking sheet to a cooling rack. Let cool completely. Gently remove the pecans from the baking sheet. Store them in an airtight container for up to two weeks.

To keep the pecans crisp, stir them together with the cranberries just before eating or packaging.

Cook's Tip on Homemade Pumpkin Pie Spice: In a small bowl, stir together 3 tablespoons ground cinnamon, 2 teaspoons ground ginger, 2 teaspoons ground nutmeg, 1 1/2 teaspoons ground allspice, and 1 1/2 teaspoons ground cloves until well blended. Store in a small jar with a tight-fitting lid, preferably in a cool, dry place. Shake the jar to blend the spice mixture before using it.

PER SERVING (WITH OPTIONAL CRANBERRIES)

calories 195	carbohydrates 9 g
total fat 18.0 g	fiber 2 g
saturated fat 1.5 g	sugars 5 g
trans fat 0.0 g	protein 3 g
polyunsaturated fat 5.5 g	DIETARY EXCHANGES
monounsaturated fat 10.0 g	1/2 other carbohydrate,
cholesterol 0 mg	1/2 lean meat, 3 fat
sodium 7 mg	

PER SERVING (WITHOUT OPTIONAL CRANBERRIES)

calories 178	sodium 7 mg
total fat 18.0 g	carbohydrates 4 g
saturated fat 1.5 g	fiber 2 g
trans fat 0.0 g	sugars 2 g
polyunsaturated fat 5.5 g	protein 3 g
monounsaturated fat 10.0 g	DIETARY EXCHANGES
cholesterol 0 mg	1/2 lean meat, 3 fat

CRUNCHY PARMESAN-GARLIC SNAP PEAS

SERVES 4

Super-quick high-heat roasting ensures that these sugar snap peas remain bright green and snappy. Punched up with Parmesan cheese, garlic powder, and a sprinkling of red pepper flakes, this crunchy snack can snap you out of a slump.

8 ounces sugar snap peas, trimmed and strings discarded (about 2 cups)
1 teaspoon olive oil
1/4 teaspoon garlic powder
2 tablespoons shredded or grated Parmesan cheese
1/4 teaspoon crushed red pepper flakes

Preheat the oven to 450°F. Line a large rimmed baking sheet with parchment paper.

In a medium bowl, stir together the peas and oil. Sprinkle the garlic powder over the peas, stirring to coat. Arrange in a single layer on the baking sheet.

Roast for 3 minutes. Remove from the oven.

Sprinkle the Parmesan over the peas. Roast for 2 to 3 minutes, or until the peas are lightly browned in spots, but still crisp. Remove from the oven. Sprinkle with the red pepper flakes.

(continued)

Cook's Tip on Sugar Snap Peas: Sugar snap peas have fibrous strings that run the length of the pea pod on both the spine and the interior curve. These should be removed before cooking. It's easy to do; simply pull the dry brown threadlike projection on the interior curve away from the pod to remove that string. Snap off a tiny portion of the tip of the pod to get a better hold on the spinal string, then pull that one away from the pod to remove it.

PER SERVING

calories 45	sodium 45 mg
total fat 2.0 g	**carbohydrates** 5 g
saturated fat 0.5 g	fiber 2 g
trans fat 0.0 g	sugars 2 g
polyunsaturated fat 0.0 g	**protein** 3 g
monounsaturated fat 1.0 g	**DIETARY EXCHANGES**
cholesterol 2 mg	1 vegetable, 1/2 fat

PIZZA-FLAVORED ROASTED CHICKPEAS

SERVES 4

Crunchy oven-roasted chickpeas seasoned with pizza flavors will do the job to satisfy your afternoon snack cravings. Or tuck a serving into school lunches instead of flavored potato chips or other packaged snacks.

> 1 15.5-ounce can no-salt-added chickpeas, rinsed and drained
> Cooking spray
> 2 teaspoons salt-free tomato, basil, and garlic seasoning blend
> 2 teaspoons garlic powder (coarse-grind preferred)
> 1/8 teaspoon pepper (freshly ground preferred)
> 1 tablespoon olive oil
> 2 tablespoons dry-pack sun-dried tomatoes, cut into matchstick-size strips and minced
> 1 tablespoon finely grated Romano cheese

Lay a triple thickness of paper towels on a large plate. Spread the chickpeas on the paper towels.

Gently roll the chickpeas around, blotting them lightly with a separate paper towel. Set aside to dry.

Move the oven rack to the top position. Preheat the oven to 450°F. Line a rimmed baking sheet with aluminum foil. Lightly spray the foil with the cooking spray. Set aside.

Meanwhile in a small bowl, stir together the seasoning blend, garlic powder, and pepper.

Once the chickpeas are dried, transfer them to a medium bowl. Add the oil, tossing to coat. Sprinkle the seasoning blend mixture over the chickpeas. Toss to coat well.

Arrange the chickpeas in a single layer on the baking sheet. Roast for 30 minutes, stirring twice.

Carefully remove the baking sheet from the oven. Stir the tomatoes together with the chickpeas. Roast for 8 to 10 minutes, or until the chickpeas are browned and crunchy, stirring twice.

Transfer the baking sheet to a cooling rack. Sprinkle the chickpeas with the Romano. Let stand for 8 to 10 minutes to serve warm or let stand to cool to room temperature.

Cook's Tip: Before cutting dried fruits or vegetables, lightly spray the knife blade with cooking spray so the fruits or vegetables won't stick to the blade.

PER SERVING

calories 154	**carbohydrates** 22 g
total fat 4.5 g	fiber 5 g
saturated fat 0.5 g	sugars 1 g
trans fat 0.0 g	**protein** 7 g
polyunsaturated fat 0.5 g	**DIETARY EXCHANGES**
monounsaturated fat 2.5 g	1 1/2 starch, 1/2 lean
cholesterol 1 mg	meat, 1/2 fat
sodium 38 mg	

SUMMER SLUSHY

SERVES 4

This super-fruity drink is a healthy way to start your morning or an easy way to add more fruit to your day.

- 2 cups frozen unsweetened strawberries or unsweetened sliced peaches
- 1 1/2 cups 100% pineapple-orange juice
- 1 large banana, sliced
- 6 ounces fat-free, sugar-free vanilla or fruit-flavored yogurt
- 2 tablespoons sugar
- 1/4 to 1/2 teaspoon coconut extract

In a food processor or blender, process all the ingredients until smooth.

Cook's Tip: For an even colder beverage, place the serving glasses in the freezer at least 30 minutes before serving.

PER SERVING

calories 149	**carbohydrates** 35 g
total fat 0.0 g	fiber 2 g
saturated fat 0.0 g	sugars 26 g
trans fat 0.0 g	**protein** 2 g
polyunsaturated fat 0.0 g	**DIETARY EXCHANGES**
monounsaturated fat 0.0 g	2 fruit, 1/2 fat free
cholesterol 1 mg	milk
sodium 32 mg	

GO FISH SNACK MIX

SERVES 16

Looking for a healthy trail mix for your kids? Try this one. Make one batch and you'll have a snack for your children and their friends all week long. It's also a perfect team snack after sports practice or a game.

- 2 1/4 cups baked whole-grain fish-shaped snack crackers
- 2/3 cup walnut halves, dry-roasted
- Cooking spray
- 3/4 teaspoon apple pie spice
- 12 ounces dried mixed fruit (any combination)

In a large nonstick saucepan or skillet, stir together the fish crackers and walnuts. Lightly spray with cooking spray. Sprinkle with the apple pie spice. Cook over medium heat for 1 minute, or until the fish crackers are slightly warmed, stirring constantly.

Stir in the dried fruit. Remove from the heat. Spread the mixture on a baking sheet or large platter to cool. Serve immediately or refrigerate in an airtight container for up to five days.

PER SERVING

calories 114	**carbohydrates** 18 g
total fat 4.0 g	fiber 2 g
saturated fat 0.5 g	sugars 8 g
trans fat 0.0 g	**protein** 2 g
polyunsaturated fat 2.5 g	**DIETARY EXCHANGES**
monounsaturated fat 1.0 g	1 fruit, 1/2 starch,
cholesterol 0 mg	1/2 fat
sodium 86 mg	

BERRY BANANA SMOOTHIE

SERVES 2

Get ready for your workout or cool down afterwards with this triple-fruit combination. It's a super-simple way to up your daily servings of fruit.

- 1 cup strawberries, hulled and halved, or raspberries
- 1 medium banana, cut into large pieces
- 1 cup 100% orange juice

In a food processor or blender, process all the ingredients until smooth.

Cook's Tip: Turn these smoothies into a sherbet-like dessert by adding 1/2 to 2 cups crushed ice.

PER SERVING

calories 133	**sodium** 3 mg
total fat 0.5 g	**carbohydrates** 32 g
saturated fat 0.0 g	fiber 3 g
trans fat 0.0 g	sugars 21 g
polyunsaturated fat 0.0 g	**protein** 2 g
monounsaturated fat 0.0 g	**DIETARY EXCHANGES**
cholesterol 0 mg	2 fruit

CINNAMON-SUGAR PITA CHIPS WITH FRUIT SALSA

SERVES 8

This is a sweet spin on the classic chips and salsa combo! Depending on which fruits are favorites at your house, you can use 2 cups of just about any fruit combination to make this family favorite. You can make the sweet, crisp pita chips up to four days ahead and store them in an airtight container at room temperature.

Chips
> 2 6-inch whole-grain pita pockets
> 2 tablespoons sugar
> 1/4 teaspoon ground cinnamon

Salsa
> 2 medium kiwifruit, peeled and diced
> 1 medium banana, diced
> 1 8-ounce can pineapple chunks in their own juice, drained and diced
> 2 teaspoons fresh lime juice

Preheat the oven to 350°F.

Cut each pita into 8 wedges. Split each wedge in half (you will have 32 pieces). Line a large baking sheet with cooking parchment. Arrange the wedges in a single layer on the parchment.

In a small bowl, stir together the sugar and cinnamon. Sprinkle over the pita wedges.

Bake for 10 to 12 minutes, or until crisp. Transfer the baking sheet to a cooling rack and let the pita chips cool completely.

Meanwhile, in a medium bowl, stir together the salsa ingredients. Serve the salsa with the chips.

PER SERVING

calories 90	sodium 82 mg
total fat 0.5 g	carbohydrates 21 g
saturated fat 0.0 g	fiber 2 g
trans fat 0.0 g	sugars 10 g
polyunsaturated fat 0.0 g	protein 2 g
monounsaturated fat 0.0 g	DIETARY EXCHANGES
cholesterol 0 mg	1 fruit, 1/2 starch

CARROT CAKE SMOOTHIE

SERVES 1

Starting with fresh carrot, this good-for-you fruit-and-vegetable smoothie has crunchy walnuts, juicy pineapple, and even a bit of fat-free cream cheese. It's the flavor of carrot cake—but without all the unwanted sugar and unhealthy fats.

> 1/2 cup unsweetened almond-coconut milk blend or 1/2 cup unsweetened almond milk and 1/8 teaspoon coconut extract
> 1 small carrot, thinly sliced
> 1 tablespoon chopped walnuts
> 1/3 cup frozen pineapple chunks
> 1 tablespoon fat-free cream cheese
> 1/4 teaspoon ground cinnamon
> 2 tablespoons chopped fresh spinach or 1 tablespoon chopped frozen spinach, thawed
> Dash of ground nutmeg

In a food processor or blender, process the almond-coconut milk, carrot, and walnuts until smooth. Add the pineapple, cream cheese, and cinnamon. Process until smooth. Add the spinach. Pulse until finely chopped.

Just before serving, lightly sprinkle the smoothie with the nutmeg.

PER SERVING

calories 139	carbohydrates 16 g
total fat 7.0 g	fiber 4 g
saturated fat 1.0 g	sugars 9 g
trans fat 0.0 g	protein 5 g
polyunsaturated fat 4.0 g	DIETARY EXCHANGES
monounsaturated fat 1.0 g	1/2 fruit, 1 vegetable,
cholesterol 2 mg	1/2 lean meat, 1 fat
sodium 255 mg	

POMEGRANATE JULEPS

SERVES 4

Chill your most festive glasses for serving this refreshing drink.

> 2 tablespoons plus 2 teaspoons pomegranate arils (seeds)
> 3 tablespoons hot water
> 1 tablespoon plus 1 teaspoon honey
> 4 sprigs of fresh mint and 4 sprigs of fresh mint, divided use
> 1 1/2 cups 100% pomegranate juice, chilled
> 1 cup 100% grapefruit juice, chilled
> 1/2 cup fresh lime juice, chilled

Put the pomegranate arils in eight sections of an ice cube tray. Fill with water and freeze.

In a small bowl or cup, stir together the hot water and honey until dissolved. Let cool.

Put 4 sprigs of mint and the cooled honey mixture in a glass pitcher. Using a muddler or a large wooden spoon, bruise the mint and combine it with the honey mixture. Stir in all the juices.

To serve, put 2 ice cubes in each glass. Pour the juice mixture over the ice cubes. Garnish with the remaining 4 sprigs of mint.

Cook's Tip on Grapefruit: Grapefruit can interact with a number of medications, including many heart medicines. Be sure to check with your doctor or pharmacist if you take any medication. In this recipe, use 100% white grape juice as an alternate ingredient if necessary.

PER SERVING

calories 112	sodium 13 mg
total fat 0.0 g	carbohydrates 29 g
saturated fat 0.0 g	fiber 1 g
trans fat 0.0 g	sugars 26 g
polyunsaturated fat 0.0 g	protein 1 g
monounsaturated fat 0.0 g	DIETARY EXCHANGES
cholesterol 0 mg	2 fruit

WATERMELON SANGRÍA

SERVES 12

The proper way to toast an outdoor Spanish feast is with sangría, a refreshing blend of fruit juices with the bubble of club soda and some sweet, fresh fruit over ice.

> 6 cups dry white wine (regular or nonalcoholic) or 100% white grape juice, chilled
> 4 cups watermelon cubes, chilled
> 1/3 cup sugar
> 3 tablespoons fresh lemon juice (about 1 medium lemon)
> 3 tablespoons fresh lime juice (about 2 medium limes)
> 5 cups club soda, chilled
> 12 medium strawberries, halved
> 2 medium limes, each cut into 6 slices

In a large glass pitcher, stir together the wine, watermelon, sugar, and both juices. Slowly pour in the club soda, stirring to combine. Serve over ice. Place 2 strawberry halves and 1 lime slice in each glass. Serve immediately.

PER SERVING

calories 123	sodium 27 mg
total fat 0.0 g	carbohydrates 12 g
saturated fat 0.0 g	fiber 1 g
trans fat 0.0 g	sugars 10 g
polyunsaturated fat 0.0 g	protein 1 g
monounsaturated fat 0.0 g	DIETARY EXCHANGES
cholesterol 0 mg	1 other carbohydrate

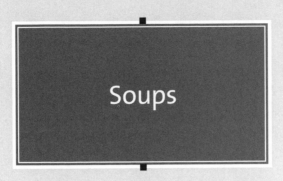

Soups

Beef Broth 35

Greek Egg and Lemon Soup
(*Avgolemono*) 35

Chicken Broth 36

Vegetable Broth 36

Peppery Cream of Carrot Soup 37

Creamy Asparagus Soup 38

Broccoli-Parmesan Soup 38

Roasted Carrot-Ginger Soup 39

Creamy Cauliflower Soup 39

Roasted Corn Soup 40

Fresh Mushroom Soup 41

Onion Soup 41

Herbed Mushroom Soup with Red
Wine 42

Kale and Orzo Soup 42

Roasted Tomato and Red Bell Pepper
Soup 43

Creamy Basil-Tomato Soup 43

Thai-Style Lemon and Spinach
Soup 44

Winter Squash Soup 44

Summer Squash Soup 45

Minestrone 46

Lentil Soup 46

Five-Minute Soup 47

Italian Vegetable Soup 47

Creamy Pumpkin Soup 48

Yogurt-Fruit Soup 48

Southwestern Cod Soup 48

Gazpacho 49

Minted Cantaloupe Soup with Fresh
Lime 50

*Tropical Minted Cantaloupe Soup
with Fresh Lime* 50

Sweet Corn Soup with Crab and
Asparagus 50

*Sweet Corn Soup with Chicken and
Asparagus* 51

New England Fish Chowder 51

Shrimp Gumbo 52

Mulligatawny Soup 52

Salad Bowl Soup 53

Chicken and Vegetable Soup 54

Chicken, Greens, and Potato Soup 54

Chile-Chicken Tortilla Soup 55

BEEF BROTH

MAKES 3 1/2 QUARTS

Roasting the bones is the key to making this beef broth so flavorful. You'll need several hours for this recipe to cook, but the investment will be worth it—a heart-healthy broth that can be used in many, many dishes. And it freezes well!

Cooking spray
6 pounds beef bones
1 teaspoon canola or corn oil
2 large carrots, sliced
2 large leeks (green and white parts), sliced
2 medium ribs of celery with leaves, coarsely chopped
1 large onion, quartered
5 quarts water
8 whole peppercorns
6 to 8 sprigs of fresh parsley
3 sprigs of fresh thyme

Preheat the oven to 400°F. Lightly spray a large baking pan with cooking spray. Put the beef bones in the pan.

Roast for 40 minutes to 1 hour, or until browned.

Meanwhile, in a stockpot, heat the oil over medium-high heat, swirling to coat the bottom. Cook the carrots, leeks, celery, and onion for 5 minutes, stirring occasionally. Reduce the heat to medium. Cook, covered, for 15 to 20 minutes, or until the leeks are limp.

Stir in the browned bones and the remaining ingredients. Increase the heat to high and bring to a boil. Reduce the heat and simmer, covered, for 4 to 5 hours. Strain the broth, discarding the solids. Cover and refrigerate for at least 8 hours so the flavors blend and the fat rises to the surface. Discard the fat before reheating the broth.

Cook's Tip on Freezing Broth: Freeze broth in airtight plastic containers for future use. For smaller amounts, freeze broth in a muffin pan or ice cube trays. Remove the frozen portions and store them in a resealable plastic freezer bag. Thaw the broth for several hours in the refrigerator or by heating it in the microwave.

PER SERVING

calories 10	sodium 30 mg
total fat 0.0 g	carbohydrates 1 g
saturated fat 0.0 g	fiber 0 g
trans fat 0.0 g	sugars 0 g
polyunsaturated fat 0.0 g	protein 2 g
monounsaturated fat 0.0 g	DIETARY EXCHANGES
cholesterol 0 mg	free

GREEK EGG AND LEMON SOUP (AVGOLEMONO)

SERVES 4

Avgolemono (ahv-goh-LEH-moh-noh) is the Greek name for this mildly tangy soup. The egg-lemon mixture creates a silky texture and beautiful appearance as you stir it into the broth.

4 cups fat-free, low-sodium chicken broth, such as on page 36
1/4 cup uncooked instant brown rice
3/4 cup egg substitute, at room temperature
1/4 cup fresh lemon juice (about 1 large lemon)

In a medium saucepan, bring the broth to a boil over medium-high heat.

Stir in the rice. Reduce the heat and simmer, covered, for 15 to 20 minutes, or until the rice is tender. Remove from the heat.

In a medium bowl, whisk together the egg substitute and lemon juice. Gradually whisk about half the broth into the egg substitute mixture. Pour the egg substitute mixture back into the remaining broth, whisking well. Return the pan to the heat.

Cook over low heat for 4 to 5 minutes, or just until the soup has thickened, whisking constantly but lightly. Don't let the soup boil.

PER SERVING

calories 57	sodium 120 mg
total fat 0.0 g	carbohydrates 7 g
saturated fat 0.0 g	fiber 0 g
trans fat 0.0 g	sugars 1 g
polyunsaturated fat 0.0 g	protein 7 g
monounsaturated fat 0.0 g	DIETARY EXCHANGES
cholesterol 0 mg	1/2 starch, 1 lean meat

CHICKEN BROTH

MAKES 4 QUARTS

Homemade broth can add so much depth of flavor to whatever you're cooking that it's really worth taking a few hours to make your own. You can skip roasting the bones, but the roasting step definitely intensifies the flavor. (See Cook's Tip on Freezing Broth, page 35, for how to always have a supply of homemade broth on hand.)

Cooking spray
4 pounds chicken bones
1 teaspoon canola or corn oil
2 medium carrots, sliced
2 medium leeks (green and white parts),
    sliced
1 large onion, quartered
1 medium rib of celery with leaves, coarsely
    chopped
2 cups dry white wine (regular or
    nonalcoholic)
5 quarts water
6 to 8 sprigs of fresh parsley
3 sprigs of fresh thyme
8 whole peppercorns
1 medium dried bay leaf

Preheat the oven to 400°F. Lightly spray a large baking pan with cooking spray. Put the chicken bones in the pan.

Roast for 1 hour, or until browned. (If you prefer a lighter-colored broth, roast the bones for only 30 to 40 minutes.)

Meanwhile, in a stockpot, heat the oil over medium-high heat, swirling to coat the bottom. Cook the carrots, leeks, onion, and celery for 5 minutes, stirring occasionally. Reduce the heat to medium. Cook, covered, for 15 to 20 minutes, or until the leeks are limp.

Stir in the wine. Increase the heat to high and bring to a boil. Boil for 5 to 10 minutes, or until the wine has evaporated.

Stir in the browned bones and the remaining ingredients. Return to a boil. Reduce the heat

and simmer, covered, for 4 to 5 hours. Strain the broth, discarding the solids. Cover and refrigerate for at least 8 hours so the flavors blend and the fat rises to the surface. Discard the fat before reheating the broth.

PER SERVING

calories 10	**sodium** 25 mg
total fat 0.0 g	**carbohydrates** 1 g
saturated fat 0.0 g	fiber 0 g
trans fat 0.0 g	sugars 0 g
polyunsaturated fat 0.0 g	**protein** 2 g
monounsaturated fat 0.0 g	**DIETARY EXCHANGES**
cholesterol 0 mg	free

VEGETABLE BROTH

MAKES 1 3/4 QUARTS

This versatile broth is a cooking essential—experiment with it as the base for other soups and vegetarian dishes and use it to replace water when you cook brown rice and other whole grains. You'll need a couple of hours for the broth to cook, but it'll be time worth spent. (See Cook's Tip on Freezing Broth, page 35, for how to ensure that you always have a supply of homemade broth on hand.)

1 teaspoon canola or corn oil
2 medium onions, quartered
2 large leeks (green and white parts), sliced
9 cups water
2 medium carrots, sliced
3 medium ribs of celery with leaves, coarsely
    chopped
3 or 4 sprigs of fresh thyme
3 large sprigs of fresh parsley
12 whole peppercorns
1 medium dried bay leaf

In a stockpot, heat the oil over medium-high heat, swirling to coat the bottom. Cook the onions and leeks for 4 to 5 minutes, stirring occasionally.

Stir in the remaining ingredients. Increase the heat to high and bring to a boil. Reduce the heat and simmer for 1 hour 15 minutes to 1 hour 30 minutes, or until reduced to about 8 cups. Strain the broth and discard the solids. Cover and refrigerate for at least 8 hours so the flavors blend.

PER SERVING

calories 5	sodium 10 mg
total fat 0.0 g	carbohydrates 1 g
saturated fat 0.0 g	fiber 0 g
trans fat 0.0 g	sugars 0 g
polyunsaturated fat 0.0 g	protein 0 g
monounsaturated fat 0.0 g	DIETARY EXCHANGES
cholesterol 0 mg	free

PEPPERY CREAM OF CARROT SOUP

SERVES 4

Using part broth and part fat-free half-and-half produces a soup that is creamy without being overwhelmingly rich. To make this vegetarian, use a fat-free, low-sodium vegetable broth, such as on page 36, instead of chicken broth.

1 teaspoon olive oil
1 pound carrots, cut into 2 x 1/2-inch pieces
3/4 cup chopped onion
2 medium garlic cloves, minced
3/4 teaspoon grated peeled gingerroot
1/4 teaspoon pepper
1/8 to 1/4 teaspoon cayenne
1/8 teaspoon ground nutmeg
1/8 teaspoon salt
2 cups fat-free, low-sodium chicken broth, such as on page 36
1 cup fat-free half-and-half

In a large, heavy saucepan, heat the oil over medium-high heat, swirling to coat the bottom. Cook the carrots and onion for 10 minutes, stirring frequently.

Stir in the garlic, gingerroot, pepper, cayenne, nutmeg, and salt. Cook for 30 seconds, stirring frequently.

Pour in the broth. Bring to a simmer, stirring frequently. Reduce the heat and simmer, covered, for 30 to 40 minutes, or until the carrots are tender, stirring occasionally.

In a food processor or blender (vent the blender lid), process the soup in batches until smooth. Carefully return the soup to the pan.

Pour in the half-and-half. Increase the heat to medium. Cook for 1 to 2 minutes, or until heated through, stirring constantly.

Cook's Tip on Whole Nutmeg: We call for ground nutmeg in our recipes because that is what most home cooks use. However, freshly grated nutmeg is more fragrant and flavorful. If you keep whole nutmeg in a tightly sealed container in a cool, dark place, it will last indefinitely. Then use a grater or rasp zester to grate only the amount needed for your recipe.

Cook's Tip on Blending Hot Liquids: Be careful when blending hot liquids. Venting the blender lid prevents heat and steam from popping off the lid. Most blender lids have a center section that can be removed. You can even place a kitchen towel over the opening to avoid splatters. Begin blending at the lowest speed and increase to the desired speed, holding the lid down firmly. If you have an immersion, or handheld, blender, you can use it instead of a blender or food processor (it will save cleanup time, too).

PER SERVING

calories 114	carbohydrates 21 g
total fat 2.0 g	fiber 3 g
saturated fat 0.5 g	sugars 11 g
trans fat 0.0 g	protein 6 g
polyunsaturated fat 0.0 g	DIETARY EXCHANGES
monounsaturated fat 1.0 g	3 vegetable, 1/2 fat-free milk
cholesterol 0 mg	
sodium 187 mg	

CREAMY ASPARAGUS SOUP

SERVES 4

Pureed rice provides creaminess, and adding the asparagus tips at the end of the cooking process gives the soup an appealing texture and a freshness.

2 teaspoons canola or corn oil
1 small onion, chopped
1 medium rib of celery, chopped
4 cups fat-free, low-sodium chicken broth, such as on page 36
10 ounces frozen asparagus spears, thawed
1/4 cup uncooked instant brown rice
Dash of pepper (white preferred)
Dash of ground nutmeg

In a large saucepan, heat the oil over medium-high heat, swirling to coat the bottom. Cook the onion and celery for about 3 minutes, or until the onion is soft, stirring frequently.

Pour in the broth. Increase the heat to high and bring to a boil.

Meanwhile, cut the tips off the asparagus and set aside. Cut the stalks into 1-inch pieces.

When the broth is boiling, stir in the asparagus pieces (not the tips) and rice. Reduce the heat and simmer, covered, for 15 minutes, or until the rice is tender.

In a food processor or blender (vent the blender lid), process the soup in batches until smooth. Carefully return the soup to the pan.

Gently stir in the asparagus tips, pepper, and nutmeg. Cook for about 5 minutes, or until heated through.

Cook's Tip on Immersion Blenders: Also called a hand blender, this wand-shaped gadget with a blender blade at the bottom has become a staple in many kitchens. If you have one, you'll find that it's especially useful when you want to make creamy soup, because you blend the soup right in the saucepan. No more burning yourself or spilling part of the soup when you transfer it from the pan to a blender or food processor and back to the pan again.

PER SERVING

calories 82	carbohydrates 11 g
total fat 2.5 g	fiber 2 g
saturated fat 0.0 g	sugars 2 g
trans fat 0.0 g	protein 5 g
polyunsaturated fat 1.0 g	DIETARY EXCHANGES
monounsaturated fat 1.5 g	1 vegetable, 1/2 starch,
cholesterol 0 mg	1/2 fat
sodium 41 mg	

BROCCOLI-PARMESAN SOUP

SERVES 6

Parmesan, parsley, and ginger set this recipe apart from traditional broccoli-cheese soup. Pair it with a fruit salad, such as Berry Explosion Salad (page 86), and a crusty whole-grain roll for a light, healthy meal.

1 teaspoon olive oil
1 cup chopped onion
1/4 cup chopped celery
2 medium garlic cloves, minced
12 ounces broccoli florets
3 cups fat-free, low-sodium chicken broth, such as on page 36
1 tablespoon chopped fresh parsley
2 cups fat-free milk
1/4 cup all-purpose flour
1/4 cup shredded or grated Parmesan cheese
1/4 teaspoon pepper
1/4 teaspoon ground ginger

In a large, heavy saucepan, heat the oil over medium-high heat, swirling to coat the bottom. Cook the onion and celery for 3 minutes, or until the onion is soft, stirring frequently.

Stir in the garlic. Cook for 30 seconds, stirring frequently.

Stir in the broccoli, broth, and parsley. Bring to a boil. Reduce the heat and simmer, covered, for 8 to 10 minutes, or until the broccoli is tender, stirring occasionally.

In a small bowl, whisk together the milk and flour. Stir into the soup. Increase the heat to medium high and bring to a boil, stirring frequently. Reduce the heat and simmer for 1 to 2 minutes, or until slightly thickened, stirring occasionally.

In a food processor or blender (vent the blender lid), process the soup in batches until slightly chunky. Carefully return the soup to the pan.

Stir in the Parmesan, pepper, and ginger.

Cook's Tip: For a change of flavor, replace the ground ginger with curry powder to taste.

PER SERVING

calories 105	**carbohydrates** 15 g
total fat 2.0 g	fiber 2 g
saturated fat 1.0 g	sugars 6 g
trans fat 0.0 g	**protein** 8 g
polyunsaturated fat 0.0 g	**DIETARY EXCHANGES**
monounsaturated fat 1.0 g	1 vegetable, 1/2 fat-
cholesterol 4 mg	free milk
sodium 127 mg	

ROASTED CARROT-GINGER SOUP

SERVES 4

Roasting the carrots deepens their sweetness, enhancing the flavors of the fresh gingerroot and cumin in this soup. Have a cup with Curried Rice and Bean Salad *(page 104) for a satisfying, palate-pleasing supper.*

    Cooking spray
    1 pound carrots, cut crosswise into 1-inch
        pieces (about 2 cups)
    3/4 cup coarsely chopped onion
    2 medium garlic cloves, minced
    2 teaspoons olive oil
    3 1/4 cups fat-free, low-sodium vegetable
        broth, such as on page 36, or fat-free,
        low-sodium chicken broth, such as on
        page 36
    1/2 teaspoon ground cumin
    1/2 teaspoon grated peeled gingerroot
    1/4 teaspoon dried thyme, crumbled
    1/8 teaspoon pepper (freshly ground
        preferred)
    2 tablespoons fat-free plain yogurt
    2 teaspoons chopped pistachios or walnuts

Preheat the oven to 425°F. Lightly spray a large rimmed baking sheet with cooking spray.

Put the carrots, onion, garlic, and oil in a large bowl. Stir to coat. Spread the carrot mixture on the baking sheet. Roast for 20 minutes, or until the carrots are almost tender and the onion is browned.

Meanwhile, in a large saucepan, whisk together the broth, cumin, gingerroot, thyme, and pepper. Bring to a boil over high heat.

Stir in the carrot mixture. Return to a boil. Reduce the heat to low. Simmer for 20 minutes, or until the carrots are very tender, stirring occasionally. Using an immersion blender, blend the soup in the pan until smooth.

Or, let the soup stand to cool to room temperature, about 20 to 30 minutes. Transfer the soup in batches to a food processor or blender. Process until smooth. Return the soup to the pan. Cook for 5 to 10 minutes, or until heated through.

Just before serving, top the soup with a dollop of yogurt. Sprinkle with the pistachios.

PER SERVING

calories 98	**sodium** 94 mg
total fat 3.0 g	**carbohydrates** 16 g
saturated fat 0.0 g	fiber 4 g
trans fat 0.0 g	sugars 7 g
polyunsaturated fat 1.0 g	**protein** 3 g
monounsaturated fat 2.0 g	**DIETARY EXCHANGES**
cholesterol 0 mg	3 vegetable, 1/2 fat

CREAMY CAULIFLOWER SOUP

SERVES 4

Cauliflower is enjoying a surge in popularity these days, and with all the culinary roles it plays—in both its raw and cooked forms—it's not surprising. Its subtle, rich flavors make this elegant soup the perfect way to lead off your next celebratory dinner.

    4 cups cauliflower florets
    1/2 cup chopped onion
    1 tablespoon fresh lemon juice
    2 tablespoons all-purpose flour
    1/4 cup fat-free milk and 2 3/4 cups fat-free
        milk, divided use
    1 medium garlic clove, minced
    1/4 cup chopped fresh basil (optional)
    2 tablespoons light tub margarine
    1/8 teaspoon salt

(continued)

In a large saucepan, add water to a depth of 1 inch. Put the cauliflower and onion in a collapsible steamer basket. Place the steamer in the pan. Make sure the water doesn't touch the bottom of the steamer. Sprinkle the lemon juice over the vegetables. Bring the water to a boil over high heat. Steam the vegetables, covered, for 8 minutes, or until the cauliflower is very tender. Remove from the heat. Carefully uncover the pan away from you (to prevent steam burns). Drain the vegetables well in a colander.

Meanwhile, put the flour in a small bowl. Add 1/4 cup milk, whisking to dissolve.

Return the cauliflower and onion to the pan. Stir in the flour mixture, garlic, and the remaining 2 3/4 cups milk. Bring just to a boil over medium-high heat, stirring occasionally. Reduce the heat and simmer for 3 minutes, or until thickened.

Using a wire whisk or potato masher, mash the cauliflower mixture to thicken it slightly. Remove from the heat. Stir in the basil, margarine, and salt.

PER SERVING

calories 133	carbohydrates 20 g
total fat 3.0 g	fiber 3 g
saturated fat 0.0 g	sugars 12 g
trans fat 0.0 g	protein 9 g
polyunsaturated fat 0.5 g	DIETARY EXCHANGES
monounsaturated fat 1.5 g	1 fat-free milk,
cholesterol 4 mg	1 vegetable, 1/2 fat
sodium 228 mg	

ROASTED CORN SOUP

SERVES 4

Roasting the corn intensifies its sweetness, making this satisfying low-calorie soup a real standout. If it's in season, try using fresh corn instead. Make this vegetarian by using vegetable broth instead of beef broth.

Cooking spray
1 cup frozen whole-kernel corn, partially thawed
1 cup fat-free, low-sodium beef broth, such as on page 35

1 cup chopped onion
1 medium garlic clove, minced
1 3/4 cups water
1 cup low-sodium mixed-vegetable juice
2 medium carrots, chopped
1/4 large red bell pepper, chopped
1/4 small green bell pepper, chopped
1 teaspoon chili powder
1/2 teaspoon ground cumin
2 tablespoons chopped fresh cilantro

Preheat the oven to 425°F.

Lightly spray a baking sheet with cooking spray. Spread the corn in a single layer on the baking sheet. Lightly spray the corn with cooking spray.

Roast for 12 to 14 minutes, or until lightly browned, stirring once halfway through. Remove from the oven.

About the time you stir the corn, stir together the broth, onion, and garlic in a medium saucepan. Cook over medium-high heat for 4 minutes.

Stir in the corn and the remaining ingredients except the cilantro. Reduce the heat to medium and cook for 15 minutes, stirring occasionally. Just before serving, stir in the cilantro.

Cook's Tip: Serving a broth-based vegetable soup such as this one with lunch or before dinner is a great way to take the edge off appetites and keep servings of higher-calorie dishes in proportion.

PER SERVING

calories 95	sodium 87 mg
total fat 0.5 g	carbohydrates 21 g
saturated fat 0.0 g	fiber 4 g
trans fat 0.0 g	sugars 8 g
polyunsaturated fat 0.5 g	protein 4 g
monounsaturated fat 0.0 g	DIETARY EXCHANGES
cholesterol 0 mg	2 vegetable, 1/2 starch

FRESH MUSHROOM SOUP

SERVES 4

Try a variety of mushrooms to make your soup more interesting. Among the choices are shiitake, portobello, oyster, cremini, and, of course, button.

> 1 teaspoon light tub margarine
> 8 ounces mushrooms, any variety, 4 ounces finely chopped and 4 ounces sliced
> 1 large onion, chopped
> 2 medium garlic cloves, minced
> 3 1/2 cups fat-free, low-sodium chicken broth, such as on page 36
> 1 5-ounce can fat-free evaporated milk
> 1/3 cup all-purpose flour
> 1 1/2 tablespoons finely chopped fresh parsley
> 1 tablespoon dry sherry (optional)
> 1/2 teaspoon grated lemon zest
> 1 teaspoon fresh lemon juice
> 1/8 teaspoon salt
> 1/8 teaspoon pepper (white preferred)

In a large saucepan, melt the margarine over medium heat, swirling to coat the bottom. Cook the mushrooms, onion, and garlic, covered, for 8 minutes, stirring occasionally. Increase the heat to high and cook, uncovered, for 2 to 3 minutes, or until the moisture evaporates.

In a medium bowl, whisk together the broth, milk, and flour. Immediately whisk into the mushroom mixture. Reduce the heat to medium high and bring to a boil, stirring occasionally. Cook for 3 to 5 minutes, or until thickened, stirring occasionally.

Stir in the remaining ingredients.

PER SERVING

calories 118	**carbohydrates** 20 g
total fat 1.0 g	fiber 2 g
saturated fat 0.0 g	sugars 9 g
trans fat 0.0 g	**protein** 8 g
polyunsaturated fat 0.0 g	**DIETARY EXCHANGES**
monounsaturated fat 0.0 g	1/2 starch, 1/2 fat-free
cholesterol 2 mg	milk, 1 vegetable
sodium 154 mg	

ONION SOUP

SERVES 6

Caramelized onions give this soup its rich flavor. Once you master the necessary technique, you can use caramelized onions to enhance the flavor of other dishes. For starters, try them in casseroles, quiches, and pizzas.

> 6 slices French bread, baguette-style (about 2 ounces total) (lowest sodium available)
> 2 tablespoons shredded or grated Parmesan cheese
> 1 teaspoon canola or corn oil
> 1 teaspoon light tub margarine
> 3 cups thinly sliced onions
> 1/2 teaspoon sugar
> 1/4 teaspoon salt
> 6 cups fat-free, low-sodium beef broth, such as on page 35
> 1/2 cup dry white wine (regular or nonalcoholic)
> 1 medium dried bay leaf
> 1/4 teaspoon dried thyme, crumbled
> 1/4 teaspoon pepper, or to taste
> 1/8 teaspoon ground nutmeg

Preheat the oven to 350°F.

Put the bread slices on a baking sheet.

Bake for 10 minutes, or until toasted. Sprinkle with the Parmesan. Bake for 1 to 2 minutes, or until the Parmesan melts. Set aside.

In a large saucepan, heat the oil and margarine over medium-high heat, swirling to coat the bottom. Cook the onions for 2 minutes, stirring occasionally. Reduce the heat to low. Cook, covered, for 5 minutes, or until the onions are soft, stirring occasionally.

Stir in the sugar and salt. Increase the heat to medium high and cook, uncovered, for 15 to 20 minutes, or until the onions are golden brown, stirring occasionally. After the first 10 minutes, stir more often to keep the onions from sticking and burning.

(continued)

Stir in the remaining ingredients. Bring to a boil. Reduce the heat and simmer, partially covered, for 15 minutes. Discard the bay leaf. Just before serving, top the soup with the toasted bread slices.

HERBED MUSHROOM SOUP WITH RED WINE

SERVES 4

The concentrated, deep flavors of onion, wine, and herbs are brought together in this any-occasion soup. For even more mushroom taste, use brown (cremini) mushrooms.

Cooking spray
2 large onions, chopped
1 pound sliced button mushrooms
1 medium garlic clove, minced
2 cups water
3/4 cup dry red wine (regular or nonalcoholic)
3 packets (1 tablespoon) salt-free instant beef bouillon
1 teaspoon dried thyme, crumbled
2 teaspoons Worcestershire sauce (lowest sodium available)
1 1/2 teaspoons sugar
1/4 teaspoon salt
1/4 teaspoon pepper
1/2 cup finely chopped fresh parsley
2 tablespoons light tub margarine

Lightly spray a Dutch oven with cooking spray. Heat over medium-high heat. Cook the onions for 3 minutes, or until soft, stirring frequently.

Stir in the mushrooms and garlic. Lightly spray the vegetables with cooking spray. Cook for 4 minutes, or until the mushrooms are soft, stirring frequently.

Stir in the water, wine, bouillon, and thyme. Increase the heat to high and bring to a boil. Reduce the heat and simmer, covered, for 15 minutes, or until the onions are very soft, stirring occasionally.

Stir in the Worcestershire sauce, sugar, salt, and pepper. Simmer, covered, for 10 minutes. Remove from the heat.

Stir in the parsley and margarine.

Cook's Tip: Adding the sugar near the end of the cooking time makes the onions taste a bit sweeter and richer.

KALE AND ORZO SOUP

SERVES 4

Very easy to make, this soup will become a fast favorite. Topped with crunchy pine nuts, it pairs well with Italian dishes, or make it an entrée by stirring in some cooked cubed or shredded chicken breast.

4 cups fat-free, low-sodium chicken broth, such as on page 36
1/2 cup water
1/4 cup plus 1 tablespoon no-salt-added tomato paste
1/2 teaspoon grated lemon zest
1/4 cup dried whole-grain orzo or pastina
8 ounces fresh kale, stems discarded and leaves chopped, or 5 ounces frozen chopped spinach, thawed and well drained
2 medium green onions, sliced
1/4 teaspoon pepper
1/8 teaspoon salt
1/4 cup pine nuts, dry-roasted

In a medium saucepan, whisk together the broth, water, and tomato paste until smooth. Add the lemon zest. Bring to a boil over medium-high heat.

Stir in the orzo. Reduce the heat to medium and cook for 5 to 7 minutes, or until the orzo is tender.

Stir in the kale and green onions. Cook for 2 to 3 minutes.

Stir in the pepper and salt. Sprinkle with the pine nuts.

Cook's Tip on Orzo: Orzo looks like, and is a good substitute for, rice, although it actually is very small pasta.

Cook's Tip on Pastina: Pastina, or "tiny pasta," is frequently used in soups. If you cannot find pastina, finely crush any type of whole-grain macaroni.

PER SERVING

calories 138	**carbohydrates** 19 g
total fat 4.5 g	fiber 3 g
saturated fat 0.5 g	sugars 4 g
trans fat 0.0 g	**protein** 9 g
polyunsaturated fat 2.0 g	**DIETARY EXCHANGES**
monounsaturated fat 1.5 g	2 vegetable, 1/2 starch,
cholesterol 0 mg	1 fat
sodium 136 mg	

ROASTED TOMATO AND RED BELL PEPPER SOUP

SERVES 4

This vibrant red soup accented with chopped fresh basil has a smoky taste from the combination of roasted red bell peppers and roasted tomatoes. Just the right amount of fresh citrus juice added at the end of the cooking process kicks up the flavor.

- 1/2 teaspoon olive oil
- 1/3 cup chopped onion
- 1 14.5-ounce can no-salt-added fire-roasted diced tomatoes, undrained
- 1/2 cup roasted red bell peppers, drained and chopped
- 1 cup water
- 1/4 cup chopped fresh basil

- 1 teaspoon fresh lemon juice
- 1/4 teaspoon pepper

In a large saucepan, heat the oil over medium-high heat, swirling to coat the bottom. Cook the onion for 3 minutes, or until beginning to soften, stirring occasionally. Stir in the tomatoes with liquid and roasted peppers. Cook for 1 minute.

Stir in the water. Increase the heat to high and bring to a boil. Reduce the heat and simmer for 20 to 25 minutes, or until the onion is soft, stirring occasionally.

In a food processor or blender (vent the blender lid), process the soup in batches until slightly smooth with some chunks remaining. Carefully return the soup to the pan. (You can also use an immersion, or handheld, blender to process the soup.)

Stir in the basil, lemon juice, and pepper. Increase the heat to medium. Cook the soup for 2 to 3 minutes, or until heated through, stirring occasionally.

PER SERVING

calories 37	**sodium** 29 mg
total fat 0.5 g	**carbohydrates** 7 g
saturated fat 0.0 g	fiber 1 g
trans fat 0.0 g	sugars 4 g
polyunsaturated fat 0.0 g	**protein** 1 g
monounsaturated fat 0.5 g	**DIETARY EXCHANGES**
cholesterol 0 mg	1 vegetable

CREAMY BASIL-TOMATO SOUP

SERVES 6

Tomato soup flavored with fresh basil has become a popular staple, but it's often packed with sodium and saturated fat. This healthier version can be ready in about 30 minutes.

(continued)

1 teaspoon olive oil

3/4 cup chopped onion

1/3 cup chopped celery

1/3 cup finely chopped carrot

2 medium garlic cloves, minced

1/2 teaspoon dried oregano, crumbled

1/8 teaspoon pepper

1 14.5-ounce can no-salt-added diced
tomatoes, undrained

1 14.5-ounce can no-salt-added stewed
tomatoes, undrained

1 cup fat-free, low-sodium chicken broth, such
as on page 36, or fat-free, low-sodium
vegetable broth, such as on page 36

1 teaspoon sugar

1/4 cup chopped fresh basil

3 tablespoons fat-free sour cream

3 tablespoons shredded or grated Parmesan
cheese

In a large saucepan, heat the oil over medium-
high heat, swirling to coat the bottom. Cook the
onion, celery, and carrot for 3 minutes, or until
the onion is soft, stirring frequently.

Stir in the garlic, oregano, and pepper. Cook for
30 seconds, stirring constantly.

Stir in the diced tomatoes with liquid, stewed tomatoes with liquid, broth, and sugar. Bring to a
simmer, stirring frequently. Reduce the heat and
simmer, covered, for 15 to 20 minutes, stirring
occasionally.

Stir in the basil.

In a food processor or blender (vent the blender
lid), process the soup in batches until almost
smooth. Carefully return the soup to the pan.

Stir in the sour cream and Parmesan. Increase
the heat to medium. Cook for 1 to 2 minutes, or
until heated through, stirring constantly.

PER SERVING

calories 79	sodium 80 mg
total fat 1.5 g	carbohydrates 12 g
saturated fat 0.5 g	fiber 2 g
trans fat 0.0 g	sugars 7 g
polyunsaturated fat 0.0 g	protein 3 g
monounsaturated fat 1.0 g	DIETARY EXCHANGES
cholesterol 3 mg	2 vegetable, 1/2 fat

THAI-STYLE LEMON AND SPINACH SOUP

SERVES 4

*So quick, so easy, so versatile! Tie it together by
pairing it with Pad Thai with Tofu and Greens
(page 359).*

3 cups fat-free, low-sodium chicken broth,
such as on page 36

2 ounces dried whole-grain vermicelli, broken
into thirds

1 ounce spinach, coarsely chopped

1/2 cup finely chopped green onions

1/2 cup finely chopped fresh cilantro

4 lemon slices

1/2 teaspoon grated peeled gingerroot

1/8 teaspoon crushed red pepper flakes

1/8 teaspoon salt

In a large saucepan over high heat, bring the
broth to a boil. Stir in the pasta. Return to a boil.
Reduce the heat and simmer, covered, for 8 minutes, or until the pasta is tender.

Stir in the remaining ingredients. Increase the
heat to high and return just to a boil. Remove
from the heat.

PER SERVING

calories 66	sodium 103 mg
total fat 0.5 g	carbohydrates 12 g
saturated fat 0.0 g	fiber 2 g
trans fat 0.0 g	sugars 1 g
polyunsaturated fat 0.0 g	protein 4 g
monounsaturated fat 0.0 g	DIETARY EXCHANGES
cholesterol 0 mg	1 starch

WINTER SQUASH SOUP

SERVES 6

*It's very easy to transform leftover cooked winter
squash or sweet potatoes into this creamy dish.
If you don't have either on hand, the Cook's Tip,
page 45, explains how to easily prepare either.*

3 cups fat-free, low-sodium chicken broth,
such as on page 36

2 cups mashed cooked winter squash (any
variety) or sweet potatoes, thawed if
frozen or well drained if canned

1 teaspoon onion powder
1/2 teaspoon garlic powder
1/2 teaspoon ground cumin
1/4 teaspoon salt
1/4 teaspoon pepper
1 cup fat-free half-and-half

In a medium saucepan, stir together all the ingredients except the half-and-half. Bring to a simmer over medium-high heat, stirring occasionally. Reduce the heat and simmer, covered, for 6 to 8 minutes.

Stir in the half-and-half. Cook for 2 to 3 minutes, or until heated through, stirring occasionally.

Cook's Tip: For 2 cups mashed roasted acorn squash, cut a 2-pound squash in half lengthwise. Discard the seeds and strings. Lightly spray the squash with cooking spray. Place the squash on a nonstick baking sheet with the cut side up. Bake at 400°F for 50 minutes to 1 hour, or until tender when tested with the tip of a sharp knife or a fork. Scoop out the flesh and mash. For 2 cups mashed sweet potatoes, cook 1 1/2 pounds sweet potatoes in boiling water for 30 minutes, or until tender. Discard the skins and mash the flesh.

Cook's Tip on Cutting Winter Squash: Some winter squash, such as butternut and acorn, are difficult to cut when raw. To make the job easy, pierce the squash several times with a fork and transfer the squash to a microwaveable plate. Microwave on 100 percent power (high) for 1 to 2 minutes. Let the squash stand for 5 minutes before cutting. Using a large, sturdy knife, cut off the stem end, then cut lengthwise from the stem end through the root end. Using a spoon, scoop out and discard the seeds and strings (or reserve the seeds and roast them).

PER SERVING

calories 63	sodium 153 mg
total fat 0.0 g	carbohydrates 13 g
saturated fat 0.0 g	fiber 2 g
trans fat 0.0 g	sugars 3 g
polyunsaturated fat 0.0 g	protein 4 g
monounsaturated fat 0.0 g	**DIETARY EXCHANGES**
cholesterol 0 mg	1 starch

SUMMER SQUASH SOUP

SERVES 5

With summer squash available year-round, you can enjoy this rice and veggie soup whenever the craving hits you.

1 teaspoon light tub margarine
1 large onion, chopped
2 medium yellow summer squash, zucchini, or a combination, diced
2 cups fat-free, low-sodium chicken broth and 2 cups fat-free, low-sodium chicken broth, such as on page 36, divided use
2 tablespoons uncooked brown rice
1 teaspoon dried thyme, crumbled
1 medium carrot, grated
1/2 cup fat-free plain yogurt

In a medium saucepan, melt the margarine over medium-high heat, swirling to coat the bottom. Cook the onion for about 3 minutes, or until soft, stirring frequently.

Stir in the squash. Cook for 5 minutes, stirring occasionally. Remove and set aside 1 cup of the mixture.

Stir 2 cups broth, the rice, and thyme into the onion mixture. Reduce the heat to medium and cook for 20 minutes, or until the rice is tender.

In a food processor or blender (vent the blender lid), process the soup in batches until smooth.

Carefully return the soup to the pan. Stir in the carrot and the remaining 2 cups broth. Cook for 5 minutes over medium-high heat, stirring occasionally. Reduce the heat to low. Stir in the reserved squash mixture. Cook for 1 to 2 minutes, stirring occasionally.

Stir in the yogurt. Cook for 1 to 2 minutes, or until the soup is heated through.

PER SERVING

calories 77	sodium 89 mg
total fat 1.0 g	carbohydrates 13 g
saturated fat 0.0 g	fiber 2 g
trans fat 0.0 g	sugars 7 g
polyunsaturated fat 0.0 g	protein 5 g
monounsaturated fat 0.0 g	**DIETARY EXCHANGES**
cholesterol 1 mg	1/2 starch, 1 vegetable

MINESTRONE

SERVES 8

One of the best things about a soup like this is that almost any combination of vegetables, beans, and pasta can be used. Use whatever you have on hand! It'll be different each time you make this recipe—but delicious every time.

2 teaspoons olive oil

1 medium onion, chopped

2 medium carrots, chopped

2 medium ribs of celery with leaves, chopped

2 medium garlic cloves, chopped, and
    1 medium garlic clove, whole, divided use

4 cups fat-free, low-sodium vegetable broth,
    such as on page 36, or fat-free, low-
    sodium beef broth, such as on page 35

1 15.5-ounce can no-salt-added navy beans,
    rinsed and drained

1 14.5-ounce can no-salt-added diced
    tomatoes, undrained

1 large potato, peeled and cubed

8 ounces green beans, trimmed and cut into
    1-inch pieces

1 small zucchini, cubed

1/2 cup dried whole-grain elbow macaroni or
    medium shell pasta

1 tablespoon dried basil, crumbled

1 teaspoon dried oregano, crumbled

1 teaspoon pepper, or to taste

1/4 teaspoon salt

1 to 2 cups water, as needed

2 tablespoons shredded or grated Parmesan
    cheese

In a stockpot, heat the oil over medium-high heat, swirling to coat the bottom. Cook the onion, carrots, celery, and chopped garlic for about 3 minutes, or until the onion is soft, stirring frequently.

Stir in the broth, navy beans, tomatoes with liquid, potato, green beans, zucchini, pasta, basil, oregano, pepper, salt, and the remaining whole garlic clove. Reduce the heat and simmer for 45 minutes.

Gradually stir in 1 cup water. Using a potato masher, slightly mash the soup ingredients. Stir

in more water as needed for the desired consistency. Just before serving, sprinkle with the Parmesan.

Cook's Tip on Potato Skins: Don't throw away potato skins—they're rich in vitamins and other nutrients. You can even use them to make a vegetable broth: Combine water and the peels of 6 or 7 raw potatoes with garlic, parsley, coarsely chopped onion, carrot, and celery to taste, then gently simmer, covered, for about 1 hour 30 minutes. Either strain the broth or, for a thicker consistency, process it in a food processor or blender (vent the blender lid) until smooth.

PER SERVING

calories 153	**carbohydrates** 29 g
total fat 2.0 g	fiber 7 g
saturated fat 0.5 g	sugars 7 g
trans fat 0.0 g	**protein** 7 g
polyunsaturated fat 0.5 g	**DIETARY EXCHANGES**
monounsaturated fat 1.0 g	1 1/2 starch,
cholesterol 1 mg	2 vegetable
sodium 151 mg	

LENTIL SOUP

SERVES 8

This legume-based soup makes an attractive orangey-red side dish to a Middle Eastern entrée, such as Falafel with Quick-Pickled Garlic Cucumbers *(page 337) or* Kibbee *(page 296).*

1 tablespoon fat-free, low-sodium
    chicken broth, such as on page 36, or
    1 tablespoon water

1 medium onion, chopped

1 medium red bell pepper, chopped

2 medium garlic cloves, chopped, or
    1 teaspoon bottled minced garlic

7 cups water

1 cup dried red lentils, sorted for stones and
    shriveled lentils, rinsed, and drained

1 1/2 teaspoons ground cumin

1/4 teaspoon ground ginger

1/4 teaspoon ground cloves

1/8 teaspoon cayenne

Pepper to taste

2 tablespoons fat-free plain Greek yogurt

In a large stockpot, heat the broth over medium-high heat, swirling to coat the bottom. Cook the onion, bell pepper, and garlic for 3 minutes, or until the onion is soft and the bell pepper is tender, stirring frequently.

Stir in the remaining ingredients except the yogurt. Bring to a boil. Reduce the heat and simmer, partially covered, for 35 to 40 minutes, or until the lentils are tender. Top each serving with a dollop of the yogurt.

PER SERVING

calories 103	carbohydrates 19 g
total fat 0.0 g	fiber 4 g
saturated fat 0.0 g	sugars 4 g
trans fat 0.0 g	protein 8 g
polyunsaturated fat 0.0 g	DIETARY EXCHANGES
monounsaturated fat 0.0 g	1 1/2 starch, 1/2 lean
cholesterol 0 mg	meat
sodium 10 mg	

FIVE-MINUTE SOUP

SERVES 6

Serve this quick-cooking soup on a busy day. It's just as fast as drive-through fast food, but much healthier.

> 4 cups fat-free, low-sodium chicken broth, such as on page 36, heated
> 2 cups shredded spinach, kale, or cabbage
> 1 medium zucchini, very thinly sliced
> 1/2 cup shredded skinless chicken breast or shredded lean meat, cooked without salt, all visible fat discarded
> 4 medium button mushrooms, sliced
> 1 medium tomato, cubed

In a large saucepan, stir together all the ingredients. Bring to a boil over medium-high heat. Reduce the heat and simmer for 5 minutes.

PER SERVING

calories 41	sodium 39 mg
total fat 0.5 g	carbohydrates 3 g
saturated fat 0.0 g	fiber 1 g
trans fat 0.0 g	sugars 1 g
polyunsaturated fat 0.0 g	protein 6 g
monounsaturated fat 0.0 g	DIETARY EXCHANGES
cholesterol 10 mg	1 lean meat

ITALIAN VEGETABLE SOUP

SERVES 8

Start your meal right with a serving's worth of veggies in this nutrient-rich side soup. Serve it as the first course to Smothered Steak with Sangría Sauce (page 258) or Chicken Marsala (page 209), or try it with Focaccia (page 443) or Kale Caesar Salad with Polenta Croutons (page 69) for a lighter meal.

> 2 tablespoons light tub margarine
> 2 large onions, coarsely chopped
> 1 1/2 cups thinly sliced carrots
> 1 1/2 cups thinly sliced celery
> 1 medium garlic clove, crushed
> 1 medium zucchini, sliced
> 3 1/2 cups fat-free, low sodium chicken broth, such as on page 36
> 1 14.5-ounce can Italian plum (Roma) tomatoes, undrained
> 1 teaspoon dried oregano, crumbled
> 1/2 teaspoon dried basil, crumbled
> 1/8 teaspoon pepper (freshly ground preferred)
> 1/4 teaspoon red hot-pepper sauce, or to taste
> 1/4 to 1/2 teaspoon salt-free all-purpose seasoning
> 1/2 cup shredded or grated Parmesan cheese (freshly grated preferred)

In a large skillet over medium-high heat, melt the margarine, swirling to coat the bottom. Cook the onions, carrots, celery, and garlic for 5 minutes, stirring frequently. Stir in the zucchini. Cook for 4 to 5 minutes, stirring occasionally. Stir in the broth and tomatoes with liquid. Stir in the remaining ingredients except the Parmesan. Bring to a boil. Reduce the heat and simmer, covered, for 8 to 12 minutes, or until the vegetables are tender-crisp.

Just before serving, sprinkle with the Parmesan.

PER SERVING

calories 86.0	sodium 235 mg
total fat 2.5 g	carbohydrates 11 g
saturated fat 1.0 g	fiber 3 g
trans fat 0.0 g	sugars 6 g
polyunsaturated fat 0.5 g	protein 5 g
monounsaturated fat 1.0 g	DIETARY EXCHANGES
cholesterol 4 mg	2 vegetable, 1/2 fat

CREAMY PUMPKIN SOUP

SERVES 8

With canned pumpkin available all year long, there's no reason not to enjoy this fall favorite during the other seasons, too. Use the leftover pumpkin to make Velvet Pumpkin Bread *(page 456) or* Slow-Cooker Pumpkin Oatmeal *(page 121).*

    2 tablespoons light tub margarine
    3 medium green onions, sliced
    2 cups canned solid-pack pumpkin (not pie
        filling)
    2 tablespoons all-purpose flour
    1/4 teaspoon ground ginger
    1/8 teaspoon ground turmeric
    1/3 cup fat-free milk and 1 2/3 cups fat-free
        milk, divided use
    4 cups fat-free, low-sodium chicken broth,
        such as on page 36
    Chopped fresh chives or parsley, to taste

In a large saucepan, melt the margarine over medium-high heat, swirling to coat the bottom. Cook the green onions for 3 minutes, or until soft, stirring frequently.

Stir in the pumpkin.

Put the flour, ginger, and turmeric in a medium bowl. Pour in 1/3 cup milk, stirring to dissolve. Stir into the pumpkin mixture until well blended.

Reduce the heat to medium. Pour the remaining 1 2/3 cups milk into the soup. Cook for 5 to 10 minutes, or until thickened, stirring constantly. Don't let the soup boil.

Pour in the broth. Cook for 3 minutes, or until almost at a boil, stirring frequently. (If the soup separates, process in a food processor or blender to restore the consistency.) Serve immediately. Garnish with the chives.

PER SERVING

calories 67	carbohydrates 10 g
total fat 1.5 g	fiber 3 g
saturated fat 0.0 g	sugars 5 g
trans fat 0.0 g	**protein** 4 g
polyunsaturated fat 0.5 g	**DIETARY EXCHANGES**
monounsaturated fat 0.5 g	1/2 other
cholesterol 1 mg	carbohydrate
sodium 65 mg	

YOGURT-FRUIT SOUP

SERVES 4

This sweet, creamy soup is a great way to start a brunch or luncheon and to take advantage of summer's bounty of juicy peaches and strawberries.

    2 cups peeled and cubed peaches (about
        4 medium)
    16 ounces fat-free plain yogurt
    1 cup strawberries, hulled
    1/2 cup fresh orange juice
    1/2 cup water
    1 tablespoon honey
    4 sprigs of fresh mint (optional)

In a food processor or blender, process all the ingredients except the mint. Pour into a glass bowl. Cover and refrigerate for at least 3 hours, or until chilled. Just before serving, garnish with the mint.

Cook's Tip: Try a wide variety of fruits in place of the fresh peaches and strawberries. For example, substitute unsweetened frozen peaches, blueberries, or mixed fruit for the fresh peaches, or use 1 to 2 medium bananas instead of the strawberries.

PER SERVING

calories 135	sodium 89 mg
total fat 0.5 g	carbohydrates 26 g
saturated fat 0.0 g	fiber 2 g
trans fat 0.0 g	sugars 24 g
polyunsaturated fat 0.0 g	**protein** 8 g
monounsaturated fat 0.0 g	**DIETARY EXCHANGES**
cholesterol 2 mg	1 fruit, 1 fat-free milk

SOUTHWESTERN COD SOUP

SERVES 4

The mild flavor of cod marries well with the intense flavors of the Southwest, including green chiles, cumin, and cilantro. This dish works well at any time of year, but it's especially comforting as the weather turns colder.

    2 cups fat-free, low-sodium chicken broth,
        such as on page 36
    1 14.5-ounce can no-salt-added diced
        tomatoes, undrained

6 small red potatoes, halved (about 6 ounces total)

1 medium carrot, sliced

1 4-ounce can chopped green chiles, drained

1 teaspoon ground cumin

2 medium garlic cloves, minced

1/4 teaspoon salt

8 ounces cod fillets, rinsed, cut into 3/4-inch cubes

2 tablespoons chopped fresh cilantro

1 teaspoon grated lime zest

1 teaspoon fresh lime juice

In a large saucepan, stir together the broth, tomatoes with liquid, potatoes, carrot, chiles, cumin, garlic, and salt. Bring to a simmer over medium-high heat, stirring occasionally. Reduce the heat and simmer, covered, for 15 minutes, or until the potatoes are tender.

Stir in the remaining ingredients. Simmer, covered, for 5 minutes, or until the fish flakes easily when tested with a fork.

PER SERVING

calories 119	carbohydrates 16 g
total fat 0.5 g	fiber 4 g
saturated fat 0.0 g	sugars 5 g
trans fat 0.0 g	protein 13 g
polyunsaturated fat 0.0 g	DIETARY EXCHANGES
monounsaturated fat 0.0 g	1/2 starch, 1 vegetable,
cholesterol 24 mg	1 1/2 lean meat
sodium 355 mg	

GAZPACHO

SERVES 6

This cold soup is versatile as well as refreshing. Enjoy it with a sandwich or fat-free cheese and crackers, use it as a salsa for dipping baked chips, or spoon it over grilled chicken or fish.

Soup

6 cups chopped tomatoes (peeled if desired) or canned no-salt-added Italian plum (Roma) tomatoes, drained

1 medium onion, coarsely chopped

1/2 medium green bell pepper, coarsely chopped

1/2 cup coarsely chopped cucumber

1 medium garlic clove, minced

3 cups no-salt-added tomato juice

1/2 cup whole-kernel corn (fresh preferred)

1/2 cup finely chopped avocado

1/4 cup red wine vinegar

2 teaspoons red hot-pepper sauce, or to taste

1/2 teaspoon sugar

1/2 teaspoon ground cumin (optional)

1/4 teaspoon salt

1/8 to 1/4 teaspoon pepper

Garnishes

1 cup finely chopped tomato

1 small to medium onion, finely chopped

1/2 medium green bell pepper, finely chopped

1/2 cup finely chopped cucumber

1/4 cup finely chopped fresh cilantro

In a food processor or blender, process the 6 cups chopped tomatoes, coarsely chopped onion, coarsely chopped bell pepper, coarsely chopped cucumber, and garlic in batches until smooth, pouring each batch into the same large bowl after it's processed.

Stir in the remaining soup ingredients. Cover and refrigerate for at least 30 minutes.

Meanwhile, put the garnishes in small individual dishes. Serve with the soup.

PER SERVING

calories 117	carbohydrates 23 g
total fat 2.5 g	fiber 6 g
saturated fat 0.5 g	sugars 14 g
trans fat 0.0 g	protein 4 g
polyunsaturated fat 0.5 g	DIETARY EXCHANGES
monounsaturated fat 1.5 g	3 vegetable, 1/2 starch,
cholesterol 0 mg	1/2 fat
sodium 134 mg	

MINTED CANTALOUPE SOUP WITH FRESH LIME

SERVES 4

Delicately sweetened melon blended with vanilla, mint, and lime—what a refreshing treat on a hot summer day!

> 4 cups diced cantaloupe
> 8 ounces fat-free vanilla yogurt
> 1/4 cup chopped fresh mint and (optional)
>   4 sprigs of fresh mint, divided use
> 1 tablespoon plus 1 teaspoon sugar
> 1 1/2 to 2 tablespoons fresh lime juice

In a food processor or blender, process the cantaloupe, yogurt, 1/4 cup mint, and sugar until smooth. Pour into a large glass bowl. Cover and refrigerate for at least 1 hour, or until well chilled.

Immediately before serving, stir in the lime juice. Garnish with the remaining sprigs of mint.

PER SERVING

calories 127	carbohydrates 28 g
total fat 0.5 g	fiber 2 g
saturated fat 0.0 g	sugars 26 g
trans fat 0.0 g	**protein** 5 g
polyunsaturated fat 0.0 g	**DIETARY EXCHANGES**
monounsaturated fat 0.0 g	1 1/2 fruit, 1/2 fat-free
cholesterol 1 mg	milk
sodium 68 mg	

TROPICAL MINTED CANTALOUPE SOUP WITH FRESH LIME

SERVES 4

Add 3 tablespoons frozen 100% orange-pineapple juice concentrate and 1 teaspoon grated peeled gingerroot and process with the cantaloupe mixture.

Time-Saver: To chill the soup quickly, put it in the freezer for 20 to 25 minutes, or until very cold, occasionally stirring at the edges with a rubber scraper. Chill the soup bowls in the refrigerator at the same time.

PER SERVING

calories 148	carbohydrates 33 g
total fat 0.5 g	fiber 2 g
saturated fat 0.0 g	sugars 31 g
trans fat 0.0 g	**protein** 5 g
polyunsaturated fat 0.0 g	**DIETARY EXCHANGES**
monounsaturated fat 0.0 g	1 1/2 fruit, 1/2 fat-free
cholesterol 1 mg	milk
sodium 68 mg	

SWEET CORN SOUP WITH CRAB AND ASPARAGUS

SERVES 8

This Cantonese-style soup is practically a meal in itself. Round out your dinner with Easy Refrigerator Rolls (page 458) and Baked Ginger Pears (page 502).

> 1 1/2 pounds asparagus spears, trimmed, cut into 1-inch pieces
> 1/4 cup water and 2 tablespoons water, divided use
> 2 tablespoons cornstarch
> 4 cups fat-free, low-sodium chicken broth, such as on page 36
> 1 14.75-ounce can no-salt-added cream-style corn
> 2 teaspoons soy sauce (lowest sodium available)
> 1/2 teaspoon salt
> 3/4 cup egg substitute
> 2 6-ounce cans crabmeat, rinsed and drained, any bits of shell and cartilage discarded
> 1/2 teaspoon toasted sesame oil
> 6 medium green onions (green part only), finely chopped
> 2 teaspoons chili garlic sauce or chili garlic paste (optional)

Put the asparagus and 1/4 cup water in a medium microwaveable dish. Microwave, covered, on 100 percent power (high) for 5 minutes, or until tender-crisp. Don't overcook. Drain well in a colander.

Meanwhile, put the cornstarch in small bowl. Add the remaining 2 tablespoons water, whisking to dissolve.

In a large saucepan, bring the broth to a boil over high heat. Stir in the corn, soy sauce, and salt. Return to a boil.

Pour the cornstarch mixture into the broth mixture, stirring constantly.

Pour the egg substitute in a thin stream into the boiling soup. Remove from the heat.

Spoon the asparagus into soup bowls. Ladle the broth mixture over the asparagus. Top with, in order, the crabmeat, sesame oil, and green onions. Dollop with the chili garlic sauce.

PER SERVING

calories 126	**carbohydrates** 16 g
total fat 1.0 g	fiber 3 g
saturated fat 0.0 g	sugars 5 g
trans fat 0.0 g	**protein** 14 g
polyunsaturated fat 0.0 g	**DIETARY EXCHANGES**
monounsaturated fat 0.0 g	1/2 starch, 1 vegetable,
cholesterol 41 mg	1 1/2 lean meat
sodium 414 mg	

SWEET CORN SOUP WITH CHICKEN AND ASPARAGUS

SERVES 8

Substitute 2 cups chopped cooked skinless chicken breast, cooked without salt, all visible fat discarded, for the crabmeat.

Cook's Tip on Asparagus: An asparagus spear has a natural bending point where the tough stem ends. Holding a spear of asparagus at the top and the bottom, bend the spear; snap it at the bending point. Discard the tough part, or save it to use in making broths and other soups.

PER SERVING

calories 151	**carbohydrates** 16 g
total fat 2.5 g	fiber 3 g
saturated fat 0.5 g	sugars 5 g
trans fat 0.0 g	**protein** 17 g
polyunsaturated fat 0.5 g	**DIETARY EXCHANGES**
monounsaturated fat 0.5 g	1/2 starch, 1 vegetable,
cholesterol 30 mg	1 1/2 lean meat
sodium 273 mg	

NEW ENGLAND FISH CHOWDER

SERVES 6

Chunks of potato and firm-fleshed fish join dainty peas in a creamy chowder that will disappear quickly from the soup pot.

> 4 cups fat-free milk
> 2 cups peeled and diced potatoes
> 1/2 teaspoon salt
> 1 teaspoon light tub margarine
> 1 cup sliced leeks (white part only)
> 1 pound cod or haddock fillets, rinsed and patted dry, cut into 1-inch pieces
> 1 cup frozen baby green peas
> 2 tablespoons finely chopped fresh parsley
> 1 tablespoon fresh lemon juice
> 1/8 teaspoon pepper (white preferred)

In a large saucepan, bring the milk, potatoes, and salt to a simmer over medium heat. Reduce the heat to low and cook, covered, for 25 to 30 minutes.

In a small nonstick skillet, melt the margarine over medium-low heat, swirling to coat the bottom. Cook the leeks for 2 to 3 minutes, or until limp.

Transfer about 1 cup potatoes and 1 cup liquid from the saucepan to a food processor or blender. Process until smooth (vent the blender lid). Return the mixture to the pan.

Stir the leeks and the remaining ingredients into the soup. Increase the heat to medium high and bring to a boil. Reduce the heat and simmer for 8 to 10 minutes, or until the fish flakes easily when tested with a fork, stirring gently and occasionally.

PER SERVING

calories 186	**carbohydrates** 22 g
total fat 1.0 g	fiber 2 g
saturated fat 0.0 g	sugars 10 g
trans fat 0.0 g	**protein** 21 g
polyunsaturated fat 0.5 g	**DIETARY EXCHANGES**
monounsaturated fat 0.5 g	1 starch, 1/2 fat-free
cholesterol 36 mg	milk, 2 lean meat
sodium 339 mg	

SHRIMP GUMBO

SERVES 6

For an inviting winter meal, try this thick gumbo with a touch of hot-pepper sauce to warm up your taste buds. Serve with Southern Raised Biscuits *(page 459).*

1 teaspoon canola or corn oil

1 pound fresh okra, trimmed and sliced, or 10 ounces frozen sliced okra, thawed

1 large onion, chopped

1/2 medium green bell pepper, chopped

1 medium rib of celery, chopped

3 medium garlic cloves, minced

1/2 teaspoon pepper, or to taste

2 cups fat-free, low-sodium chicken broth, such as on page 36

1 14.5-ounce can no-salt-added diced tomatoes, undrained

2 medium dried bay leaves

1 cup uncooked brown rice

1 tablespoon cornstarch

2 tablespoons water

1 pound raw medium shrimp, peeled, rinsed, and patted dry

1 tablespoon gumbo filé powder (optional)

1/8 teaspoon red hot-pepper sauce, or to taste

In a stockpot, heat the oil over medium-high heat, swirling to coat the bottom. Cook the okra, onion, bell pepper, celery, garlic, and pepper for 5 minutes, stirring frequently.

Stir in the broth, tomatoes with liquid, and bay leaves. Increase the heat to high and bring to a boil. Reduce the heat and simmer, covered, for 45 minutes.

Meanwhile, prepare the rice using the package directions, omitting the salt and margarine. Set aside.

Put the cornstarch in a small bowl. Add the water, stirring to dissolve. Stir into the gumbo. Cook for 1 minute, or until thickened, stirring constantly.

Stir in the shrimp. Increase the heat to high and bring to a low boil. Reduce the heat and simmer, covered, for 3 to 5 minutes, or until the shrimp are pink on the outside. Don't overcook, or the shrimp will become rubbery.

Discard the bay leaves. Stir in the filé powder and hot-pepper sauce. Serve the gumbo over the rice.

PER SERVING

calories 256	**carbohydrates** 39 g
total fat 3.0 g	fiber 6 g
saturated fat 0.5 g	sugars 6 g
trans fat 0.0 g	**protein** 19 g
polyunsaturated fat 1.0 g	**DIETARY EXCHANGES**
monounsaturated fat 1.0 g	1 1/2 starch,
cholesterol 121 mg	3 vegetable, 2 lean
sodium 595 mg	meat

MULLIGATAWNY SOUP

SERVES 8

This hearty and warming entrée soup is charged with the flavors of a curry. With a variety of spices, fruit, potatoes, and legumes, this spicy chicken soup is based on the classic dish from southern India.

1 tablespoon curry powder

1 teaspoon ground cumin

1/2 teaspoon paprika

1/2 teaspoon ground cinnamon

1/2 teaspoon ground turmeric

1/2 teaspoon dried thyme, crumbled

1/4 teaspoon ground coriander

1/4 teaspoon pepper (freshly ground preferred)

1/8 teaspoon cayenne (optional)

2 tablespoons canola or corn oil

1 large onion, chopped

1 tablespoon minced peeled gingerroot (about 1-inch piece)

3 medium garlic cloves, minced

1 pound boneless, skinless chicken breasts, all visible fat discarded, cut into 1-inch pieces

2 small tart apples, such as Granny Smith, Braeburn, or Jonagold, cut into 1/2-inch cubes

1 cup dried red lentils, sorted for stones and shriveled lentils, rinsed, and drained

1 large sweet potato, peeled and cut into
    1/2-inch cubes
4 cups fat-free, low-sodium chicken broth,
    such as on page 36
1/2 cup lite coconut milk
2 tablespoons chopped fresh cilantro
    (optional)

In a small bowl, stir together the curry powder, cumin, paprika, cinnamon, turmeric, thyme, coriander, pepper, and cayenne. Set aside.

In a Dutch oven or large saucepan, heat the oil over medium-high heat, swirling to coat the bottom. Cook the onion for 3 minutes, or until soft, stirring frequently. Stir in the ginger and garlic. Cook for 2 to 3 minutes, stirring frequently. Stir in the curry powder mixture. Cook for 2 to 3 minutes, or just until fragrant, stirring constantly.

Stir in the chicken, apples, lentils, and sweet potato. Cook for 2 to 3 minutes, stirring constantly to combine well.

Stir in the broth. Bring to a boil. Reduce the heat to medium low. Simmer for 25 to 30 minutes, or until the lentils are tender and the chicken is no longer pink in the center.

Gradually stir in the coconut milk. If desired, transfer 2 to 3 cups of the soup to a food processor or blender (vent the blender lid). Process until smooth and creamy. Carefully return the processed soup to the pot, stirring to combine. Cook for 5 to 8 minutes, or until heated through. Garnish with the cilantro.

Cook's Tip on Coconut Milk: Use the canned lite coconut milk in the ethnic section of your grocery store rather than the refrigerated coconut milk found in the dairy section for the recipes in this book, which is more of a beverage than an ingredient.

PER SERVING

calories 267	carbohydrates 33 g
total fat 6.0 g	fiber 7 g
saturated fat 1.0 g	sugars 10 g
trans fat 0.0 g	**protein** 22 g
polyunsaturated fat 1.5 g	**DIETARY EXCHANGES**
monounsaturated fat 2.5 g	1 1/2 starch, 1/2 fruit,
cholesterol 36 mg	2 1/2 lean meat
sodium 109 mg	

SALAD BOWL SOUP

SERVES 4

If you like creamy tomato soup, then you're going to enjoy this Mexican-influenced version. Protein-packed chicken and fiber-filled legumes along with avocado rich in healthy fats are the delicioso complements in this fast-to-make and hearty soup.

18 ounces spicy low-sodium mixed-vegetable
    juice
1 cup canned no-salt-added chickpeas, rinsed
    and drained
2 medium tomatoes, seeded and coarsely
    chopped
3/4 cup cubed cooked skinless chicken breast,
    cooked without salt, all visible fat
    discarded
1 medium avocado, peeled and mashed, and
    (optional) 1/4 medium avocado, peeled
    and cut into 4 thin slices, divided use
1/4 cup fat-free plain Greek yogurt
1/8 teaspoon salt

In a large saucepan, stir together the vegetable juice, chickpeas, tomatoes, and chicken. Bring to a boil over high heat. Reduce the heat and simmer for about 5 minutes, stirring occasionally.

Stir in the mashed avocado, yogurt, and salt.

Serve immediately. Garnish with the remaining avocado slices.

PER SERVING

calories 238	carbohydrates 25 g
total fat 9.0 g	fiber 8 g
saturated fat 1.5 g	sugars 8 g
trans fat 0.0 g	**protein** 16 g
polyunsaturated fat 1.0 g	**DIETARY EXCHANGES**
monounsaturated fat 5.5 g	2 vegetable, 1 starch,
cholesterol 22 mg	1 1/2 lean meat, 1 fat
sodium 199 mg	

CHICKEN AND VEGETABLE SOUP

SERVES 4

This all-in-one meal cooks together all in one pot, making cleanup one less thing to worry about. Enjoy with Spinach Salad with Kiwifruit and Raspberries *(page 67).*

Cooking spray
1 pound boneless, skinless chicken breasts, all visible fat discarded, cut into bite-size pieces
1 medium zucchini, thinly sliced
1 medium red bell pepper, chopped
1 3/4 cups fat-free, low-sodium chicken broth, such as on page 36
2 ounces dried whole-grain fettuccine, broken into thirds
1/2 cup frozen whole-kernel corn
1/2 cup water
1/2 teaspoon dried thyme, crumbled
4 or 5 medium green onions, finely chopped
1/4 cup finely chopped fresh parsley
1 tablespoon olive oil
1/2 teaspoon salt
1/4 teaspoon pepper
2 tablespoons shredded or grated Parmesan cheese

Lightly spray a Dutch oven with cooking spray. Cook the chicken over medium-high heat for 2 to 3 minutes, or until no longer pink on the outside, stirring constantly (the chicken won't be done at this point). Transfer to a plate.

Lightly spray the Dutch oven with cooking spray. Cook the zucchini and bell pepper for 2 minutes, or until just beginning to brown lightly on the edges, stirring constantly.

Stir in the broth, pasta, corn, water, and thyme. Increase the heat to high and bring to a boil. Reduce the heat and simmer, covered, for 10 minutes, or until the pasta is al dente (has some bite).

Stir in the chicken and any accumulated juices. Cook for 3 minutes, or until the chicken is no longer pink in the center. Remove from the heat.

Stir in the remaining ingredients except the Parmesan. Just before serving, sprinkle with the Parmesan.

PER SERVING

calories 278	**carbohydrates** 22 g
total fat 7.5 g	fiber 4 g
saturated fat 1.5 g	sugars 5 g
trans fat 0.0 g	**protein** 29 g
polyunsaturated fat 1.0 g	**DIETARY EXCHANGES**
monounsaturated fat 3.5 g	1 starch, 1 vegetable,
cholesterol 74 mg	3 lean meat
sodium 498 mg	

CHICKEN, GREENS, AND POTATO SOUP

SERVES 4

Chicken and mustard greens add protein and additional nutrients to this hearty main-dish soup. The potato puree makes the soup thick and creamy. Leek, dillweed, and thyme supply accents of savory flavor.

2 1/2 cups fat-free, low-sodium chicken broth, such as on page 36
3 medium potatoes, peeled and cut into 1/2-inch pieces
2 teaspoons canola or corn oil
1 medium leek, sliced (white part only), or 9 medium green onions, sliced (white part only)
4 medium garlic cloves, minced
10 ounces boneless, skinless chicken breasts, all visible fat discarded, cut into bite-size pieces
1 12-ounce can fat-free evaporated milk
5 ounces frozen mustard greens, thawed and well drained
1 teaspoon chopped fresh dillweed or 1/4 teaspoon dried dillweed, crumbled
1 teaspoon chopped fresh thyme or 1/4 teaspoon dried thyme, crumbled
1/4 teaspoon salt
1/8 teaspoon pepper

In a Dutch oven, bring the broth and potatoes to a boil over medium-high heat. Reduce the heat and simmer, covered, for 20 minutes, or until the potatoes are tender. Don't drain. Remove from the heat and let cool slightly.

In a food processor or blender (vent the blender lid), process the broth mixture (in batches if necessary) until smooth. Set aside.

Wipe the Dutch oven with paper towels. Pour in the oil, swirling to coat the bottom. Heat over medium heat. Cook the leek for 5 minutes, stirring occasionally.

Stir in the garlic. Cook for 1 minute, stirring occasionally.

Stir in the chicken. Cook for 5 minutes, or until the chicken is no longer pink in the center, stirring frequently.

Stir in the broth mixture and the remaining ingredients. Reduce the heat to low and cook for about 3 minutes, or until heated through, stirring occasionally.

PER SERVING

calories 295	carbohydrates 36 g
total fat 4.5 g	fiber 4 g
saturated fat 0.5 g	sugars 13 g
trans fat 0.0 g	protein 27 g
polyunsaturated fat 1.0 g	DIETARY EXCHANGES
monounsaturated fat 2.0 g	1 starch, 1 fat-free milk,
cholesterol 49 mg	1 vegetable, 2 lean
sodium 375 mg	meat

CHILE-CHICKEN TORTILLA SOUP

SERVES 8

This entrée soup is a smart way to use up leftover chicken. Tex-Mex Cucumber Salad *(page 78) makes a simple accompaniment.*

1 teaspoon canola or corn oil
1/2 cup chopped onion
2 medium garlic cloves, minced
4 cups fat-free, low-sodium chicken broth, such as on page 36
1 15.5-ounce can no-salt-added pinto beans, rinsed and drained
1 14.5-ounce can no-salt-added crushed tomatoes, undrained

1 cup cubed cooked skinless chicken breast, cooked without salt, all visible fat discarded
2 fresh Anaheim or poblano peppers, diced (see Cook's Tip on Handling Hot Chiles, page 24)
1 teaspoon ground cumin
1 teaspoon chili powder and 1/2 teaspoon chili powder, divided use
1/2 teaspoon dried oregano, crumbled
1/4 teaspoon salt
1/8 teaspoon pepper
Cooking spray
8 6-inch corn tortillas, halved and cut into 1/4-inch strips
2 medium green onions, thinly sliced

In a large nonstick saucepan, heat the oil over medium-high heat, swirling to coat the bottom. Cook the onion and garlic for about 3 minutes, or until the onion is soft, stirring frequently.

Stir in the broth, beans, tomatoes with liquid, chicken, peppers, cumin, 1 teaspoon chili powder, oregano, salt, and pepper. Bring to a boil. Reduce the heat and simmer, covered, for 20 to 25 minutes, stirring occasionally.

Meanwhile, preheat the oven to 350°F. Lightly spray a baking sheet with cooking spray.

Arrange the tortilla strips in a single layer on the baking sheet. Lightly spray with cooking spray. Sprinkle the remaining 1/2 teaspoon chili powder over the strips.

Bake for 10 minutes, or until crisp.

Just before serving, sprinkle the soup with the tortilla strips and green onions.

PER SERVING

calories 142	carbohydrates 20 g
total fat 2.0 g	fiber 4 g
saturated fat 0.5 g	sugars 4 g
trans fat 0.0 g	protein 11 g
polyunsaturated fat 0.5 g	DIETARY EXCHANGES
monounsaturated fat 1.0 g	1 starch, 1 vegetable,
cholesterol 15 mg	1 lean meat
sodium 138 mg	

ASIAN CHICKEN SOUP

SERVES 6

Serve this fast-cooking soup with Sweet-and-Sour Spring Rolls *(page 23).*

4 cups fat-free, low-sodium chicken broth, such as on page 36

1 1/2 cups cooked skinless chicken breast, cooked without salt, all visible fat discarded, cut into thin slivers

1 cup rice noodles

4 medium green onions, thinly sliced diagonally

1 teaspoon grated peeled gingerroot

1/8 teaspoon salt

1/4 teaspoon Worcestershire sauce (lowest sodium available)

Pour the broth into a large saucepan. Stir in the remaining ingredients except the Worcestershire sauce. Cook over medium-high heat for 6 to 8 minutes, or until heated through, stirring occasionally.

Just before serving, stir in the Worcestershire sauce.

PER SERVING

calories 158	carbohydrates 21 g
total fat 1.5 g	fiber 1 g
saturated fat 0.5 g	sugars 1 g
trans fat 0.0 g	protein 13 g
polyunsaturated fat 0.5 g	**DIETARY EXCHANGES**
monounsaturated fat 0.5 g	1 1/2 starch, 1 1/2 lean
cholesterol 30 mg	meat
sodium 99 mg	

VIETNAMESE BEEF AND RICE NOODLE SOUP

SERVES 6

Tender beef in a flavorful broth and a spike of lime just before serving characterize this classic Vietnamese soup known as pho (FUH). It's traditionally served with garnishes to be added by each diner, such as Thai basil, chopped green onions, matchstick-size strips of fresh snow peas, or shredded carrots.

4 cups water (if using rice noodles)

4 ounces dried rice noodles or dried whole-grain angel hair pasta

3 cups fat-free, low-sodium beef broth, such as on page 35

2 cups fat-free, low-sodium chicken broth, such as on page 36

2 1/4-inch-thick slices unpeeled gingerroot

1 teaspoon grated lime zest

1/4 teaspoon sugar

1/8 teaspoon ground allspice

1 pound boneless sirloin steak, all visible fat discarded, cut into slivers

1 teaspoon toasted sesame oil

1/3 cup loosely packed coarsely chopped fresh cilantro or mint

1 large lime, cut into 6 wedges

If using the rice noodles, in a medium saucepan, bring the water to a boil over high heat. Stir in the noodles. Remove from the heat and let the noodles soak in the hot water for 3 to 4 minutes, or until tender. If using the angel hair pasta, prepare using the package directions, omitting the salt. Drain well in a colander.

Rinse the pan. Put the broths, gingerroot, lime zest, sugar, and allspice in the pan, whisking to combine. Bring to a simmer over medium-high heat. Reduce the heat and simmer for 2 to 3 minutes, or until the broth is infused with ginger flavor, stirring occasionally.

Stir in the beef and oil. Return to a simmer and simmer for 2 to 4 minutes, or until the beef is the desired doneness. Discard the gingerroot.

Put the noodles in bowls. Ladle the broth mixture over the noodles. Sprinkle with the cilantro. Squeeze the lime into the soup, or serve the lime wedges on the side.

Cook's Tip: Because the gingerroot is removed before the soup is served, there's no need to peel it; the thin skin won't affect the flavor.

calories 184	**sodium** 71 mg
total fat 4.0 g	**carbohydrates** 16 g
saturated fat 1.5 g	fiber 0 g
trans fat 0.0 g	sugars 0 g
polyunsaturated fat 0.5 g	**protein** 20 g
monounsaturated fat 2.0 g	**DIETARY EXCHANGES**
cholesterol 40 mg	1 starch, 2 lean meat

PER SERVING (WITH ANGEL HAIR PASTA)

calories 183	**sodium** 69 mg
total fat 4.5 g	**carbohydrates** 15 g
saturated fat 1.5 g	fiber 2 g
trans fat 0.0 g	sugars 1 g
polyunsaturated fat 0.5 g	**protein** 21 g
monounsaturated fat 2.0 g	**DIETARY EXCHANGES**
cholesterol 40 mg	1 starch, 2 lean meat

MEXICAN CHICKEN SOUP

SERVES 8

This soup is a fiesta in a bowl. Balance out the mild heat from the chiles with a side of Spinach-Chayote Salad with Orange Vinaigrette (page 68).

1 2 1/2- to 3-pound chicken, skin and all visible fat discarded, cut into serving pieces

2 15.5-ounce cans no-salt-added black beans

1 14.5-ounce can Italian plum (Roma) tomatoes, undrained

2 4-ounce cans diced green chiles, drained

1/2 cup chopped onion

1 medium garlic clove, minced

Cooking spray

8 6-inch corn tortillas, halved and cut into 1/4-inch strips

1/2 cup finely chopped avocado

1/4 cup snipped fresh cilantro

2 medium limes, cut into 4 wedges each

Put the chicken in large stockpot, adding enough water to cover. Bring to a boil over medium-high heat. Reduce the heat and simmer for 25 minutes, or until the chicken is tender and no longer pink in the center.

Using a slotted spoon, transfer the chicken to a plate. Discard the bones. Cut the chicken into bite-size pieces. Return to the pot. Stir in the beans, tomatoes with liquid, chiles, onion, and garlic. Simmer for 15 minutes, or until the onion is soft and the soup is warmed through.

Meanwhile, preheat the oven to 350°F. Lightly spray a baking sheet with cooking spray.

Arrange the tortilla strips in a single layer on the baking sheet. Lightly spray with cooking spray. Bake for 10 minutes, or until crisp.

Just before serving, sprinkle the soup with the avocado, cilantro, and tortilla strips. Serve with the lime wedges.

PER SERVING

calories 226	**carbohydrates** 28 g
total fat 2.5 g	fiber 7 g
saturated fat 0.5 g	sugars 5 g
trans fat 0.0 g	**protein** 22 g
polyunsaturated fat 0.5 g	**DIETARY EXCHANGES**
monounsaturated fat 0.5 g	1 1/2 starch,
cholesterol 47 mg	1 vegetable, 2 1/2 lean
sodium 262 mg	meat

BEEF BARLEY SOUP

SERVES 6

Served with Baked Curried Fruit (page 425) and Whole-Wheat Muffins (page 465), this filling soup makes a meal that will help drive away the winter chill.

2 teaspoons canola or corn oil

1 pound bottom round steak, all visible fat discarded, cut into bite-size pieces

1 medium onion, chopped

4 cups fat-free, low-sodium beef broth, such as on page 35

4 cups water

1/2 cup uncooked pearl barley

1 medium dried bay leaf

1/2 teaspoon salt and 1/4 teaspoon salt, divided use

1/4 teaspoon pepper

2 medium potatoes, peeled and diced

3 medium carrots, sliced crosswise

2 medium ribs of celery, thickly sliced on the diagonal

2 teaspoons dried thyme, crumbled

(continued)

In a Dutch oven, heat the oil over medium heat, swirling to coat the bottom. Cook the beef pieces for 10 minutes, or until browned, stirring occasionally.

Stir in the onion. Cook for 4 minutes, stirring occasionally.

Stir in the broth, water, barley, bay leaf, 1/2 teaspoon salt, and pepper. Increase the heat to high and bring to a boil. Reduce the heat and simmer, covered, for 1 hour, or until the beef is tender.

Stir in the potatoes, carrots, celery, thyme, and the remaining 1/4 teaspoon salt. Increase the heat to medium high and bring to a boil. Reduce the heat and simmer, partially covered, for 20 to 25 minutes, or until the vegetables are tender. Discard the bay leaf before serving the soup.

PER SERVING

calories 252	carbohydrates 28 g
total fat 5.5 g	fiber 6 g
saturated fat 1.5 g	sugars 4 g
trans fat 0.0 g	**protein** 22 g
polyunsaturated fat 1.0 g	**DIETARY EXCHANGES**
monounsaturated fat 3.0 g	1 1/2 starch,
cholesterol 45 mg	1 vegetable, 2 lean
sodium 410 mg	meat

JAPANESE UDON NOODLE SOUP WITH TOFU

SERVES 4

This hearty soup is a one-bowl meal that will please and satisfy. Follow the Japanese, and use your largest, deepest bowls for serving. The rich-tasting broth is filled with noodles, "meaty" fried tofu, and colorful vegetables.

14 ounces light firm tofu, drained and patted dry, cut into 16 1-inch pieces

2 tablespoons plain rice vinegar

2 teaspoons soy sauce (lowest sodium available)

2 teaspoons canola or corn oil

4 ounces dried udon noodles

4 cups fat-free, low-sodium vegetable broth, such as on page 36

3/4 cup small broccoli florets

3/4 cup shiitake mushrooms, stems discarded, caps sliced

1/2 cup frozen edamame or frozen green peas

1/4 cup diagonally sliced carrots

2 teaspoons minced peeled gingerroot

1 large garlic clove, minced

2 hard-boiled eggs, halved

Arrange the tofu on a large shallow plate. Drizzle the vinegar and soy sauce over the tofu pieces. Cover and refrigerate for 30 minutes, turning occasionally.

In a large nonstick skillet, heat the oil over medium-high heat, swirling to coat the bottom. Drain the tofu, reserving the marinade. Cook the tofu for 5 minutes, or until golden, turning to brown on all sides. Transfer to a large plate. Cover to keep warm.

Meanwhile, prepare the noodles using the package directions, omitting the salt. Drain well in a colander.

In a large saucepan, bring the broth and reserved marinade to a boil over medium-high heat. Stir in the remaining ingredients except the eggs. Reduce the heat to medium. Cook for 3 minutes, or until the vegetables are tender-crisp. Pile the noodles in the center of large soup bowls. Top with the tofu. Pour in the broth mixture. Garnish with the egg halves. (They will float on the surface of the soup.)

Cook's Tip on Udon Noodles: Udon noodles are thick white Japanese noodles usually made from wheat. If they're unavailable, you can substitute whole-grain spaghetti or linguine.

PER SERVING

calories 256	carbohydrates 26 g
total fat 8.0 g	fiber 4 g
saturated fat 1.0 g	sugars 3 g
trans fat 0.0 g	**protein** 20 g
polyunsaturated fat 3.0 g	**DIETARY EXCHANGES**
monounsaturated fat 3.5 g	1 1/2 starch, 2 lean
cholesterol 93 mg	meat
sodium 197 mg	

TUSCAN KALE AND CANNELLINI BEAN SOUP

SERVES 8

This hearty soup will fill you up on a cold winter's night. Just add some crusty whole-grain bread, such as Whole-Wheat French Bread *(page 443), for dunking.*

- 1 tablespoon olive oil
- 3 medium leeks (white and pale green parts), coarsely chopped
- 1 large sweet onion, such as Vidalia, Maui, or Oso Sweet, coarsely chopped
- 4 15.5-ounce cans no-salt-added cannellini beans, undrained
- 6 cups water
- 2 cups fat-free, low-sodium chicken broth, such as on page 36
- 2 medium dried bay leaves
- 6 cups chopped kale, any large stems discarded
- 4 medium ribs of celery, including leaves, cut into 1/2-inch pieces
- 2 medium carrots, chopped
- 1 cup coarsely chopped fresh Italian (flat-leaf) parsley
- 2 tablespoons chopped fresh basil and 1 cup chopped fresh basil, divided use
- 1 tablespoon finely chopped fresh thyme, or 1 teaspoon dried thyme, crumbled
- 1 tablespoon fresh rosemary, or 1 teaspoon dried rosemary, crushed
- 1 tablespoon fresh lemon juice
- 1/2 teaspoon salt
- 1/2 teaspoon pepper, or to taste

In a large stockpot, heat the oil over medium-low heat, swirling to coat the bottom. Cook the leeks and onion, covered, for 10 minutes, stirring occasionally.

Stir in the beans with liquid, water, broth, and bay leaves. Increase the heat to high and bring to a boil. Reduce the heat and simmer, covered, for 30 minutes.

Stir in the kale, celery, carrots, parsley, 2 table-spoons basil, thyme, rosemary, lemon juice, salt, and pepper. Simmer, covered, for about 45 min-utes, or until the celery and carrots are very tender, stirring occasionally. Add hot water if needed. Remove from the heat. Discard the bay leaves.

In a food processor or blender (vent the blender lid), process 1 1/2 to 2 cups of soup and the re-maining 1 cup basil until smooth. Stir the pro-cessed mixture back into the soup.

PER SERVING

calories 258	carbohydrates 44 g
total fat 4.0 g	fiber 12 g
saturated fat 0.5 g	sugars 6 g
trans fat 0.0 g	protein 14 g
polyunsaturated fat 1.5 g	DIETARY EXCHANGES
monounsaturated fat 2.0 g	2 starch, 3 vegetable,
cholesterol 0 mg	1 lean meat
sodium 284 mg	

BLACK BEAN SOUP

SERVES 8

As the Brazilians do with feijoada, *a popular black bean stew, this entrée soup is served with an as-sortment of optional garnishes, including sliced green onions and segments of fresh orange.*

- 1 teaspoon olive oil
- 1 medium onion, chopped
- 2 medium garlic cloves, minced
- 1 1/2 quarts water
- 3 15.5-ounce cans no-salt-added black beans, undrained
- 1 8-ounce can no-salt-added tomato sauce
- 1/4 cup dry sherry or fresh orange juice and (optional) 2 tablespoons dry sherry or fresh orange juice, divided use
- 1 teaspoon dried oregano, crumbled
- 1 teaspoon dried thyme, crumbled
- 1 teaspoon white vinegar
- 1 medium dried bay leaf
- 1 sprig of fresh parsley
- 3/4 teaspoon salt
- 1/8 teaspoon ground cloves (optional)
- Chopped cilantro, thinly sliced green onions, chopped cucumber, and/or peeled and seeded orange segments (optional)
- Dash of red hot-pepper sauce (optional)

(continued)

In a stockpot, heat the oil over medium-high heat, swirling to coat the bottom. Cook the onion and garlic for 3 minutes, or until the onion is soft, stirring frequently.

Stir in the water, beans with liquid, tomato sauce, 1/4 cup sherry, the oregano, thyme, vinegar, bay leaf, parsley, salt, and cloves. Bring to a simmer. Reduce the heat and simmer, covered, for 30 minutes. Stir in the remaining 2 tablespoons sherry. Discard the bay leaf.

For a smooth soup, in a food processor or blender (vent the blender lid), process the soup in batches. For a thicker texture, using a potato masher, mash some of the beans in the soup.

Serve the soup with the garnishes.

PER SERVING

calories 166	sodium 228 mg
total fat 0.5 g	carbohydrates 29 g
saturated fat 0.0 g	fiber 7 g
trans fat 0.0 g	sugars 7 g
polyunsaturated fat 0.0 g	protein 10 g
monounsaturated fat 0.5 g	**DIETARY EXCHANGES**
cholesterol 0 mg	2 starch, 1 lean meat

HOT-AND-SOUR SOUP

SERVES 4

Always a favorite, this soup gets a protein boost from both tofu and strips of pork, making it a filling Asian meal. If you want, add a handful of chopped snow peas, chopped broccoli florets, shredded carrots, or sliced water chestnuts for extra crunch and color.

2 cups wate

2 cups fat-free, low-sodium vegetable broth, such as on page 36, or fat-free, low-sodium chicken broth, such as on page 36

2 boneless center-cut pork chops (about 4 ounces each), all visible fat discarded, sliced into 2 x 1/4-inch strips

1/2 teaspoon sugar

1/2 teaspoon grated peeled gingerroot

2 cups thinly sliced button mushrooms

14 ounces light firm tofu, well drained, patted dry, and cut into 1/4-inch cubes

6 ounces snow peas, ends trimmed, halved on the diagonal

1 8-ounce can sliced water chestnuts, rinsed and drained

1 teaspoon cornstarch

3 tablespoons soy sauce (lowest sodium available)

3 tablespoons plain rice vinegar

1 teaspoon chili garlic paste or chili garlic sauce, or 1/8 teaspoon crushed red pepper flakes

1/2 teaspoon toasted sesame oil

1/4 cup thinly sliced green onions

In a large saucepan, stir together the water, broth, pork, sugar, and gingerroot. Bring to a boil over medium-high heat.

Stir in the mushrooms. Reduce the heat and simmer, covered, for 10 minutes, or until soft and the pork is no longer pink on the outside, stirring occasionally.

Stir in the tofu, snow peas, and water chestnuts. Cook for 1 to 2 minutes, or just until the snow peas are tender-crisp, stirring occasionally.

Put the cornstarch in a small bowl. Add the soy sauce and vinegar, whisking to dissolve. Whisk into the soup. Cook for 1 minute, or until the soup thickens slightly. Remove from the heat.

Stir in the chili garlic paste and oil. Just before serving, sprinkle with the green onions.

Cook's Tip on Chili Garlic Paste and Chili Garlic Sauce: Two staples of Asian cooking, spicy chili garlic paste and chili garlic sauce, differ a bit but are almost always interchangeable. In addition to chopped chiles and garlic, the paste includes vinegar. Look for both products in the Asian section of the grocery store and in Asian markets when you want to heighten the flavor of soups, stir-fries, and dipping sauces.

calories 181	**carbohydrates** 14 g
total fat 5.0 g	fiber 4 g
saturated fat 1.0 g	sugars 5 g
trans fat 0.0 g	**protein** 21 g
polyunsaturated fat 2.0 g	**DIETARY EXCHANGES**
monounsaturated fat 1.5 g	1/2 starch, 1 vegetable,
cholesterol 29 mg	2 1/2 lean meat
sodium 417 mg	

LENTIL CHILI SOUP

SERVES 6

Try this robust entrée soup that gets its full-bodied flavor from beer and a wide variety of seasonings. Partner it with Herb Bread *(page 444).*

1 teaspoon canola or corn oil

2 medium onions, chopped

1 medium green bell pepper, finely chopped

3 medium garlic cloves, minced

3 1/2 cups fat-free, low-sodium vegetable broth, such as on page 36

1 1/2 cups dried lentils, sorted for stones and shriveled lentils, rinsed, and drained

12 ounces beer (light or nonalcoholic)

1 1/4 cups water and 1/2 to 1 cup water, as needed, divided use

1 6-ounce can no-salt-added tomato paste

2 1/2 to 3 tablespoons chili powder

1 1/2 teaspoons ground cumin

1 teaspoon salt-free all-purpose seasoning blend

1 teaspoon sugar

1/4 teaspoon cayenne

1/2 cup grated fat-free Cheddar cheese

3 or 4 medium green onions, thinly sliced

In a stockpot, heat the oil over medium-high heat, swirling to coat the bottom. Cook the onions, bell pepper, and garlic for 10 minutes, stirring frequently.

Stir in the broth, lentils, beer, 1 1/4 cups water, the tomato paste, chili powder, cumin, seasoning blend, sugar, and cayenne. Increase the heat to high and bring to a boil. Reduce the heat and simmer, partially covered, for 35 to 40 minutes, or until the lentils are tender, stirring occasion-

ally. Gradually stir in the remaining 1/2 to 1 cup water as needed for the desired consistency.

Just before serving, sprinkle with the Cheddar and green onions.

calories 285	**carbohydrates** 49 g
total fat 1.5 g	fiber 11 g
saturated fat 0.0 g	sugars 12 g
trans fat 0.0 g	**protein** 20 g
polyunsaturated fat 0.5 g	**DIETARY EXCHANGES**
monounsaturated fat 0.5 g	2 starch, 3 vegetable,
cholesterol 2 mg	1 1/2 lean meat
sodium 159 mg	

SPLIT PEA SOUP

SERVES 4

Easy to prepare, homemade split pea soup is much lower in sodium than the canned version. This vegetarian version is flavorful even without the usual ham.

1 cup dried split peas, sorted for stones and shriveled peas, rinsed, and drained

1 teaspoon canola or corn oil

1 small onion, chopped

4 cups water

3 medium ribs of celery with leaves, chopped

1 medium carrot, chopped

1/2 cup chopped fresh parsley

1 teaspoon pepper, or to taste

1/2 teaspoon dried marjoram, crumbled

1/2 teaspoon dried thyme, crumbled

1/2 teaspoon dried basil, crumbled

1/2 teaspoon celery seeds

1/4 teaspoon salt

1 medium dried bay leaf

Soak the split peas using the package directions.

In a large saucepan, heat the oil over medium-high heat, swirling to coat the bottom. Cook the onion for 5 minutes, or until lightly browned, stirring frequently.

Stir in the peas and the remaining ingredients. Bring to a simmer. Reduce the heat and simmer,

(continued)

covered, for 1 hour to 1 hour 30 minutes, or until the peas are tender, stirring occasionally. Discard the bay leaf before serving the soup.

Cook's Tip: If you like lots of texture, serve this soup as is. For a little less texture, use a potato masher to blend the ingredients. For an even smoother texture, process the soup in batches in a food processor or blender (vent the blender lid) until it's the desired consistency.

PER SERVING

calories 208	**carbohydrates** 36 g
total fat 2.0 g	fiber 15 g
saturated fat 0.0 g	sugars 7 g
trans fat 0.0 g	**protein** 13 g
polyunsaturated fat 0.5 g	**DIETARY EXCHANGES**
monounsaturated fat 1.0 g	2 starch, 1 vegetable,
cholesterol 0 mg	1 lean meat
sodium 202 mg	

NAVY BEAN SOUP

SERVES 4

Made without the traditional ham hocks to reduce sodium, this vegetarian soup is still substantial and satisfying. Serve it with Rye Bread (page 445).

Cooking spray
1 large onion, chopped
2 medium ribs of celery, thinly sliced
2 medium carrots, finely chopped
2 medium garlic cloves, minced
1 15.5-ounce can no-salt-added navy beans, rinsed and drained
1 3/4 cups fat-free, low-sodium vegetable broth, such as on page 36
1/2 cup water
1 teaspoon ground cumin
1/2 teaspoon dried tarragon, crumbled
1/2 cup finely chopped green onions
1/4 cup finely chopped fresh parsley
2 teaspoons olive oil (extra-virgin preferred)

Lightly spray a Dutch oven with cooking spray. Put the onion, celery, carrots, and garlic in the pot. Lightly spray the vegetables and garlic with cooking spray. Cook over medium-high heat

for 3 minutes, or until the onion is soft, stirring frequently.

Stir in the beans, broth, water, cumin, and tarragon. Increase the heat to high and bring to a boil. Reduce the heat and simmer, covered, for 15 minutes, or until the carrots are tender. Remove from the heat.

Stir in the green onions, parsley, and oil.

PER SERVING

calories 165	**carbohydrates** 28 g
total fat 2.5 g	fiber 7 g
saturated fat 0.5 g	sugars 9 g
trans fat 0.0 g	**protein** 8 g
polyunsaturated fat 0.5 g	**DIETARY EXCHANGES**
monounsaturated fat 1.5 g	1 starch, 2 vegetable,
cholesterol 0 mg	1/2 lean meat
sodium 60 mg	

CURRIED PUMPKIN SOUP

SERVES 6

In addition to providing protein for this entrée soup, tofu contributes to its creaminess. Serve it at home as an entrée, tote it to work for a satisfying lunch, or serve small portions as a starter course for dinner with friends.

1 teaspoon olive oil
1/4 cup chopped shallots
2 15-ounce cans solid-pack pumpkin (not pie filling)
2 cups fat-free, low-sodium vegetable broth, such as on page 36
12 ounces light firm tofu, drained, patted dry, and chopped
1 12-ounce can fat-free evaporated milk
2 tablespoons pure maple syrup
2 teaspoons curry powder
1/4 teaspoon salt
1/8 teaspoon cayenne (optional)
1/4 cup unsalted shelled pepitas (pumpkin seeds), dry-roasted
2 tablespoons chopped fresh cilantro

In a large saucepan, heat the oil over medium-low heat, swirling to coat the bottom. Cook the shallots for 2 to 3 minutes, or until soft, stirring occasionally.

Stir in the pumpkin, broth, tofu, milk, maple syrup, curry powder, salt, and cayenne.

In a food processor or blender (vent the blender lid), process the soup in batches until smooth. Carefully return the soup to the pan.

Cook, still over medium-low heat, for 20 to 30 minutes, or until the soup is heated through, stirring occasionally.

Just before serving, sprinkle with the pepitas and cilantro.

Cook's Tip on Pepitas: Popular in Mexican cooking, pepitas are small green pumpkin seeds without the hull. Look for them in the Hispanic section of the supermarket.

PER SERVING

calories 188	carbohydrates 25 g
total fat 5.0 g	fiber 7 g
saturated fat 0.5 g	sugars 17 g
trans fat 0.0 g	**protein** 14 g
polyunsaturated fat 2.0 g	**DIETARY EXCHANGES**
monounsaturated fat 1.5 g	1 starch, 1/2 fat-free
cholesterol 3 mg	milk, 1 lean meat
sodium 202 mg	

BAKED POTATO SOUP

SERVES 4

Finished with a sprinkling of Cheddar and turkey bacon crumbles, this creamy, low-fat soup is like enjoying a loaded baked potato. And you can use the leftover potato skins for Mexican Potato Skins *(page 25).*

> 2 8-ounce baking potatoes (russet preferred), pierced in several places
> 2 slices turkey bacon
> 1 1/2 tablespoons canola or corn oil
> 1 medium bunch green onions, white and pale green parts chopped and 1/4 cup chopped dark green parts (keep dark green parts separate), divided use
> 2 1/2 tablespoons all-purpose flour

> 1 3/4 cups fat-free, low-sodium chicken broth, such as on page 36
> 1 1/2 cups fat-free milk
> 1/2 cup fat-free sour cream
> 2 tablespoons low-fat Cheddar cheese

Preheat the oven to 425°F.

Bake the potatoes on the oven rack for 1 hour 15 minutes, or until slightly overdone (the skins will be crisp and will crackle slightly when you gently squeeze the potatoes, using an oven mitt or tongs). Transfer to a cooling rack. Let stand for 15 to 20 minutes, or until cool enough to handle. Halve the potatoes lengthwise, then halve crosswise (to make 4 quarters each). Using a spoon, scoop out the flesh, leaving about an 1/8-inch shell. Reserve the skins for another use. Cut the scooped-out flesh into bite-size pieces. Set aside.

In a Dutch oven or large skillet, cook the bacon over medium heat for 8 minutes, or until lightly browned, turning frequently. Transfer to a small plate. When cool enough to handle, crumble onto the plate. Set aside.

Reduce the heat to medium low. In the same pot, heat the oil, swirling to coat the bottom. Cook the white and pale green parts of the green onions for 3 to 4 minutes, or until beginning to soften, stirring occasionally.

Sprinkle the flour over the green onions. Cook for 1 minute, stirring frequently.

Slowly whisk in the broth until the flour is dissolved. Whisk in the milk. Increase the heat to medium high and bring to a boil. Reduce the heat and simmer for 5 minutes, stirring occasionally.

Stir in the potato pieces. Return to a simmer and simmer for 2 to 3 minutes.

Whisk in the sour cream by spoonfuls. Stir in the remaining 1/4 cup chopped dark green onions. Cook for 2 to 3 minutes to heat through, but don't boil.

Just before serving, sprinkle with the Cheddar and bacon.

(continued)

Cook's Tip on Potatoes: Potatoes are a great source of potassium and other important nutrients. The baked potato has gotten a bad reputation because of the company it keeps—the standard toppings of full-fat cheese and sour cream, butter, and regular bacon add calories and unhealthy fats.

PER SERVING

calories 254
total fat 7.5 g
  saturated fat 1.0 g
  trans fat 0.0 g
  polyunsaturated fat 2.0 g
  monounsaturated fat 4.0 g
cholesterol 13 mg
sodium 231 mg

carbohydrates 36 g
  fiber 2 g
  sugars 8 g
protein 12 g
DIETARY EXCHANGES
  2 starch, 1/2 fat-free milk, 1/2 lean meat, 1 fat

Salads and Salad Dressings

Spinach Salad with Chickpeas and Cider Vinaigrette 67

Spinach Salad with Kiwifruit and Raspberries 67

Arugula Salad with Roasted Beets and Pomegranate Vinaigrette 67

Spinach-Chayote Salad with Orange Vinaigrette 68

Kale Caesar Salad with Polenta Croutons 69

Fattoush Salad 70

Greek Village Salad *(Horiatiki)* 71

Hot and Spicy Arugula and Romaine Salad 71

Watermelon and Feta Salad with Honey-Lemon Vinaigrette 72

Cucumber and Mango Salad with Lime Dressing 72

Marinated Fresh Asparagus, Tomato, and Hearts of Palm Salad 73

Beet Salad with Red Onions 74

Roasted Beet Salad 74

Broccoli Salad 75

Brussels Sprouts Caesar-Style 75

Shaved Brussels Sprouts Salad 76

Moroccan Farro, Carrot, and Date Salad 76

Carrot-Raisin Salad 77

Cauliflower Salad 77

Zesty Corn Relish 78

Tex-Mex Cucumber Salad 78

Spiralized Cucumbers with Yogurt-Dill Dressing 79

Green Bean and Tomato Toss 79

Marinated Green Beans 80

Caprese Salad with Grilled Zucchini 80

Marinated Tomato Salad 81

Herbed Tomato Orzo Salad 81

Grilled Tomato-Peach Salad 82

Dijon-Marinated Vegetable Medley 82

Parsnip Salad with Jícama and Apple 83

Jícama Slaw 83

Warm Red Cabbage Salad 83

Asian Coleslaw 84

SPINACH SALAD WITH CHICKPEAS AND CIDER VINAIGRETTE

SERVES 10

Jazz up an ordinary spinach salad with legumes, extra veggies, and mild, crumbly cheese to make it extraordinary. The creaminess of the chickpeas and the queso fresco (fresh cheese), as well as the crispness of the beets and the crunch of the seeds, elevates this salad to a new level—both in flavor and in nutrition.

16 ounces spinach, stems discarded and leaves torn into bite-size pieces
2/3 cup cooked chickpeas, cooked without salt
4 ounces queso fresco or farmer cheese
1/2 cup sliced button mushrooms
1/2 cup sliced beets

Dressing

1/4 cup plus 2 tablespoons olive oil (extra-virgin preferred)
1 1/2 tablespoons cider vinegar
1/4 teaspoon sugar
1/4 teaspoon pepper (freshly ground preferred)
1/8 teaspoon salt

■ ■ ■

1/3 cup unsalted shelled pumpkin or sunflower seeds

In a large bowl, toss together the spinach, chickpeas, queso fresco, mushrooms, and beets.

In a small bowl, whisk together the dressing ingredients. Pour the dressing and sprinkle the pumpkin seeds over the salad, tossing gently to coat.

PER SERVING

calories 144	carbohydrates 7 g
total fat 11.5 g	fiber 2 g
saturated fat 2.0 g	sugars 1 g
trans fat 0.0 g	protein 5 g
polyunsaturated fat 2.0 g	DIETARY EXCHANGES
monounsaturated fat 7.0 g	1/2 other
cholesterol 4 mg	carbohydrate, 1/2 lean
sodium 87 mg	meat, 2 fat

SPINACH SALAD WITH KIWIFRUIT AND RASPBERRIES

SERVES 4

The red raspberries contrast beautifully with the dark green spinach leaves in this quick and easy salad that's perfect during grilling season.

1 1/2 tablespoons white wine vinegar
1 tablespoon all-fruit seedless raspberry spread
1 1/2 tablespoons canola or corn oil
4 ounces spinach, torn into bite-size pieces
2 medium kiwifruit, peeled and sliced
1/2 cup raspberries

Put the vinegar and raspberry spread In a blender or mini food processor. Add the oil in a stream, processing constantly until blended.

In a large bowl, combine the spinach, half the kiwifruit, and half the raspberries. Pour the dressing over the salad, tossing to coat. Top with the remaining kiwifruit and raspberries. Serve immediately.

PER SERVING

calories 94	sodium 24 mg
total fat 5.5 g	carbohydrates 11 g
saturated fat 0.5 g	fiber 3 g
trans fat 0.0 g	sugars 6 g
polyunsaturated fat 1.5 g	protein 1 g
monounsaturated fat 3.5 g	DIETARY EXCHANGES
cholesterol 0 mg	1 fruit, 1 fat

ARUGULA SALAD WITH ROASTED BEETS AND POMEGRANATE VINAIGRETTE

SERVES 4

Bitter arugula contrasts beautifully with the sweet beets and fruity dressing. If you're in a rush, you can use packaged steamed baby beets.

4 medium beets, stems trimmed to about 1 inch
Cooking spray
2 teaspoons cumin seeds

(continued)

Dressing

> 2 tablespoons frozen 100% orange juice
>   concentrate
> 1 tablespoon balsamic vinegar
> 2 teaspoons olive oil (extra-virgin preferred)
> 2 medium garlic cloves, finely chopped
> 1 teaspoon honey
> 1/3 cup 100% pomegranate juice

■ ■ ■

> 4 ounces baby arugula
> 1 medium red onion, halved lengthwise, each
>   half cut crosswise into 1/4-inch slices
> 1 large seedless orange, peeled and
>   segmented
> 1 tablespoon sliced almonds, dry-roasted

Preheat the oven to 375°F.

Place each beet on a separate piece of aluminum foil large enough to enclose the beet. Lightly spray the beets with cooking spray. Sprinkle the cumin seeds over the beets. Wrap tightly. Transfer to a baking sheet.

Roast for 40 to 45 minutes, or until the beets are tender when pierced with a fork. Carefully unwrap the packets away from you (to prevent steam burns). Let stand for 5 to 10 minutes, or just until cool enough to handle. Wearing disposable plastic gloves (to keep from staining your fingers), peel off the skins using your fingers or a paring knife. Discard the skins, including any cumin seeds that stick to them. Cut each beet crosswise into 1/4-inch slices. Set aside.

Meanwhile, in a small bowl, whisk together the dressing ingredients except the pomegranate juice. Whisk in the pomegranate juice.

In a medium bowl, toss together the arugula and onion.

When the beets are ready, pour half the dressing over the arugula mixture, tossing gently to coat. Mound the arugula mixture on plates. Arrange the beet slices and orange segments on top. Drizzle with the remaining dressing. Sprinkle with the almonds. Serve immediately for the best texture.

Cook's Tip: When you buy fresh beets, don't throw away the beet greens. They're packed with vitamins. Use them as you would spinach, either cut into slivers and steamed or cooked quickly in a small amount of olive oil. You can even toss them with your favorite whole-grain pasta.

PER SERVING

calories 140	carbohydrates 26 g
total fat 3.5 g	fiber 5 g
saturated fat 0.5 g	sugars 20 g
trans fat 0.0 g	protein 4 g
polyunsaturated fat 0.5 g	DIETARY EXCHANGES
monounsaturated fat 2.0 g	2 vegetable, 1 fruit,
cholesterol 0 mg	1/2 fat
sodium 77 mg	

SPINACH-CHAYOTE SALAD WITH ORANGE VINAIGRETTE
SERVES 10

If you've ever wondered how to use the pale-green, pear-shaped chayote squash, this salad—large enough for a small family gathering—is one option. Chayote, a member of the gourd family, is a good source of potassium and has a mild taste that melds the flavors of cucumber and zucchini.

Dressing

> 1/2 teaspoon grated orange zest
> 1/2 cup fresh orange juice
> 2 tablespoons canola or corn oil
> 2 tablespoons sugar
> 1 1/2 tablespoons white wine vinegar
> 1 tablespoon fresh lemon juice

Salad

> 1 medium chayote squash, peeled, seeded,
>   and thinly sliced
> 1 11-ounce can mandarin oranges in juice, well
>   drained
> 6 to 8 ounces spinach or other salad greens,
>   torn into bite-size pieces
> 1 small cucumber, thinly sliced
> 2 tablespoons sliced green onions

In a small bowl, whisk together the dressing ingredients until the sugar is dissolved.

In a large bowl, stir together the chayote and 2 tablespoons dressing. Let stand for 5 to 10 minutes.

Add the remaining salad ingredients to the chayote, tossing well. Pour the remaining dressing over the salad, tossing to coat.

Cook's Tip on Chayote: *Chayote* (chay-OH-tay or kay-OH-tay), a mild-flavored summer squash, has many names. It's called *mirliton* in Louisiana, *christophine* in France and the Caribbean, and *custard marrow* in Britain. A vegetable peeler works well to remove the skin except at the puckered end, which requires a sharp knife. After peeling the squash, halve it lengthwise to remove its seed. Use chayote raw in salads, cook it like other summer squash, or stuff and bake it like acorn squash. In the West Indies, it's used in pies as we use apples and even combined with the same spices.

PER SERVING

calories 61	**sodium** 18 mg
total fat 3.0 g	**carbohydrates** 8 g
saturated fat 0.0 g	fiber 1 g
trans fat 0.0 g	sugars 6 g
polyunsaturated fat 1.0 g	**protein** 1 g
monounsaturated fat 2.0 g	**DIETARY EXCHANGES**
cholesterol 0 mg	1/2 fruit, 1/2 fat

KALE CAESAR SALAD WITH POLENTA CROUTONS

SERVES 4

Here's a nontraditional Caesar-style salad that's made with kale instead of romaine. It's tossed with a lighter version of a Caesar dressing that complements the taste of the slightly peppery greens. Serve on chilled salad plates for maximum flavor.

Cooking spray

Croutons
    3 cups water
    1 cup fine yellow cornmeal
    1/2 teaspoon pepper (freshly ground preferred)

Dressing
    2 tablespoons shredded or grated Parmesan cheese
    2 tablespoons cider vinegar
    1 tablespoon fresh lemon juice
    1 tablespoon olive oil (extra-virgin preferred)
    1 medium garlic clove, finely minced
    1/2 teaspoon Dijon mustard (lowest sodium available)
    1/2 teaspoon Worcestershire sauce (lowest sodium available)
    1/8 teaspoon pepper (freshly ground preferred)

■ ■ ■

    1 12-ounce bunch kale, stems and ribs discarded, torn into bite-size pieces
    1 cup grape tomatoes, halved lengthwise (optional)

Prepare the polenta at least 3 hours before serving time.

Lightly spray an 8-inch square baking dish with cooking spray. Set aside.

In a large saucepan, bring the water to boil over high heat. Reduce the heat to medium. Using a long-handled whisk, carefully whisk the water to create a swirl. Slowly pour the cornmeal in a steady stream into the swirl, whisking constantly. After all the cornmeal is added, reduce the heat to low. Simmer for 20 minutes, or until the mixture is very thick, whisking frequently. Remove from the heat. Stir in the pepper.

Spoon the cooked polenta into the baking dish. Using a metal spatula lightly sprayed with cooking spray, smooth the top. Refrigerate, uncovered, for at least 45 minutes, or until thoroughly chilled and solid. The polenta can be prepared in advance and chilled for up to 24 hours. Cover it with plastic wrap once it's cold and solid.

Preheat the oven to 400°F. Line a rimmed baking sheet with aluminum foil. Lightly spray the foil with cooking spray. Set aside.

(continued)

Remove the chilled polenta from the refrigerator, inverting it onto a cutting board. Using a sharp knife lightly sprayed with cooking spray, slice the polenta into 1 x 1-inch pieces. Using a small metal spatula or knife, carefully transfer the pieces to the baking sheet. Bake for 55 minutes to 1 hour, or until the croutons are crisp and golden, turning occasionally. Transfer the baking sheet to a cooling rack and let cool for at least 30 minutes. Set aside until just before serving time.

In a small bowl, whisk together the dressing ingredients. Pour over the kale. Using your fingertips, gently massage the dressing into the kale until the leaves are just softened. Transfer the salad to plates. Top each serving with the croutons and tomatoes.

Cook's Tip: Dry the kale very well by putting it in a salad spinner, or pat it dry with several paper towels. Water droplets clinging to the leaves will prevent the dressing from tenderizing the kale. Be sure to massage the kale leaves with the dressing for a few minutes before using them. This softens them and mellows any bitter flavor.

Cook's Tip: You'll have plenty of extra croutons, so use them on other salads, in soups, and even just for snacking. Store them in an airtight container and refrigerate for up to two days or freeze them in an airtight container for up to two months. To reheat them, bake the room-temperature croutons in a 350°F oven for 10 to 15 minutes, or until slightly crisp.

PER SERVING

calories 145	carbohydrates 22 g
total fat 5.5 g	fiber 3 g
saturated fat 1.0 g	sugars 2 g
trans fat 0.0 g	protein 6 g
polyunsaturated fat 1.0 g	DIETARY EXCHANGES
monounsaturated fat 3.0 g	1/2 starch, 2 vegetable,
cholesterol 2 mg	1 fat
sodium 96 mg	

FATTOUSH SALAD
SERVES 4

Fattoush is a Middle Eastern salad featuring crisped pita bread mixed with greens and vegetables. In this version, the pita is seasoned before toasting to intensify the flavor, and the salad is dressed with a vinaigrette brightened with lemony sumac, a popular Middle Eastern spice.

> Cooking spray
> 1 6-inch whole-grain pita pocket, split and cut into 1 1/2 by 1/4-inch strips
> 1 teaspoon celery seeds
> 1/2 teaspoon garlic powder
> 1/4 teaspoon paprika

Dressing
> 1 teaspoon grated lemon zest
> 2 tablespoons fresh lemon juice
> 2 tablespoons white wine vinegar
> 2 teaspoons olive oil (extra-virgin preferred)
> 1 teaspoon honey
> 1 teaspoon ground sumac, or 1 teaspoon grated lemon zest
> 1 medium garlic clove, minced
> 1/4 teaspoon salt
> 1/8 teaspoon pepper

■ ■ ■

> 2 cups torn romaine
> 1 cup unpeeled diced English, or hothouse, cucumber
> 4 medium radishes, thinly sliced
> 1 medium Italian plum (Roma) tomato, chopped
> 2 medium green onions, thinly sliced
> 2 tablespoons chopped Italian (flat-leaf) parsley
> 1 tablespoon chopped fresh mint
> 1 tablespoon chopped fresh cilantro

Preheat the oven to 350°F. Lightly spray a large baking sheet with cooking spray.

Arrange the pita strips in a single layer on the baking sheet. Lightly spray the tops with cooking spray. In a small bowl, stir together the celery seeds, garlic powder, and paprika. Sprinkle the mixture over the pita strips. Bake for 6 to 7 minutes, or until crisp. Remove from the oven. Let cool for 10 minutes.

In a large bowl, whisk together the dressing ingredients.

Add the pita strips and the remaining ingredients, tossing gently to coat.

Cook's Tip on Sumac: A useful and unusual seasoning to have on hand, sumac works well with everything from chicken and fish to salads and rice dishes. As a bonus, its deep red color adds visual appeal. You can find it at Middle Eastern markets or in your grocery store's spice section or bulk spice section (allowing you to buy a small amount to see if you like it).

PER SERVING

calories 93	carbohydrates 15 g
total fat 3.0 g	fiber 3 g
saturated fat 0.5 g	sugars 4 g
trans fat 0.0 g	**protein** 3 g
polyunsaturated fat 0.5 g	**DIETARY EXCHANGES**
monounsaturated fat 2.0 g	1/2 starch, 1 vegetable,
cholesterol 0 mg	1/2 fat
sodium 236 mg	

GREEK VILLAGE SALAD (HORIATIKI)

SERVES 4

Authentic Greek salads contain no lettuce and use only the freshest vegetables available. Horiatiki salad is also called "peasant salad." It's popular everywhere in Greece; the vegetables are coarsely chopped to give the salad a rustic look.

Dressing

    1 tablespoon olive oil (extra-virgin preferred)

    1 1/2 teaspoons fresh lemon juice

    1 1/2 teaspoons red wine vinegar

    1/4 teaspoon dried oregano, crumbled

    1/4 teaspoon pepper

Salad

    2 medium cucumbers, peeled, halved lengthwise, and sliced

    2 medium red or green bell peppers, coarsely chopped

2 cups halved cherry or grape tomatoes

1/2 cup slivered red onion

1 ounce fat-free feta cheese, crumbled

3 tablespoons chopped kalamata olives

■ ■ ■

1 medium lemon, cut into 4 wedges (optional)

In a small bowl, whisk together the dressing ingredients.

In a large bowl, toss together the salad ingredients. Pour the dressing over the salad, tossing to coat. Serve with the lemon wedges.

Cook's Tip on Olive Oil: Use the best-quality olive oil you can for salads and other uncooked dishes. Since the oil isn't heated, its flavor components don't break down; therefore, the deep, fruity notes of a superior oil are really prominent.

PER SERVING

calories 112	**sodium** 240 mg
total fat 6.0 g	**carbohydrates** 13 g
saturated fat 1.0 g	fiber 3 g
trans fat 0.0 g	sugars 7 g
polyunsaturated fat 1.0 g	**protein** 4 g
monounsaturated fat 4.0 g	**DIETARY EXCHANGES**
cholesterol 0 mg	3 vegetable, 1 fat

HOT AND SPICY ARUGULA AND ROMAINE SALAD

SERVES 4

This salad combines jicama, also called Mexican potato, with peppery arugula, crunchy romaine, and several staples of Asian cooking. The result? Greens with an attitude.

Dressing

    1 1/2 tablespoons soy sauce (lowest sodium available)

    1 tablespoon white wine vinegar

    2 1/2 teaspoons toasted sesame oil

    1 1/2 teaspoons sugar

    1 teaspoon hot chili oil

(continued)

Salad

    1 head romaine, torn into pieces
    4 cups baby arugula, torn into pieces
    6 medium radishes, thinly sliced
    1/2 cup matchstick-size jícama strips
    4 medium green onions, thinly sliced

In a small bowl, whisk together the dressing ingredients until the sugar is dissolved.

In a large bowl, toss together the salad ingredients. Pour the dressing over the salad, tossing gently to coat. Serve immediately for the best texture.

PER SERVING

calories 95	sodium 172 mg
total fat 4.5 g	carbohydrates 12 g
saturated fat 0.5 g	fiber 5 g
trans fat 0.0 g	sugars 6 g
polyunsaturated fat 2.0 g	protein 3 g
monounsaturated fat 2.0 g	DIETARY EXCHANGES
cholesterol 0 mg	2 vegetable, 1 fat

WATERMELON AND FETA SALAD WITH HONEY-LEMON VINAIGRETTE

SERVES 4

Juicy watermelon and feta cheese crown a salad of spicy arugula and crisp spinach. A drizzle of a sweet-tart vinaigrette perfectly complements all the flavors.

    8 cups baby spinach or baby arugula (half
        spinach and half arugula preferred)
    2 medium hothouse, or English, cucumbers,
        peeled and seeded, cut into 1/2-inch
        cubes
    1 small red onion, halved and thinly sliced

Dressing

    2 teaspoons grated lemon zest
    1/4 cup fresh lemon juice (about 1 large lemon)
    3 tablespoons canola or corn oil (canola oil
        preferred)
    1 tablespoon honey
    1/8 teaspoon pepper (freshly ground
        preferred)

■ ■ ■

    2 cups cubed seedless watermelon
    1/4 cup crumbled fat-free feta cheese
    Chiffonade of fresh mint (about 8 mint
        leaves, or 1/4 cup loosely packed mint
        leaves)

In a large bowl, gently toss together the spinach mixture, cucumbers, and onion.

In a small bowl, whisk together the dressing ingredients. Pour over the salad, tossing to coat.

Transfer the salad to plates. Top each serving with the watermelon. Sprinkle with the feta and mint. Serve immediately.

Cook's Tip on Chiffonades: To cut herbs or lettuce into a chiffonade, stack the leaves into a neat pile (no more than 8 leaves at a time). Roll up the pile lengthwise into a tight cylinder. Using a sharp knife, cut the cylinder crosswise to create thin strips.

Cook's Tip: To save time and money, buy small quantities of ready-to-eat cut watermelon.

PER SERVING

calories 179	sodium 186 mg
total fat 11.0 g	carbohydrates 18 g
saturated fat 1.0 g	fiber 3 g
trans fat 0.0 g	sugars 12 g
polyunsaturated fat 3.0 g	protein 5 g
monounsaturated fat 6.5 g	DIETARY EXCHANGES
cholesterol 0 mg	1 fruit, 1 vegetable, 2 fat

CUCUMBER AND MANGO SALAD WITH LIME DRESSING

SERVES 6

Cucumber and mango combine to make a crunchy, spicy-sweet salad with a refreshing mix of flavors and textures. Its island flavors pair well with entrées such as Coconut-Rum Baked Fish (page 157) or Caribbean Grilled Chicken Kebabs (page 202).

Dressing

    1 teaspoon grated lime zest
    2 tablespoons fresh lime juice
    1 tablespoon olive oil (extra-virgin preferred)

1 teaspoon honey

1/2 teaspoon ground cumin

1/4 teaspoon salt

Salad

1 cup uncooked quinoa, rinsed and drained

1 large mango, thinly sliced

1 large cucumber (English, or hothouse, preferred), halved lengthwise and crosswise, seeded, and cut into thin strips

1 medium red bell pepper, thinly sliced

1/4 cup chopped fresh cilantro

1 teaspoon seeded and minced fresh jalapeño (see Cook's Tip on Handling Hot Chiles, page 24)

In a small bowl, whisk together the dressing ingredients. Set aside.

Prepare the quinoa using the package directions, omitting the salt. Transfer to a large bowl. Fluff with a fork.

Stir the remaining ingredients into the cooked quinoa. Pour the dressing over the salad, tossing gently to coat.

Cook's Tip: For the most eye-catching salad, cut the mango, cucumber, and bell pepper into slices that are about the same size.

PER SERVING

calories 178	carbohydrates 31 g
total fat 4.5 g	fiber 4 g
saturated fat 0.5 g	sugars 12 g
trans fat 0.0 g	protein 5 g
polyunsaturated fat 1.0 g	DIETARY EXCHANGES
monounsaturated fat 2.0 g	1 1/2 starch, 1/2 fruit,
cholesterol 0 mg	1/2 fat
sodium 102 mg	

MARINATED FRESH ASPARAGUS, TOMATO, AND HEARTS OF PALM SALAD

SERVES 6

This simple salad is perfect for springtime, when fresh asparagus is in season. The light dressing enhances the flavor of the vegetables.

Salad

8 ounces asparagus spears, trimmed and cut into 2-inch pieces

1 pound Italian plum (Roma) tomatoes, cut into 1/4-inch slices

1 14-ounce can hearts of palm, rinsed and drained

1/4 cup thinly sliced onion

Dressing

1/4 cup red wine vinegar

2 tablespoons dry red wine (regular or nonalcoholic)

2 teaspoons sugar

1/4 teaspoon pepper

In a medium saucepan, steam the asparagus for 3 minutes, or until tender-crisp. Immediately transfer to a shallow glass casserole dish.

Gently stir in the tomatoes, hearts of palm, and onion.

In a small bowl, whisk together the dressing ingredients until the sugar is dissolved. Pour over the asparagus mixture. Cover and refrigerate for 30 minutes, stirring occasionally.

Cook's Tip: You can make this salad up to 24 hours in advance, but don't add the hearts of palm until about 30 minutes before serving. They become discolored from the wine if added sooner.

Cook's Tip on Hearts of Palm: Hearts of palm, which really do come from palm trees, taste somewhat like artichokes. They're actually the core—the central growing part—of the palm. Sometimes the outer layer of the larger pieces is a bit tough. Make a small slit in that layer and peel it off before using the more tender inner part.

PER SERVING

calories 44	sodium 165 mg
total fat 0.5 g	carbohydrates 8 g
saturated fat 0.0 g	fiber 3 g
trans fat 0.0 g	sugars 4 g
polyunsaturated fat 0.0 g	protein 3 g
monounsaturated fat 0.0 g	DIETARY EXCHANGES
cholesterol 0 mg	2 vegetable

BEET SALAD WITH RED ONIONS

SERVES 4

A beet is a sweet root veggie that naturally pairs well with pungent and acidic foods, such as the onion, vinegar, ginger, and orange used in this recipe. Enjoy this salad with Ginger-Walnut Salmon and Asparagus (page 146).

    6 cups water
    1 pound beets, stems trimmed to about 1 inch
    1/4 large red onion, sliced
    2 tablespoons red wine vinegar
    2 tablespoons canola or corn oil
    1 1/2 tablespoons soy sauce (lowest sodium
        available)
    2 teaspoons grated peeled gingerroot
    1 teaspoon grated orange zest
    1/4 teaspoon pepper, or to taste (freshly
        ground preferred)

In a large saucepan, bring the water to a boil over high heat. Add the beets. Reduce the heat and simmer for 35 to 40 minutes, or until the beets are tender (when easily pierced with a fork). Drain the beets. Set aside until cool enough to handle.

When the beets have cooled, peel them and discard the stems. Cut into thin slices.

In a medium bowl, stir together the beets and onion.

In a food processor or blender, process the remaining ingredients until smooth. Pour over the beet mixture, tossing lightly to coat. Cover and refrigerate for at least 1 hour before serving.

Cook's Tip on Beets: Peel beets under running water to prevent the beet juice from staining your hands or wear disposable plastic gloves.

PER SERVING

calories 105	sodium 206 mg
total fat 7.0 g	carbohydrates 10 g
saturated fat 0.5 g	fiber 3 g
trans fat 0.0 g	sugars 7 g
polyunsaturated fat 2.0 g	protein 2 g
monounsaturated fat 4.5 g	**DIETARY EXCHANGES**
cholesterol 0 mg	2 vegetable, 1 1/2 fat

ROASTED BEET SALAD

SERVES 4

Peppery arugula is the perfect complement to the sweet beets and tangy citrus of this jewel-toned salad. The pomegranate vinaigrette is also delicious on green salads.

    Cooking spray
    1 pound beets
Dressing
    1 1/2 tablespoons white wine vinegar
    1 1/2 teaspoons olive oil (extra-virgin
        preferred)
    1 1/2 teaspoons 100% pomegranate juice or
        fresh orange juice
    1 teaspoon pure maple syrup or honey
    1/2 teaspoon grated lime zest

■ ■ ■

    4 cups arugula
    4 medium clementines, sectioned
    1/4 cup pomegranate arils (seeds)
    Sprigs of fresh mint (optional)

Preheat the oven to 350°F. Lightly spray a shallow baking pan with cooking spray.

Cut off all but 1 to 2 inches of the stems from the beets. Arrange the beets in a single layer on the baking pan. Lightly spray the beets with cooking spray.

Roast the beets for about 1 hour, or until they can be pierced easily with the tip of a sharp knife. Let cool slightly. Peel the beets, discarding the skin (see Cook's Tip on Beets). Coarsely chop the beets (you should have about 3 cups). Transfer to a medium bowl.

In a small bowl, whisk together the dressing ingredients. Pour over the beets, tossing gently to coat. Refrigerate, covered, for 2 to 24 hours, tossing occasionally.

Just before serving, arrange the arugula on plates. Gently stir the clementines into the beet mixture. Using a slotted spoon, transfer the beet mixture onto the arugula. Sprinkle each serving with the pomegranate arils. Garnish with the mint.

Time-Saver: Fresh roasted beets give this salad a delicious concentrated beet flavor. However, if you don't have time to roast fresh beets, you can use two 15-ounce cans or jars of sliced beets, rinsed and drained, instead. Or buy pre-steamed baby beets.

BROCCOLI SALAD

SERVES 8

Include this healthier, lighter version of a classic salad on your party buffet. The combo of fresh broccoli with crisp turkey bacon, sweet raisins, and a creamy, lemony dressing will appeal to everyone.

Dressing
- 1/4 cup light mayonnaise
- 1/4 cup fat-free plain Greek yogurt
- 1 tablespoon fresh lemon juice
- 1 teaspoon sugar
- 1/4 teaspoon pepper (freshly ground preferred)

■ ■ ■

- 1/2 pound broccoli crowns, broken into florets and stems trimmed (about 2 cups)
- 3 slices turkey bacon, cooked and crumbled
- 1/3 cup raisins
- 1/2 small red onion, halved and thinly sliced
- 2 tablespoons plus 2 teaspoons finely chopped unsalted cashews, dry-roasted

In a small bowl, whisk together the dressing ingredients until the sugar is dissolved.

In a large bowl, combine the remaining ingredients except the cashews. Pour the dressing over the salad, tossing to combine. Cover and chill for 15 minutes. Just before serving, sprinkle with the cashews.

BRUSSELS SPROUTS CAESAR-STYLE

SERVES 4

Vitamin-rich brussels sprouts are teamed with a Caesar style dressing, crisp homemade croutons, and juicy tomato slices. This is a practical way to use up leftover Roasted Brussels Sprouts *(page 378).*

- Olive oil cooking spray
- 4 ounces brussels sprouts, trimmed, halved lengthwise, and loose outer leaves discarded
- 1 slice whole-grain bread (lowest sodium available), cut into 3/4-inch cubes
- 1/4 teaspoon garlic powder

Dressing
- 1 tablespoon shredded or grated Parmesan cheese
- 1 1/2 teaspoons Dijon mustard (lowest sodium available)
- 1 1/2 teaspoons fresh lemon juice
- 1 1/2 teaspoons Worcestershire sauce (lowest sodium available)
- 1 1/2 teaspoons white wine vinegar
- 1 teaspoon olive oil
- 1/2 teaspoon sugar
- 1/8 teaspoon pepper

■ ■ ■

- 2 medium Italian plum (Roma) tomatoes, thinly sliced

(continued)

Preheat the oven to 350°F. Lightly spray a rimmed baking sheet with cooking spray.

Arrange the brussels sprouts in a single layer on the baking sheet. Lightly spray with cooking spray. Bake for 30 minutes.

Put the bread cubes on the baking sheet around the brussels sprouts. Lightly spray the cubes with cooking spray. Sprinkle the garlic powder over the cubes.

Bake for 5 minutes, or until the brussels sprouts are tender with lightly browned edges and the bread cubes are golden brown. Transfer the baking sheet to a cooling rack. Let cool.

In a small bowl, whisk together the dressing ingredients until the sugar is dissolved.

Arrange the tomatoes in a single layer on plates. Arrange the brussels sprouts on top. Drizzle with the dressing. Sprinkle with the croutons.

Cook's Tip on Brussels Sprouts: Miniature versions of cabbage, brussels sprouts provide significant amounts of vitamin C and beta-carotene, and are a good vegetable source of protein. Choose sprouts that are heavy for their size and have compact heads without yellow outer leaves. For more even cooking, choose sprouts of about the same size.

PER SERVING

calories 51	sodium 106 mg
total fat 2.0 g	carbohydrates 8 g
saturated fat 0.5 g	fiber 2 g
trans fat 0.0 g	sugars 3 g
polyunsaturated fat 0.0 g	protein 2 g
monounsaturated fat 1.0 g	DIETARY EXCHANGES
cholesterol 1 mg	1 vegetable, 1/2 fat

SHAVED BRUSSELS SPROUTS SALAD

SERVES 4

This recipe gives you a fresh take on brussels sprouts, which have a mild cabbage-like flavor when eaten raw. The sweet and tangy dressing perfectly complements the juicy crispness of pears and nutty crunch of toasted walnuts.

Dressing
> 1/4 cup red wine vinegar
> 1 tablespoon Dijon mustard (lowest sodium available)
> 2 teaspoons olive oil (extra-virgin preferred)
> 1 teaspoon light brown sugar
> 1 medium garlic clove, minced
> 1/4 teaspoon salt
> 1/8 teaspoon pepper

■ ■ ■

> 8 ounces brussels sprouts, shredded or grated
> 1 medium carrot, shredded
> 1/4 medium red onion, cut into thin strips
> 1 medium pear, such as Bartlett, Anjou, or Bosc, thinly sliced
> 2 tablespoons chopped walnuts, dry-roasted

In a medium bowl, whisk together the dressing ingredients until the sugar is dissolved.

Add the remaining ingredients, tossing gently to coat (using two large serving spoons works well for this).

PER SERVING

calories 114	carbohydrates 17 g
total fat 5.0 g	fiber 5 g
saturated fat 0.5 g	sugars 9 g
trans fat 0.0 g	protein 3 g
polyunsaturated fat 2.0 g	DIETARY EXCHANGES
monounsaturated fat 2.0 g	1/2 fruit, 2 vegetable,
cholesterol 0 mg	1 fat
sodium 250 mg	

MOROCCAN FARRO, CARROT, AND DATE SALAD

SERVES 4

Farro, once called emmer, is an ancient strain of wheat. Used in pasta and soups, its popularity is increasing throughout the world, but especially in Italy, where it was renamed "farro." Its nutty flavor and toothsome texture partner beautifully with sweet carrots and warm spices.

Dressing
> 1 teaspoon grated orange zest
> 1/4 cup fresh orange juice

1 1/2 tablespoons honey

1 tablespoon fresh lemon juice

2 teaspoons canola or corn oil

1/4 teaspoon ground cinnamon

1/8 teaspoon ground cumin

1/8 teaspoon pepper (freshly ground preferred)

■ ■ ■

1 cup uncooked pearled or semi-pearled farro

1 cup shredded carrots (about 3 medium carrots)

1/4 cup chopped dates

1/4 cup minced fresh mint

1/4 unsalted, shelled, chopped pistachio nuts (optional)

In a small bowl, whisk together the dressing ingredients. Set aside.

Prepare the farro using the package directions, omitting the salt. Transfer to a large bowl and let cool to room temperature. Fluff with a fork.

Add the carrots and dates to the farro, stirring to combine. Pour the dressing over the farro mixture, tossing well to combine. Cover and refrigerate for 1 hour so the flavors blend.

Just before serving, sprinkle with the mint and pistachios. Toss well. Serve cold or at room temperature.

Cook's Tip: Save time and purchase pre-shredded carrots at the supermarket. Use any leftover carrots in green salads, meat loaf, or spaghetti sauce.

PER SERVING

calories 268	sodium 53 mg
total fat 2.5 g	carbohydrates 53 g
saturated fat 0.0 g	fiber 5 g
trans fat 0.0 g	sugars 16 g
polyunsaturated fat 0.5 g	protein 8 g
monounsaturated fat 1.5 g	DIETARY EXCHANGES
cholesterol 0 mg	2 1/2 starch, 1 fruit

CARROT-RAISIN SALAD

SERVES 6

The tanginess from the yogurt and citrus in this dish is a perfect pairing for the sweetness of the carrots and raisins. Enjoy with Grilled Tempeh Burgers *(page 364) or* Grilled Lemongrass Flank Steak *(page 249).*

2 cups shredded carrots

1/4 cup raisins

1/4 cup fat-free plain Greek yogurt

1 tablespoon fresh lemon juice

2 tablespoons chopped pecans, dry-roasted

In a medium bowl, stir together the carrots and raisins.

In a small bowl, whisk together the yogurt and lemon juice. Pour over the carrot mixture, stirring to coat. Just before serving, sprinkle with the pecans.

PER SERVING

calories 57	carbohydrates 10 g
total fat 2.0 g	fiber 2 g
saturated fat 0.0 g	sugars 6 g
trans fat 0.0 g	protein 2 g
polyunsaturated fat 0.5 g	DIETARY EXCHANGES
monounsaturated fat 1.0 g	1/2 fruit, 1 vegetable,
cholesterol 0 mg	1/2 fat
sodium 30 mg	

CAULIFLOWER SALAD

SERVES 4

Visually appealing and full of crunch, this salad is tossed with a nutty, lemony dressing. Enjoy it with a bowl of Slow-Cooker Chicken Noodle Soup *(page 108) for a nutritious lunch.*

1 cup shredded carrots

1 cup sliced cauliflower florets (1/4- to 1/2-inch pieces)

1 cup spinach, leaves torn into bite-size pieces

Pepper to taste (freshly ground preferred)

Dressing

1/3 cup walnut oil

2 tablespoons fresh lemon juice

1/4 teaspoon salt-free lemon pepper

1/8 teaspoon salt

(continued)

■ ■ ■

1/4 cup chopped pecans, dry-roasted

In a large salad bowl, toss together the carrots, cauliflower, spinach, and pepper. Cover and refrigerate for 30 minutes.

Meanwhile, in a medium bowl, whisk together the dressing ingredients. Just before serving, pour the dressing over the salad, tossing to coat. Sprinkle with the pecans.

Cook's Tip: For even more color, look for purple cauliflower to use in this salad.

PER SERVING

calories 232	**sodium** 106 mg
total fat 24.0 g	**carbohydrates** 6 g
saturated fat 2.0 g	fiber 2 g
trans fat 0.0 g	sugars 2 g
polyunsaturated fat 13.0 g	**protein** 2 g
monounsaturated fat 7.0 g	**DIETARY EXCHANGES**
cholesterol 0 mg	1 vegetable, 5 fat

ZESTY CORN RELISH

SERVES 8

Serve this corn and bell pepper combination on leaf lettuce as a light side salad, or use small portions as a condiment at your next barbecue.

1 tablespoon olive oil
3 cups fresh corn kernels or frozen whole-kernel corn, thawed
1 medium red bell pepper, finely diced
1/4 cup minced red onion
1/2 medium fresh jalapeño, seeds and ribs discarded, minced (see Cook's Tip on Handling Hot Chiles, page 24)
2 tablespoons dry white wine (regular or nonalcoholic) (optional)
6 medium fresh basil leaves, finely chopped, or 1/2 teaspoon dried basil, crumbled
3 or 4 sprigs of fresh cilantro, coarsely chopped, or 1/8 teaspoon dried coriander seeds, crushed
3 sprigs of fresh thyme, stems discarded, or 1/2 to 1 teaspoon dried thyme, crumbled
2 teaspoons fresh lime juice

1 small garlic clove, crushed
1/4 teaspoon salt
1/4 teaspoon pepper, or to taste

In a large skillet, heat the oil over medium heat, swirling to coat the bottom. Cook the corn, bell pepper, onion, and jalapeño for about 3 minutes, or until the corn and bell pepper are tender. Remove the skillet from the heat. Let the mixture cool for about 10 minutes.

Stir in the remaining ingredients. Transfer to a glass dish. Cover and refrigerate for 30 minutes to two days.

PER SERVING

calories 70	**sodium** 82 mg
total fat 2.5 g	**carbohydrates** 12 g
saturated fat 0.5 g	fiber 2 g
trans fat 0.0 g	sugars 4 g
polyunsaturated fat 0.5 g	**protein** 2 g
monounsaturated fat 1.5 g	**DIETARY EXCHANGES**
cholesterol 0 mg	1 starch, 1/2 fat

TEX-MEX CUCUMBER SALAD

SERVES 4

A delicious, easy way to serve garden vegetables, this salad is a great companion to grilled fish or poultry, such as Grilled Pineapple-Lime Salmon *(page 150) or* Spicy Grilled Chicken *(page 195).*

1 medium cucumber, peeled, seeded, and diced
1 medium tomato, seeded and diced
1/3 cup picante sauce (lowest sodium available)
2 medium green onions, finely chopped
2 tablespoons chopped fresh cilantro
1 tablespoon fresh lime juice
1 tablespoon olive oil (extra-virgin preferred)
1 medium garlic clove, minced

In a small bowl, stir together all the ingredients. Serve immediately for peak flavor.

Cook's Tip on Seeding Cucumbers: To seed cucumbers easily, halve them lengthwise and run the tip of a teaspoon down the center.

calories 55	sodium 94 mg
total fat 3.5 g	carbohydrates 5 g
saturated fat 0.5 g	fiber 1 g
trans fat 0.0 g	sugars 3 g
polyunsaturated fat 0.5 g	protein 1 g
monounsaturated fat 2.5 g	DIETARY EXCHANGES
cholesterol 0 mg	1 vegetable, 1 fat

SPIRALIZED CUCUMBERS WITH YOGURT-DILL DRESSING

SERVES 6

The ability to slice and shred a range of vegetables into ribbons has long been possible with a julienne peeler, but the technique has been made popular with a spiralizer, a gadget that creates vegetables ribbons, or "noodles," in a variety of thicknesses. This creamy salad is a calming complement to a dish with some heat such as Grilled Salmon with Cilantro Sauce *(page 150).*

> 3 medium cucumbers (English, or hothouse, preferred), peeled, seeded, and spiralized or cut into ribbons with a vegetable peeler, then cut into smaller pieces
> 1 small onion, finely chopped
> 1/2 cup fat-free plain yogurt
> 2 tablespoons chopped fresh dillweed
> 1 teaspoon sugar
> 1 teaspoon fresh lemon juice
> 1/2 teaspoon pepper (freshly ground preferred)

In a medium bowl, stir together the cucumbers and onion.

In a small bowl, whisk together the remaining ingredients until the sugar is dissolved. Pour the dressing over the cucumber mixture, tossing to coat. Cover and refrigerate until cold.

PER SERVING

calories 35	sodium 19 mg
total fat 0.0 g	carbohydrates 6 g
saturated fat 0.0 g	fiber 1 g
trans fat 0.0 g	sugars 5 g
polyunsaturated fat 0.0 g	protein 2 g
monounsaturated fat 0.0 g	DIETARY EXCHANGES
cholesterol 0 mg	1 vegetable

GREEN BEAN AND TOMATO TOSS

SERVES 4

Fresh and pretty, this heart-friendly salad is a welcome addition on the picnic table or the kitchen table or even the buffet table.

> 8 ounces green beans, trimmed
> 4 ounces grape tomatoes
> 3 tablespoons fresh lemon juice (about 1 medium lemon)
> 2 tablespoons olive oil (extra-virgin preferred)
> 1 tablespoon Dijon mustard (lowest sodium available)
> 1/4 teaspoon pepper
> 1/8 teaspoon salt

In a medium saucepan, steam the green beans for 5 minutes, or until just tender-crisp.

Meanwhile, fill a medium bowl with ice water.

When the green beans are cooked, using a slotted spoon, immediately plunge them into the ice water to stop the cooking process. Drain well in a colander. Transfer to an 8-inch square glass baking dish or other glass dish large enough to hold the green beans in a single layer.

Sprinkle the tomatoes over the green beans.

In a small glass bowl, whisk together the remaining ingredients. Pour over the green bean mixture, tossing to coat. Cover and refrigerate for 1 to 2 hours, or until well chilled, tossing occasionally. Just before serving, drain the salad, discarding the marinade.

PER SERVING

calories 91	sodium 156 mg
total fat 7.5 g	carbohydrates 7 g
saturated fat 1.0 g	fiber 2 g
trans fat 0.0 g	sugars 3 g
polyunsaturated fat 1.0 g	protein 2 g
monounsaturated fat 5.0 g	DIETARY EXCHANGES
cholesterol 0 mg	1 vegetable, 1 1/2 fat

MARINATED GREEN BEANS

SERVES 4

This version of the classic dish marinates for just 30 minutes so it'll be ready about the same time as an entrée. If you don't have tarragon vinegar, you can use cider vinegar instead, but be sure to use fresh green beans.

8 ounces green beans, trimmed
1/4 cup thinly sliced red onion
2 tablespoons sugar
2 tablespoons tarragon vinegar
1 tablespoon walnut oil (optional)
1/4 teaspoon salt
1/4 teaspoon pepper
2 tablespoons finely chopped walnuts, dry-roasted

In a medium saucepan, steam the green beans for 5 minutes, or until just tender-crisp.

Meanwhile, fill a medium bowl with ice water.

When the green beans are cooked, using a slotted spoon, immediately plunge them into the ice water to stop the cooking process. Drain well in a colander.

Transfer the green beans to a medium bowl. Add the remaining ingredients except the walnuts, tossing gently to coat. Refrigerate for 30 minutes, tossing occasionally.

Just before serving, sprinkle with the walnuts. Toss gently.

Cook's Tip: This salad is best if eaten within 1 hour of combining the ingredients.

PER SERVING

calories 69	carbohydrates 12 g
total fat 2.5 g	fiber 2 g
saturated fat 0.5 g	sugars 9 g
trans fat 0.0 g	**protein** 2 g
polyunsaturated fat 2.0 g	**DIETARY EXCHANGES**
monounsaturated fat 0.5 g	1 vegetable, 1/2 other
cholesterol 0 mg	carbohydrate, 1/2 fat
sodium 149 mg	

CAPRESE SALAD WITH GRILLED ZUCCHINI

SERVES 4

Drizzled with zesty balsamic vinaigrette, this vibrant salad features the colors of the Italian flag. The grilled squash adds an intriguing smokiness to this classic dish. It's a great use for grilled zucchini left over after your last cookout.

Dressing
2 tablespoons balsamic vinegar
2 tablespoons frozen 100% apple juice concentrate, thawed
2 teaspoons Dijon mustard (lowest sodium available)
1 teaspoon olive oil (extra-virgin preferred)
1 medium garlic clove, minced

■ ■ ■

1 teaspoon olive oil
2 medium zucchini, halved lengthwise
4 medium Italian plum (Roma) tomatoes, cored, each cut crosswise into 8 slices
2 ounces fat-free mozzarella cheese, cut into 16 small, thin slices
16 medium fresh basil leaves (as uniform in size as possible)
1/4 teaspoon pepper

In a small bowl, whisk together the dressing ingredients. Cover and refrigerate.

Preheat the grill on medium high.

Lightly brush the oil on both sides of the zucchini. Grill the zucchini for 5 minutes on each side, or until tender. Place the zucchini with the cut side up on a serving platter. Let cool slightly.

Arrange 8 overlapping tomato slices on each zucchini half. Tuck 4 mozzarella slices and 4 basil leaves between the tomato slices, as follows: tomato slice, mozzarella slice, tomato slice, basil leaf, repeating the pattern until all are used. Drizzle with the dressing. Sprinkle with the pepper. Serve immediately.

Cook's Tip: This dish is also delicious with portobello mushrooms in place of the zucchini.

calories 96	carbohydrates 13 g
total fat 3.0 g	fiber 2 g
saturated fat 0.5 g	sugars 9 g
trans fat 0.0 g	protein 7 g
polyunsaturated fat 0.5 g	DIETARY EXCHANGES
monounsaturated fat 1.5 g	1 vegetable, 1/2 fruit,
cholesterol 2 mg	1 lean meat
sodium 163 mg	

MARINATED TOMATO SALAD

SERVES 6

This is the perfect salad for summer, when toma-toes and mint are at their best. Stir leftovers into cooked whole-grain pasta, or spoon them onto crisp whole-wheat baguette slices for a summery version of bruschetta.

> 1/4 cup olive oil (extra-virgin preferred)
> 2 tablespoons balsamic vinegar or red wine vinegar
> 12 medium grape tomatoes (yellow preferred), halved
> 1/4 cup thinly sliced red onion
> 6 kalamata olives, chopped
> 4 medium beefsteak tomatoes, thickly sliced
> 1/4 cup chopped fresh mint
> 1/4 teaspoon pepper, or to taste (freshly ground preferred)
> 1/8 teaspoon salt

In a medium bowl, whisk together the oil and vinegar. Stir in the grape tomatoes, onion, and olives. Let stand, covered, for about 20 minutes, stirring occasionally.

Arrange the sliced tomatoes on a serving plat-ter. Spoon the grape tomato mixture over the sliced tomatoes. Sprinkle with the mint, pepper, and salt.

PER SERVING

calories 119	sodium 125 mg
total fat 10.5 g	carbohydrates 6 g
saturated fat 1.5 g	fiber 2 g
trans fat 0.0 g	sugars 4 g
polyunsaturated fat 1.0 g	protein 1 g
monounsaturated fat 7.5 g	DIETARY EXCHANGES
cholesterol 0 mg	1 vegetable, 2 fat

HERBED TOMATO ORZO SALAD

SERVES 4

Flecks of red, purple, black, and green add visual ap-peal to this fresh-tasting pasta salad. The Mediter-ranean flavors pair well with grilled fish or chicken.

> 2 ounces dried whole-grain orzo
> 1 medium tomato, seeded and diced
> 1/3 cup finely chopped red onion
> 6 kalamata olives, finely chopped
> 1 1/2 teaspoons cider vinegar
> 1/2 medium garlic clove, minced
> 1 teaspoon dried basil, crumbled
> 1/2 teaspoon dried oregano, crumbled
> 1 ounce fat-free feta cheese, crumbled (about 1/4 cup)
> 1/16 teaspoon salt

Prepare the orzo using the package directions, omitting the salt. Drain in a colander. Rinse with cold water until completely cooled. Drain well.

Meanwhile, in a medium bowl, stir together the tomato, onion, olives, vinegar, garlic, basil, and oregano.

Add the orzo to the tomato mixture, tossing gently to combine.

Sprinkle with the feta and salt. Toss gently.

Cook's Tip: Be sure to remove the seeds and liq-uidy center before chopping the tomato so they don't dilute the intense flavors of this salad.

PER SERVING

calories 89	sodium 241 mg
total fat 2.0 g	carbohydrates 15 g
saturated fat 0.0 g	fiber 3 g
trans fat 0.0 g	sugars 2 g
polyunsaturated fat 0.5 g	protein 4 g
monounsaturated fat 1.0 g	DIETARY EXCHANGES
cholesterol 0 mg	1 starch

GRILLED TOMATO-PEACH SALAD

SERVES 6

Two of summer's best gifts are ripe tomatoes and juicy peaches. Add an extra dimension to these favorites by tossing them on the grill. Layer the mouthwatering results with fresh herbs and soft mozzarella.

Cooking spray
2 cups cherry tomatoes (assorted colors if available)
2 medium peaches, cut into 1 1/4-inch wedges
1 teaspoon canola or corn oil
3 tablespoons fresh mozzarella pearls
1 tablespoon coarsely chopped fresh basil
1 tablespoon coarsely chopped fresh mint
1 teaspoon balsamic vinegar

Lightly spray the grill rack with cooking spray. Preheat the grill on high.

In a large bowl, toss together the tomatoes, peaches, and oil.

Grill the tomatoes and peaches for 2 to 3 minutes, or until lightly charred, turning once halfway through.

Arrange the tomatoes and peaches on a serving platter. Place the mozzarella on the tomatoes and peaches. Sprinkle with the basil and mint. Drizzle with the vinegar.

Cook's Tip on Mozzarella: If you can't find pearl-size fresh mozzarella, chop fresh mozzarella into 1/2-inch pieces.

PER SERVING

calories 57	carbohydrates 9 g
total fat 2.0 g	fiber 2 g
saturated fat 1.0 g	sugars 6 g
trans fat 0.0 g	**protein** 2 g
polyunsaturated fat 0.0 g	**DIETARY EXCHANGES**
monounsaturated fat 1.0 g	1/2 fruit, 1 vegetable,
cholesterol 4 mg	1/2 fat
sodium 10 mg	

DIJON-MARINATED VEGETABLE MEDLEY

SERVES 4

This multicolored salad will brighten any dinner plate. It can be put together in minutes, but be sure to plan ahead so it has time to chill in the refrigerator before serving.

Dressing
1/4 to 1/2 cup balsamic vinegar plus water to make 3/4 cup
2 tablespoons Dijon mustard (lowest sodium available)
2 tablespoons chopped fresh basil or
  2 teaspoons dried basil, crumbled
1 tablespoon chopped fresh thyme or
  1 teaspoon dried thyme, crumbled
1 tablespoon olive oil (extra-virgin preferred)
2 medium garlic cloves, minced
1 teaspoon sugar
1/4 teaspoon pepper (white preferred)

Salad
2 cups chopped tomatoes
1/2 cup chopped red onion
3/4 cup frozen whole-kernel corn, thawed
3/4 cup frozen cut green beans, thawed
3/4 cup canned no-salt-added black beans, rinsed and drained

■ ■ ■

4 large lettuce leaves

In a medium bowl, whisk together the dressing ingredients until the sugar is dissolved.

In a large bowl, gently toss together the salad ingredients. Pour in the dressing, tossing gently to coat. Cover and refrigerate for 4 to 8 hours, tossing occasionally. Drain the salad, discarding the dressing. Spoon the salad onto the lettuce.

PER SERVING

calories 174	carbohydrates 30 g
total fat 4.5 g	fiber 5 g
saturated fat 0.5 g	sugars 13 g
trans fat 0.0 g	**protein** 6 g
polyunsaturated fat 0.5 g	**DIETARY EXCHANGES**
monounsaturated fat 2.5 g	1 1/2 starch,
cholesterol 0 mg	1 vegetable, 1/2 fat
sodium 195 mg	

PARSNIP SALAD WITH JÍCAMA AND APPLE

SERVES 4

Potassium-rich parsnips are related to carrots and parsley. They have an earthy, sweet flavor that's complemented by the nutty overtones of the jícama in this creamy slaw-like salad.

1/3 cup fat-free sour cream
1 1/2 tablespoons fresh lemon juice
1 tablespoon chopped fresh parsley
3/4 teaspoon sugar
3 medium parsnips, peeled and shredded
1 cup matchstick-size jícama strips
1 tablespoon finely chopped onion
1 unpeeled medium apple (Delicious preferred)
1/3 cup golden raisins (optional)

In a large bowl, whisk together the sour cream, lemon juice, parsley, and sugar until the sugar is dissolved.

Stir in the parsnips, jícama, and onion. Cover and refrigerate for 2 hours.

Just before serving, chop the apple. Stir the apple and raisins into the salad. Serve immediately.

PER SERVING

calories 126	sodium 28 mg
total fat 0.5 g	carbohydrates 29 g
saturated fat 0.0 g	fiber 7 g
trans fat 0.0 g	sugars 12 g
polyunsaturated fat 0.0 g	protein 3 g
monounsaturated fat 0.0 g	DIETARY EXCHANGES
cholesterol 3 mg	1 1/2 starch, 1/2 fruit

JÍCAMA SLAW

SERVES 4

A refreshing blend of citrus combines with the crunch of the juicy white flesh of the jícama to produce a salad that's a great palate cleanser. A native of Mexico, jícama can be briefly stir-fried or peeled, sliced, and served raw as a snack.

Dressing
1 tablespoon canola or corn oil
1/4 teaspoon grated lemon zest
1 tablespoon fresh lemon juice
1/4 teaspoon grated lime zest
1 tablespoon fresh lime juice
1/4 teaspoon grated orange zest
1 tablespoon fresh orange juice
1 teaspoon honey
1/4 teaspoon chili powder
1/8 teaspoon salt
1/8 teaspoon pepper

■ ■ ■

1 small jícama (about 1/2 pound), peeled and cut into matchstick-size strips
1/4 medium red bell pepper, diced
1 medium green onion, thinly sliced
2 sprigs of fresh cilantro, coarsely chopped

In a large bowl, whisk together the dressing ingredients.

Add the remaining ingredients, tossing to coat. Serve immediately.

PER SERVING

calories 67	sodium 80 mg
total fat 3.5 g	carbohydrates 9 g
saturated fat 0.5 g	fiber 3 g
trans fat 0.0 g	sugars 4 g
polyunsaturated fat 1.0 g	protein 1 g
monounsaturated fat 2.0 g	DIETARY EXCHANGES
cholesterol 0 mg	1/2 starch, 1 fat

WARM RED CABBAGE SALAD

SERVES 8

If you're looking for a twist on a traditional coleslaw, try this one. Sautéing the vegetables for just a few minutes brings out their natural sweet flavors. Cooking the dressing ingredients allows the sweetness of the brown sugar, the tartness of the apple juice, the acidity of the vinegar, and the bite of the mustard to blend together, creating a thick, warm dressing that coats the slaw.

(continued)

2 tablespoons canola or corn oil

1 cup finely chopped onion

1/2 cup diced celery

1 1/3 cups diced carrots

1 cup diced red bell pepper

3 cups shredded red cabbage

1 1/2 cups 100% apple juice

1/4 cup firmly packed brown sugar

2 tablespoons Dijon mustard (lowest sodium available)

3 tablespoons cornstarch

1/2 cup cider vinegar

1/4 teaspoon salt

In a large nonstick skillet, heat the oil over medium-high heat, swirling to coat the bottom. Cook the onion, celery, carrots, and bell pepper for 3 minutes, or until the onion is soft, stirring occasionally. Stir in the cabbage. Cook, covered, for 5 minutes.

In a small bowl, whisk together the remaining ingredients until the sugar is dissolved. Pour over the onion mixture, stirring to coat. Cook over medium heat for 3 to 5 minutes, or until the sauce is thickened, stirring constantly.

PER SERVING

calories 128	**carbohydrates** 22 g
total fat 4.0 g	fiber 2 g
saturated fat 0.5 g	sugars 15 g
trans fat 0.0 g	**protein** 1 g
polyunsaturated fat 1.0 g	**DIETARY EXCHANGES**
monounsaturated fat 2.0 g	1 vegetable, 1 other
cholesterol 0 mg	carbohydrate, 1 fat
sodium 180 mg	

ASIAN COLESLAW

SERVES 10

You can make this salad a day ahead, and there's no mayonnaise to worry about—perfect picnic or potluck fare. Try it with Grilled Lemongrass Flank Steak *(page 249) or* Teriyaki Halibut *(page 145).*

Dressing

2 tablespoons soy sauce (lowest sodium available)

2 tablespoons plain rice vinegar

1 tablespoon finely grated peeled gingerroot or 1 teaspoon ground ginger

2 teaspoons toasted sesame oil

1 medium garlic clove, finely chopped

1/4 teaspoon crushed red pepper flakes

Slaw

1 small head of napa cabbage (about 2 pounds), thinly sliced

2 medium carrots, coarsely grated

1 medium red bell pepper, thinly sliced

2 medium green onions, thinly sliced diagonally

In a large bowl, whisk together the dressing ingredients.

Add the slaw ingredients, tossing to coat. Serve at room temperature or cover and refrigerate until needed, tossing again just before serving.

Cook's Tip on Napa Cabbage: Napa, or Chinese, cabbage has long, crinkly, cream-colored leaves with pale green tips. It's delicious in salads, soups, and stir-fries. You can store napa cabbage in the vegetable bin of your refrigerator for up to five days.

Time-Saver: Use a food processor for the slicing and grating. The salad won't be as pretty, but the preparation will be fast.

PER SERVING

calories 41	**sodium** 102 mg
total fat 1.0 g	**carbohydrates** 6 g
saturated fat 0.0 g	fiber 2 g
trans fat 0.0 g	sugars 3 g
polyunsaturated fat 0.5 g	**protein** 2 g
monounsaturated fat 0.5 g	**DIETARY EXCHANGES**
cholesterol 0 mg	1 vegetable

CONFETTI COLESLAW

SERVES 12

This tangy coleslaw, with a vinegar-based dressing, is excellent with barbecued entrées. It makes a cool accompaniment to Jerk Chicken *(page 196) or* Grilled Tempeh Burgers *(page 364).*

Dressing

1/3 cup white wine vinegar

1/4 cup sugar

1 tablespoon canola or corn oil

1 tablespoon honey

1/4 teaspoon salt

1/4 teaspoon pepper (coarsely ground preferred)

Slaw

12 ounces green cabbage, shredded (about 4 cups)

8 ounces red cabbage, shredded (about 3 cups)

4 medium green onions, thinly sliced

1/2 medium red bell pepper, diced

1/2 medium green bell pepper, diced

In a large bowl, whisk together the dressing ingredients until the sugar is dissolved.

Add the slaw ingredients, tossing to coat. Cover and refrigerate for at least 30 minutes.

PER SERVING

calories 53	carbohydrates 10 g
total fat 1.5 g	fiber 2 g
saturated fat 0.0 g	sugars 8 g
trans fat 0.0 g	protein 1 g
polyunsaturated fat 0.5 g	**DIETARY EXCHANGES**
monounsaturated fat 0.5 g	1 vegetable, 1/2 other
cholesterol 0 mg	carbohydrate
sodium 61 mg	

GARDEN VEGETABLE SALAD IN GARLICKY VINAIGRETTE

SERVES 15

A hybrid of a salad and a coleslaw, this side dish uses cabbage rather than lettuce along with traditional garden salad vegetables. Tossed with a garlicky, sweet vinaigrette, it's a delicious salad-coleslaw combo, and because it serves so many, it's perfect for your next summer barbecue with family and friends.

1 medium head green cabbage, thinly sliced

2 medium cucumbers, thinly sliced

2 medium green bell peppers, diced

2 large carrots, thinly sliced crosswise into rounds

12 small radishes, trimmed and thinly sliced

1/4 cup canola or corn oil

2 tablespoons vinegar

1 tablespoon sugar

1 teaspoon garlic powder

1 teaspoon paprika

Pepper to taste (freshly ground preferred)

In a large salad bowl, toss together the cabbage, cucumbers, bell peppers, carrots, and radishes.

In a small bowl, whisk together the remaining ingredients until the sugar is dissolved. Pour over the vegetables, tossing to coat. Cover and refrigerate until serving time. This salad will keep for a week in the refrigerator.

PER SERVING

calories 63	sodium 19 mg
total fat 4.0 g	carbohydrates 7 g
saturated fat 0.5 g	fiber 2 g
trans fat 0.0 g	sugars 4 g
polyunsaturated fat 1.0 g	protein 1 g
monounsaturated fat 2.5 g	**DIETARY EXCHANGES**
cholesterol 0 mg	1 vegetable, 1 fat

VEGETABLE SALAD IN HONEY DIJON CREAMY VINAIGRETTE

SERVES 8

This cold veggie dish is ideal in the heat of summer as an accompaniment to sandwiches or burgers.

Dressing

1/4 cup fat-free plain yogurt

2 tablespoons red wine vinegar

2 tablespoons Dijon mustard (lowest sodium available)

2 teaspoons honey

1 teaspoon canola or corn oil

1/2 teaspoon pepper (coarsely ground preferred)

1/4 teaspoon salt

■ ■ ■

2 large carrots, sliced on the diagonal

8 ounces snow peas, trimmed and cut on the diagonal

16 grape tomatoes

4 ounces medium button mushrooms, quartered

3 to 4 small radishes, thinly sliced

(continued)

In a medium bowl, whisk together the dressing ingredients.

In a large saucepan, steam the carrots and snow peas for 3 to 4 minutes, or until tender-crisp. Plunge them into a bowl of ice water to stop the cooking process. Drain well in a colander. Pat dry with paper towels and transfer to a shallow glass bowl.

Stir in the tomatoes, mushrooms, and radishes.

Pour the dressing over the salad, tossing gently to coat. Cover and refrigerate for 30 minutes to 4 hours.

PER SERVING

calories 45	sodium 136 mg
total fat 1.0 g	carbohydrates 8 g
saturated fat 0.0 g	fiber 2 g
trans fat 0.0 g	sugars 5 g
polyunsaturated fat 0.5 g	protein 2 g
monounsaturated fat 0.5 g	DIETARY EXCHANGES
cholesterol 0 mg	2 vegetable

BERRY EXPLOSION SALAD

SERVES 4

Sweet and tangy flavors are infused in this salad, making every bite "explode" with freshness. Enjoy with a grilled entrée, such as Grilled Meat Loaf *(page 274).*

> 2 cups berries, such as blueberries, raspberries, blackberries, or sliced hulled strawberries, or a combination
> 1/2 medium mango, cubed
> 4 fresh mint leaves, finely chopped
> 1 tablespoon light brown sugar
> 1/2 medium kiwifruit, peeled and halved
> 1/2 cup fat-free, sugar-free vanilla yogurt
> 1/2 teaspoon grated lemon zest
> 2 tablespoons sliced almonds, dry-roasted

Put the berries and mango in a large bowl.

In a small bowl, stir together the mint and brown sugar. Using the back of a spoon, mash the mixture. Add to the berry mixture. Using two spoons, toss gently.

In a separate small bowl, mash the kiwifruit with a fork. Stir in the yogurt and lemon zest.

Sprinkle the berry mixture with the almonds. Top with the yogurt dressing, or serve the dressing on the side.

Cook's Tip on Mint: Mashing the mint "bruises" it, bringing out its full flavor. You can use a mortar and pestle for this step if you have one; otherwise, a spoon works just fine.

PER SERVING

calories 123	sodium 24 mg
total fat 2.0 g	carbohydrates 26 g
saturated fat 0.0 g	fiber 3 g
trans fat 0.0 g	sugars 21 g
polyunsaturated fat 0.5 g	protein 3 g
monounsaturated fat 1.0 g	DIETARY EXCHANGES
cholesterol 1 mg	1 1/2 fruit, 1/2 fat

WINTER FRUIT SALAD WITH SPINACH AND GORGONZOLA

SERVES 6

The beauty of this salad lies not only in the presentation but also in the fact that you can prepare the fruit mixture ahead, then assemble the salad quickly at the last minute. The juices of the cooked fruit mingle with the raspberry vinegar for a simple yet sensational dressing.

> 2 medium Granny Smith or Gala apples, peeled and thinly sliced
> 2 medium Bosc or Bartlett pears, peeled and thinly sliced
> 1/4 cup 100% cranberry juice
> 2 tablespoons light brown sugar
> 4 ounces baby spinach
> 3 tablespoons walnut halves, dry-roasted
> 3 tablespoons raspberry vinegar or red wine vinegar
> 2 tablespoons crumbled Gorgonzola cheese
> 1/4 teaspoon pepper

In a medium saucepan, bring the apples, pears, cranberry juice, and brown sugar to a simmer over medium-high heat. Reduce the heat and simmer, covered, for 5 to 6 minutes, or until the fruit is tender. Transfer the fruit with juices to a medium bowl. Let cool for 5 to 10 minutes.

Put the spinach in a large serving bowl or on a platter. Spoon the fruit mixture with juices over the spinach. Sprinkle with the remaining ingredients.

GINGER-INFUSED WATERMELON AND MIXED BERRIES

SERVES 4

The watermelon absorbs the sweet and tart flavors of the liquid mixture in this summery salad.

2 cups bite-size watermelon cubes
1 cup strawberries, hulled and quartered
1/2 cup blueberries
1/4 cup 100% white grape juice
2 tablespoons fresh lemon juice
1 tablespoon sugar
2 teaspoons grated peeled gingerroot
4 ounces spring greens, torn into bite-size pieces, or 4 whole Bibb lettuce leaves (optional)

In a medium bowl, stir together all the ingredients except the spring greens until the sugar is dissolved. Place the greens on salad plates Spoon the watermelon mixture over the greens. Serve immediately for peak flavors and texture.

Cook's Tip: Omit the spring greens or lettuce leaves and spoon the watermelon mixture into wine goblets or dessert dishes for a refreshing, light dessert.

POTATO SALAD WITH PEPPER AND PARSLEY

SERVES 6

This backyard-barbecue staple is often packed with saturated fat and sodium. This recipe uses light mayonnaise, then adds chopped veggies for extra color and crunch.

2 cups diced cooked red potatoes (about 3 medium)
1 medium rib of celery, chopped
2 tablespoons chopped fresh parsley
1 tablespoon chopped onion
1 tablespoon chopped red bell pepper
1 1/2 teaspoons cider vinegar
1 teaspoon dry mustard
1/2 teaspoon celery seeds
1/8 teaspoon salt
1/8 teaspoon pepper
1/4 cup light mayonnaise
1 medium red bell pepper, cut into 12 strips, or 1 to 2 tablespoons pimiento, drained (optional)

In a large bowl, gently toss together the potatoes, celery, parsley, onion, bell pepper, vinegar, mustard, celery seeds, salt, and pepper.

Stir in the mayonnaise. Arrange the bell pepper strips on top of the salad. Cover and refrigerate for several hours.

Cook's Tip: If you prefer a more mustard-based potato salad, omit the dry mustard and replace 2 tablespoons of the mayonnaise with yellow mustard (lowest sodium available).

ROASTED GERMAN POTATO SALAD

SERVES 4

Red potatoes are roasted until golden brown in this updated version of a perennial favorite. They are then tossed with smoky turkey bacon, onion, and fresh spinach to create the perfect side dish for cookouts and casual dinners.

Cooking spray
12 ounces baby red potatoes (about 5), cut into eighths (about 1-inch pieces)
1/2 teaspoon olive oil and 1/2 teaspoon olive oil, divided use
2 slices turkey bacon, chopped
3/4 cup chopped onion
1 cup loosely packed spinach, stems discarded
1/4 teaspoon caraway seeds

Dressing
1 tablespoon chopped fresh chives
2 teaspoons olive oil (extra-virgin preferred)
1 teaspoon cider vinegar
1/2 teaspoon spicy brown mustard
1/4 teaspoon pepper

Preheat the oven to 425°F. Lightly spray a small rimmed baking sheet with cooking spray.

Put the potatoes in a medium bowl. Lightly spray the potatoes with cooking spray. Stir to coat. Arrange in a single layer on the baking sheet.

Roast for 25 minutes, or until the potatoes are golden brown and tender when pierced with the tip of a sharp knife.

Meanwhile, in a medium nonstick skillet, heat 1/2 teaspoon oil over medium heat, swirling to coat the bottom. Cook the bacon for 2 minutes, stirring occasionally.

Stir in the onion and the remaining 1/2 teaspoon oil. Cook for 3 to 4 minutes, or until the bacon is lightly browned and the onion is soft, stirring frequently.

Add the spinach. Cook for 2 to 3 minutes, or until the spinach is wilted. Remove from the heat.

Stir in the caraway seeds. Cover to keep warm.

In a small bowl, whisk together the dressing ingredients.

In a medium bowl, toss together the potatoes, bacon mixture, and dressing. Serve warm.

PER SERVING

calories 126	**sodium** 155 mg
total fat 5.0 g	**carbohydrates** 17 g
saturated fat 1.0 g	fiber 2 g
trans fat 0.0 g	sugars 2 g
polyunsaturated fat 1.0 g	**protein** 4 g
monounsaturated fat 3.0 g	**DIETARY EXCHANGES**
cholesterol 5 mg	1 starch, 1 fat

TABBOULEH

SERVES 10

Tabbouleh, a fresh-tasting salad made with bulgur, parsley, and vegetables and seasoned with lemon juice and mint, originated in the Middle East. It is particularly good with roasted or grilled meats, or with Middle Eastern dishes such as Chicken Gyros with Tzatziki Sauce *(page 223).*

Salad
1/2 cup uncooked instant (fine-grain) bulgur
2 cups chopped fresh parsley
1 medium red bell pepper, diced
1 medium cucumber, peeled, seeded, and chopped
4 medium green onions, finely chopped
1/3 cup chopped fresh mint
1/2 teaspoon pepper
1/4 teaspoon salt

■ ■ ■

1/4 cup plus 2 tablespoons fresh lemon juice (about 2 medium lemons)
2 tablespoons olive oil (extra-virgin preferred)
1 to 2 medium garlic cloves, crushed or minced
20 cherry tomatoes, quartered

Prepare the bulgur using the package directions. Transfer to a large bowl. Fluff with a fork.

Gently stir the remaining salad ingredients into the bulgur.

In a small bowl, whisk together the lemon juice, oil, and garlic. Pour over the salad, tossing gently to coat. Cover and refrigerate for 3 to 4 hours.

Just before serving, stir in the tomatoes.

Cook's Tip on Bulgur: Bulgur, which has a nutty flavor and texture, is wheat kernels that have been steamed, dried, and coarsely broken or ground into grain.

PER SERVING

calories 73	carbohydrates 10 g
total fat 3.0 g	fiber 3 g
saturated fat 0.5 g	sugars 2 g
trans fat 0.0 g	protein 2 g
polyunsaturated fat 0.5 g	**DIETARY EXCHANGES**
monounsaturated fat 2.0 g	1/2 starch, 1 vegetable,
cholesterol 0 mg	1/2 fat
sodium 73 mg	

VEGGIE COUSCOUS SALAD

SERVES 8

Fresh basil and feta team with a medley of vegetables and couscous in a refreshing Mediterranean-inspired side salad. It pairs well with Greek Fish Fillets (page 139) or Saffron-Scented Grilled Chicken (page 201).

Dressing

1/3 cup water

1/4 cup plus 2 tablespoons cider vinegar

1 1/2 tablespoons sugar

1 tablespoon plus 1 teaspoon canola or corn oil

1 medium garlic clove, minced

1/4 teaspoon salt

Salad

2/3 cup uncooked whole-wheat couscous

6 ounces frozen artichoke hearts, thawed, drained, and chopped

1/2 cup diced zucchini

1/2 cup quartered grape tomatoes

1/3 cup diced red bell pepper

1/4 cup finely chopped red onion

3 to 4 tablespoons chopped fresh basil

1 ounce fat-free feta cheese

In a small bowl, whisk together the dressing ingredients. Set aside.

Prepare the couscous using the package directions, omitting the salt. Pour into a medium bowl. Fluff lightly with a fork.

Gently stir in the dressing and the remaining salad ingredients. Serve immediately or cover and refrigerate for several hours.

PER SERVING

calories 130	carbohydrates 21 g
total fat 4.5 g	fiber 4 g
saturated fat 0.0 g	sugars 4 g
trans fat 0.0 g	protein 4 g
polyunsaturated fat 1.5 g	**DIETARY EXCHANGES**
monounsaturated fat 2.0 g	1 starch, 1 vegetable,
cholesterol 0 mg	1/2 fat
sodium 192 mg	

WILD RICE SALAD WITH CRANBERRY VINAIGRETTE

SERVES 4

The fall flavors in this side dish make it a perfect addition to a holiday brunch or buffet table, or serve it with a turkey dinner, such as Roasted Garlic–Lemon Turkey Breast (page 233). If it's a bit too tart for your liking, add just a hint of sugar.

1/3 cup uncooked wild rice

1/3 cup chopped mixed dried fruit

1/4 cup thinly sliced celery

1/4 cup 100% cranberry juice

3 tablespoons finely chopped red onion

2 tablespoons finely chopped pecans, dry-roasted

2 teaspoons red wine vinegar

1/2 teaspoon grated peeled gingerroot

1/2 teaspoon toasted sesame oil

1/2 teaspoon sugar (optional)

(continued)

Prepare the rice using the package directions, omitting the salt and margarine. Transfer to a medium bowl and let cool to room temperature.

Gently stir in the remaining ingredients.

MEXICAN STREET VENDOR CORN-AND-BEAN SALAD

SERVES 6

This salad recipe was inspired by the popular grilled corn on the cob (elote) that's sold by street vendors all over Mexico. The corn is slathered with mayonnaise, seasoned with chili powder and lime juice, and then rolled in cheese. Our salad derivative adds hearty black beans, has a lighter dressing, and is much neater to eat.

> 1 teaspoon canola or corn oil
> 2 1/4 cups frozen whole-kernel corn, thawed
> 1 1/4 cups canned no-salt-added black beans, rinsed and drained
> 1/3 cup sliced green onions
> 3 tablespoons chopped fresh cilantro
> 3 tablespoons light mayonnaise
> 1 1/2 teaspoons grated lime zest
> 1 1/2 tablespoons fresh lime juice
> 3/4 teaspoon chili powder
> 1 tablespoon finely shredded Cotija cheese or crumbled queso fresco

In a large nonstick skillet, heat the oil over medium-high heat, swirling to coat the bottom. Cook the corn for 4 to 5 minutes, or until lightly browned, stirring frequently. Transfer to a large bowl. Stir in the beans, green onions, and cilantro.

In a small bowl, whisk together the remaining ingredients except the cheese. Stir the mayonnaise mixture into the salad. Sprinkle with the cheese. Serve at room temperature, or cover and refrigerate for 1 hour to serve chilled.

Cook's Tip: This salad can be made up to 10 hours in advance. Cover and refrigerate it until serving time.

THREE-BEAN SALAD

SERVES 14

Tired of bringing traditional salads or slaws to get-togethers with family and friends? This recipe serves a crowd, so try it at your next barbecue or potluck supper. The kidney, green, and yellow beans make this salad stand out on a buffet table.

> 10 ounces frozen or 1 pound fresh green beans, trimmed and halved
> 10 ounces frozen or 1 pound fresh yellow beans, trimmed and halved
> 1/2 cup cider vinegar
> 1/2 cup sugar
> 1/3 cup canola or corn oil
> 1/2 teaspoon pepper (freshly ground preferred)
> 1 medium garlic glove, minced
> 1 15.5-ounce can no-salt-added kidney beans, rinsed and drained
> 1 medium red onion, thinly sliced
> 1/2 medium bell pepper, any color, chopped

In a large saucepan, steam the green and yellow beans for 6 to 8 minutes, or just until tender-crisp. Transfer to a colander. Rinse with cold water to stop the cooking process. Let cool to room temperature. Drain well. Dry on paper towels.

Meanwhile, in a small saucepan, heat the vinegar and sugar over medium heat, stirring until the sugar is dissolved. Stir in the oil, pepper, and garlic.

In a large bowl, add the green and yellow beans, kidney beans, onion, bell pepper, vinegar, and dressing, tossing to combine.

Cover and chill for 6 hours or overnight so the flavors blend.

PER SERVING

calories 122	carbohydrates 16 g
total fat 5.5 g	fiber 3 g
saturated fat 0.5 g	sugars 9 g
trans fat 0.0 g	protein 3 g
polyunsaturated fat 1.5 g	DIETARY EXCHANGES
monounsaturated fat 3.5 g	1/2 starch, 1/2 other
cholesterol 0 mg	carbohydrate, 1 fat
sodium 26 mg	

MARINATED PASTA SALAD

SERVES 8

This is a wonderful make-ahead dish to take to potlucks or backyard barbecues and a great way to add vegetables to your diet. To make this a vegetarian entrée, double the serving size and sprinkle each serving with 1 ounce of fat-free feta cheese.

  8 ounces dried whole-grain pasta, such as rotini, farfalle, or ziti (3 to 4 cups)
  8 ounces fresh asparagus (6 to 10 spears) or 10 ounces frozen asparagus, thawed and patted dry, cut into 1-inch pieces

Dressing
  1/4 cup fresh lemon juice (about 1 large lemon)
  1/4 cup olive oil (extra-virgin preferred)
  2 tablespoons Dijon mustard (lowest sodium available)
  1 garlic clove, minced
  1/8 teaspoon salt
  1/8 teaspoon pepper

■ ■ ■

  1/2 medium red bell pepper, very thinly sliced
  1/2 cup very thinly sliced zucchini

  1/2 cup finely chopped red onion
  1 medium rib of celery, thinly sliced

Prepare the pasta using the package directions, omitting the salt. Drain well in a colander. Set aside to let cool. Transfer to a large bowl.

Meanwhile, in a large saucepan, steam the asparagus for 5 minutes, or until tender-crisp. Plunge into a bowl of ice water to stop the cooking process. Drain well in a colander.

In a small bowl, whisk together the dressing ingredients.

Add the asparagus, remaining ingredients, and the dressing to the pasta, tossing to combine. Cover and refrigerate for 2 to 8 hours.

PER SERVING

calories 182	carbohydrates 25 g
total fat 8.0 g	fiber 4 g
saturated fat 1.0 g	sugars 3 g
trans fat 0.0 g	protein 5 g
polyunsaturated fat 1.0 g	DIETARY EXCHANGES
monounsaturated fat 5.0 g	1 1/2 starch,
cholesterol 0 mg	1 vegetable, 1/2 fat
sodium 119 mg	

SIXTEEN-BEAN SALAD

SERVES 4

Here's one way to eat your soup with a fork! Using a dried soup mix provides real variety with a minimum of effort and expense.

  1 cup 16-bean soup mix, sorted for stones and shriveled beans, rinsed, and drained
  1/2 cup chopped tomato
  1/3 medium red bell pepper, chopped
  1/3 medium yellow bell pepper, chopped
  3 medium green onions, thinly sliced
  1/4 cup salsa (lowest sodium available), such as Salsa Cruda (page 437)
  1 tablespoon chopped fresh cilantro
  1/8 teaspoon pepper
  4 ounces mixed salad greens, torn into bite-size pieces

(continued)

Prepare the beans using the package directions, omitting the salt, discarding the seasoning packet, and cooking until the beans are just tender. Drain and let cool for about 30 minutes, or until room temperature. Transfer to a large bowl.

Add the remaining ingredients except the salad greens, tossing gently. Cover and refrigerate for 4 hours, stirring occasionally. Spoon over the salad greens.

Cook's Tip: For a really quick lunch, wrap some of the leftovers minus the salad greens in a whole-wheat tortilla (look for the lowest sodium available). Zap the wrap in the microwave until warm.

PER SERVING

calories 188	carbohydrates 34 g
total fat 1.0 g	fiber 5 g
saturated fat 0.0 g	sugars 4 g
trans fat 0.0 g	protein 11 g
polyunsaturated fat 0.5 g	DIETARY EXCHANGES
monounsaturated fat 0.5 g	2 starch, 1 vegetable,
cholesterol 0 mg	1/2 lean meat
sodium 80 mg	

GREEK PASTA SALAD

SERVES 8

Feta cheese and fresh dillweed enhance this pasta-vegetable combo. Serve with pita bread and Greek Egg and Lemon Soup (Avgolemono) *(page 35).*

Salad

   12 ounces dried whole-wheat rotini

   9 ounces frozen artichoke hearts, thawed, drained, and chopped

   1 medium red bell pepper, diced

   2/3 cup seeded and diced cucumber

   8 kalamata olives, chopped

   4 medium green onions, thinly sliced

   4 ounces fat-free feta cheese, crumbled

Dressing

   1/2 cup fat-free cottage cheese

   1/2 cup fat-free plain Greek yogurt

   1/4 cup light mayonnaise

   1/4 cup thinly sliced green onions (green part only)

   2 tablespoons fresh lemon juice

   1 to 2 tablespoons finely chopped fresh dillweed

   1/4 teaspoon pepper

Prepare the pasta using the package directions, omitting the salt. Drain well in a colander. Transfer to a large bowl.

Stir in the remaining salad ingredients.

In a food processor or blender, process the cottage cheese, yogurt, mayonnaise, 1/4 cup green onions, and the lemon juice until smooth. Stir in the dillweed and pepper. Pour over the pasta mixture, tossing to coat. Cover and refrigerate for about 30 minutes, or until chilled.

PER SERVING

calories 237	carbohydrates 41 g
total fat 3.5 g	fiber 7 g
saturated fat 0.5 g	sugars 3 g
trans fat 0.0 g	protein 13 g
polyunsaturated fat 1.5 g	DIETARY EXCHANGES
monounsaturated fat 1.0 g	2 1/2 starch, 1 lean
cholesterol 3 mg	meat
sodium 430 mg	

SESAME-GINGER PASTA SALAD WITH EDAMAME

SERVES 4

This Asian-inspired vinaigrette blends soy sauce and rice vinegar with pops of flavor from fresh ginger and sesame oil. Try it with a cup of Thai-Style Lemon and Spinach Soup *(page 44).*

Salad

   12 ounces dried whole-grain angel hair pasta

   1 cup frozen shelled edamame

   1 large cucumber (English, or hothouse, preferred), halved lengthwise, seeded, and sliced crosswise

   4 medium green onions, thinly sliced

   1 medium red bell pepper, cut into short, thin strips

   1/2 cup chopped fresh cilantro

Dressing

   3 tablespoons plain rice vinegar

   2 tablespoons soy sauce (lowest sodium available)

1 tablespoon canola or corn oil

1 1/2 teaspoons grated peeled gingerroot

1/2 teaspoon toasted sesame oil

1/8 teaspoon cayenne

Prepare the pasta using the package directions, omitting the salt and adding the edamame during the last 3 minutes of cooking. Drain in a colander. Rinse with cold water until cool. Drain well. Transfer to a large bowl.

Stir in the remaining salad ingredients.

In a small bowl, whisk together the dressing ingredients. Pour over the salad, tossing to coat.

PER SERVING

calories 426	carbohydrates 74 g
total fat 8.5 g	fiber 13 g
saturated fat 0.5 g	sugars 9 g
trans fat 0.0 g	protein 17 g
polyunsaturated fat 3.0 g	**DIETARY EXCHANGES**
monounsaturated fat 4.0 g	4 1/2 starch,
cholesterol 0 mg	1 vegetable, 1 lean
sodium 206 mg	meat

SALMON AND ORZO SALAD

SERVES 4

Made with petite pasta, crunchy cucumbers, pre-cooked salmon, and a burst of lemon, this dish gives you a variation on classic tuna pasta salad.

8 ounces dried whole-grain orzo

2 5-ounce vacuum-sealed pouches boneless, skinless pink salmon, flaked

1/2 cup light mayonnaise

1/4 medium English, or hothouse, cucumber, or 1/2 medium cucumber, peeled, seeded, and diced

2 medium green onions, thinly sliced

1 teaspoon grated lemon zest

2 tablespoons fresh lemon juice

1 teaspoon dried dillweed, crumbled

1/2 teaspoon salt-free lemon pepper, or 1/4 teaspoon pepper and 1/2 teaspoon grated lemon zest

Prepare the orzo using the package directions, omitting the salt. Drain in a colander. Rinse with

cold water until cool. Drain well. Transfer to a medium bowl. Let cool for 10 minutes.

Gently stir in the remaining ingredients. Serve immediately or cover and refrigerate for up to three days.

PER SERVING

calories 360	carbohydrates 46 g
total fat 11.0 g	fiber 7 g
saturated fat 2.0 g	sugars 3 g
trans fat 0.0 g	protein 20 g
polyunsaturated fat 6.0 g	**DIETARY EXCHANGES**
monounsaturated fat 2.5 g	3 starch, 2 lean meat,
cholesterol 35 mg	1 fat
sodium 618 mg	

SALMON AND SPRING GREENS WITH TANGY-SWEET DRESSING

SERVES 4

The Anaheim pepper adds a gentle heat to this salad that blends well with the bite of red onion and the tender salmon.

3/4 cup dried whole-grain rotini (about 2 ounces)

1/4 cup red wine vinegar

2 tablespoons sugar

2 tablespoons Dijon mustard (coarse-grain preferred, lowest sodium available)

1 tablespoon canola or corn oil

5 ounces spring greens

1/4 cup thinly sliced red onion

1 medium fresh Anaheim or poblano pepper, seeds and ribs discarded, cut into thin rounds (see Cook's Tip on Handling Hot Chiles, page 24)

2 5-ounce vacuum-sealed pouches boneless, skinless pink salmon, flaked

Prepare the pasta using the package directions, omitting the salt. Drain in a colander. Rinse with cold water until cool. Drain well.

Meanwhile, in a small bowl, whisk together the vinegar, sugar, mustard, and oil until the sugar is dissolved.

(continued)

Arrange the spring greens on plates. Top with the pasta, onion, and Anaheim pepper. Pour the dressing over the salad. Top with the salmon.

Cook's Tip: A serrated knife is helpful when slicing the Anaheim pepper.

PER SERVING

calories 215	**carbohydrates** 23 g
total fat 7.0 g	fiber 4 g
saturated fat 1.5 g	sugars 10 g
trans fat 0.0 g	**protein** 15 g
polyunsaturated fat 2.0 g	**DIETARY EXCHANGES**
monounsaturated fat 2.5 g	1 starch, 1 vegetable,
cholesterol 25 mg	2 lean meat
sodium 523 mg	

MEDITERRANEAN TUNA SALAD

SERVES 4

The pomegranate seeds add a hint of texture, a touch of tartness, and pop of color, and the nuts bring an earthiness to modernize this classic creamy tuna salad. Enjoy it on a bed of lettuce or open face on a whole-wheat English muffin half.

Dressing
- 1/3 cup fat-free sour cream
- 3 tablespoons plain rice vinegar
- 1 tablespoon sugar
- 1 teaspoon olive oil (extra-virgin preferred)
- 1/8 teaspoon salt

Salad
- 1 15.5-ounce can no-salt-added cannellini beans, rinsed and drained
- 1 4.5-ounce can very low sodium albacore tuna, packed in water, drained and flaked
- 1 cup grape tomatoes, halved
- 1/2 cup chopped cucumber
- 1/2 cup chopped red onion
- 1/4 cup chopped walnuts
- 2 tablespoons pomegranate arils (seeds)
- 1 1/2 teaspoons dried oregano, crumbled
- 1/4 teaspoon pepper

In a small bowl, whisk together the dressing ingredients until the sugar is dissolved.

In a medium bowl, stir together the salad ingredients. Gently stir in the dressing. Refrigerate for 15 minutes so the flavors blend.

PER SERVING

calories 237	**carbohydrates** 28 g
total fat 7.5 g	fiber 6 g
saturated fat 0.5 g	sugars 9 g
trans fat 0.0 g	**protein** 17 g
polyunsaturated fat 4.0 g	**DIETARY EXCHANGES**
monounsaturated fat 2.0 g	1 1/2 starch,
cholesterol 17 mg	1 vegetable, 2 lean
sodium 149 mg	meat

CURRIED TUNA SALAD

SERVES 4

Mild tuna steps up a notch with an unexpected sweet curry mayonnaise and a bright pop of island fruit. Serve scooped into romaine leaves.

Salad
- 1/2 cup light mayonnaise
- 1 tablespoon plus 1 teaspoon sugar
- 2 teaspoons curry powder
- 1/8 teaspoon cayenne
- 2 4.5-ounce cans very low sodium albacore tuna, packed in water, drained and flaked
- 1/2 small pineapple, chopped, shell reserved
- 1 8-ounce can sliced water chestnuts, drained
- 1 medium red bell pepper, chopped
- 1 1/2 medium ribs of celery, chopped

■ ■ ■

- 2 tablespoons finely chopped pecans, dry-roasted

In a medium bowl, whisk together the mayonnaise, sugar, curry powder, and cayenne.

Stir in the remaining salad ingredients.

For an attractive presentation, spoon the salad into the reserved pineapple shell. Sprinkle with the pecans.

Cook's Tip: You can substitute 8 ounces chopped cooked boneless, skinless chicken breast (cooked without salt) for the tuna.

MEXICAN SHRIMP SALAD

SERVES 6

If you like spicy, you'll love this dish. Ingredients marry during the 2-hour chilling time to bring this dish alive with flavor. Enjoy some Edamame Guacamole *(page 15) or* Tortilla Pinwheels *(page 17) for a complete fiesta!*

    2 1/2 quarts water
    1 pound raw medium shrimp, unpeeled,
        rinsed
    2 teaspoons liquid crab-and-shrimp-boil
        seasoning
    1/2 cup light mayonnaise
    1/3 cup fat-free plain yogurt
    2 teaspoons bottled white horseradish,
        drained
    1/2 cup sliced green onions
    2 tablespoons chili sauce
    1 teaspoon chili powder
    1/2 teaspoon grated lime zest
    1 tablespoon chopped fresh cilantro
        (optional)
    Red hot-pepper sauce to taste
    6 cups chopped romaine

In a large saucepan, bring the water to a boil. Stir in the shrimp and liquid seasoning. Return to a boil. Remove from the heat and set aside for 5 minutes. Drain in a colander. Rinse with cold water. Peel, devein, and cut the shrimp in half horizontally to retain their C shape.

In a medium bowl, whisk together the remaining ingredients. Add shrimp, stirring to coat. Cover and refrigerate at least 2 hours to allow flavors to blend. Just before serving, put the romaine on plates. Spoon the shrimp salad onto the romaine.

CHICKEN AND VEGETABLE PASTA SALAD

SERVES 6

This light savory entrée salad pairs well with a cup of soup, such as Creamy Cauliflower Soup *(page 39) or* Fresh Mushroom Soup *(page 41).*

Salad
    8 ounces dried whole-grain penne
    2 cups diced cooked skinless chicken breast,
        cooked without salt, all visible fat
        discarded
    1/2 medium cucumber, peeled, seeded, and
        diced
    1 medium rib of celery, diced
    1/2 cup sliced water chestnuts, drained
    1/4 medium green bell pepper, diced
    2 medium green onions, sliced
    1/4 cup chopped pimiento, drained and
        patted dry
    1/4 cup light mayonnaise

■ ■ ■

    2 tablespoons capers, drained
    1/4 teaspoon paprika

Prepare the pasta using the package directions, omitting the salt. Drain well in a colander. Rinse with cold water until cool. Drain well. Transfer to a large bowl.

Gently stir in the remaining salad ingredients.

Sprinkle with the capers and paprika.

(continued)

Cook's Tip: If you prefer, substitute two 4.5-ounce cans very low sodium albacore tuna, packed in water, drained and flaked, for the chicken.

PER SERVING

calories 257	sodium 218 mg
total fat 5.5 g	carbohydrates 32 g
saturated fat 1.0 g	fiber 6 g
trans fat 0.0 g	sugars 3 g
polyunsaturated fat 2.5 g	protein 20 g
monounsaturated fat 1.5 g	DIETARY EXCHANGES
cholesterol 43 mg	2 starch, 2 lean meat

CAJUN CHICKEN SALAD

SERVES 4

A bed of mixed salad greens piled high with roasted red bell peppers, mushrooms, and chicken is a perfect no-cook entrée on a hot summer night. Serve with Yogurt-Fruit Soup (page 48) as a side or Spiced Skillet Bananas (page 503) or Frozen Banana-Orange Push-Ups (page 504) for dessert.

Dressing
> 1/4 cup plus 2 tablespoons cider vinegar
> 1 tablespoon olive oil (extra-virgin preferred)
> 3 medium garlic cloves, minced
> 1 1/2 teaspoons sugar
> 1/2 teaspoon red hot-pepper sauce

Salad
> 8 ounces button mushrooms, sliced
> 1 7.2-ounce jar roasted red bell peppers, drained and thinly sliced, or 1 large red bell pepper, roasted and thinly sliced
> 3 medium green onions, chopped
> 1 pound cooked skinless chicken breast, cooked without salt, all visible fat discarded, cut into thin strips
> 6 ounces mixed salad greens, torn into bite-size pieces

In a small bowl, whisk together the dressing ingredients until the sugar is dissolved.

In a large shallow glass baking dish, stir together the mushrooms, roasted peppers, and green onions. Pour in the dressing, tossing to coat. Let stand for 20 minutes.

Stir the chicken into the mushroom mixture. Spoon over the salad greens.

Cook's Tip: You can make the mushroom mixture up to 8 hours in advance. Cover and refrigerate it until serving time.

PER SERVING

calories 281	carbohydrates 11 g
total fat 9.0 g	fiber 2 g
saturated fat 2.0 g	sugars 4 g
trans fat 0.0 g	protein 38 g
polyunsaturated fat 1.5 g	DIETARY EXCHANGES
monounsaturated fat 4.0 g	2 vegetable, 4 lean meat
cholesterol 96 mg	
sodium 212 mg	

CHICKEN AND SNOW PEA SALAD

SERVES 6

This Asian-inspired salad packs fruit and vegetables into one entrée. It's quick to assemble, but be sure to do it a few hours ahead so the flavors can reach their peak. Meanwhile, consider making Chai-Spiced Flans with Blueberries (page 496) or Ginger-Berry Wonton Baskets (page 500) for dessert.

> 6 ounces snow peas, trimmed, or 6 ounces frozen snow peas, thawed
> 2 11-ounce cans mandarin oranges (canned in light syrup), drained
> 1 pound cooked chicken breast, cooked without salt, all visible fat discarded, cubed
> 1/4 cup finely chopped red onion
> 1/4 cup thinly sliced water chestnuts
> 1/2 cup light mayonnaise
> 1/2 cup sugar-free, fat-free vanilla yogurt
> 1 teaspoon grated peeled gingerroot
> 1 teaspoon grated lime zest
> 1/4 teaspoon salt
> Dash of white pepper

Using paper towels, blot the snow peas and oranges dry.

In a large bowl, stir together the chicken, snow peas, oranges, onion, and water chestnuts.

In a small bowl, whisk together the remaining ingredients. Pour over the chicken mixture, stirring gently (a rubber spatula works well for this). Be careful to avoid breaking the oranges. Cover and refrigerate for several hours.

ASIAN CHICKEN AND RICE SALAD

SERVES 8

Classic mayo-based chicken salad gets a global makeover with Asian-inspired flavors in this recipe. In a ring mold, this salad is a worthy centerpiece for a brunch. For a fancier presentation, spoon individual servings into hollowed-out bell peppers.

Salad

    3/4 cup uncooked brown rice

    1 1/2 pounds diced cooked skinless chicken breasts, cooked without salt, all visible fat discarded

    10 ounces frozen green peas, thawed

    4 medium green onions, sliced

    1 medium rib of celery, diced

    2 tablespoons diced green bell pepper

Dressing

    1/4 cup plain rice vinegar

    2 tablespoons canola or corn oil

    2 tablespoons dry sherry

    1 tablespoon soy sauce (lowest sodium available)

    1 tablespoon Dijon mustard (lowest sodium available)

    1/4 teaspoon hot chili oil (optional)

    1/8 teaspoon ground ginger

■ ■ ■

    Cooking spray (if using ring mold)

    Sprigs of fresh cilantro (optional)

Prepare the rice using the package directions, omitting the salt and margarine. Transfer to a large bowl and let cool to room temperature.

Gently stir in the remaining salad ingredients.

In a small bowl, whisk together the dressing ingredients. Pour over the salad, tossing to coat.

If using a ring mold, lightly spray with cooking spray. Spoon the salad into the mold, packing firmly. If you prefer, leave the salad in the large bowl. Cover the mold or the bowl and refrigerate for at least 30 minutes. Turn the salad out onto the serving platter, or mound the salad on plates or in hollowed-out bell peppers. Garnish with the cilantro.

GRILLED FLANK STEAK SALAD WITH SWEET-AND-SOUR SESAME DRESSING

SERVES 4

If you plan ahead, you'll have some reserved Grilled Lemongrass Flank Steak to use in this salad of colorful, crisp vegetables and earthy wild rice. A sweet-and-sour dressing harmonizes with the flavors.

    2/3 cup uncooked wild rice

Dressing

    2 tablespoons fresh lemon juice

    2 tablespoons plain rice vinegar

    1 tablespoon light brown sugar

    1 tablespoon toasted sesame seeds

    1 tablespoon Chinese plum sauce

    1/2 teaspoon grated lemon zest

■ ■ ■

(continued)

4 cups shredded napa cabbage (12 to 16 ounces)

4 medium asparagus spears, trimmed and cooked

8 cherry tomatoes (yellow preferred)

1/2 medium cucumber, thinly sliced

1/2 medium red bell pepper, thinly sliced

1/2 medium red onion, thinly sliced

6 ounces grilled flank steak (warm or chilled), as from Grilled Lemongrass Flank Steak (page 249), thinly sliced diagonally across the grain, or 6 ounces grilled flank steak (warm or chilled), all visible fat discarded

Prepare the rice using the package directions, omitting the salt and margarine. Transfer to a large bowl. Cover and refrigerate until chilled.

In a medium bowl, whisk together the dressing ingredients until the sugar is dissolved.

Spread the cabbage on a platter. Mound the rice in the center of the cabbage. Decoratively arrange the asparagus, tomatoes, cucumber, bell pepper, and onion on the cabbage. Lay the beef slices on the rice. Drizzle the dressing over all.

PER SERVING

calories 271	carbohydrates 33 g
total fat 6.0 g	fiber 4 g
saturated fat 2.0 g	sugars 9 g
trans fat 0.0 g	protein 21 g
polyunsaturated fat 1.0 g	DIETARY EXCHANGES
monounsaturated fat 2.5 g	2 starch, 1 vegetable,
cholesterol 30 mg	2 lean meat
sodium 68 mg	

CHICKEN SALAD WITH APPLE AND PINEAPPLE

SERVES 4

If you have extra cooked chicken, this is a simple dish to throw together quickly. A light curry-mayo dressing marries the sweet tart fruit flavors. Pair this salad with Roasted Carrot-Ginger Soup (page 39).

2 cups diced cooked skinless chicken breast, cooked without salt, all visible fat discarded

2 medium apples, diced

1 cup pineapple chunks, canned in their own juice, drained

1/4 cup chopped almonds

3 tablespoons light mayonnaise

3/4 teaspoon curry powder

In a large bowl, toss together all the ingredients. Serve on salad greens.

PER SERVING

calories 255	sodium 153 mg
total fat 9.5 g	carbohydrates 20 g
saturated fat 1.5 g	fiber 4 g
trans fat 0.0 g	sugars 14 g
polyunsaturated fat 3.5 g	protein 24 g
monounsaturated fat 4.0 g	DIETARY EXCHANGES
cholesterol 63 mg	1 1/2 fruit, 3 lean meat

LAYERED TACO SALAD WITH TORTILLA CHIPS

SERVES 4

Taco salad—served in a fried tortilla shell—is a staple in many Mexican restaurants, but it's often loaded with saturated fat and salt. Try this version to keep it healthy without sacrificing any of the familiar flavors.

1 teaspoon canola or corn oil

8 ounces extra-lean ground beef

3/4 teaspoon ground cumin

8 ounces romaine, shredded

1/2 15.5-ounce can no-salt-added kidney beans, rinsed and drained

1/2 medium green bell pepper, thinly sliced lengthwise and cut into 2-inch pieces

1/2 cup fat-free sour cream

1/3 cup medium or hot picante sauce (lowest sodium available)

1 cup grape tomatoes, quartered

1 1/2 ounces shredded low-fat sharp Cheddar cheese

1/4 cup chopped fresh cilantro

2 ounces baked unsalted tortilla chips, slightly crushed

In a large nonstick skillet, heat the oil over medium-high heat, swirling to coat the bottom. Cook the beef for 4 to 5 minutes, or until browned on the outside and no longer pink in the center, stirring occasionally to turn and break up the beef. Remove the skillet from the heat.

Stir in the cumin. Spoon the beef mixture in a thin layer onto a large plate and let cool, about 8 minutes.

Meanwhile, spread the romaine in an 11 x 7 x 2-inch glass baking dish. Sprinkle with the beans and bell pepper.

In a small bowl, whisk together the sour cream and picante sauce. Spoon over the salad.

Sprinkle the beef mixture over the salad. If not serving immediately, cover and refrigerate for up to 2 hours. Just before serving, top with the remaining ingredients.

Cook's Tip: For a change, use no-salt-added black beans instead of kidney beans and substitute salsa verde (lowest sodium available) for the picante sauce. Or use one of the salsas in this book, such as Salsa Cruda (page 437) or Tomatillo-Cilantro Salsa with Lime (page 438).

PER SERVING

calories 266	carbohydrates 33 g
total fat 5.5 g	fiber 5 g
saturated fat 1.5 g	sugars 7 g
trans fat 0.0 g	**protein** 23 g
polyunsaturated fat 0.5 g	**DIETARY EXCHANGES**
monounsaturated fat 2.0 g	2 starch, 1 vegetable,
cholesterol 38 mg	2 1/2 lean meat
sodium 236 mg	

SOUTHWESTERN PORK SALAD

SERVES 6

This salad is particularly delicious if you use the Cuban Black Beans *recipe in this book instead of the canned variety. Serve with* Roasted Corn Soup *(page 40).*

2 cups cubed cooked pork tenderloin, cooked without salt, all visible fat discarded
1 cup Cuban Black Beans (page 332) or canned no-salt-added black beans, rinsed and drained if canned
4 medium green onions, finely chopped

1/2 medium green or red bell pepper, chopped
1 small garlic clove, minced
Dressing
1/4 cup chopped fresh parsley
1/4 cup cider vinegar
2 tablespoons canola or corn oil
1 1/2 tablespoons sugar
2 teaspoons olive oil (extra-virgin preferred)
1/2 teaspoon dried oregano, crumbled
1/2 teaspoon dry mustard

■ ■ ■

3 cups salad greens
1 cup cherry tomatoes, quartered
6 medium black olives, chopped
1 medium orange, cut into 6 slices (optional)
18 green grapes (optional)

In a large bowl, stir together the pork, beans, green onions, bell pepper, and garlic.

In a small bowl, whisk together the dressing ingredients until the sugar is dissolved. Pour over the pork mixture, tossing to coat. Cover and refrigerate for at least 30 minutes, stirring occasionally.

Just before serving, spread the salad greens on plates. Gently stir the tomatoes and olives into the pork mixture. Spoon over the greens. Garnish with the orange slices and grapes.

PER SERVING

calories 202	carbohydrates 15 g
total fat 8.5 g	fiber 4 g
saturated fat 1.0 g	sugars 7 g
trans fat 0.0 g	**protein** 16 g
polyunsaturated fat 2.0 g	**DIETARY EXCHANGES**
monounsaturated fat 5.0 g	1/2 starch, 1 vegetable,
cholesterol 35 mg	2 lean meat
sodium 71 mg	

WARM ORZO SALAD WITH BLACK BEANS AND HAM

SERVES 4

Bright yellow pasta swirled with color from bell peppers and punctuated with black beans—this curry-like salad is as beautiful as it is flavorful.

1 cup dried whole-grain orzo or pastina

2 teaspoons olive oil and 2 teaspoons olive oil, divided use

1 medium onion, diced

1 medium garlic clove, minced

2 large red or yellow bell peppers or a combination, diced

1/2 cup dry white wine (regular or nonalcoholic)

1/2 to 1 cup frozen whole-kernel corn, thawed

2 tablespoons red wine vinegar

1 teaspoon ground cumin

1/2 teaspoon ground turmeric

1/8 to 1/4 teaspoon crushed red pepper flakes

1 15.5-ounce can no-salt-added black beans, rinsed and drained

4 ounces lower-sodium, low-fat ham, all visible fat discarded, minced (about 1 cup)

Prepare the orzo using the package directions, omitting the salt. Drain well in a colander. Set aside.

Meanwhile, in a large nonstick skillet, heat 2 teaspoons oil over medium-high heat, swirling to coat the bottom. Cook the onion and garlic for 3 minutes, stirring occasionally.

Reduce the heat to medium. Stir in the bell peppers. Cook for 2 to 3 minutes.

Pour in the wine. Cook for 5 minutes, or until the peppers are very soft and most of the wine has evaporated.

Stir in the corn. Cook for 2 minutes, or just until heated through. Remove from the heat.

In a large bowl, whisk together the vinegar, cumin, turmeric, red pepper flakes, and the remaining 2 teaspoons oil.

Stir in the beans, ham, onion mixture, and orzo. Serve warm or at room temperature.

PER SERVING

calories 405	carbohydrates 64 g
total fat 7.0 g	fiber 12 g
saturated fat 1.0 g	sugars 12 g
trans fat 0.0 g	**protein** 18 g
polyunsaturated fat 1.0 g	**DIETARY EXCHANGES**
monounsaturated fat 4.0 g	4 starch, 1 vegetable,
cholesterol 12 mg	1 lean meat
sodium 244 mg	

CHEF'S SALAD

SERVES 4

A traditional chef's salad is chock full of cheese, meats, egg, and garden vegetables placed over iceberg lettuce and tossed with a high-calorie dressing. This version provides all the same variety and flavor, but with healthier ingredients. Enjoy with a cup of soup, such as Creamy Basil-Tomato Soup (page 43).

8 cups mixed salad greens, torn

1 cup chopped cucumber

1 medium carrot, sliced crosswise into rounds

8 tomato slices

2 large hard-boiled eggs, peeled and cut into slices

1 cup sliced medium green onions

3 ounces fat-free Cheddar cheese, cut into thin strips

3 ounces low-fat Swiss cheese, cut into thin strips

3 ounces lower-sodium, low-fat ham, all visible fat discarded, cut into thin strips

1/2 medium avocado, diced

Dressing

1/4 cup plus 2 tablespoons balsamic vinegar

2 tablespoons olive oil (extra-virgin preferred)

1 medium garlic clove, minced

1/2 teaspoon Dijon mustard (lowest sodium available)

Arrange the salad greens on salad plates. Scatter the cucumber and carrot over the greens. Top with the tomato and egg slices. Sprinkle with the green onions.

Arrange the cheese and ham strips on the salads. Sprinkle with the avocado.

In a small bowl, whisk together the dressing ingredients. Pour the dressing over the salad or serve it on the side.

EIGHT-LAYER SALAD

SERVES 4

A creamy, slightly sweet dressing coats layers of different colors and textures in this refreshing entrée salad that will appeal to even the choosy ones in the family.

Dressing
- 3 tablespoons light mayonnaise
- 3 tablespoons fat-free sour cream
- 2 tablespoons sugar
- 2 tablespoons water
- 1 1/2 tablespoons fresh lemon juice
- 1 teaspoon yellow mustard (lowest sodium available)

Salad
- 4 ounces mustard greens or baby kale, massaged
- 2 cups bite-size pieces torn romaine
- 1 medium carrot, peeled into thin ribbons
- 1/2 medium cucumber, chopped
- 1 medium tomato, chopped
- 3 medium radishes, thinly sliced
- 1 cup shredded or grated fat-free Cheddar cheese
- 1 cup green peas, thawed if frozen

In a small bowl, whisk together the dressing ingredients until the sugar is dissolved. Set aside.

In a glass trifle bowl or 11 x 7 x 2-inch glass baking dish, layer the salad ingredients in the order listed. Spoon the dressing over all. Serve immediately or cover and refrigerate for up to 4 hours.

Cook's Tip on Carrot Ribbons: Make thin strips of carrot (carrot ribbons) by running a vegetable peeler down the length of the carrot, letting the ribbons fall into a small bowl. Turn the carrot frequently as you work. Repeat until the carrot is too small to use.

DOUBLE SPINACH TORTELLINI SALAD

SERVES 6

If spinach is one of your favorite vegetables, then you're going to love this duet of spinach tortellini and chopped spinach. Serve it with Creamy Basil-Tomato Soup *(page 43).*

Salad
- 9 ounces fresh spinach-and-cheese tortellini
- 10 ounces frozen chopped spinach
- 1 medium zucchini, thinly sliced
- 1 medium yellow summer squash, thinly sliced
- 1 large carrot, thinly sliced
- 1 large yellow or red tomato, diced

Dressing
- 1/2 cup fat-free, low-sodium chicken broth, such as on page 36
- 1/3 cup white wine vinegar
- 1 tablespoon olive oil
- 2 teaspoons sugar
- 2 medium garlic cloves, minced
- 1 teaspoon dried oregano, crumbled
- 1 teaspoon dried basil, crumbled
- 1/4 teaspoon pepper

■ ■ ■

1/2 cup pine nuts, dry-roasted

(continued)

Prepare the tortellini using the package directions, omitting the salt. Drain well in a colander. Transfer to a large bowl. Let cool for 10 minutes.

Meanwhile, prepare the spinach using the package directions, omitting the salt and margarine. Drain well and squeeze dry.

Add the spinach and the remaining salad ingredients to the tortellini. Toss gently to combine.

In a small bowl, whisk together the dressing ingredients until the sugar is dissolved. Pour over the tortellini mixture, tossing gently to coat. Sprinkle with the pine nuts. Serve immediately.

Or, cover and refrigerate for up to three days. Sprinkle with the pine nuts just before serving.

PER SERVING

calories 213	carbohydrates 24 g
total fat 10.5 g	fiber 4 g
saturated fat 3.0 g	sugars 6 g
trans fat 0.0 g	protein 10 g
polyunsaturated fat 3.0 g	DIETARY EXCHANGES
monounsaturated fat 4.0 g	1 starch, 1 vegetable,
cholesterol 10 mg	1/2 lean meat, 1 1/2 fat
sodium 157 mg	

ITALIAN FARRO SALAD WITH ARTICHOKES

SERVES 6

Farro adds a delicious nutty flavor that matches well with the sweetness of the vegetables in this tasty salad.

Salad

 8 ounces uncooked pearled or semi-pearled farro (about 1 1/4 cups)
 9 ounces frozen artichoke hearts, thawed, patted dry, and halved lengthwise
 4 medium Italian plum (Roma) tomatoes, halved lengthwise and thinly sliced
 1 cup frozen green peas, thawed
 1/4 cup diced red onion

Dressing

 2 tablespoons shredded or grated Parmesan cheese
 2 tablespoons fresh lemon juice

 1 tablespoon chopped fresh basil or
  1 teaspoon dried basil, crumbled
 1 tablespoon olive oil (extra-virgin preferred)
 1 medium garlic clove, minced
 1/2 teaspoon sugar
 1/4 teaspoon salt
 1/8 teaspoon pepper

Prepare the farro using the package directions, omitting the salt. Transfer to a large bowl and let cool to room temperature. Fluff with a fork.

Gently stir in the remaining salad ingredients until the sugar is dissolved.

In a food processor or blender, process the dressing ingredients for about 20 seconds. Pour over the salad. Using a rubber scraper, stir gently. Cover and refrigerate for several hours.

Cook's Tip: If you can't find farro, use Arborio rice, which absorbs more flavor than other rice.

PER SERVING

calories 206	sodium 197 mg
total fat 3.0 g	carbohydrates 35 g
saturated fat 0.5 g	fiber 7 g
trans fat 0.0 g	sugars 3 g
polyunsaturated fat 0.5 g	protein 9 g
monounsaturated fat 2.0 g	DIETARY EXCHANGES
cholesterol 1 mg	2 starch, 1 vegetable

CURRIED FREEKEH SALAD WITH CRANBERRIES AND ALMONDS

SERVES 4

Freekeh (FREE-kah) is a wheat grain common to the Middle East that's harvested while still green, roasted over an open fire, then threshed and sundried. It has more protein than quinoa and twice the fiber. If you can't find it, you can always use quinoa instead.

 1 cup uncooked freekeh or quinoa, rinsed and drained
 2 tablespoons soy sauce (lowest sodium available)
 1 tablespoon cider vinegar
 1 tablespoon honey

1/2 teaspoon curry powder

1/4 teaspoon crushed red pepper flakes, or to taste

1 8-ounce can sliced water chestnuts, drained

1/2 medium green bell pepper, chopped

1 medium rib of celery, finely chopped

1/2 cup sweetened dried cranberries or dried mixed fruit

1/2 teaspoon grated orange zest

1 cup sliced almonds, dry-roasted

Prepare the freekeh using the package directions, omitting the salt. Remove from the heat and let cool. Fluff with a fork.

Meanwhile, in a small bowl, whisk together the soy sauce, vinegar, honey, curry powder, and red pepper flakes.

In a large bowl, stir together the remaining ingredients except the almonds.

Gently stir in the cooled freekeh, then the soy sauce mixture. Sprinkle with the almonds.

Time-Saver: A quick way to cool cooked freekeh, quinoa, and any other grain is to spread it in a thin layer on a baking sheet or large piece of aluminum foil on a cooling rack. Let it stand for 5 to 10 minutes.

PER SERVING

calories 321	carbohydrates 46 g
total fat 13.0 g	fiber 9 g
saturated fat 1.5 g	sugars 17 g
trans fat 0.0 g	protein 9 g
polyunsaturated fat 3.0 g	**DIETARY EXCHANGES**
monounsaturated fat 7.5 g	2 starch, 1 fruit, 1 lean
cholesterol 0 mg	meat, 1 1/2 fat
sodium 209 mg	

ARTICHOKE AND HEARTS OF PALM SALAD

SERVES 4

Here's a salad with lots of heart—tender hearts of artichoke and palm—gently tossed with fresh citrus juices and cilantro, sitting on a bed of whole grains. If you prefer, use only the artichokes or the hearts of palm and double the amount.

2 teaspoons olive oil and 2 teaspoons olive oil (extra-virgin preferred), divided use

1 large shallot, minced

3 cups water

3/4 cup uncooked pearled or semi-pearled farro, rinsed and drained

1/4 teaspoon pepper (freshly ground preferred)

9 ounces frozen artichoke hearts, thawed and drained

1/2 14-ounce can hearts of palm, rinsed, drained, and cut into 1/2-inch pieces

1/2 cup thinly sliced red onion

1/2 cup chopped red bell pepper

1/4 cup chopped fresh cilantro

1/4 cup fresh orange juice

2 tablespoons fresh lime juice

1 1/2 tablespoons sugar

1 tablespoon fresh lemon juice

1/8 teaspoon crushed red pepper flakes

In a medium saucepan, heat 2 teaspoons oil over medium-high heat, swirling to coat the bottom. Cook the shallot for 1 to 2 minutes, stirring constantly. Pour in the water. Increase the heat to high and bring to a boil. Stir in the farro. Reduce the heat and simmer for 15 minutes, or until the farro is tender. Drain well in a fine-mesh sieve. Transfer the farro mixture to a large bowl. Fluff with a fork. Stir in the pepper. Set aside to cool.

Meanwhile, in a medium bowl, stir together the remaining ingredients including the remaining 2 teaspoons oil, tossing gently to coat.

Transfer the farro to a large serving platter. Spoon the artichoke mixture onto the farro.

PER SERVING

calories 250	carbohydrates 42 g
total fat 5.0 g	fiber 8 g
saturated fat 0.5 g	sugars 8 g
trans fat 0.0 g	protein 8 g
polyunsaturated fat 0.5 g	**DIETARY EXCHANGES**
monounsaturated fat 3.5 g	2 vegetable,
cholesterol 0 mg	2 carbohydrate, 1/2 fat
sodium 233 mg	

CURRIED RICE AND BEAN SALAD

SERVES 6

Make this your Meatless Monday entrée, accompanied by Easy Refrigerator Rolls (page 458) and fresh tomato and cucumber slices.

1 cup uncooked brown rice

Dressing
- 1/4 cup light mayonnaise
- 1/4 cup fat-free plain yogurt
- 2 teaspoons curry powder
- Pepper to taste

■ ■ ■

- 1 15.5-ounce can no-salt-added kidney beans, rinsed and drained
- 2 medium ribs of celery, diced
- 4 medium green onions, chopped
- 1/2 medium green bell pepper, diced
- 1/4 cup chopped fresh parsley

Prepare the rice using the package directions, omitting the salt and margarine. Let cool.

Meanwhile, in a small bowl, whisk together the dressing ingredients.

In a large bowl, stir together the rice, beans, celery, green onions, bell pepper, and parsley. Pour the dressing over the salad, stirring to coat.

PER SERVING

calories 219	carbohydrates 40 g
total fat 3.5 g	fiber 5 g
saturated fat 0.5 g	sugars 3 g
trans fat 0.0 g	**protein** 8 g
polyunsaturated fat 2.0 g	DIETARY EXCHANGES
monounsaturated fat 1.0 g	2 1/2 starch, 1/2 lean
cholesterol 4 mg	meat
sodium 116 mg	

BARLEY AND ASPARAGUS SALAD WITH FETA CHEESE

SERVES 4

Barley, a whole grain, combines well with vegetables in this vegetarian entrée. Enjoy with Greek Egg and Lemon Soup (Avgolemono) (page 35).

- 2 cups water
- 1/2 cup uncooked quick-cooking barley
- 4 ounces asparagus spears, trimmed and cut into 2-inch pieces
- 2 ounces spring greens, coarsely chopped
- 2 tablespoons cider vinegar
- 1 tablespoon capers, drained
- 1 tablespoon olive oil (extra-virgin preferred)
- 2 teaspoons dried basil, crumbled
- 1/2 teaspoon dried rosemary, crushed
- 1 cup grape tomatoes, quartered
- 4 ounces fat-free feta cheese, crumbled

In a medium saucepan, bring the water to a boil over high heat. Stir in the barley. Reduce the heat and simmer, covered, for 8 minutes.

Stir in the asparagus. Cook for 2 minutes. Drain the barley mixture in a colander. Rinse with cold water until cool. Drain well.

Meanwhile, in a medium bowl, toss together the spring greens, vinegar, capers, oil, basil, and rosemary.

Add the tomatoes, feta, and barley mixture, tossing gently.

Cook's Tip: Try using a rubber scraper to toss ingredients. It will keep them from bruising.

PER SERVING

calories 175	carbohydrates 27 g
total fat 4.0 g	fiber 6 g
saturated fat 0.5 g	sugars 4 g
trans fat 0.0 g	**protein** 10 g
polyunsaturated fat 0.5 g	DIETARY EXCHANGES
monounsaturated fat 2.5 g	1 1/2 starch,
cholesterol 0 mg	1 vegetable, 1 lean
sodium 522 mg	meat

COUSCOUS SALAD

SERVES 4

Couscous rehydrates so quickly that it makes this lemony entrée salad come together without much of a wait.

- 3/4 cup uncooked whole-wheat couscous
- 1 cup shredded fat-free mozzarella cheese
- 1 cup diced tomatoes

1/2 cup finely chopped fresh parsley

12 kalamata olives, finely chopped

1 teaspoon grated lemon zest

2 tablespoons fresh lemon juice

1/2 medium garlic clove, minced

1/4 teaspoon crushed red pepper flakes

1/8 teaspoon salt

2 cups coarsely chopped baby spinach

Prepare the couscous using the package directions. Fluff with a fork. Spread the couscous in a thin layer on a baking sheet or large piece of aluminum foil on a cooling rack. Let stand for 5 to 10 minutes, or until cooled.

Meanwhile, in a large bowl, stir together the remaining ingredients except the spinach. Add the couscous, tossing gently. Add the spinach, tossing gently.

PER SERVING

calories 253	carbohydrates 41 g
total fat 4.0 g	fiber 7 g
saturated fat 0.5 g	sugars 2 g
trans fat 0.0 g	protein 16 g
polyunsaturated fat 0.5 g	**DIETARY EXCHANGES**
monounsaturated fat 2.5 g	2 1/2 starch,
cholesterol 5 mg	1 vegetable, 1 1/2 lean
sodium 482 mg	meat

ZESTY TOMATO DRESSING

SERVES 10; 2 TABLESPOONS PER SERVING

Fresh lemon juice and red wine vinegar make this Italian-inspired dressing a good choice over fresh spinach or romaine leaves.

1 cup no-salt-added tomato juice

2 medium green onions, thinly sliced

2 tablespoons fresh lemon juice

2 tablespoons red wine vinegar

1 teaspoon dried parsley, crumbled

1 teaspoon sugar

1/2 teaspoon dried oregano, crumbled

1/2 teaspoon dry mustard

1/2 teaspoon soy sauce (lowest sodium available)

1/4 teaspoon pepper

In a medium glass bowl, whisk together the ingredients until the sugar is dissolved. Cover and refrigerate for up to three days.

Cook's Tip: A standard serving of salad dressing is 2 tablespoons.

PER SERVING

calories 10	sodium 10 mg
total fat 0.0 g	carbohydrates 2 g
saturated fat 0.0 g	fiber 0 g
trans fat 0.0 g	sugars 2 g
polyunsaturated fat 0.0 g	protein 0 g
monounsaturated fat 0.0 g	**DIETARY EXCHANGES**
cholesterol 0 mg	free

POPPY SEED DRESSING WITH KIWIFRUIT

SERVES 8; 2 TABLESPOONS PER SERVING

Serve this delicately sweet dressing over a crisp lettuce and jicama salad, seasonal fresh fruit, or fat-free frozen vanilla or strawberry yogurt.

3/4 cup 100% pineapple juice

1 tablespoon cornstarch

2 medium kiwifruit, peeled and coarsely diced

2 tablespoons honey

1 tablespoon fresh lime juice

1 teaspoon poppy seeds

In a small saucepan, whisk together the pineapple juice and cornstarch. Bring to a boil over medium-high heat, whisking occasionally. Reduce the heat and simmer for 3 to 4 minutes, or until the mixture thickens, whisking occasionally. Spoon into a small bowl. Let cool at room temperature for 5 minutes. Cover and refrigerate until chilled, or at least 15 minutes.

In a food processor or blender, process the pineapple juice mixture, kiwifruit, honey, and lime juice until smooth. Pour into a glass bowl or jar.

Stir in the poppy seeds. Cover and refrigerate for up to five days.

Cook's Tip on Kiwifruit: Choose kiwifruit that yields to gentle pressure (it shouldn't be soft or mushy). If the kiwifruit is extremely firm, let it

(continued)

stand on the counter for a few days to ripen. Although the fuzzy skin is almost always removed, it is edible, as are the tiny black seeds.

PER SERVING

calories 45	carbohydrates 11 g
total fat 0.0 g	fiber 1 g
saturated fat 0.0 g	sugars 8 g
trans fat 0.0 g	protein 0 g
polyunsaturated fat 0.0 g	**DIETARY EXCHANGES**
monounsaturated fat 0.0 g	1/2 fruit, 1/2 other
cholesterol 0 mg	carbohydrate
sodium 2 mg	

CHUNKY CUCUMBER AND GARLIC DRESSING

SERVES 6; 2 TABLESPOONS PER SERVING

Be as cool as a cucumber on a hot summer day and serve this dressing on your favorite salad or on a grilled chicken, pork, or beef pita sandwich. It even makes a tasty dip when served with fresh veggies or whole-grain pita wedges.

> 1/2 cup fat-free plain yogurt
> 1/2 medium cucumber, peeled, seeded, and chopped
> 1 tablespoon sugar
> 1 tablespoon canola or corn oil
> 1/2 teaspoon dried minced onion
> 1/4 teaspoon garlic powder
> 1/4 teaspoon pepper
> 1 tablespoon red wine vinegar

In a small glass bowl, whisk the yogurt until smooth.

Whisk in the remaining ingredients except the vinegar.

Gradually whisk in the vinegar until combined. Cover and refrigerate the dressing for at least 4 hours.

PER SERVING

calories 43	sodium 16 mg
total fat 2.5 g	carbohydrates 4 g
saturated fat 0.0 g	fiber 0 g
trans fat 0.0 g	sugars 4 g
polyunsaturated fat 0.5 g	protein 1 g
monounsaturated fat 1.5 g	**DIETARY EXCHANGES**
cholesterol 0 mg	1/2 fat

LEMON DRESSING

SERVES 8; 2 TABLESPOONS PER SERVING

Tangy and flavorful, this dressing is a rousing accompaniment for spinach salads and other fresh vegetables, such as asparagus and green beans.

> 1/2 cup fresh lemon juice (about 2 large lemons)
> 2 tablespoons water
> 1 tablespoon chopped fresh parsley
> 1 tablespoon chopped fresh oregano
> 1 tablespoon olive oil (extra-virgin preferred)
> 1 tablespoon honey
> 1 tablespoon Dijon mustard (lowest sodium available)
> 2 medium garlic cloves, minced
> 1/2 teaspoon fennel seeds, crushed

In a small glass bowl, whisk together all the ingredients. Cover and refrigerate for up to three days.

Cook's Tip on Fennel: Known primarily as an Italian spice and herb, fennel has a delicate anise flavor. The two main kinds of fennel both have feathery fronds and celery-like stems. Garden, or common, fennel produces the fennel seed that's used as a spice. Fennel seeds resemble caraway seeds and are usually ground before they're used. Florence fennel, or finocchio, is prized for the thickened leaf stalks that form a bulb at the base. The bulb and stems of both kinds can be used as a vegetable, raw or cooked, much as celery is used. The fronds can be chopped and used for flavoring. Add them to cooked dishes at the last minute so the flavor doesn't dissipate.

PER SERVING

calories 31	sodium 39 mg
total fat 2.0 g	carbohydrates 4 g
saturated fat 0.0 g	fiber 0 g
trans fat 0.0 g	sugars 3 g
polyunsaturated fat 0.0 g	protein 0 g
monounsaturated fat 1.0 g	**DIETARY EXCHANGES**
cholesterol 0 mg	1/2 fat

Special Section: Slow-Cooker Recipes

SLOW-COOKER CHICKEN NOODLE SOUP

SERVES 4

There's nothing better than enjoying a steaming bowl of chicken noodle soup when the weather is rainy and cool or you've had a rough day at work. Full of hearty, tender root vegetables and melt-in-your-mouth chicken, this slow-cooked soup is a bowl of comfort.

2 small parsnips, sliced

1 medium onion, coarsely chopped

1 medium carrot, sliced

1 1/4 pounds bone-in chicken thighs, skin and all visible fat discarded

1 leek (white and light green parts), sliced

3 large garlic cloves, finely chopped

2 sprigs of fresh thyme or 1/2 teaspoon dried thyme, crumbled

1/4 teaspoon pepper

4 cups fat-free, low-sodium chicken broth, such as on page 36

■ ■ ■

2 ounces dried whole-grain egg noodles

1/4 cup chopped fresh parsley

In a 3- to 4 1/2-quart round or oval slow cooker, layer, in order, the parsnips, onion, carrot, chicken, leek, garlic, sprigs of thyme, and pepper. Pour in the broth. Cook, covered, on low for 8 to 10 hours or on high for 4 to 5 hours, or until chicken is no longer pink in the center and the parsnips and carrot are tender.

Quickly transfer the chicken to a cutting board.

Stir the noodles and parsley into the broth mixture. Re-cover the slow cooker. If using the low setting, change it to high. Cook, covered for 15 minutes, or until the pasta is tender.

Meanwhile, using one or two forks, shred the chicken. When the pasta is tender, stir the chicken into the broth mixture. Discard the sprigs of thyme before serving the soup.

PER SERVING

calories 229

total fat 6.0 g

   saturated fat 2.0 g

   trans fat 0.0 g

   polyunsaturated fat 1.0 g

   monounsaturated fat 2.0 g

cholesterol 90 mg

sodium 112 mg

carbohydrates 24 g

   fiber 5 g

   sugars 7 g

protein 20 g

DIETARY EXCHANGES

   1 starch, 2 vegetable,

   2 1/2 lean meat

SLOW-COOKER CHICKEN SOUP WITH MATZO BALLS

SERVES 4

1/4 cup matzo meal

1 large egg

1 tablespoon canola or corn oil

1 tablespoon seltzer water, sparkling water, club soda, or tonic water

1/4 teaspoon baking powder

Follow the directions for Slow-Cooker Chicken Noodle Soup, eliminating the noodles and parsley.

In a small bowl, stir together all the ingredients until smooth. Cover and refrigerate the mixture for 30 minutes.

About 45 minutes before the soup is finished cooking, in a large saucepan, bring 4 cups of water to a gentle boil over medium-high heat. With wet hands, roll the matzo mixture between your palms into twelve 1-inch balls. Transfer to a large plate. When the water is just boiling, gently slide the balls into the water. Reduce the heat and simmer, covered, for 30 minutes, or until almost doubled in size and slightly firm to the touch. Transfer the matzo balls to the soup.

Cook's Tip: For even more flavorful matzo balls, cook them in 3 cups fat-free, low-sodium chicken broth, such as on page 36.

PER SERVING

calories 288
total fat 11.0 g
  saturated fat 2.0 g
  trans fat 0.0 g
  polyunsaturated fat 2.0 g
  monounsaturated fat 5.0 g
cholesterol 136 mg
sodium 150 mg

carbohydrates 26 g
  fiber 5 g
  sugars 7 g
protein 22 g
DIETARY EXCHANGES
  1 starch, 2 vegetable,
  2 1/2 lean meat, 1/2 fat

PER SERVING

calories 212
total fat 2.5 g
  saturated fat 0.5 g
  trans fat 0.0 g
  polyunsaturated fat 1.0 g
  monounsaturated fat 1.0 g
cholesterol 50 mg

sodium 84 mg
carbohydrates 28 g
  fiber 2 g
  sugars 2 g
protein 19 g
DIETARY EXCHANGES
  2 starch, 2 lean meat

TURKEY AND RICE SOUP

SERVES 6

This slow-cooker soup gives you twice the rice— wild and brown—and is a good way to use leftover holiday turkey. Enjoy it with Cranberry Bread *(page 455).*

- 2 cups chopped cooked turkey breast, cooked without salt (about 8 ounces), all visible fat discarded
- 1 cup chopped butternut squash or carrots
- 1 cup sliced button mushrooms
- 1 medium rib of celery, sliced
- 1/2 cup uncooked wild rice
- 1 1/2 teaspoons dried savory, crumbled; or
  - 1 teaspoon dried thyme, crumbled, and
  - 1/2 teaspoon dried sage
- 1/2 teaspoon pepper
- 4 cups water
- 2 cups fat-free, low-sodium chicken broth, such as on page 36
- 1 cup uncooked instant brown rice
- 1/4 cup plus 2 tablespoons fat-free sour cream

In a 3- to 4 1/2-quart round or oval slow cooker, stir together the turkey, squash, mushrooms, celery, wild rice, savory, and pepper. Stir in the water and broth. Cook, covered, on low for 6 to 7 hours or on high for 3 to 4 hours, or until the squash and wild rice are tender.

If using the low setting, change it to high. Stir in the brown rice. Cook for 30 minutes, or until the brown rice is tender. Stir a dollop of sour cream into each serving.

ITALIAN WEDDING SOUP

SERVES 4

This comforting soup starts with homemade turkey meatballs spiked with the sweet flavor of fennel, a common seasoning in Italian sausage. As it gently simmers in the slow cooker, the broth becomes infused with the flavors of the vegetables. Parmesan-Herb Breadsticks *(page 451) complete your Italian feast.*

- 1/2 cup fat-free milk
- 4 slices whole-grain French bread (lowest sodium available), torn into pieces
- 1 pound ground skinless turkey breast
- 1 teaspoon fennel seeds, crushed
- 1 teaspoon dried basil, crumbled
- 1 teaspoon onion powder
- 1 teaspoon garlic powder
- 1/4 teaspoon pepper
- 4 cups fat-free, low-sodium chicken broth, such as on page 36
- 1 medium onion, cut into 3/4-inch pieces
- 2 medium ribs of celery, cut into 1/2-inch slices
- 2 medium garlic cloves, minced
- 1 teaspoon dried oregano, crumbled
- 1/2 teaspoon smoked paprika

■ ■ ■

- 4 cups coarsely chopped Swiss chard, tough stems discarded
- 2 ounces dried whole-grain pastina or other small pasta
- 2 ounces shredded or grated Parmesan cheese (about 1/2 cup)

(continued)

Pour the milk into a medium bowl. Place the pieces of bread in the milk. Let stand for 5 minutes, or until the bread has absorbed the milk.

Add the turkey, fennel seeds, basil, onion powder, garlic powder, and pepper. Using your hands or a spoon, combine the ingredients until well blended. Using 1 level tablespoon of the turkey mixture for each, shape into 16 meatballs, each about 3/4 inch in diameter. Transfer the meatballs to a 3- to 4 1/2-quart round or oval slow cooker. Pour in the broth.

Gently stir in the onion, celery, garlic, oregano, and paprika. Cook, covered, on low for 5 to 7 hours or on high for 2 1/2 to 3 1/2 hours, gently stirring once or twice.

Stir in the Swiss chard. Cook, covered, on low for 1 hour or on high for 30 minutes, or until the meatballs are no longer pink in the center.

When the soup is almost done, prepare the pasta using the package directions, omitting the salt.

Spoon the pasta into serving bowls. Ladle the soup over the pasta. Sprinkle with the Parmesan.

PER SERVING

calories 359	carbohydrates 32 g
total fat 6.5 g	fiber 6 g
saturated fat 3.0 g	sugars 7 g
trans fat 0.0 g	**protein** 42 g
polyunsaturated fat 1.0 g	**DIETARY EXCHANGES**
monounsaturated fat 2.0 g	1 1/2 starch,
cholesterol 88 g	1 vegetable, 5 lean
sodium 538 mg	meat

SLOW-COOKED POSOLE VERDE WITH PORK

SERVES 5

Posole *is the Spanish word for hominy, and those corn kernels are the main ingredient in this rich and flavorful Mexican stew. It can be prepared* rojo *(red—with tomatoes) or* verde *(green—with tomatillos), as in this version. Serve it with an array of traditional garnishes, such as diced onion, shredded Cotija cheese, sliced fresh jalapeño, diced avocado,*

or chopped fresh cilantro. Warm corn tortillas are a perfect accompaniment so you can better enjoy the delicious broth.

   Cooking spray
   1 tablespoon olive oil and 1 teaspoon oil, divided use
   1 pound boneless pork chops, all visible fat discarded, cut into 1-inch cubes
   3 large onions, chopped
   6 medium garlic cloves, minced
   1 small fresh jalapeño, halved, seeds and ribs discarded (optional; see Cook's Tip on Handling Hot Chiles, page 24)
   1 1/2 teaspoons ground cumin
   1 teaspoon oregano, crumbled (Mexican oregano preferred)
   1/4 teaspoon pepper (freshly ground preferred)
   1 pound medium tomatillos, papery husks and stems discarded, coarsely chopped (about 4 cups)
   1/2 cup water (as needed)
   4 cups fat-free, low sodium chicken broth, such as on page 36, or fat-free, low-sodium vegetable broth, such as on page 36
   Juice of 1 medium lime and 1 medium lime, cut into 8 wedges, divided use
   3 1/2 cups cooked hominy or 2 15-ounce cans hominy, rinsed and drained

Lightly spray a 5- to 7-quart round or oval slow cooker with cooking spray. Set aside.

In a large nonstick skillet, heat the 1 tablespoon oil over medium-high heat, swirling to coat the bottom. Cook the pork for 5 minutes, or until browned on all sides, stirring occasionally. Spoon into the slow cooker.

In the same skillet, still over medium-high heat, heat the remaining 1 teaspoon oil, swirling to coat the bottom. Cook the onions for 3 to 5 minutes, or until soft, stirring frequently. Stir in the garlic, jalapeño, cumin, oregano, and pepper. Cook for 1 to 2 minutes, or until fragrant, stirring constantly. Remove from the heat.

In a large bowl, stir together the onion mixture and tomatillos until well blended. Spoon half this mixture into a food processor or blender, adding the water to the work bowl as needed. Process until finely chopped (but don't purée until smooth). Transfer the mixture to the slow cooker. Repeat with the remaining half of the mixture.

Stir the broth and lime juice into the pork mixture in the slow cooker. Cook, covered, on low for 4 hours.

Quickly stir in the hominy and re-cover the slow cooker. Cook for 30 minutes, or until the hominy is tender and the pork is no longer pink in the center.

Cook's Tip on Dried Hominy: Dried hominy has a better texture and is lower in sodium than canned hominy. It's important to follow the package directions when cooking dried hominy because these directions vary by brand. For best results, cook the hominy until just tender and al dente (has some bite).

Cook's Tip on Tomatillos: Tomatillos look like small green tomatoes and have a parchment-like outer covering, which should be discarded. Their taste has notes of lemon, apple, and herb. You can find tomatillos in your grocery store's produce department or at Hispanic markets. They can be eaten raw but are more commonly cooked.

PER SERVING

calories 363	carbohydrates 47 g
total fat 8.5 g	fiber 5 g
saturated fat 2.0 g	sugars 11 g
trans fat 0.0 g	protein 27 g
polyunsaturated fat 1.0 g	DIETARY EXCHANGES
monounsaturated fat 4.5 g	2 starch, 3 vegetable,
cholesterol 53 mg	3 lean meat
sodium 87 mg	

SLOW-COOKER DILLED CHICKEN WITH RICE, GREEN BEANS, AND CARROTS

SERVES 4

This slow-cooker dish is truly a one-pot meal—even the instant brown rice is added to the crock during the last half-hour of cooking.

> 2 medium carrots, chopped
> 1 cup frozen cut green beans
> 1 medium onion, chopped
> 1 medium rib of celery, sliced
> 1 1/2 teaspoons dried dillweed, crumbled
> 1/8 teaspoon cayenne or 1/4 teaspoon pepper
> 4 boneless, skinless chicken breast halves (about 4 ounces each), all visible fat discarded
> 1 10.75-ounce can low-fat condensed cream of chicken soup (lowest sodium available)
> 1 cup water
> 2 cups uncooked instant brown rice

In a 3- to 4 1/2-quart round or oval slow cooker, stir together the carrots, green beans, onion, celery, dillweed, and cayenne. Place the chicken on the vegetables.

In a small bowl, whisk together the soup and water. Pour over the chicken. Cook, covered, on low for 5 to 6 hours or on high for 2 1/2 to 3 hours, or until the chicken is no longer pink in the center and the carrots and green beans are tender.

If using the low setting, change it to high. Stir in the rice. Cook for 30 minutes, or until the rice is tender.

PER SERVING

calories 380	carbohydrates 49 g
total fat 6.0 g	fiber 5 g
saturated fat 1.5 g	sugars 6 g
trans fat 0.0 g	protein 30 g
polyunsaturated fat 1.5 g	DIETARY EXCHANGES
monounsaturated fat 2.0 g	2 1/2 starch,
cholesterol 76 mg	2 vegetable, 3 lean
sodium 509 mg	meat

SLOW-COOKER CIOPPINO

SERVES 4

Often made with shellfish and the catch of the day, cioppino (chuh-PEE-no) originated in San Francisco and lends itself to just about any combination of your favorite seafood. San Franciscans usually eat it with crusty sourdough bread (but try to use whole-grain sourdough, if you can find it).

2 cups fat-free, low-sodium chicken broth, such as on page 36
1 14.5-ounce can no-salt-added diced tomatoes, undrained
2 medium potatoes, peeled and cut into 3/4-inch cubes
1/2 medium onion, cut into 3/4-inch cubes
1/2 medium yellow or green bell pepper, cut into 3/4-inch squares
1/2 cup 1 x 1/2-inch carrot sticks
1 large rib of celery, cut into 1/2-inch slices
2 medium garlic cloves, minced
1 teaspoon olive oil
1/2 teaspoon dried basil, crumbled
1/2 teaspoon dried oregano, crumbled
1/2 teaspoon fennel seeds, crushed (optional)
1/8 teaspoon salt
1/4 teaspoon pepper
1/4 teaspoon crushed red pepper flakes (optional)
8 ounces fish fillets, such as cod, red snapper, halibut, or a combination, rinsed, patted dry, and cut into 1-inch cubes
8 ounces raw medium shrimp, peeled, rinsed, and patted dry
2 tablespoons chopped fresh parsley

In a 3- to 4 1/2-quart round or oval slow cooker, stir together the broth, tomatoes with liquid, potatoes, onion, bell pepper, carrots, celery, garlic, oil, basil, oregano, fennel seeds, salt, pepper, and red pepper flakes. Cook, covered, on low for 7 to 9 hours or on high for 3 to 4 hours, or until the vegetables are tender. About 10 minutes before the end of the cooking time if using high or 20 minutes before if using low, stir in the fish, shrimp, and parsley.

PER SERVING

calories 217
total fat 2.5 g
  saturated fat 0.5 g
  trans fat 0.0 g
  polyunsaturated fat 0.5 g
  monounsaturated fat 1.0 g
cholesterol 114 mg
sodium 589 mg

carbohydrates 24 g
  fiber 4 g
  sugars 7 g
protein 25 g
DIETARY EXCHANGES
  1 starch, 2 vegetable,
  3 lean meat

SLOW-COOKER THYME-GARLIC CHICKEN WITH COUSCOUS

SERVES 4

A fresh spinach and tomato couscous mixture is the bed for citrusy chicken breasts that are cooked low and slow.

1 teaspoon dried thyme, crumbled
1/4 teaspoon salt
4 boneless, skinless chicken breast halves (about 4 ounces each), all visible fat discarded
1 teaspoon grated orange zest
1/2 cup fresh orange juice
1 tablespoon balsamic vinegar
4 medium garlic cloves, minced
1 cup uncooked whole-wheat couscous
2 cups shredded spinach, stems discarded (about 2 ounces)
1 medium tomato, seeded and chopped

Sprinkle the thyme and salt over both sides of the chicken. Transfer to a 3- to 4 1/2-quart round or oval slow cooker.

In a small bowl, stir together the orange zest, orange juice, vinegar, and garlic. Pour over the chicken. Cook, covered, on low for 4 to 5 hours or on high for 2 to 2 1/2 hours, or until the chicken is no longer pink in the center.

About 10 minutes before the chicken is finished cooking, prepare the couscous using the package directions, omitting the salt and oil.

Add the spinach and tomato to the couscous, stirring until the spinach is wilted. Serve the chicken over the couscous. If desired, spoon a little of the cooking liquid on top.

Cook's Tip on Couscous: If your supermarket doesn't have whole-wheat couscous, look in the ethnic food sections or bulk food bins of natural food supermarkets. Almost all couscous takes only about 5 minutes to prepare; avoid any brand that calls for long steaming.

PER SERVING

calories 372	carbohydrates 52 g
total fat 4.0 g	fiber 8 g
saturated fat 1.0 g	sugars 4 g
trans fat 0.0 g	protein 33 g
polyunsaturated fat 1.0 g	DIETARY EXCHANGES
monounsaturated fat 1.0 g	3 1/2 starch, 3 lean
cholesterol 73 mg	meat
sodium 292 mg	

CHICKEN SOFRITO

SERVES 4

Sofrito is one of the foundations of Caribbean cooking. It's a sauce consisting of tomatoes, onions, peppers, garlic, and herbs. This slow-cooker version eliminates the need to make the sauce ahead of time. Traditionally, it's served over rice.

1 cup chopped onion

1/2 cup coarsely chopped green bell pepper

1/2 cup coarsely chopped red bell pepper

3 large garlic cloves, chopped

4 bone-in chicken thighs, skin and all visible fat discarded (about 1 1/4 pounds)

1 14.5-ounce can no-salt-added diced tomatoes, undrained

1/8 teaspoon cayenne

■ ■ ■

1/3 cup chopped fresh cilantro

3 tablespoons coarsely chopped pitted green olives, drained

1 tablespoon fresh lemon juice

In a 3- to 4 1/2-quart round or oval slow cooker, layer the onion, both bell peppers, and garlic. Place the chicken on the vegetables. Top with the tomatoes with liquid. Sprinkle the cayenne over all. Cook, covered, on low for 8 to 9 hours or on high for 4 to 4 1/2 hours, or until the chicken is no longer pink in the center and the bell peppers are tender.

Stir in the cilantro, olives, and lemon juice. Using a slotted spatula, transfer the chicken to plates. Spoon the vegetable mixture over the chicken.

Cook's Tip: For a more stewlike consistency, quickly transfer the chicken thighs to a cutting board at the end of the cooking time. Remove and discard the bones and cut the chicken into pieces. Stir the chicken pieces into the vegetable mixture with the cilantro, olives, and lemon juice.

PER SERVING

calories 207	carbohydrates 12 g
total fat 8.0 g	fiber 2 g
saturated fat 2.0 g	sugars 6 g
trans fat 0.0 g	protein 21 g
polyunsaturated fat 1.5 g	DIETARY EXCHANGES
monounsaturated fat 3.5 g	2 vegetable, 3 lean
cholesterol 110 mg	meat
sodium 280 mg	

SLOW-COOKED CHICKEN ITALIAN STYLE

SERVES 4

Your home will be filled with the comforting aromas of an Italian kitchen when you prepare this meal. Fennel seed gives a hint of Italian sausage in this dish without the extra sodium or saturated fat.

4 skinless chicken breast halves with bone (about 6 ounces each), all visible fat discarded

1 14.5-ounce can no-salt-added diced tomatoes, undrained

9 ounces frozen artichoke hearts, thawed and drained

1 8-ounce can no-salt-added tomato sauce

2 tablespoons sliced green olives (not stuffed with pimiento), rinsed and drained

1 teaspoon dried oregano, crumbled

1/2 teaspoon fennel seed

1/4 teaspoon pepper

(continued)

8 ounces sliced brown (cremini) mushrooms
2 cups frozen green beans, thawed

Put the chicken in a 3- to 4 1/2-quart round or oval slow cooker.

Stir in the tomatoes with liquid, artichoke hearts, tomato sauce, olives, oregano, fennel seed, and pepper. Cook, covered, on low for 7 hours or on high for 3 hours, or until the chicken is no longer pink in the center.

Stir in the mushrooms. Place the green beans on top; don't stir (this will help keep the tomatoes' acid from changing the color of the green beans). Cook, covered, on low for 2 hours or on high for 1 hour, or until the mushrooms are soft and the green beans are cooked through. Stir before serving.

PER SERVING

calories 269	carbohydrates 21 g
total fat 4.5 g	fiber 9 g
saturated fat 1.0 g	sugars 9 g
trans fat 0.0 g	**protein** 35 g
polyunsaturated fat 1.0 g	**DIETARY EXCHANGES**
monounsaturated fat 1.5 g	4 vegetable, 4 lean
cholesterol 87 mg	meat
sodium 376 mg	

SLOW-COOKER WHITE CHILI

SERVES 6

You can easily stretch this low-and-slow cooking dish to serve more people by ladling it over brown rice or bulgur. Tortilla Pinwheels *(page 17) or* Jalapeño Poppers *(page 24) make great starters.*

Chili
1 pound dried navy or great northern beans, sorted for stones and shriveled beans, rinsed and drained
1 pound skinless chicken thighs with bone, all visible fat discarded
6 cups fat-free, low-sodium chicken broth, such as on page 36
2 4-ounce cans chopped green chiles, drained

1 medium onion, chopped
4 medium garlic cloves, minced
1 medium fresh jalapeño, seeds and ribs discarded, minced (see Cook's Tip on Handling Hot Chiles, page 24)
2 teaspoons ground cumin
2 teaspoons dried oregano, crumbled
1/4 teaspoon cayenne
1/8 to 1/4 teaspoon ground cloves

■ ■ ■

1/4 cup plus 2 tablespoons salsa (lowest sodium available), such as Salsa Cruda (page 437)
1/4 cup plus 2 tablespoons fat-free sour cream

In the order listed, put the chili ingredients in a 3- to 4 1/2-quart round or oval slow cooker. Don't stir. Cook, covered, on high for 10 hours, or until the beans and chicken are tender.

Transfer the chicken to a cutting board. Discard the bones. Separate the chicken into bite-size pieces. Stir the chicken into the chili. Just before serving, dollop with the salsa and sour cream.

PER SERVING

calories 388	carbohydrates 55 g
total fat 5.5 g	fiber 20 g
saturated fat 1.5 g	sugars 7 g
trans fat 0.0 g	**protein** 31 g
polyunsaturated fat 1.5 g	**DIETARY EXCHANGES**
monounsaturated fat 1.5 g	3 1/2 starch,
cholesterol 41 mg	1 vegetable, 3 lean
sodium 279 mg	meat

SLOW-COOKER BRISKET STEW

SERVES 4

Slow cooking creates this succulent meat and veggie bowl of goodness. Serve as is or over egg noodles or Twice-Baked Potatoes *(page 398) to soak up all the juices.*

2 medium carrots, cut into 1-inch pieces
1 medium onion, cut into 1/2-inch wedges
1 medium green bell pepper, cut into 1-inch squares

1 medium rib of celery, cut into 1-inch pieces

1 1-pound flat-cut beef brisket, all visible fat discarded

1/4 cup dry sherry or dry red wine (regular or nonalcoholic)

1 packet (1 teaspoon) salt-free instant beef bouillon

1 teaspoon dried oregano, crumbled

2 tablespoons no-salt-added tomato paste

1 tablespoon sugar

1 tablespoon cider vinegar

2 teaspoons Worcestershire sauce (lowest sodium available)

1/2 teaspoon salt

1/4 teaspoon dried basil, crumbled

Put the carrots, onion, bell pepper, and celery in a 3- to 4 1/2-quart round or oval slow cooker. Place the roast on top. Pour in the sherry and sprinkle the bouillon and oregano over all.

Cook, covered, on high for 6 hours, or until the beef is tender when tested with a fork. Transfer the roast to a cutting board, leaving the carrot mixture in the slow cooker. Let the roast stand for 10 minutes before slicing.

In a small bowl, whisk together the remaining ingredients until the sugar is dissolved. Stir into the carrot mixture. Return the sliced roast to the slow cooker to heat for 5 minutes.

Cook's Tip: Purchase a brisket that weighs about 2 1/2 pounds. After you trim all the fat, the roast should weigh about 2 pounds. Cut it in half and freeze one piece to use later.

PER SERVING

calories 214	carbohydrates 15 g
total fat 4.5 g	fiber 3 g
saturated fat 1.5 g	sugars 10 g
trans fat 0.0 g	**protein** 26 g
polyunsaturated fat 0.5 g	**DIETARY EXCHANGES**
monounsaturated fat 2.0 g	2 vegetable, 3 lean
cholesterol 74 mg	meat
sodium 429 mg	

SHREDDED BEEF SOFT TACOS

SERVES 8

Let your slow cooker work on dinner while you're at your job or running errands. Then give your family a Mexican feast of sirloin, onions, and bell peppers with cumin, all wrapped in warm tortillas. Serve with plenty of napkins!

1 1/2 pounds boneless top sirloin steak or sirloin tip roast, all visible fat discarded

3 large onions, chopped

1 medium green bell pepper, chopped

1/2 cup no-salt-added ketchup

1/4 cup dry red wine (regular or nonalcoholic)

2 tablespoons cider vinegar

6 medium garlic cloves, minced

2 packets (2 teaspoons) salt-free instant beef bouillon

2 medium dried bay leaves

3/4 teaspoon liquid smoke

1/2 teaspoon ground cumin and 1/2 teaspoon ground cumin, divided use

1/2 teaspoon red hot-pepper sauce

1/4 teaspoon pepper

1 teaspoon sugar (dark brown preferred)

8 8-inch whole-wheat tortillas (lowest sodium available)

4 medium Italian plum (Roma) tomatoes, chopped

6 cups shredded romaine

1/2 cup fat-free sour cream

Put the beef in a 3- to 4 1/2-quart round or oval slow cooker. Add the onions and bell pepper.

In a medium bowl, whisk together the ketchup, wine, vinegar, garlic, bouillon, bay leaves, liquid smoke, 1/2 teaspoon cumin, the hot-pepper sauce, and pepper. Pour into the slow cooker.

Cook, covered, on low for 9 hours, or until the beef is tender. Transfer the beef to a cutting board. Discard the bay leaves.

Using two forks, shred the beef. Return to the slow cooker to stand (the heat should be off).

(continued)

Stir in the sugar and the remaining 1/2 teaspoon cumin until the sugar is dissolved. Let stand, covered, for 1 hour so the flavors blend.

Warm the tortillas using the package directions.

Spoon the beef mixture down the center of each tortilla. Top with the tomatoes, romaine, and sour cream.

PER SERVING

calories 335	fiber 6 g
total fat 5.5 g	sugars 15 g
saturated fat 1.5 g	**protein** 26 g
trans fat 0.0 g	**DIETARY EXCHANGES**
polyunsaturated fat 1.5 g	2 starch, 2 vegetable,
monounsaturated fat 2.5 g	1/2 other
cholesterol 48 mg	carbohydrate, 3 lean
sodium 419 mg	meat
carbohydrates 44 g	

SLOW-COOKER ROUND STEAK WITH MUSHROOMS AND TOMATOES

SERVES 4

Browning the steak strips in olive oil before placing them in the slow cooker adds a more robust flavor to the final dish.

> Cooking spray
> 1 teaspoon garlic powder
> 1/4 teaspoon cayenne
> 1/8 teaspoon pepper
> 1 pound boneless top round steak, all visible fat discarded, cut into 2 x 1-inch strips
> 1 tablespoon olive oil
> 1 14.5-ounce can no-salt-added stewed tomatoes, undrained
> 8 ounces button mushrooms, sliced
> 1/2 medium sweet onion, such as Vidalia, Maui, or Oso Sweet, chopped
> 1 medium green or red bell pepper, chopped
> 1/4 cup water and 2 tablespoons cold water, divided use
> 1/4 cup picante sauce (lowest sodium available)
> 2 tablespoons vinegar
> 1 tablespoon Worcestershire sauce (lowest sodium available)
> 1 tablespoon chopped fresh parsley
> 2 teaspoons dried oregano, crumbled
> 3 medium garlic cloves, minced
> 1 1/2 teaspoons light brown sugar
> 1 tablespoon cornstarch
> 3 ounces dried whole-grain fettuccine
> 1/4 cup chopped green onions (optional)

Lightly spray a 3- to 4 1/2-quart round or oval slow cooker with cooking spray.

In a small bowl, stir together the garlic powder, cayenne, and pepper. Sprinkle over the top of the beef.

In a large nonstick skillet, heat the oil over medium-high heat, swirling to coat the bottom. Cook the beef for 5 to 7 minutes, or until browned, stirring frequently. Transfer to the slow cooker.

In a large bowl, stir together the tomatoes with liquid, mushrooms, onion, bell pepper, 1/4 cup water, the picante sauce, vinegar, Worcestershire sauce, parsley, oregano, garlic, and brown sugar. Stir into the beef mixture. Cook, covered, on low for 6 to 7 hours, or until the beef is tender. (If you're in a hurry, you can cook the mixture on high for 3 hours to 3 hours 30 minutes, but the beef won't be quite as tender.)

Put the cornstarch in a small bowl. Add the remaining 2 tablespoons water, whisking to dissolve. Stir into the beef mixture. Cook, covered, on high for 10 to 15 minutes, or until slightly thickened.

Meanwhile, prepare the pasta using the package directions, omitting the salt. Drain well in a colander. Serve topped with the beef mixture and green onions.

Cook's Tip on Slow Cookers: Lifting the lid of a slow cooker to take a quick peek increases the time needed to finish cooking the dish. Because most slow-cooker recipes don't require stirring, taking that peek usually isn't necessary.

calories 327	**carbohydrates** 34 g
total fat 7.0 g	fiber 6 g
saturated fat 1.5 g	sugars 11 g
trans fat 0.0 g	**protein** 32 g
polyunsaturated fat 1.0 g	**DIETARY EXCHANGES**
monounsaturated fat 4.0 g	1 1/2 starch,
cholesterol 58 mg	2 vegetable, 3 lean
sodium 172 mg	meat

BEEF STEW

SERVES 4

This dish cooked low and slow gets high marks for flavor. Browning the meat caramelizes it, providing an even deeper richness. Serve with Yogurt Dinner Rolls (page 459) to soak up all the stew's goodness.

    2 teaspoons canola or corn oil
    1 pound boneless sirloin steak, all visible fat
        discarded, cut into 1-inch cubes
    4 medium carrots, chopped
    2 medium potatoes, cut into eighths
    2 medium tomatoes, chopped
    1 cup chopped onion
    1/2 cup water
    1/2 cup diced celery
    1 cup dark beer (regular or nonalcoholic)
    1/4 cup chopped fresh parsley
    2 medium garlic cloves, minced
    1/2 teaspoon pepper (freshly ground
        preferred)
    1/4 teaspoon salt
    1/4 teaspoon smoked paprika
    1/2 teaspoon ground cardamom

■ ■ ■

    2 tablespoons all-purpose flour
    2 tablespoons cold water

In a large nonstick skillet, heat the oil over medium-high heat, swirling to coat the bottom. Cook the beef for 5 minutes, or until browned on all sides, stirring frequently. Transfer the beef and any accumulated juices to a 3- to 4 1/2-quart round or oval slow cooker.

Stir in the carrots, potatoes, tomatoes, onion, water, celery, beer, parsley, garlic, pepper, salt,

paprika, and cardamom. Cook, covered, on low for 8 to 10 hours or on high for 5 to 6 hours, or until the beef and vegetables are tender.

Put the flour in a small bowl. Add the water, whisking to dissolve. Quickly uncover the slow cooker and stir in the flour mixture. Re-cover the slow cooker. If using the low setting, change it to high. Cook for about 10 minutes, or until the stew has slightly thickened.

calories 343	**carbohydrates** 39 g
total fat 5.5 g	fiber 5 g
saturated fat 1.5 g	sugars 8 g
trans fat 0.0 g	**protein** 30 g
polyunsaturated fat 1.0 g	**DIETARY EXCHANGES**
monounsaturated fat 3.0 g	1 1/2 starch,
cholesterol 58 mg	3 vegetable, 3 lean
sodium 437 mg	meat

SLOW-COOKER CHILI

SERVES 6

This classic is perfect for the slow cooker. It's served over spaghetti—just like the Cincinnati version.

    Cooking spray
Chili
    1 pound extra-lean ground beef
    1 cup chopped onion
    1 medium green bell pepper, chopped
    3 large garlic cloves, minced
    1 15.5-ounce can no-salt-added kidney beans,
        rinsed and drained
    1 14.5-ounce can no-salt-added diced
        tomatoes, undrained
    1 8-ounce can no-salt-added tomato sauce
    2 to 3 tablespoons chili powder
    2 tablespoons water
    1 teaspoon sugar (optional)
    1/2 teaspoon dried basil, crumbled
    1/2 teaspoon pepper
    1/4 teaspoon salt

■ ■ ■

    6 ounces dried whole-grain spaghetti
    2 tablespoons shredded or grated Parmesan
        cheese

(continued)

Lightly spray a large, heavy skillet and a 3- to 4 1/2-quart round or oval slow cooker with cooking spray.

In the skillet, cook the beef over medium-high heat for 8 to 10 minutes, or until no longer pink, stirring occasionally to turn and break up the beef. Using a slotted spoon, transfer the beef to the slow cooker.

Wipe the skillet with paper towels. Lightly spray with cooking spray. Cook the onion and bell pepper over medium-high heat for 3 minutes, or until the onion is soft, stirring frequently.

Stir in the garlic. Cook for 30 seconds, stirring frequently.

Stir the remaining chili ingredients and onion mixture into the beef. Cook, covered, on low for 8 to 10 hours or on high for 4 to 5 hours.

Shortly before serving time, prepare the spaghetti using the package directions, omitting the salt. Drain well in a colander. Serve topped with the chili and Parmesan.

Cook's Tip: To prep the chili up to a day in advance, combine all the chili ingredients in the slow cooker as directed, but don't cook. Remove the insert from the slow cooker, cover, and refrigerate. When you are ready to cook the chili, place the insert in the slow cooker (the slow cooker should be off). Proceed as directed.

PER SERVING

calories 323	carbohydrates 44 g
total fat 5.5 g	fiber 9 g
saturated fat 2.0 g	sugars 8 g
trans fat 0.0 g	**protein** 27 g
polyunsaturated fat 1.0 g	**DIETARY EXCHANGES**
monounsaturated fat 2.0 g	2 starch, 3 vegetable,
cholesterol 43 mg	3 lean meat
sodium 255 mg	

SLOW-COOKER PORK ROAST WITH ORANGE CRANBERRY SAUCE

SERVES 8

This fork-tender pork roast features a savory, slightly tart sauce. You can enjoy it any time of year, but it'll be especially popular during the summer, because you don't need to heat up the kitchen.

Cooking spray
1 2-pound boneless pork loin roast, all visible fat discarded
1 14-ounce can whole-berry cranberry sauce
2 teaspoons grated orange zest
1 cup fresh orange juice
1/2 cup water
2 medium shallots, coarsely chopped
2 tablespoons cider vinegar
1 tablespoon fresh rosemary, coarsely chopped, or 1 teaspoon dried rosemary, crushed
1/4 teaspoon pepper

Lightly spray a 3- to 4 1/2-quart round or oval slow cooker with cooking spray. Put the remaining ingredients in the slow cooker. Cook, covered, on low for 8 to 10 hours or on high for 4 to 5 hours, or until the pork is tender and registers 145°F on an instant-read thermometer.

Transfer the pork to a cutting board, reserving the sauce. Let stand for 3 minutes before slicing.

Spoon the sauce over the pork slices or serve it on the side.

Cook's Tip: If you have leftover pork, try chopping some and combining it with whole-wheat pasta and broccoli with the sauce spooned on top. Or add a small amount of Dijon mustard (lowest sodium available) to the sauce and use it as a dipping sauce for a sandwich of pork slices on whole-grain bread or buns (lowest sodium available).

PER SERVING

calories 206	**carbohydrates** 23 g
total fat 3.0 g	fiber 1 g
saturated fat 1.0 g	sugars 15 g
trans fat 0.0 g	**protein** 22 g
polyunsaturated fat 0.5 g	**DIETARY EXCHANGES**
monounsaturated fat 1.0 g	1 1/2 other
cholesterol 60 mg	carbohydrate, 3 lean
sodium 59 mg	meat

HARVEST PORK STEW

SERVES 4

This stew combines subtle spices and mild pork tenderloin with the sweetness of apples and sweet potatoes. While the meal slow cooks, prepare a dark green, leafy salad as a side dish and Pumpkin Custards *(page 497) for dessert.*

1 pound pork tenderloin, all visible fat discarded, cut into 1-inch cubes

2 teaspoons ground ginger

1/4 teaspoon salt

1/4 teaspoon cayenne

Cooking spray

3 medium garlic cloves, finely chopped

1 tablespoon cider vinegar

3/4 pound sweet potatoes, peeled and cut into 1-inch cubes

2 medium unpeeled Granny Smith apples, cut into 1-inch cubes

1 8-ounce red onion, halved lengthwise and cut crosswise into 1/2-inch slices

1 tablespoon cornstarch

1/2 teaspoon paprika

1/4 teaspoon ground nutmeg

1/2 cup 100% apple cider

1/2 cup fat-free, low-sodium chicken broth, such as on page 36

Put the pork in a medium bowl.

In a small bowl, stir together the ginger, salt, and cayenne. Sprinkle over the pork. Using your fingertips, gently press the mixture so it adheres to the pork.

Lightly spray a medium skillet with cooking spray. Cook the pork over medium-high heat for 3 to 5 minutes, or until browned on all sides, stirring frequently.

Lightly spray a 3- to 4 1/2-quart round or oval slow cooker with cooking spray. Transfer the pork to the slow cooker. Sprinkle the garlic over the pork. Using a spoon, press the garlic into the pork. Drizzle the vinegar over the pork, turning to coat.

Put the sweet potatoes, apples, and onion in the slow cooker. Using a large spoon or tongs, gently combine.

In a measuring cup (this works well for easy pouring), stir together the cornstarch, paprika, and nutmeg. Pour in the apple cider and broth, stirring until the cornstarch is dissolved. Pour into the slow cooker. Gently stir. Cook, covered, on low for 7 hours, or until the pork is tender. (The high setting isn't recommended for this recipe.)

Cook's Tip on Cider Vinegar: The cider vinegar helps tenderize the lean pork tenderloin.

PER SERVING

calories 300	**carbohydrates** 42 g
total fat 3.0 g	fiber 6 g
saturated fat 1.0 g	sugars 20 g
trans fat 0.0 g	**protein** 27 g
polyunsaturated fat 0.5 g	**DIETARY EXCHANGES**
monounsaturated fat 1.0 g	1 starch, 1 1/2 fruit,
cholesterol 74 mg	1 vegetable, 3 lean
sodium 263 mg	meat

SLOW-COOKER CHILE VERDE PORK CHOPS

SERVES 4

In this tangy take on a Mexican classic, tomatillos, lime, and fresh cilantro put the verde in this dish. Serve with Tex-Mex Cucumber Salad *(page 78) and* Mexican Fried Rice *(page 421).*

(continued)

1 teaspoon ground cumin

1/4 teaspoon salt

1/4 teaspoon pepper

4 boneless center-cut pork loin chops (about 4 ounces each), all visible fat discarded

2 teaspoons olive oil

1 pound tomatillos, papery husks discarded, chopped

1 medium onion, chopped

1 teaspoon grated lime zest

1 tablespoon fresh lime juice

4 medium garlic cloves, minced

2 tablespoons chopped fresh cilantro

In a small bowl, stir together the cumin, salt, and pepper. Sprinkle over the pork. Using your fingertips, gently press the mixture so it adheres to the pork.

In a large nonstick skillet, heat the oil over medium heat, swirling to coat the bottom. Cook the pork for 2 minutes on each side, or until lightly browned.

In a 3- to 4 1/2-quart round or oval slow cooker, stir together the remaining ingredients except the cilantro. Add the pork, spooning some sauce over it. Cook, covered, on low for 4 to 5 hours or on high for 2 to 3 hours, or until the tomatillos are tender and the pork is no longer pink on the outside. Transfer the pork to plates. Using a slotted spoon, spoon the tomatillo mixture on top. Sprinkle with the cilantro.

PER SERVING

calories 198	carbohydrates 11 g
total fat 8.5 g	fiber 3 g
saturated fat 2.0 g	sugars 7 g
trans fat 0.0 g	protein 20 g
polyunsaturated fat 1.5 g	DIETARY EXCHANGES
monounsaturated fat 3.5 g	2 vegetable, 3 lean
cholesterol 57 mg	meat
sodium 188 mg	

SLOW-COOKER CHICKPEA STEW

SERVES 6

Toasted cumin seeds impart a slightly smoky flavor to this hearty vegetarian stew. Fattoush Salad (page 70) makes an excellent starter while you wait for the stew to cook low and slow.

2 15.5-ounce cans no-salt-added chickpeas, rinsed and drained

1 14.5-ounce can no-salt-added diced tomatoes, undrained

8 ounces unpeeled red potatoes, coarsely chopped

1 medium zucchini, quartered lengthwise and sliced

1 medium onion, chopped

1 medium garlic clove, minced

1 teaspoon cumin seeds and 1 teaspoon cumin seeds, dry-roasted, divided use

1/2 teaspoon paprika

1/8 teaspoon cayenne or 1/4 teaspoon pepper

3 cups fat-free, low-sodium vegetable broth, such as on page 36, or water

In a 3- to 4 1/2-quart round or oval slow cooker, stir together the chickpeas, tomatoes with liquid, potatoes, zucchini, onion, garlic, 1 teaspoon cumin seeds, the paprika, and cayenne. Pour in the broth, stirring to combine. Cook, covered, on low for 8 to 9 hours or on high for 4 1/2 to 5 hours, or until the potatoes are tender. Sprinkle with the remaining 1 teaspoon cumin seeds.

Cook's Tip on Dry-Roasting Cumin Seeds: Add an extra dimension of flavor to cumin seeds by spreading them in a skillet and cooking them over medium heat for 2 to 3 minutes, or until they are toasted and aromatic, shaking the skillet occasionally. Transfer the seeds to a plate immediately so they don't burn.

PER SERVING

calories 208	carbohydrates 39 g
total fat 1.5 g	fiber 8 g
saturated fat 0.0 g	sugars 6 g
trans fat 0.0 g	protein 10 g
polyunsaturated fat 0.5 g	DIETARY EXCHANGES
monounsaturated fat 0.5 g	2 starch, 1 vegetable,
cholesterol 0 mg	1/2 lean meat
sodium 58 mg	

SOUTHERN-STYLE BLACK-EYED PEAS

SERVES 12 AS A SIDE DISH; SERVES 6 AS AN ENTRÉE

Seasoning the peas with lean ham instead of the traditional salt pork reduces the saturated fat and sodium. If you want to cook this dish faster, use the stovetop directions.

1 pound dried black-eyed peas, sorted for stones and shriveled peas, rinsed, and drained

5 to 7 cups water

4 ounces smoke-flavored lower-sodium, low-fat ham, all visible fat discarded, diced

1/2 medium onion, diced

1 medium carrot, thinly sliced

1 small fresh serrano pepper, seeds and ribs discarded, thinly sliced (optional; see Cook's Tip on Handling Hot Chiles, page 24)

SLOW-COOKER DIRECTIONS

Place the peas in a 3 to 4 1/2-quart round or oval slow cooker. Pour in 5 cups of water to cover. Stir in the remaining ingredients. Cook, covered, on low for 8 to 10 hours, or until the peas are tender.

STOVETOP DIRECTIONS

Place the peas in a large saucepan or Dutch oven. Pour in 7 cups of water to cover. Stir in the remaining ingredients. Bring to a boil over high heat. Skim off any foam.

Reduce the heat to medium low and simmer, covered, for 2 hours, or until the peas are tender.

PER SERVING (ENTRÉE)

calories 273	sodium 181 mg
total fat 2.0 g	carbohydrates 46 g
saturated fat 0.5 g	fiber 14 g
trans fat 0.0 g	sugars 9 g
polyunsaturated fat 0.5 g	protein 20 g
monounsaturated fat 0.5 g	DIETARY EXCHANGES
cholesterol 8 mg	4 1/2 starch, 2 lean meat

PER SERVING (SIDE DISH)

calories 136	carbohydrates 23 g
total fat 1.0 g	fiber 7 g
saturated fat 0.5 g	sugars 4 g
trans fat 0.0 g	protein 10 g
polyunsaturated fat 0.5 g	DIETARY EXCHANGES
monounsaturated fat 0.0 g	1 1/2 starch, 1 lean meat
cholesterol 4 mg	
sodium 91 mg	

SLOW-COOKER PUMPKIN OATMEAL

SERVES 8

Wake up and smell the oatmeal. This pumpkin-spiced cereal cooks while you sleep, so all you need to do is rise and shine, and then sprinkle it with walnuts.

Cooking spray

Oatmeal

2 cups uncooked oatmeal (steel-cut oats preferred)

1/3 cup light brown sugar

1 1/2 tablespoons ground cinnamon

3/4 teaspoon ground nutmeg

1 cup canned solid-pack pumpkin (not pie filling)

6 cups water

1 cup fat-free half-and-half

1 cup raisins

1 teaspoon vanilla extract

∎ ∎ ∎

1/4 cup plus 1 1/2 tablespoons chopped walnuts, dry-roasted

Lightly spray a 3- to 4 1/2-quart round or oval slow cooker with cooking spray.

In a large bowl, stir together the oatmeal, brown sugar, cinnamon, and nutmeg. Stir in the pumpkin. Gradually stir in the water and half-and-half. Stir in the raisins and vanilla.

(continued)

Ladle the mixture into the slow cooker. Cook, covered, on low for 7 1/2 to 8 1/2 hours. Just before serving, sprinkle with the walnuts.

Cook's Tip: Refrigerate any leftover oatmeal for up to three days. Put the desired amount in a microwaveable bowl. Microwave it, covered, on 100 percent power (high), adding a bit of fat-free milk as necessary for the desired consistency. (The chilled oatmeal will have thickened.)

Cook's Tip on Steel-Cut Oats: Steel-cut oats, also known as Irish oats or pinhead oats, are better than rolled oats for use in slow-cooker recipes because they can withstand the longer cooking time without getting mushy.

PER SERVING

calories 326	carbohydrates 61 g
total fat 6.5 g	fiber 11 g
saturated fat 0.5 g	sugars 25 g
trans fat 0.0 g	**protein** 10 g
polyunsaturated fat 3.5 g	**DIETARY EXCHANGES**
monounsaturated fat 1.5 g	2 starch, 1 fruit, 1 other
cholesterol 0 mg	carbohydrate, 1 fat
sodium 42 mg	

SMOKY PULLED PORK WITH BARBECUE SAUCE

SERVES 8

Slow cook this melt-in-your-mouth pork and enjoy it with a sweet smoky sauce. Serve with Southern-Style Greens *(page 391) and* Southern Raised Biscuits *(page 459).*

Rub

1 tablespoon paprika

1 tablespoon chili powder

1 tablespoon ground cumin

1 tablespoon garlic powder

1 tablespoon salt-free all-purpose seasoning blend

1 tablespoon brown sugar (light or dark)

1 tablespoon Worcestershire sauce (lowest sodium available)

1 teaspoon pepper (freshly ground preferred)

1 teaspoon dry mustard

1 teaspoon onion powder

1/4 teaspoon cayenne (optional)

∎ ∎ ∎

1 4-pound boneless pork loin roast, all visible fat discarded

6 large garlic cloves, slivered (optional)

Sauce

1 teaspoon olive oil

1 medium onion, chopped

2 medium garlic cloves, minced

1 8-ounce can no-salt-added tomato sauce

1 cup diet root beer

2 tablespoons no-salt-added tomato paste

2 tablespoons cider vinegar

2 teaspoons brown sugar (light or dark)

1 teaspoon chili powder

1 teaspoon dry mustard

1/4 teaspoon red hot-pepper sauce (optional)

1/4 teaspoon liquid smoke (optional)

∎ ∎ ∎

Cooking spray

3 large onions, thinly sliced

12 ounces diet root beer

In a small bowl, stir together the rub ingredients. Set aside.

Using the tip of a sharp paring knife, make 1-inch-deep slits that are evenly spaced all over the pork roast. Using your fingers, push the garlic slivers deep into the pork.

Sprinkle the rub all over the pork. Using your fingertips, gently press the mixture so it adheres to the pork. Place the pork in a shallow dish. Cover with plastic wrap and refrigerate for at least 1 hour, or up to 24 hours.

Lightly spray the inside of a 5- to 7-quart round or oval slow cooker with cooking spray. Spread half the sliced onions on the bottom. Remove the pork from the refrigerator. Transfer to the slow cooker, placing it on the bed of onions. Scatter the remaining sliced onions over the pork. Pour the root beer over the pork and onions.

Cook, covered, on low for about 7 hours. The pork should register 145°F on an instant-read thermometer and easily pull apart when tested with two forks. Carefully transfer the pork to a platter. Let stand for 3 minutes (if necessary, remove and discard any kitchen twine). Using two forks, pull and shred the pork, chopping up any large pieces.

Just about 20 minutes before the pork is finished cooking, in a medium saucepan, heat the oil over medium-high heat, swirling to coat the bottom. Cook the onion for 3 minutes, or until soft, stirring frequently. Stir in the garlic. Cook for 1 to 2 minutes, stirring constantly. Stir in the remaining sauce ingredients. Increase the heat to high and bring just to a boil, stirring frequently. Reduce the heat and simmer for 8 to 10 minutes, or until the desired thickness, stirring occasionally.

Return the shredded pork to the slow cooker. Stir to combine with the cooking liquid and onions. Serve with the warm sauce on the side or poured over the pork.

Cook's Tip: You can prepare and cook the sauce in advance. Cover and refrigerate it in an airtight container for up to three days.

PER SERVING

calories 371
total fat 10.0 g
   saturated fat 3.0 g
   trans fat 0.0 g
   polyunsaturated fat 1.5 g
   monounsaturated fat 4.0 g
cholesterol 134 mg
sodium 159 mg

carbohydrates 18 g
   fiber 4 g
   sugars 11 g
protein 51 g
DIETARY EXCHANGES
   2 vegetable. 1/2 other carbohydrate, 7 lean meat

Seafood

CURRIED FILLETS AMANDINE

SERVES 4

This fish takes next to no time at all to prepare and get on the table. Complement the curry flavor in this dish by serving it with Gingered Carrots (page 381).

1/4 cup all-purpose flour
2 teaspoons curry powder
Pepper to taste (freshly ground preferred)
4 fresh or frozen fish fillets, such as sole (about 4 ounces each), thawed if frozen, rinsed and patted dry
2 teaspoons light tub margarine
1/3 cup chopped slivered almonds, dry-roasted

In a small bowl, stir together the flour, curry powder, and pepper. Sprinkle over the fish. Using your fingertips, gently press the mixture so it adheres to the fish.

In a large skillet, melt the margarine over medium heat, swirling to coat the bottom. Cook the fish for about 6 minutes, turning once halfway through, or until it flakes easily when tested with a fork and is slightly browned. Transfer to a serving platter.

Spoon the almonds over the fish.

PER SERVING

calories 194	sodium 108 mg
total fat 7.0 g	carbohydrates 9 g
saturated fat 0.5 g	fiber 2 g
trans fat 0.0 g	sugars 0 g
polyunsaturated fat 1.5 g	protein 24 g
monounsaturated fat 3.5 g	DIETARY EXCHANGES
cholesterol 54 mg	1/2 starch, 3 lean meat

FILLETS IN LEMON DRESSING

SERVES 4

Citrus brightens up any fish, and an abundance of lemon plays a starring role in this dish. Tartness also complements many vegetables, so pair this entrée with Creamy Asparagus Soup (page 38) or Mediterranean Lima Beans (page 393).

Cooking spray

Dressing
2 teaspoons canola or corn oil
2 tablespoons grated onion
1 tablespoon finely chopped celery
4 slices whole-wheat toast (lowest sodium available), cut into 1/2-inch cubes
1 1/2 teaspoons grated lemon zest
Juice of 1 medium lemon
1 tablespoon chopped fresh parsley
Pepper to taste (freshly ground preferred)
Dash of ground nutmeg

■ ■ ■

4 firm white fish fillets (about 4 ounces each), rinsed and patted dry
1/2 teaspoon paprika

Preheat the oven to 375°F. Lightly spray an 8-inch square glass baking dish with cooking spray.

In a medium skillet, heat the oil over medium heat, swirling to coat the bottom. Cook the onion and celery for 3 minutes, or until the onion is almost soft, stirring occasionally. Stir in the remaining dressing ingredients. Cook for 3 minutes, or until heated through, stirring to combine.

Put 2 fish fillets in the baking dish. Spread all the dressing over the fish. Top with the remaining 2 fillets. Sprinkle the paprika over all.

Bake for 20 minutes, or until the fish flakes easily when tested with a fork.

PER SERVING

calories 189	sodium 176 mg
total fat 4.0 g	carbohydrates 13 g
saturated fat 0.5 g	fiber 2 g
trans fat 0.0 g	sugars 2 g
polyunsaturated fat 1.0 g	protein 24 g
monounsaturated fat 2.0 g	DIETARY EXCHANGES
cholesterol 49 mg	1 starch, 3 lean meat

GINGER-SOY FILLETS

SERVES 4

This lightly pan-seared fish is finished with a tangy, sweet, Asian-inflected sauce. Serve the fish on a bed of steamed spinach or over whole-grain pasta.

> 2 tablespoons all-purpose flour
> 4 firm white fish fillets (about 4 ounces each), rinsed and patted dry
> 1 tablespoon canola or corn oil
> 2 tablespoons sherry or fresh orange juice
> 1 teaspoon ground ginger
> 1 teaspoon soy sauce (lowest sodium available)
> 1/2 teaspoon sugar
> 1 medium garlic clove, minced
> 2 medium tomatoes, chopped
> 1 tablespoon chopped fresh parsley
> 2 teaspoons chopped chives or green onions (green part only)
> Pepper to taste (freshly ground preferred)

Put the flour in a shallow dish. Dip the fish in the flour, turning to coat and gently shaking off any excess. Transfer to a plate.

In a large, heavy skillet, heat the oil over medium-high heat, swirling to coat the bottom. Cook the fish for 4 minutes, or until slightly browned, turning once halfway through.

In a 1-cup measuring cup, whisk together the sherry, ginger, soy sauce, sugar, and garlic with enough water to make 1 cup. Pour over the fish. Cook, covered, for 6 minutes.

Sprinkle the remaining ingredients over the fish. Cook, uncovered, for 3 minutes, or until the fish flakes easily when tested with a fork.

PER SERVING

calories 161	**carbohydrates** 7 g
total fat 4.5 g	fiber 1 g
saturated fat 0.5 g	sugars 2 g
trans fat 0.0 g	**protein** 21 g
polyunsaturated fat 1.5 g	**DIETARY EXCHANGES**
monounsaturated fat 2.5 g	1/2 other
cholesterol 49 mg	carbohydrate, 3 lean
sodium 97 mg	meat

CRISPY BAKED FILLETS

SERVES 4

It's easy to get in your omega-3s with this shake-and-bake fish recipe; you can have it on the table within 15 minutes from start to finish. Whip up Tartar Sauce (page 428) and Confetti Coleslaw (page 84) to accompany this dish.

> Cooking spray
> 4 mild white fish fillets (about 4 ounces each) (about 1/2 inch thick), rinsed and patted dry
> Pepper to taste (freshly ground preferred)
> 2 tablespoons canola or corn oil
> 1/3 cup cornflake crumbs

Preheat the oven to 400°F. Lightly spray a large shallow baking dish with cooking spray.

Put the fish on a large plate. Sprinkle the pepper over the fish.

Put the oil in a large shallow dish. Pour the corn-flake crumbs into a separate large shallow dish. Arrange the plate, dishes, and the baking dish in a row, assembly-line fashion. Dip the fish in the oil, then in the crumbs, turning to coat at each step and gently shaking off any excess. Place the fish in the baking dish.

Bake for 5 minutes, or until the fish flakes easily when tested with a fork.

PER SERVING

calories 182	**sodium** 109 mg
total fat 8.0 g	**carbohydrates** 6 g
saturated fat 0.5 g	fiber 0 g
trans fat 0.0 g	sugars 1 g
polyunsaturated fat 2.0 g	**protein** 21 g
monounsaturated fat 4.5 g	**DIETARY EXCHANGES**
cholesterol 49 mg	1/2 starch, 3 lean meat

CRISPY FISH WITH FENNEL SEEDS

SERVES 4

This mild fish gets its licorice flavor from the fennel and its crispiness from whole-grain cereal. Serve with Roasted Brussels Sprouts *(page 378) or* Crunchy Broccoli Casserole *(page 376).*

1 cup all-purpose flour
2 large egg whites, lightly beaten using a fork
1 1/4 cups whole-grain wheat and barley
    nugget cereal
1 tablespoon dried fennel seeds
4 mild white fish fillets (about 4 ounces each)
    (about 1/2 inch thick), rinsed and patted
    dry
1 medium lemon, cut into 4 wedges

Preheat the oven to 400°F.

Put the flour in a medium shallow dish. Put the egg whites in a separate medium shallow dish. In a third medium shallow dish, stir together the cereal and fennel seeds. Set the dishes and a baking sheet in a row, assembly-line fashion.

Dip the fish in the flour, then in the egg whites, and finally in the cereal mixture, turning to coat at each step and gently shaking off any excess. Using your fingertips, gently press the coating so it adheres to the fish.

Transfer to the baking sheet. Bake for 5 minutes, or until the fish flakes easily when tested with a fork. Serve with the lemon wedges.

Cook's Tip for Baking Fish: As a good rule of thumb, let fish bake about 10 minutes per inch of thickness, measuring at its thickest point.

PER SERVING

calories 227	sodium 242 mg
total fat 1.5 g	carbohydrates 31 g
saturated fat 0.5 g	fiber 3 g
trans fat 0.0 g	sugars 3 g
polyunsaturated fat 0.5 g	protein 23 g
monounsaturated fat 0.5 g	**DIETARY EXCHANGES**
cholesterol 43 mg	2 starch, 3 lean meat

QUINOA-CRUSTED FISH WITH PLUM CHUTNEY

SERVES 4

A sweet-and-sour chutney harmonizes beautifully with mild halibut encrusted with the delicate crunch of toasted quinoa. Try this with steamed broccolini or sautéed spinach.

1 teaspoon grated orange zest
1/4 cup fresh orange juice
1/4 teaspoon salt
1/8 teaspoon pepper
4 halibut fillets (about 4 ounces each), rinsed
    and patted dry
1/2 cup uncooked quinoa (red preferred),
    rinsed and drained

Chutney
1 cup fat-free, low-sodium chicken broth, such
    as on page 36
1/3 cup chopped dried plums
1/2 cup fresh orange juice
2 tablespoons chopped red onion
2 tablespoons red wine vinegar
1 tablespoon light brown sugar
1 teaspoon grated peeled gingerroot

■ ■ ■

2 large egg whites, beaten until frothy

In a shallow dish, whisk together the orange zest, 1/4 cup orange juice, salt, and pepper. Add the fish, turning to coat. Cover and refrigerate for 30 minutes, turning once halfway through.

Preheat the oven to 300°F.

Prepare the quinoa using the package directions, omitting the salt. Transfer to a medium bowl. Fluff with a fork.

Spread the quinoa in an even layer on a large, rimmed, nonstick baking sheet or a large baking sheet lined with cooking parchment. Bake for 25 to 30 minutes, or until slightly toasted. Transfer the quinoa to a shallow dish, stirring to break up any large pieces. Wipe the baking sheet with paper towels.

(continued)

Meanwhile, in a small saucepan, stir together the chutney ingredients. Bring to a simmer over medium heat. Reduce the heat and simmer for 10 to 12 minutes, or until the plums are tender, stirring occasionally. Remove from the heat. Cover to keep warm. Set aside.

Increase the oven temperature to 400°F. Line the baking sheet with cooking parchment.

Pour the egg whites into a shallow bowl. Put the bowl, the dish with the quinoa, and the baking sheet in a row, assembly-line fashion. Dip the fish in the egg whites, then in the quinoa, turning to coat at each step and gently shaking off any excess. Place the fish on the baking sheet. Bake for 11 to 13 minutes, or until the fish flakes easily when tested with a fork.

Serve the fish with the chutney.

PER SERVING

calories 239	**carbohydrates** 27 g
total fat 3.0 g	fiber 2 g
saturated fat 0.5 g	sugars 11 g
trans fat 0.0 g	**protein** 26 g
polyunsaturated fat 1.0 g	**DIETARY EXCHANGES**
monounsaturated fat 1.0 g	1 starch, 1 fruit, 3 lean
cholesterol 56 mg	meat
sodium 239 mg	

FISH AND CHIPS

SERVES 4

Enjoy fish and chips without the guilt. The secret to these crisp yet tender baked chips (also known as french fries) is that they're double-cooked. The potatoes are first blanched in boiling water and then baked until golden brown. The fish is spread with a garlic-caper tartar sauce and sprinkled with panko for a light, crisp crust.

Cooking spray
2 russet potatoes (about 6 ounces each), peeled and cut lengthwise into 1/2-inch strips
1 teaspoon olive oil
1/4 teaspoon salt (coarse sea salt preferred)
1/4 teaspoon pepper
1/4 cup light mayonnaise
2 teaspoons small capers, drained

1 small garlic clove, minced
1 1-pound cod fillet, rinsed and patted dry, cut into 4 pieces
2 tablespoons whole-wheat panko (Japanese-style bread crumbs)

Preheat the oven to 425°F. Lightly spray a small rimmed baking sheet with cooking spray.

Fill a medium pot halfway with water. Bring to a boil over high heat. Boil the potatoes for 30 seconds to 1 minute, or until partially cooked. Transfer to paper towels to drain. Blot dry.

In a medium bowl, stir together the potatoes, oil, salt, and pepper. Arrange the potatoes in a single layer on the baking sheet. Roast for 18 to 20 minutes, or until lightly browned.

Meanwhile, in a small bowl, stir together the mayonnaise, capers, and garlic to make tartar sauce.

Line a separate small rimmed baking sheet with aluminum foil. Lightly spray the foil with cooking spray.

Arrange the fish on the foil. Spread the tartar sauce over each fillet. Sprinkle the panko over the tartar sauce. Lightly spray the fillets with cooking spray.

Roast the fish (along with the potatoes) for the final 10 minutes of roasting time, or until the fish flakes easily when tested with a fork and the potatoes are golden brown and tender when pierced with the tip of a sharp knife. Serve with the remaining tartar sauce.

Cook's Tip: For a traditional condiment of British origin, serve this entrée with malt vinegar.

PER SERVING

calories 203	**sodium** 387 mg
total fat 5.0 g	**carbohydrates** 18 g
saturated fat 1.0 g	fiber 2 g
trans fat 0.0 g	sugars 1 g
polyunsaturated fat 3.0 g	**protein** 20 g
monounsaturated fat 2.0 g	**DIETARY EXCHANGES**
cholesterol 48 mg	1 starch, 3 lean meat

SEARED FISH WITH ROSEMARY AÏOLI

SERVES 4

Aïoli (ay-OH-lee or I-OH-lee) *is basically may-onnaise with herbs and fresh garlic. The use of a particular herb is generally what makes the big difference. Rosemary is the choice for this assertive entrée!*

Aïoli
- 1/4 cup fat-free sour cream
- 2 tablespoons fat-free milk
- 2 tablespoons light mayonnaise
- 1 medium garlic clove, minced
- 1/4 teaspoon dried rosemary, crushed
- 1/4 teaspoon salt

■ ■ ■

- 1/2 teaspoon paprika
- 1/4 teaspoon pepper
- 1/8 teaspoon salt
- 4 mild fish fillets, such as tilapia (about 4 ounces each), rinsed and patted dry

In a small bowl, whisk together the aïoli ingredients.

In a separate small bowl, stir together the paprika, pepper, and the remaining 1/8 teaspoon salt. Sprinkle over both sides of the fish. Using your fingertips, gently press the mixture so it adheres to the fish.

Heat a large nonstick skillet over medium-high heat. Cook the fish for 3 minutes on each side, or until it flakes easily when tested with a fork. Serve with the aïoli.

PER SERVING

calories 147	sodium 358 mg
total fat 3.5 g	carbohydrates 4 g
saturated fat 1.0 g	fiber 0 g
trans fat 0.0 g	sugars 1 g
polyunsaturated fat 1.5 g	protein 24 g
monounsaturated fat 1.0 g	DIETARY EXCHANGES
cholesterol 62 mg	3 lean meat

FISH FILLETS WITH ZESTY ROSEMARY OIL

SERVES 4

Just a hint of cider vinegar is added to heighten the flavor impact of this already-tasty fish dish. The sauce is very intense, so a little goes a long way.

- 4 mild fish fillets, such as tilapia (about 4 ounces each), rinsed and patted dry
- 1 teaspoon grated lemon zest
- 1 tablespoon fresh lemon juice
- 1 tablespoon olive oil (extra-virgin preferred)
- 1/2 teaspoon cider vinegar
- 1/2 medium garlic clove, minced
- 1/4 teaspoon salt
- 1/8 teaspoon dried rosemary, crushed

Heat a large nonstick skillet over medium heat. Cook the fish for 3 minutes on each side, or until it flakes easily when tested with a fork.

Meanwhile, in a small bowl, whisk together the remaining ingredients. Drizzle the sauce over the fish.

PER SERVING

calories 141	sodium 205 mg
total fat 5.5 g	carbohydrates 1 g
saturated fat 1.0 g	fiber 0 g
trans fat 0.0 g	sugars 0 g
polyunsaturated fat 1.0 g	protein 23 g
monounsaturated fat 3.0 g	DIETARY EXCHANGES
cholesterol 57 mg	3 lean meat

FISH WITH ZESTY MERINGUE TOPPING

SERVES 4

High direct heat cooks the fish quickly and cara-melizes it for a rich flavor. While the broiler is still on, use it to cook Basil Roasted Peppers *(page 397).*

(continued)

Cooking spray

4 mild white fish fillets with skin (about
  5 ounces each), rinsed and patted dry

1 tablespoon light tub margarine, melted

1/2 teaspoon pepper (freshly ground
  preferred)

2 tablespoons tartar sauce, such as on
  page 428, or bottled tartar sauce
  (lowest sodium available)

2 tablespoons light mayonnaise

1 large egg white, beaten until stiff

Preheat the broiler. Lightly spray a shallow baking dish with cooking spray.

Put the fish with the skin side down in the baking dish. Brush the margarine over the fish. Sprinkle the pepper over the fish.

Broil about 4 inches from the heat for 10 minutes, or until the fish flakes easily when tested with a fork.

Meanwhile, gently fold the tartar sauce and mayonnaise into the egg white. When the fish is done, remove it from the oven. Spread the tartar sauce mixture over the fish. Broil for 2 minutes, or until the topping is golden brown.

PER SERVING

calories 149	sodium 201 mg
total fat 7.5 g	carbohydrates 1 g
saturated fat 1.0 g	fiber 0 g
trans fat 0.0 g	sugars 0 g
polyunsaturated fat 2.5 g	protein 19 g
monounsaturated fat 1.5 g	DIETARY EXCHANGES
cholesterol 48 mg	3 lean meat

WHITE FISH FILLETS WITH ASPARAGUS

SERVES 4

A rich topping elevates fish and veggies to a new level of goodness. Try with Lemon-Basil Rice *(page 420).*

Cooking spray

4 mild white fish fillets, such as catfish or
  cod (about 4 ounces each), rinsed and
  patted dry

1 tablespoon fresh lemon juice

1/2 teaspoon pepper

12 medium spears of asparagus, cooked

Topping

1/3 cup fat-free sour cream

1/3 cup fat-free plain yogurt

2 teaspoons minced green onions (green part
  only)

2 teaspoons bottled white horseradish,
  drained

1/2 teaspoon dried dillweed, crumbled

1 large egg white

■ ■ ■

2 tablespoons chopped fresh parsley

Preheat the broiler. Lightly spray a broiler pan and rack with cooking spray.

Place the fish on the broiler rack. Pour the lemon juice over the fish. Sprinkle the pepper over the fish. Lightly spray the top of the fish with cooking spray.

Broil about 6 inches from the heat for 4 minutes on each side, or until the fish almost flakes when tested with a fork. Remove from the broiler. Place 3 spears of asparagus on each fillet.

Meanwhile, in a small bowl, whisk together the topping ingredients except the egg white.

In a separate small bowl, beat the egg white until stiff peaks form (the peaks won't fall when the beaters are lifted). Fold into the topping mixture. Spread over each fillet to cover the fish and asparagus.

Broil about 6 inches from the heat for 1 to 2 minutes, or until the topping is golden brown.

Sprinkle with the parsley.

Cook's Tip on Beating Egg Whites: Even a single drop of egg yolk will prevent egg whites from forming peaks when beaten, so separate eggs very carefully. If you're using more than one egg, crack just one egg and drain the white into a small bowl. Pour the yolk into a separate bowl. Pour the white into the mixing bowl. Repeat with the remaining eggs. That way you won't spoil the entire bowl of whites if a yolk breaks. If you do get a speck of yolk in the white, you can blot the yolk up with the corner of a paper towel.

PER SERVING

calories 160	carbohydrates 9 g
total fat 3.5 g	fiber 2 g
saturated fat 1.0 g	sugars 5 g
trans fat 0.0 g	protein 23 g
polyunsaturated fat 1.0 g	DIETARY EXCHANGES
monounsaturated fat 1.0 g	1/2 other
cholesterol 70 mg	carbohydrate, 3 lean
sodium 108 mg	meat

GINGER BROILED FISH

SERVES 4

Fresh ginger and wine are a winning combination in this simple fish dish. Serve it on a bed of Asian Spinach and Mushrooms *(page 403).*

Cooking spray
1/2 cup dry white wine (regular or
    nonalcoholic)
1 medium green onion, chopped
1 1/2 teaspoons soy sauce (lowest sodium
    available)
1 teaspoon grated peeled gingerroot
1 teaspoon bottled white horseradish,
    drained
1 teaspoon canola or corn oil
4 halibut or other fish fillets or steaks (about
    4 ounces each), 3/4 inch thick, rinsed
    and patted dry

Preheat the broiler. Lightly spray a broilerproof baking dish with cooking spray.

In a small bowl, stir together the remaining ingredients except the fish.

Put the baking dish under the broiler for 1 to 2 minutes. Remove from the broiler.

Arrange the fish in a single layer in the preheated dish. Pour the wine mixture over the fish.

Broil the fish about 2 inches from the heat for 5 minutes on each side, or until the fish flakes easily when tested with a fork.

Cook's Tip on Gingerroot: You can find gingerroot in the produce section. Choose a root with smooth skin. To keep it from drying out, peel just as much as you need to grate, keeping a "handle" with the peel left on. Wrap leftover unpeeled gingerroot in a paper towel and refrigerate it in a resealable plastic bag for up to three weeks. For longer storage, wrap peeled gingerroot in aluminum foil and place it in a resealable plastic bag in the freezer for up to three months.

PER SERVING

calories 111	sodium 100 mg
total fat 2.0 g	carbohydrates 1 g
saturated fat 0.5 g	fiber 0 g
trans fat 0.0 g	sugars 1 g
polyunsaturated fat 0.5 g	protein 21 g
monounsaturated fat 1.0 g	DIETARY EXCHANGES
cholesterol 56 mg	3 lean meat

BROILED MARINATED FISH STEAKS

SERVES 6

The assertiveness of tarragon vinegar boosts the flavor of mild fish. Serve these steaks with frenchcut green beans and Spinach Salad with Kiwifruit and Raspberries *(page 67).*

1/3 cup tarragon vinegar
2 teaspoons pepper, or to taste
2 teaspoons canola or corn oil
1 teaspoon Worcestershire sauce (lowest
    sodium available)
1 medium dried bay leaf
1 1/2 pounds fish steaks, such as swordfish or
    halibut (about 1 inch thick), rinsed and
    patted dry
Cooking spray

In a large shallow dish, stir together the vinegar, pepper, oil, Worcestershire sauce, and bay leaf. Add the fish, turning to coat. Cover and refrigerate for at least 30 minutes, turning occasionally.

Preheat the broiler. Lightly spray a broiler pan and rack with cooking spray.

(continued)

Drain the fish, discarding the marinade. Place the fish on the rack. Broil about 3 inches from the heat for 5 minutes. Carefully turn over the fish. Broil for about 5 minutes, or until the fish flakes easily when tested with a fork.

PER SERVING

calories 143	sodium 84 mg
total fat 6.5 g	carbohydrates 0 g
saturated fat 1.5 g	fiber 0 g
trans fat 0.0 g	sugars 0 g
polyunsaturated fat 1.0 g	protein 19 g
monounsaturated fat 3.0 g	DIETARY EXCHANGES
cholesterol 65 mg	3 lean meat

MEDITERRANEAN FISH

SERVES 6

You can use almost any fish fillets—thick or thin—in this dish. Try it with Risotto Milanese (page 423) and fresh steamed carrots, or serve it on a bed of steamed spinach or arugula.

Cooking spray
1 medium onion, thinly sliced
1 1/2 pounds fish fillets (thin or thick), such as tilapia or salmon, rinsed and patted dry, cut into serving pieces as necessary
2 large tomatoes, sliced
6 ounces button mushrooms, sliced
1/2 medium green bell pepper, sliced
1/4 cup chopped fresh parsley
1/2 cup dry white wine (regular or nonalcoholic)
2 tablespoons fresh lemon juice
1 teaspoon chopped fresh dillweed or 1/4 teaspoon dried dillweed, crumbled
Pepper to taste
1/2 cup plain dry bread crumbs (lowest sodium available)
1 tablespoon olive oil
1/2 teaspoon dried basil, crumbled

Preheat the oven to 350°F. Lightly spray a 13 x 9 x 2-inch glass baking dish with cooking spray.

Arrange the onion in the baking dish. Place the fish on the onion.

In a medium bowl, stir together the tomatoes, mushrooms, bell pepper, and parsley. Spoon over the fish.

In a small bowl, whisk together the wine, lemon juice, dillweed, and pepper. Pour over the tomato mixture.

Bake thinner fish, such as tilapia, covered, for 15 minutes. If using thicker fish, such as halibut, add about 5 minutes.

Meanwhile, in a small bowl, stir together the bread crumbs, oil, and basil. Sprinkle over the fish mixture after the baking time in the previous step.

Bake, uncovered, for 5 to 10 minutes, or until the fish flakes easily when tested with a fork.

PER SERVING

calories 207	carbohydrates 13 g
total fat 5.0 g	fiber 2 g
saturated fat 1.0 g	sugars 5 g
trans fat 0.0 g	protein 26 g
polyunsaturated fat 1.0 g	DIETARY EXCHANGES
monounsaturated fat 2.5 g	1/2 starch, 1 vegetable,
cholesterol 57 mg	3 lean meat
sodium 133 mg	

FISH IN CRAZY WATER

SERVES 4

Cooks in Italian coastal villages add vegetables and wine to the fish's poaching liquid, making something they call acqua pazza, or "crazy water." It's crazy easy and crazy good. Serve with farro or brown rice.

1/4 teaspoon salt
4 mild fish steaks or fillets, such as halibut (about 4 ounces each), rinsed and patted dry
1 cup white wine (regular or nonalcoholic)
1 cup fat-free, low-sodium chicken broth, such as on page 36
1 medium yellow bell pepper, chopped
2 Italian plum (Roma) tomatoes, chopped
1 tablespoon capers, drained and crushed
1 tablespoon olive oil
3 medium garlic cloves, minced

1/4 teaspoon crushed red pepper flakes

1/4 cup chopped fresh parsley

Sprinkle the salt over the fish.

In a large skillet, stir together the remaining ingredients except the parsley. Bring to a boil over high heat. Reduce the heat and simmer for 5 minutes, stirring occasionally.

Add the fish, turning to coat. Increase the heat to medium high and return to a simmer. Reduce the heat and simmer, partially covered, for 10 to 11 minutes, or until the fish flakes easily when tested with a fork.

Using a slotted spatula, transfer the fish to plates. Using a slotted spoon, spoon the vegetables and capers over the fish. Sprinkle with the parsley.

PER SERVING

calories 195	**carbohydrates** 5 g
total fat 5.0 g	fiber 1 g
saturated fat 1.0 g	sugars 2 g
trans fat 0.0 g	**protein** 23 g
polyunsaturated fat 1.0 g	**DIETARY EXCHANGES**
monounsaturated fat 3.0 g	1 vegetable, 3 lean
cholesterol 56 mg	meat
sodium 300 mg	

FISH STEW

SERVES 6

A delicacy from the West Indies, this fragrant stew is a refreshing change from the usual baked fish. Serve it with crusty whole grain bread and a green salad tossed with Lemon Dressing (page 106).

1/4 cup fresh lemon juice (1 to 2 medium lemons)

1 1/2 pounds fish fillets, at least 3/4 inch thick, such as salmon or halibut, rinsed and patted dry, cut into 2-inch cubes

8 medium green onions, thinly sliced

1 cup chopped tomatoes

1 pound unpeeled red potatoes, cut into 1/2-inch cubes

1 1/2 cups water

1/2 cup chopped fresh parsley

1/4 cup no-salt-added ketchup

3 medium garlic cloves, minced, or

1 1/2 teaspoons bottled minced garlic

1 1/2 teaspoons minced fresh gingerroot or 1/2 teaspoon ground ginger

Sprinkle the lemon juice over the fish. Set aside.

In a large saucepan, cook the green onions over medium-high heat for 1 minute, or until wilted.

Stir in the tomatoes. Cook for 2 to 3 minutes, or until reduced almost to a pulp.

Add the remaining ingredients except the fish. Reduce the heat and simmer, covered, for 10 minutes.

Add the fish. Simmer, covered, for 10 to 15 minutes, or until the fish is almost cooked. Simmer, uncovered, for 4 to 5 minutes, or until the stew thickens slightly.

PER SERVING

calories 188	**carbohydrates** 21 g
total fat 1.0 g	fiber 3 g
saturated fat 0.0 g	sugars 6 g
trans fat 0.0 g	**protein** 22 g
polyunsaturated fat 0.5 g	**DIETARY EXCHANGES**
monounsaturated fat 0.0 g	1 starch, 1 vegetable,
cholesterol 49 mg	3 lean meat
sodium 88 mg	

FISH TACOS WITH WATERMELON-MANGO PICO DE GALLO

SERVES 4

Fish tacos are a great way to get your omega-3s with a side of spice. This version includes a margarita-style marinade and fresh, fruity pico de gallo.

Pico de Gallo

2 1/2 cups diced seedless watermelon

1 cup diced mango

1/4 small red onion, finely chopped

1 medium fresh jalapeño, seeds and ribs discarded, finely chopped (see Cook's Tip on Handling Hot Chiles, page 24)

2 tablespoons coarsely chopped fresh cilantro

1 1/2 to 2 tablespoons fresh lime juice

(continued)

∎ ∎ ∎

1 tablespoon tequila or dry white wine
    (regular or nonalcoholic) (optional)
1 teaspoon grated lime zest
1 tablespoon fresh lime juice
1 teaspoon canola or corn oil
1 pound firm fish fillets, such as mahi mahi,
    rinsed and patted dry, cut into 3/4-inch
    cubes
8 6-inch corn tortillas

In a medium glass bowl, stir together the pico de gallo ingredients. Set aside.

In a separate medium glass bowl, whisk together the tequila, lime zest, the remaining 1 tablespoon lime juice, and the oil. Add the fish, turning to coat. Cover and refrigerate for 10 to 30 minutes.

In a large nonstick skillet, cook the fish with the marinade over medium-high heat for 4 to 6 minutes, or until the fish flakes easily when tested with a fork and most of the liquid has evaporated. Using a slotted spatula, transfer the fish to a large plate.

Meanwhile, warm the tortillas using the package directions.

Put the fish on the tortillas. Top with the pico de gallo.

PER SERVING

calories 228	**carbohydrates** 28 g
total fat 3.0 g	fiber 3 g
saturated fat 0.5 g	sugars 12 g
trans fat 0.0 g	**protein** 24 g
polyunsaturated fat 1.0 g	**DIETARY EXCHANGES**
monounsaturated fat 1.0 g	1 starch, 1 fruit, 3 lean
cholesterol 83 mg	meat
sodium 147 mg	

MUSHROOM-STUFFED FISH ROLLS
SERVES 6

Herbed fresh vegetables fill these baked fish rolls and a light paprika-spiked sauce tops them to add color and flavor. Serve with Brown Rice Pilaf with Summer Squash *(page 404) and steamed or roasted veggies.*

Cooking spray
1 teaspoon light tub margarine
12 ounces button mushrooms, finely diced
8 medium green onions, thinly sliced
1/2 medium red bell pepper, diced
2 tablespoons finely chopped fresh parsley
    and 2 tablespoons finely chopped fresh
    parsley, divided use
1/4 teaspoon salt
1/4 teaspoon pepper
6 thin mild fish fillets, such as sole or
    flounder, (about 4 ounces each), rinsed
    and patted dry
2 to 3 tablespoons fresh lemon juice (about
    1 medium lemon)
1/2 cup dry white wine (regular or
    nonalcoholic)
2 tablespoons all-purpose flour
2 tablespoons water
3/4 teaspoon paprika

Preheat the oven to 350°F. Lightly spray a 9-inch round or square baking pan with cooking spray.

In a large nonstick skillet, melt the margarine over medium heat, swirling to coat the bottom. Cook the mushrooms, green onions, bell pepper, and 2 tablespoons parsley for 3 to 5 minutes, or until the red bell pepper is tender, stirring occasionally.

Sprinkle the salt and pepper over the fish. Spoon the mushroom mixture evenly down the center of each fillet. Starting at a short side, roll up the fish jelly-roll style. Secure with wooden toothpicks. Transfer the fish to the baking pan. Sprinkle the lemon juice over the fish. Pour the wine over all.

Bake, covered, for 25 to 35 minutes, or until the fish flakes easily when tested with a fork. Using a slotted spoon, transfer the fish to a platter. Remove the toothpicks. Cover to keep warm. Pour the cooking liquid into a small saucepan.

In a small bowl, whisk together the flour, water, and paprika. Whisk into the cooking liquid. Cook over medium heat for 2 to 3 minutes, or until thickened, whisking constantly. Spoon over the fish. Sprinkle with the remaining 2 tablespoons parsley.

PER SERVING

calories 161	**carbohydrates** 8 g
total fat 2.0 g	fiber 2 g
saturated fat 0.5 g	sugars 3 g
trans fat 0.0 g	**protein** 24 g
polyunsaturated fat 0.5 g	**DIETARY EXCHANGES**
monounsaturated fat 0.5 g	1 vegetable, 3 lean
cholesterol 54 mg	meat
sodium 207 mg	

FISH FILLETS IN FOIL

SERVES 4

Cooking fish in aluminum foil packets keeps the filling and the fillets moist and minimizes mess. Custom-design your dinner by replacing the mushroom sauce with one of the variations that follow.

> Cooking spray
> 4 thin fish fillets, such as sole or flounder, (about 4 ounces each), rinsed and patted dry
> 1/2 teaspoon pepper

Sauce
> 1 teaspoon light tub margarine
> 1 tablespoon chopped shallots or green onions
> 8 ounces button mushrooms, chopped
> 3 tablespoons dry white wine (regular or nonalcoholic)
> 1 tablespoon chopped fresh parsley
> 1 tablespoon fresh lemon juice

Preheat the oven to 400°F. Lightly spray eight 8-inch square pieces of heavy-duty aluminum foil with cooking spray.

Place the fish in the center of the sprayed side of four of the foil squares. Sprinkle the pepper over the fish.

In a medium nonstick skillet, melt the margarine over medium-high heat, swirling to coat the bottom. Cook the shallots for 2 to 3 minutes, or until soft, stirring occasionally.

Stir in the mushrooms. Cook for 5 minutes, stirring occasionally.

Stir in the wine, parsley, and lemon juice. Cook for 2 to 3 minutes, or until most of the liquid has evaporated. Spoon over the fish. Place one of the remaining foil squares over each serving with the sprayed side down. Wrap the foil loosely (this leaves room for the heat to circulate inside) and seal the edges tightly. Transfer to a large baking sheet.

Bake the packets for 20 minutes. Using the tines of a fork, carefully open a packet away from you (to prevent steam burns). If the fish flakes easily when tested with the fork, carefully open the remaining packets and serve. If the fish isn't cooked enough, reclose the open packet and bake all the packets for 3 to 5 minutes.

In place of the mushroom sauce, use any of the variations listed below and on page 138. Amounts of all the ingredients except the margarine may be changed to suit individual preferences. Use the margarine to dot each serving.

PER SERVING

calories 130	**sodium** 104 mg
total fat 2.0 g	**carbohydrates** 3 g
saturated fat 0.5 g	fiber 1 g
trans fat 0.0 g	sugars 1 g
polyunsaturated fat 0.5 g	**protein** 23 g
monounsaturated fat 0.5 g	**DIETARY EXCHANGES**
cholesterol 54 mg	3 lean meat

FISH FILLETS WITH KALE AND GARLIC

> Kale, fresh or frozen, thawed and squeezed dry if frozen
> Balsamic vinegar or red wine vinegar
> Crushed red pepper flakes
> Garlic, minced
> 1 teaspoon light tub margarine

(continued)

FISH FILLETS WITH TOMATILLO, CILANTRO, AND LIME

Tomatillo, papery husks discarded, or tomato, thinly sliced or chopped
Green onions, thinly sliced
Fresh cilantro, chopped
Fresh lime juice
1 teaspoon light tub margarine

FISH FILLETS WITH DILL AND CUCUMBERS

Cucumber, thinly sliced
Fresh lemon juice
Fresh dillweed and/or parsley, chopped
1 teaspoon light tub margarine

FISH FILLETS WITH THYME AND CELERY

Celery, thinly sliced
Fresh lemon juice
Thyme, fresh and chopped, or dried and crumbled
1 teaspoon light tub margarine

FISH FILLETS WITH CURRIED VEGETABLES

Green onions, thinly sliced
Carrots, very thinly sliced
Curry powder
Green bell pepper, thinly sliced
1 teaspoon light tub margarine

STOVETOP FISH WITH VEGETABLE RICE MEXICAN STYLE

SERVES 4

Cumin-seasoned fillets and turmeric rice tossed with fresh vegetables, cilantro, and lemon are a winning combination for nights when you don't want to use your oven.

1/2 cup uncooked instant brown rice
1/2 teaspoon ground turmeric (optional)
1 1/2 teaspoons ground cumin
1 teaspoon paprika
1/4 teaspoon salt and 1/4 teaspoon salt, divided use
1/4 teaspoon cayenne
4 tilapia or other mild fish fillets (about 4 ounces each), rinsed and patted dry
Cooking spray
1 cup finely chopped green bell pepper or fresh poblano pepper, seeds and ribs discarded (see Cook's Tip on Handling Hot Chiles, page 24)
2 medium Italian plum (Roma) tomatoes, chopped
1/3 cup chopped fresh cilantro
1 teaspoon grated lemon zest
3 tablespoons fresh lemon juice (about 1 medium lemon)
1 tablespoon olive oil (extra-virgin preferred)

Prepare the rice using the package directions, omitting the salt and margarine and adding the turmeric.

Meanwhile, in a small bowl, stir together the cumin, paprika, 1/4 teaspoon salt, and cayenne. Sprinkle over one side of the fish. Using your fingertips, gently press the mixture so it adheres to the fish.

Lightly spray a large skillet with cooking spray. Heat over high heat. Cook the fish for 1 minute on each side. Reduce the heat to medium. Turn over the fish again. Cook for 2 minutes. Turn over the fish. Cook for 1 minute, or until it flakes easily when tested with a fork. Transfer to plates.

In a medium bowl, stir together the bell pepper, tomatoes, cilantro, lemon zest, lemon juice, oil, and the remaining 1/4 teaspoon salt.

Spoon the rice beside the fish. Top the rice with the bell pepper mixture.

PER SERVING

calories 202	**carbohydrates** 13 g
total fat 6.0 g	fiber 2 g
saturated fat 1.0 g	sugars 2 g
trans fat 0.0 g	**protein** 25 g
polyunsaturated fat 1.0 g	**DIETARY EXCHANGES**
monounsaturated fat 3.0 g	1/2 starch, 1 vegetable,
cholesterol 57 mg	3 lean meat
sodium 357 mg	

GREEK FISH FILLETS

SERVES 4

It doesn't get much easier than this, from the simple seasonings to the simple cleanup. Serve with Greek Village Salad *(Horiatiki) (page 71) and roasted red potatoes.*

1 teaspoon dried oregano, crumbled
1 teaspoon salt-free lemon pepper
1/4 teaspoon paprika
1/4 teaspoon salt
4 thin fish fillets, such as tilapia, (about
    4 ounces each), rinsed and patted dry
Cooking spray
1 tablespoon plus 1 teaspoon olive oil (extra-
    virgin preferred)
1 medium lemon, cut into 4 wedges

Preheat the broiler.

In a small bowl, stir together the oregano, lemon pepper, paprika, and salt.

Put the fish on a nonstick baking sheet. Lightly spray the top of the fish with cooking spray. Sprinkle the oregano mixture over the fish.

Broil about 4 inches from the heat with the seasoned side up for 5 minutes, or until the fish flakes easily when tested with a fork. Transfer to plates.

Drizzle the fish with the oil. Serve with the lemon wedges.

PER SERVING

calories 153	sodium 205 mg
total fat 6.5 g	carbohydrates 1 g
saturated fat 1.5 g	fiber 0 g
trans fat 0.0 g	sugars 0 g
polyunsaturated fat 1.0 g	protein 23 g
monounsaturated fat 4.0 g	DIETARY EXCHANGES
cholesterol 57 mg	3 lean meat

ARCTIC CHAR IN PARCHMENT

SERVES 4

Cooking in parchment paper or aluminum foil packets is one of the simplest and best ways to prepare fish. Here, the fillets cook on a pallet of fresh vegetables with lemon slices and tarragon, creating aromatic juices that can be soaked up with a whole grain, such as quinoa or brown rice.

2/3 cup sliced zucchini (1 small)
1/4 cup thinly sliced carrot (1 small)
1 1-pound arctic char or salmon, skin
    discarded, rinsed and patted dry, cut
    into 4 pieces
2/3 cup sugar snap peas (about 4 ounces),
    trimmed and halved diagonally
1 small leek, sliced (light green and white
    parts only)
1 tablespoon plus 1 teaspoon coarsely
    chopped fresh tarragon or 1 teaspoon
    dried tarragon, crumbled
1/8 teaspoon salt
1/8 teaspoon pepper
Cooking spray
4 lemon slices, about 1/4 inch thick, halved

Preheat the oven to 425°F.

Cut four 12-inch-square pieces of cooking parchment or heavy-duty aluminum foil. Fold each square in half. Cut into half-moon shapes. Open and place the zucchini and carrots next to the fold lines. Place the fish on the zucchini and carrots. Arrange the peas and leek on the fish. Sprinkle the tarragon, salt, and pepper over the fish. Lightly spray with cooking spray. Top with the lemon slices. Close and tightly fold and pleat the edges together to seal the packets securely. Transfer to a large rimmed baking sheet.

Bake the packets for 10 minutes, or until the parchment is lightly browned and puffed. Carefully (to prevent steam burns) cut a slit in one packet. The fish should flake easily when tested with a fork. If the fish isn't cooked enough, carefully reclose the packet and bake for an additional 3 to 5 minutes.

(continued)

Cook's Tip: Fresh dillweed or chives can be used in place of the tarragon.

PER SERVING

calories 167	**sodium** 128 mg
total fat 4.0 g	**carbohydrates** 7 g
saturated fat 1.0 g	fiber 2 g
trans fat 0.0 g	sugars 3 g
polyunsaturated fat 1.0 g	**protein** 24 g
monounsaturated fat 2.0 g	**DIETARY EXCHANGES**
cholesterol 51 mg	1 vegetable, 3 lean meat

BRONZED CATFISH WITH REMOULADE SAUCE

SERVES 4

The bronzing technique used in this recipe is similar to the blackening used for dishes such as blackened redfish. To get that bronzed look, however, the fish is cooked at a more moderate temperature so the seasonings don't burn.

Sauce
  2 medium green onions, thinly sliced
  1 small rib of celery, finely chopped
  2 tablespoons chopped fresh parsley
  2 tablespoons no-salt-added ketchup
  1 tablespoon Creole mustard or coarse-grain
    Dijon mustard (lowest sodium available)
  1 tablespoon red wine vinegar
  2 teaspoons Worcestershire sauce (lowest
    sodium available)
  2 teaspoons olive oil (extra-virgin preferred)
  1 medium garlic clove, minced
  1/2 teaspoon paprika
  1/4 teaspoon salt

■ ■ ■

  4 catfish fillets (about 4 ounces each), rinsed
    and patted dry
  Cooking spray
  1 tablespoon plus 1 teaspoon salt-free Creole
    or Cajun seasoning blend

In a medium glass bowl, stir together the sauce ingredients. Cover and refrigerate for up to three days.

Lightly spray both sides of the fish with cooking spray. Sprinkle the seasoning blend over both sides of the fish.

Heat a nonstick skillet over medium-high heat. Cook the fish for 5 minutes, or until the bottom is golden brown. Turn over the fish. Cook for 4 to 5 minutes, or until the bottom is browned and the fish flakes easily when tested with a fork. Serve topped with the sauce.

PER SERVING

calories 144	**sodium** 279 mg
total fat 5.5 g	**carbohydrates** 4 g
saturated fat 1.0 g	fiber 1 g
trans fat 0.0 g	sugars 2 g
polyunsaturated fat 1.0 g	**protein** 19 g
monounsaturated fat 2.5 g	**DIETARY EXCHANGES**
cholesterol 66 mg	3 lean meat

CRISPY CAJUN CATFISH NUGGETS

SERVES 4

If you like fried popcorn shrimp, you'll love these crisp morsels of catfish. They're baked at a high temperature to create a crispy texture that tastes "fried," but is much healthier for you. The dipping sauce is a variation of a tradition cocktail sauce.

  Cooking spray
  3 tablespoons yellow cornmeal
  1/2 teaspoon chili powder
  1/2 teaspoon ground cumin
  1/4 teaspoon salt
  1/4 teaspoon garlic powder
  1/8 teaspoon pepper
  1 pound catfish fillets, rinsed and patted dry,
    cut into 1/2-inch cubes
  1/4 cup egg substitute
  1/2 cup cornflake crumbs (about 1 heaping
    cup cornflakes)
Sauce
  1/4 cup no-salt-added ketchup
  2 tablespoons white wine vinegar
  2 tablespoons fresh lemon juice
  1 tablespoon honey
  1 tablespoon bottled white horseradish,
    drained

Preheat the oven to 400°F. Lightly spray a baking sheet with cooking spray.

In a large shallow dish, stir together the corn-meal, chili powder, cumin, salt, garlic powder, and pepper. Add the fish, turning gently to coat.

Put the egg substitute and cornflake crumbs in two separate shallow dishes. Set the dishes and a large baking sheet in a row, assembly-line fashion. Working in batches, dip the fish in the egg substitute, then in the cornflake crumbs, turning to coat at each step and gently shaking off any excess. Transfer the fish to the baking sheet, arranging it in a single layer. Lightly spray the top with cooking spray.

Bake for 7 to 8 minutes, or until the fish flakes easily when tested with a fork.

Meanwhile, in a small bowl, whisk together the sauce ingredients. Serve with the fish.

PER SERVING

calories 213	carbohydrates 25 g
total fat 3.5 g	fiber 1 g
saturated fat 1.0 g	sugars 8 g
trans fat 0.0 g	**protein** 22 g
polyunsaturated fat 1.0 g	**DIETARY EXCHANGES**
monounsaturated fat 1.0 g	1 starch, 1/2 other
cholesterol 66 mg	carbohydrate, 3 lean
sodium 333 mg	meat

CATFISH WITH ZESTY SLAW TOPPING

SERVES 4

A New Orleans favorite gets a lean update with crispy baked catfish and a broccoli-slaw topping, kicked up with Cajun or Creole seasoning and horseradish. Serve with Oven-Fried Onion Rings *(page 395), which can bake along with the fish.*

Cooking spray
1/4 cup white whole-wheat flour
1 teaspoon salt-free spicy all-purpose
    seasoning blend
1/4 cup egg substitute, lightly beaten with
    a fork
3/4 cup cornflake crumbs
1 pound catfish fillets, rinsed and patted dry,
    cut into 1-inch cubes

Slaw
    4 cups packaged broccoli slaw or shredded
        green cabbage
    1 medium carrot, shredded
    2 medium green onions, thinly sliced
    2 tablespoons light mayonnaise
    1 teaspoon white wine vinegar
    1 teaspoon bottled white horseradish,
        drained
    1/2 teaspoon salt-free Creole or Cajun
        seasoning blend

Preheat the oven to 400°F. Lightly spray a baking sheet with cooking spray.

In a shallow dish, stir together the flour and spicy seasoning blend. Put the egg substitute and cornflake crumbs in two separate shallow dishes. Set the dishes and the baking sheet in a row, assembly-line fashion. Working in batches, dip the fish cubes in the flour mixture, then in the egg substitute (a slotted spoon works well for this), and finally in the cornflake crumbs, turning to coat at each step and gently shaking off any excess. Transfer the cubes to the baking sheet, spacing them at least 1 inch apart. Lightly spray the top of the cubes with cooking spray.

Bake for 10 to 12 minutes, or until the fish flakes easily when tested with a fork. Transfer the baking sheet to a cooling rack. Let cool for 5 minutes.

Meanwhile, in a medium bowl, stir together the slaw ingredients. Serve over the fish.

PER SERVING

calories 252	carbohydrates 28 g
total fat 5.0 g	fiber 4 g
saturated fat 1.0 g	sugars 5 g
trans fat 0.0 g	**protein** 24 g
polyunsaturated fat 2.5 g	**DIETARY EXCHANGES**
monounsaturated fat 1.5 g	1 1/2 starch,
cholesterol 68 mg	1 vegetable, 3 lean
sodium 306 mg	meat

COD BAKED WITH VEGETABLES

SERVES 6

This one-dish comfort meal preserves the mildness of cod yet is full of flavor from fresh veggies and herbs. And with just a baking dish and a small bowl, cleanup is a snap!

Cooking spray
10 to 12 ounces red potatoes, cut into 1-inch
    cubes
2 medium carrots, sliced crosswise in 1/4-inch
    pieces
2 tablespoons light tub margarine, melted
2 tablespoons fresh lemon juice
1/4 teaspoon salt and 1/4 teaspoon salt,
    divided use
1/4 teaspoon pepper and 1/4 teaspoon
    pepper, divided use
1 1/2 pounds cod fillets, rinsed and patted dry,
    cut into 2-inch cubes
4 medium green onions, sliced
2 tablespoons chopped fresh parsley or
    2 teaspoons dried parsley, crumbled
1 tablespoon finely chopped fresh dillweed or
    1 teaspoon dried dillweed, crumbled

Preheat the oven to 400°F. Lightly spray a 13 x 9 x 2-inch glass baking dish with cooking spray.

Put the potatoes and carrots in the baking dish.

In a small bowl, stir together the margarine, lemon juice, 1/4 teaspoon salt, and 1/4 teaspoon pepper. Pour over the potatoes and carrots.

Bake, covered, for 25 minutes.

Put the fish in a medium bowl. Sprinkle the green onions, the remaining 1/4 teaspoon salt, and the remaining 1/4 teaspoon pepper over the fish. Gently stir into the potato mixture. Sprinkle the parsley and dillweed over all.

Bake, covered, for 15 to 20 minutes, or until the fish flakes easily when tested with a fork.

Cook's Tip: If you're in a hurry, you can cook this dish in your microwave oven. Prepare the potatoes, carrots, and margarine mixture as directed.

Microwave, covered, on 100 percent power (high) for 8 to 10 minutes. Add the remaining ingredients and microwave, covered and vented, on 100 percent power (high) for 5 to 7 minutes.

PER SERVING

calories 151	**carbohydrates** 13 g
total fat 2.5 g	fiber 2 g
saturated fat 0.0 g	sugars 3 g
trans fat 0.0 g	**protein** 19 g
polyunsaturated fat 0.5 g	**DIETARY EXCHANGES**
monounsaturated fat 1.0 g	1/2 starch, 1 vegetable,
cholesterol 43 mg	3 lean meat
sodium 315 mg	

COD AND VEGETABLES IN LEMONY CREAM SAUCE

SERVES 4

Baby carrots, pearl onions, red potatoes, and mild-flavored cod are enveloped in a velvety sauce. Serve this dish with a delicate salad, such as Spinach Salad with Kiwifruit and Raspberries *(page 67).*

8 small red potatoes, halved
1 1/2 cups baby carrots
1 1/2 cups fat-free, low-sodium chicken broth,
    such as on page 36
1 cup frozen pearl onions, thawed
1 teaspoon salt-free all-purpose seasoning
1/2 cup fat-free half-and-half
2 1/2 tablespoons all-purpose flour
2 tablespoons chopped fresh parsley
1 teaspoon grated lemon zest
1 medium garlic clove, minced
4 cod fillets (about 4 ounces each), rinsed
    and patted dry

In a large skillet, stir together the potatoes, carrots, broth, onions, and seasoning blend. Bring to a simmer over medium-high heat, stirring occasionally. Reduce the heat and simmer, covered, for 10 minutes, or until the potatoes and carrots are tender and the onions are soft.

In a small bowl, whisk together the remaining ingredients except the fish (there may be a few lumps). Stir into the potato mixture. Simmer, covered, for 2 to 3 minutes, or until thickened, stirring occasionally.

Place the fish in the skillet, spacing the fillets evenly. Spoon the potato mixture on top. Simmer, covered, for 8 to 10 minutes, or until the fish flakes easily when tested with a fork.

PER SERVING

calories 269	carbohydrates 38 g
total fat 1.5 g	fiber 3 g
saturated fat 0.0 g	sugars 8 g
trans fat 0.0 g	protein 27 g
polyunsaturated fat 0.5 g	DIETARY EXCHANGES
monounsaturated fat 0.0 g	2 starch, 2 vegetable,
cholesterol 49 mg	3 lean meat
sodium 146 mg	

FLOUNDER-CRABMEAT ROLLS

SERVES 8

If you're a seafood lover, you'll enjoy this duet—a mild white fish and shellfish—all in one meal. Serve with Baked Okra Bites *(page 394) and a dark green, leafy salad.*

Cooking spray

8 flounder fillets (about 4 ounces each), rinsed and patted dry, pounded to 1/2-inch thickness

1 6-ounce can lump crabmeat, rinsed, drained, and flaked

1/2 cup whole-wheat panko (Japanese-style bread crumbs)

4 ounces button mushrooms, chopped

3 tablespoons chopped onion

1 tablespoon chopped fresh parsley

1/4 teaspoon salt

Sauce

1 1/2 cups fat-free milk

1/4 cup dry white wine (regular or nonalcoholic)

2 1/2 tablespoons cornstarch

2 ounces low-fat mozzarella cheese, shredded (about 1/2 cup)

■ ■ ■

1/2 to 3/4 teaspoon paprika

Preheat the oven to 400°F. Lightly spray a shallow 13 x 9 x 2-inch baking dish with cooking spray.

Place the fish fillets on a work surface. In a medium bowl, stir together the crabmeat, panko, mushrooms, onion, parsley, and salt. Spread the mixture over the fish fillets. Starting at a short side, roll up the fish jelly-roll style. Secure with wooden toothpicks if desired. Place the rolls with the seam side down in the baking dish.

In a medium bowl, whisk together the milk and wine. Put the cornstarch in a small bowl. Add a small amount of the milk mixture, whisking to dissolve. Pour the remaining milk mixture into a medium saucepan. Gradually whisk in the cornstarch mixture. Cook for about 5 minutes over medium heat, whisking gently until the mixture thickens. Add the mozzarella. Cook for 2 minutes, or until melted, whisking occasionally.

Pour the sauce over the rolls. Sprinkle with the paprika.

Bake for 25 to 30 minutes, or until the fish flakes easily when tested with a fork.

PER SERVING

calories 164	sodium 569 mg
total fat 3.0 g	carbohydrates 9 g
saturated fat 1.0 g	fiber 1 g
trans fat 0.0 g	sugars 3 g
polyunsaturated fat 0.5 g	protein 23 g
monounsaturated fat 1.0 g	DIETARY EXCHANGES
cholesterol 75 mg	1/2 starch, 3 lean meat

FLOUNDER ROULADES

SERVES 4

Nestled inside these mild white fish roll-ups is a fresh herb, citrus, and vegetable filling. Serve these on top of a bed of whole grains, such as Lemon-Basil Rice *(page 420).*

(continued)

Cooking spray

2 teaspoons olive oil and 2 teaspoons olive oil, divided use

8 ounces brown (cremini) mushrooms, chopped

2 medium green onions, thinly sliced

4 flounder, tilapia, or catfish fillets (about 4 ounces each), rinsed and patted dry

1 medium lemon, cut into 4 wedges

3/4 teaspoon chopped fresh tarragon and 2 teaspoons chopped fresh tarragon, divided use

1/4 teaspoon salt

1/4 teaspoon pepper

10 ounces frozen chopped spinach, thawed and squeezed dry

2 medium roasted red bell peppers, drained if bottled, halved

Preheat the oven to 350°F. Lightly spray a 13 x 9 x 2-inch glass baking dish with cooking spray.

In a medium skillet, heat 2 teaspoons oil over medium-high heat, swirling to coat the bottom. Cook the mushrooms and green onions for 2 to 3 minutes, or until soft, stirring frequently.

Put the fish on a flat surface. Squeeze 1 lemon wedge over each fillet. Sprinkle 3/4 teaspoon tarragon, the salt, and pepper on the fish. Spoon the spinach on the fish. Place a bell pepper half on the spinach. Spoon the mushroom mixture over the bell pepper halves. Starting with a short side, roll up the fish fillets jelly-roll style. Secure with wooden toothpicks. Place with the seam side down in the baking dish. Spoon the remaining 2 teaspoons oil over the fish.

Bake for 20 to 25 minutes, or until the fish flakes easily when tested with a fork. Just before serving, sprinkle with the remaining 2 teaspoons tarragon.

HADDOCK WITH TOMATOES AND GINGER
SERVES 6

A citrusy tomato sauce with an Asian flair tops mild haddock fillets. Serve with stir-fried veggies, such as Vegetable Stir-Fry (page 414), and brown rice.

Cooking spray

3 tablespoons all-purpose flour

Dash of pepper

6 haddock fillets (about 4 ounces each), rinsed and patted dry

1 tablespoon canola or corn oil

1 tablespoon grated peeled gingerroot

2 medium garlic cloves, minced

2 cups chopped tomatoes

2 or 3 medium green onions, sliced

1 cup fresh orange juice

1/2 cup dry white wine (regular or nonalcoholic)

1 1/2 tablespoons cornstarch

1 tablespoon soy sauce (lowest sodium available)

1 tablespoon chopped fresh parsley

Preheat the oven to 350°F. Lightly spray a 13 x 9 x 2-inch glass baking dish with cooking spray.

In a shallow dish, stir together the flour and pepper. Dip the fish in the flour mixture, turning to coat and gently shaking off any excess. Transfer the fish to a plate.

In a large nonstick skillet, heat the oil over medium-high heat, swirling to coat the bottom. Cook the fish for 1 minute on each side. Transfer to the baking dish, leaving any remaining oil in the skillet.

Bake for 10 to 15 minutes, or until the fish flakes easily when tested with a fork.

Meanwhile, in the same skillet, cook the gingerroot and garlic over medium heat for 2 to 3 minutes, stirring occasionally. Stir in the tomatoes and green onions. Bring to a simmer. Reduce the heat and simmer for 3 to 4 minutes.

In a small bowl, whisk together the remaining four ingredients except the parsley. Stir into the gingerroot mixture. Increase the heat to medium high and cook for 2 to 3 minutes, or until thickened, stirring constantly. Stir in the parsley. Just before serving, spoon the sauce over the fish.

PER SERVING

calories 178	**carbohydrates** 13 g
total fat 3.0 g	fiber 1 g
saturated fat 0.5 g	sugars 6 g
trans fat 0.0 g	**protein** 20 g
polyunsaturated fat 1.0 g	**DIETARY EXCHANGES**
monounsaturated fat 1.5 g	1 other carbohydrate,
cholesterol 61 mg	3 lean meat
sodium 314 mg	

TERIYAKI HALIBUT

SERVES 8

Savory teriyaki-glazed fish is even better when it's topped with juicy, sweet caramelized pineapple. Prepare some brown rice and steam bright-green sugar snap peas, such as Stir-Fried Sugar Snap Peas (page 402), to serve with the fish.

Marinade
  1/2 cup dry white wine (regular or nonalcoholic)
  3 tablespoons soy sauce (lowest sodium available)
  1 tablespoon light brown sugar
  1 teaspoon all-purpose flour
  1 teaspoon canola or corn oil
  1/2 teaspoon dry mustard

■ ■ ■

8 halibut fillets (about 4 ounces each), rinsed and patted dry
Cooking spray

8 slices pineapple, canned in its own juice, drained

In a small saucepan, whisk together the marinade ingredients. Bring to a boil over medium-high heat. Reduce the heat and simmer for 3 minutes. Pour into a large shallow glass dish. Cover and refrigerate for 30 minutes to 1 hour.

Add the fish to the marinade, turning to coat. Refrigerate for 15 minutes.

Preheat the broiler. Lightly spray a broiler pan and rack with cooking spray.

Transfer the fish to the broiler rack. Pour the marinade into a small saucepan. Bring to a boil over medium-high heat. Boil for 5 minutes. Brush the fish with the hot marinade, discarding any that isn't used.

Broil the fish about 5 to 6 inches from the heat for 5 minutes. Turn over the fish. Top with the pineapple. Broil for about 5 minutes, or until the fish flakes easily when tested with a fork.

Cook's Tip: Seafood doesn't need to marinate for long. Too much marinating time can cause it to become rubbery or mushy.

PER SERVING

calories 161	**sodium** 230 mg
total fat 2.0 g	**carbohydrates** 11 g
saturated fat 0.5 g	fiber 1 g
trans fat 0.0 g	sugars 9 g
polyunsaturated fat 0.5 g	**protein** 22 g
monounsaturated fat 1.0 g	**DIETARY EXCHANGES**
cholesterol 56 mg	1 fruit, 3 lean meat

HALIBUT AND VEGETABLES IN WHITE WINE SAUCE

SERVES 8

This entrée provides protein and vegetables all in one dish. To round out the meal, serve it with a simple whole grain such as quinoa, farro, or Apricot Bulgur with Pine Nuts (page 416) and a dark, leafy green salad with Lemon Dressing (page 106).

(continued)

Cooking spray

2/3 cup thinly sliced onion

8 halibut fillets (about 4 ounces each), rinsed and patted dry

1/2 cup sliced button or brown (cremini) mushrooms

1/3 cup chopped tomato

1/4 cup chopped green bell pepper

1/4 cup chopped fresh parsley

3 tablespoons chopped pimiento

1/2 cup dry white wine (regular or nonalcoholic)

2 tablespoons fresh lemon juice

1/4 teaspoon chopped fresh dillweed

Pepper to taste (freshly ground preferred)

2 medium lemons, each cut into 4 wedges

Preheat the oven to 350°F. Lightly spray a baking dish with cooking spray.

Put the onion in the baking dish. Place the fish on top.

In a medium bowl, stir together the mushrooms, tomato, bell pepper, parsley, and pimiento. Spoon over the fish.

In a small bowl, whisk together the wine, lemon juice, dillweed, and pepper. Pour over the fish and vegetables. Bake, covered, for 25 to 30 minutes, or until the fish flakes easily when tested with a fork. Serve with the lemon wedges.

PER SERVING

calories 123	sodium 81 mg
total fat 1.5 g	carbohydrates 2 g
saturated fat 0.5 g	fiber 1 g
trans fat 0.0 g	sugars 1 g
polyunsaturated fat 0.5 g	protein 22 g
monounsaturated fat 0.5 g	DIETARY EXCHANGES
cholesterol 56 mg	3 lean meat

GINGER-WALNUT SALMON AND ASPARAGUS

SERVES 4

Walnuts add a bit of crunch and earthiness to this salmon and asparagus dish. Preparation is fast, and because the fish cooks in aluminum foil packets, cleanup is a breeze.

Cooking spray

12 medium asparagus spears (about 1 pound), trimmed

4 salmon fillets with skin (about 5 ounces each), rinsed and patted dry

2 tablespoons honey

1 tablespoon Worcestershire sauce (lowest sodium available)

1 tablespoon cornstarch

2 teaspoons light brown sugar

2 teaspoons grated peeled gingerroot

1/4 cup chopped walnuts

Preheat the oven to 450°F.

Lightly spray four 15 x 12-inch sheets of aluminum foil with cooking spray. Place 3 asparagus spears in the center of each. Top with the fish with the skin side down.

In a small bowl, whisk together the honey, Worcestershire sauce, cornstarch, brown sugar, and gingerroot until the cornstarch and brown sugar are dissolved. Using a pastry brush, spread over the top and sides of the fish. Sprinkle the walnuts over the fish. Wrap the foil loosely around the fish and vegetables (this leaves room for the heat to circulate inside) and seal the edges tightly. Transfer the packets to a large baking sheet.

Bake for 20 minutes. Using the tines of a fork, carefully open a packet away from you (to avoid steam burns). If the fish is cooked to the desired doneness, carefully open the remaining packets and serve. If the fish isn't cooked enough, reclose the open packet and bake all the packets for 3 to 5 minutes more. Transfer the fish and asparagus to plates, discarding the fish skin if desired (tongs work well for this). Spoon the sauce over all.

PER SERVING

calories 287	carbohydrates 19 g
total fat 10.5 g	fiber 3 g
saturated fat 1.5 g	sugars 14 g
trans fat 0.0 g	protein 30 g
polyunsaturated fat 4.5 g	DIETARY EXCHANGES
monounsaturated fat 2.5 g	1 vegetable, 1 other
cholesterol 60 mg	carbohydrate,
sodium 118 mg	3 1/2 lean meat

BAKED SALMON WITH CUCUMBER RELISH

SERVES 4

This attractive salmon dish has two crisscrossed toppings, one a fiery cucumber-based relish and the other a tangy yogurt and lemon mixture. Serve on a bed of steamed spinach or arugula.

Cooking spray
4 salmon fillets (about 4 ounces each), rinsed and patted dry
1/4 teaspoon pepper
1/8 teaspoon salt and 1/8 teaspoon salt, divided use
1/2 cup fat-free plain yogurt
1 teaspoon grated lemon zest
1 tablespoon fresh lemon juice
1/2 medium cucumber, peeled, seeded, and chopped
1/4 cup finely chopped red onion
1 medium fresh jalapeño, seeds and ribs discarded, finely chopped (see Cook's Tip on Handling Hot Chiles, page 24)

Preheat the oven to 400°F. Line a large baking sheet with aluminum foil. Lightly spray with cooking spray.

Put the fish on the baking sheet. Sprinkle the pepper and 1/8 teaspoon salt over the fish.

Bake for 20 minutes, or to the desired doneness.

Meanwhile, in a small bowl, whisk together the yogurt, lemon zest, lemon juice, and the remaining 1/8 teaspoon salt.

In a medium bowl, stir together the cucumber, onion, and jalapeño.

Transfer the fish to a small platter. Spoon the yogurt mixture diagonally over each piece of fish. Spoon the cucumber mixture diagonally in the other direction over the fish.

PER SERVING

calories 171	**carbohydrates** 5 g
total fat 5.0 g	fiber 1 g
saturated fat 1.0 g	sugars 3 g
trans fat 0.0 g	**protein** 25 g
polyunsaturated fat 1.0 g	**DIETARY EXCHANGES**
monounsaturated fat 1.5 g	1/2 other
cholesterol 53 mg	carbohydrate, 3 lean
sodium 255 mg	meat

SALMON WITH CUCUMBER-DILL SAUCE

SERVES 4

Cucumber is a complementary pairing with salmon, and so is dill, so why not put all three together? Serve this light entrée warm, at room temperature, or chilled.

4 salmon fillets (about 4 ounces each), rinsed and patted dry
1 cup dry white wine (regular or nonalcoholic)
2 medium dried bay leaves
2 tablespoons finely chopped fresh dillweed or 2 teaspoons dried dillweed, crumbled
Pepper to taste

Sauce

2 medium cucumbers, peeled, halved lengthwise, seeded, and cut into 1/2-inch slices
1 medium rib of celery, including leaves, cut into 1/2-inch slices
3 tablespoons chopped fresh dillweed or 1 tablespoon dried dillweed, crumbled
1 teaspoon olive oil (extra-virgin preferred)
1/4 teaspoon salt
Pepper to taste

Preheat the oven to 350°F.

Put the fish in a glass baking dish. Pour the wine over the fish. Add the bay leaves. Sprinkle the dillweed and pepper over the fish. Cover tightly with aluminum foil.

Bake the fish for 8 to 10 minutes, or until the desired doneness. Remove from the oven. Cover to keep warm.

Put the sauce ingredients in a large saucepan. Pour in enough water to barely cover the vegetables. Bring to a boil over high heat. Boil, covered, for about 30 minutes, or until the celery is very tender, stirring occasionally.

In a food processor or blender (vent the blender lid), process the sauce until smooth.

(continued)

Spoon half the sauce onto a platter. Place the fish on the sauce, discarding the bay leaves. Spoon the remaining sauce over the fish.

PER SERVING

calories 171	sodium 242 mg
total fat 6.5 g	carbohydrates 3 g
saturated fat 1.0 g	fiber 1 g
trans fat 0.0 g	sugars 2 g
polyunsaturated fat 1.0 g	protein 24 g
monounsaturated fat 2.5 g	DIETARY EXCHANGES
cholesterol 53 mg	3 lean meat

SALMON FILLETS WITH MANGO-STRAWBERRY SALSA

SERVES 4

The fruity salsa in this recipe is perfect not only over salmon but also over grilled chicken and pork, or as a dip for heart-healthy chips.

Salsa
  1/2 medium mango, finely chopped, or 1/2 cup frozen mango slices, thawed and finely chopped
  1/2 cup strawberries, hulled and finely chopped
  1/4 medium fresh poblano pepper, seeds and ribs discarded, finely chopped (see Cook's Tip on Handling Hot Chiles, page 24)
  1 tablespoon fresh lime juice
  1 teaspoon grated peeled gingerroot

■ ■ ■

  2 tablespoons fresh lime juice
  1 1/2 teaspoons salt-free jerk seasoning blend
  1/4 teaspoon salt
  4 salmon fillets (about 4 ounces each), rinsed and patted dry
  1 teaspoon canola or corn oil

In a small bowl, stir together the salsa ingredients. Set aside.

Sprinkle the remaining 2 tablespoons lime juice, seasoning blend, and salt over one side of the fish. Using your fingertips, gently press the mixture so it adheres to the fish.

In a large nonstick skillet, heat the oil over medium-high heat, swirling to coat the bottom. Cook the fish with the seasoned side down for 3 minutes. Turn over the fish. Cook for 3 minutes, or to the desired doneness. Serve the fish with the seasoned side up and the salsa on the side.

Cook's Tip on Homemade Salt-Free Jerk Seasoning Blend: If you want to make your own salt-free jerk seasoning blend, stir together 3/4 teaspoon ground allspice, 1/4 teaspoon ground cinnamon, 1/4 teaspoon garlic powder, and 1/4 teaspoon dried thyme, crumbled. That mixture will give you 1 1/2 teaspoons for the blend.

PER SERVING

calories 191	sodium 232 mg
total fat 6.5 g	carbohydrates 9 g
saturated fat 1.0 g	fiber 1 g
trans fat 0.0 g	sugars 7 g
polyunsaturated fat 1.5 g	protein 24 g
monounsaturated fat 2.5 g	DIETARY EXCHANGES
cholesterol 52 mg	1/2 fruit, 3 lean meat

BROILED SALMON WITH MINTY CITRUS RELISH

SERVES 4

A delightfully minty fruit relish dresses up just-about-foolproof broiled salmon. The acidic sweetness of the citrus is a perfect complement to the richness of the fish.

  Cooking spray
  4 salmon fillets (about 4 ounces each), rinsed and patted dry
  1/4 teaspoon salt
  1/4 teaspoon pepper
Relish
  1 1/2 cups grapefruit and orange sections, finely chopped
  1/4 cup finely chopped red onion
  2 tablespoons chopped fresh mint
  1 teaspoon sugar
  1/4 teaspoon crushed red pepper flakes

Preheat the broiler. Lightly spray a broiler pan and rack with cooking spray.

Put the fish in the pan. Sprinkle the salt and pepper over the fish.

Broil for 5 minutes on each side, or to the desired doneness.

Meanwhile, in a medium bowl, stir together the relish ingredients. Spoon on top of the fish.

Cook's Tip on Grapefruit: Grapefruit can interact with a number of medications, including many heart medicines. Be sure to check with your doctor or pharmacist if you take any medication. If necessary, use only orange sections in the salsa.

PER SERVING

calories 184	**sodium** 233 mg
total fat 5.0 g	**carbohydrates** 10 g
saturated fat 1.0 g	fiber 2 g
trans fat 0.0 g	sugars 8 g
polyunsaturated fat 1.0 g	**protein** 24 g
monounsaturated fat 1.5 g	**DIETARY EXCHANGES**
cholesterol 52 mg	1 fruit, 3 lean meat

BROILED SALMON OVER GARDEN-FRESH CORN AND BELL PEPPERS

Serves 4

Celebrate summer with a dish that marries seasonal local corn, bell peppers, and garden-grown basil and mint with the rich taste of salmon. Serve this dish with brown rice, whole-wheat couscous, or quinoa, and dinner is ready!

Cooking spray
4 salmon fillets (about 4 ounces each), about 1 inch thick, rinsed and patted dry
1 tablespoon chopped fresh basil and 3 tablespoons chopped fresh basil, divided use
1 teaspoon chopped fresh mint and 1 teaspoon chopped fresh mint, divided use
1/8 teaspoon salt and 1/8 teaspoon salt, divided use
1/8 teaspoon pepper and 1/8 teaspoon pepper, divided use
2 teaspoons olive oil
1/2 cup coarsely chopped red onion
3/4 cup chopped bell peppers
2 cups corn kernels, cut from 3 or 4 medium ears of corn, husks and silk discarded

Preheat the broiler. Line a baking sheet with aluminum foil. Lightly spray the foil with cooking spray.

Put the fish on the baking sheet. Sprinkle 1 tablespoon basil, 1 teaspoon mint, 1/8 teaspoon salt, and 1/8 teaspoon pepper over the top of the fish. Lightly spray with cooking spray.

In a large nonstick skillet, heat the oil over medium heat, swirling to coat the bottom. Cook the onion for 1 minute, stirring frequently. Stir in the bell peppers. Cook for 1 minute, stirring frequently. Stir in the corn. Cook for 5 to 6 minutes, or until the onion is soft and the vegetables are tender-crisp, stirring occasionally. Remove from the heat.

Stir in the remaining 3 tablespoons basil, 1 teaspoon mint, 1/8 teaspoon salt, and 1/8 teaspoon pepper.

Meanwhile, broil the fish about 4 to 6 inches from the heat for 5 to 8 minutes, or until the desired doneness.

Transfer the onion mixture to plates. Top with the fish.

Cook's Tip: Look for packages of sweet baby bell peppers in red, orange, and yellow so you'll have an assortment of colors for this recipe.

PER SERVING

calories 245	**sodium** 245 mg
total fat 8.5 g	**carbohydrates** 17 g
saturated fat 1.5 g	fiber 2 g
trans fat 0.0 g	sugars 6 g
polyunsaturated fat 1.5 g	**protein** 27 g
monounsaturated fat 3.5 g	**DIETARY EXCHANGES**
cholesterol 53 mg	1 starch, 3 lean meat

GRILLED PINEAPPLE-LIME SALMON

SERVES 6

Once the salmon soaks up the pineapple-lime marinade flavors, it's ready in almost no time. For a simple meal, grill some vegetables along with the fish. You can even grill halved peaches or serve Grilled Pineapple (page 502) for dessert.

Marinade
> 6 ounces 100% pineapple juice
> 1/2 cup finely chopped onion
> 1/2 teaspoon grated lime zest
> 2 tablespoons fresh lime juice
> 1 tablespoon grated peeled gingerroot
> 1 tablespoon soy sauce (lowest sodium available)
> 2 medium garlic cloves, minced
> 1 teaspoon hot chili oil (optional)
> 1 teaspoon canola or corn oil

■ ■ ■

> 6 salmon steaks or fillets (about 4 ounces each), rinsed and patted dry
> Cooking spray

In a large shallow glass dish, stir together the marinade ingredients. Add the fish, turning to coat. Cover and refrigerate for 15 minutes to 1 hour, turning occasionally.

Lightly spray the grill rack or a broiler pan and rack with cooking spray. Preheat the grill on medium high or preheat the broiler.

Drain the fish, discarding the marinade. Grill or broil about 4 inches from the heat for 5 to 7 minutes on each side, or to the desired doneness.

Cook's Tip on Hot Chili Oil: This is vegetable oil flavored with hot red chiles. Commonly used in Chinese cuisine, it can be very spicy. You can make your own by steeping crushed red pepper flakes in canola or corn oil.

PER SERVING

calories 146
total fat 5.0 g
   saturated fat 1.0 g
   trans fat 0.0 g
   polyunsaturated fat 1.0 g
   monounsaturated fat 1.5 g
cholesterol 52 mg

sodium 150 mg
carbohydrates 0 g
   fiber 0 g
   sugars 0 g
protein 23 g
DIETARY EXCHANGES
   3 lean meat

GRILLED SALMON WITH CILANTRO SAUCE

SERVES 4

With its fresh and slightly crunchy sauce, this fish dish pairs swimmingly with a cool and refreshing cucumber salad such as Cucumber and Mango Salad with Lime Dressing *(page 72).*

> Cooking spray

Sauce
> 1 cup tightly packed fresh cilantro
> 1/4 cup sliced almonds, dry-roasted
> 1/4 cup shredded or grated Parmesan cheese
> 1/4 cup cold water
> 2 tablespoons thinly sliced green onions
> 1 tablespoon plus 2 teaspoons fresh lime juice
> 1 tablespoon olive oil (extra-virgin preferred)
> 1 small garlic clove, chopped
> 1/2 medium fresh jalapeño, seeds and ribs discarded, chopped (see Cook's Tip on Handling Hot Chiles, page 24)

■ ■ ■

> 1/2 teaspoon ground cumin
> 1/4 teaspoon ground coriander
> 1/4 teaspoon salt
> Pinch of cayenne
> 4 salmon fillets with skin (about 5 ounces each), rinsed and patted dry

Lightly spray the grill rack with cooking spray. Preheat the grill on medium high.

Meanwhile, in a food processor or blender, process the sauce ingredients until chunky. Cover and refrigerate until ready to serve.

In a small bowl, stir together the cumin, coriander, salt, and cayenne. Sprinkle the mixture onto the flesh side of the fish. Using your fingertips, gently press the mixture so it adheres to the fish.

Grill the fish for 5 to 7 minutes on each side, or to the desired doneness. Remove the skin if desired (tongs work well for this). Serve the fish with the sauce.

Cook's Tip: Grill salmon with the skin still on so it doesn't fall apart when you turn it on the grill. The skin comes off easily once the fish is cooked.

PER SERVING

calories 256	sodium 332 mg
total fat 13.5 g	carbohydrates 3 g
saturated fat 2.5 g	fiber 1 g
trans fat 0.0 g	sugars 1 g
polyunsaturated fat 2.0 g	protein 30 g
monounsaturated fat 6.5 g	DIETARY EXCHANGES
cholesterol 63 mg	3 1/2 lean meat, 1 fat

SESAME-ORANGE SALMON

SERVES 4

A light crust of sesame seeds and an orange glaze dress up salmon in an entrée that's so easy to prepare, you can serve it any weeknight. The Asian flavors pair well with Vegetable Stir-Fry (page 414) or Stir-Fried Sugar Snap Peas (page 402).

Cooking spray
4 salmon fillets with skin (about 5 ounces each) or 4 skinless salmon fillets (about 4 ounces each), rinsed and patted dry
2 tablespoons fresh orange juice and 1/2 cup fresh orange juice, divided use
3 tablespoons sesame seeds
1 tablespoon grated orange zest
1/4 teaspoon salt-free lemon pepper
1 teaspoon soy sauce (lowest sodium available)
1/2 teaspoon toasted sesame oil

Preheat the oven to 425°F. Line a 13 x 9 x 2-inch baking pan with aluminum foil. Lightly spray with cooking spray.

Place the fish in the pan with the skin side down. Brush the top of the fish with 2 tablespoons orange juice.

In a small bowl, stir together the sesame seeds, orange zest, and lemon pepper. Sprinkle over the top of the fish.

Bake for 10 to 12 minutes, or until the fish is cooked to the desired doneness. Remove the skin if desired (tongs work well for this).

Meanwhile, pour the remaining 1/2 cup orange juice into a small saucepan. Cook over medium high heat for 4 minutes, or until reduced by about half (to 1/4 cup). Remove from the heat.

Whisk in the soy sauce and sesame oil. Drizzle over the fish.

Cook's Tip on Toasted Sesame Oil: Widely used in Asian and Indian cuisines, this polyunsaturated oil is also called Asian sesame oil or fragrant toasted sesame oil.

PER SERVING

calories 235	carbohydrates 5 g
total fat 10.5 g	fiber 1 g
saturated fat 2.0 g	sugars 4 g
trans fat 0.0 g	protein 29 g
polyunsaturated fat 3.0 g	DIETARY EXCHANGES
monounsaturated fat 3.5 g	1/2 fruit, 3 1/2 lean
cholesterol 60 mg	meat
sodium 134 mg	

SALMON CAKES WITH CREOLE AÏOLI

SERVES 4

Skip the tartar sauce this time and serve these salmon cakes with a spicy aïoli—similar to mayonnaise, but garlicky. It's also supremely good with grilled fish or chicken.

(continued)

Cooking spray

Salmon Cakes

 1 5-ounce vacuum-sealed pouch boneless,
   skinless pink salmon, flaked

 1/2 cup whole-wheat panko (Japanese-style
   bread crumbs)

 1/2 cup finely chopped red bell pepper

 1/4 cup finely chopped green bell pepper

 2 large egg whites

 2 tablespoons fat-free milk

 1 small fresh jalapeño, finely chopped
   (optional; see Cook's Tip on Handling
   Hot Chiles, page 24)

Aïoli

 1/3 cup fat-free sour cream

 2 tablespoons light mayonnaise

 2 teaspoons Dijon mustard (coarse-grain
   preferred) (lowest sodium available)

 1 teaspoon Louisiana-style hot-pepper sauce

 1/2 medium garlic clove, minced

Preheat the oven to 375°F. Lightly spray a baking sheet with cooking spray.

In a medium bowl, stir together the salmon cake ingredients. Form into 8 patties, each about 2 1/2 inches in diameter and about 1/2 inch thick. Arrange the cakes on the baking sheet. Lightly spray the tops with cooking spray.

Bake for about 22 minutes, or until the cakes are golden brown.

Meanwhile, in a small bowl, whisk together the aïoli ingredients. Serve with the salmon cakes.

PER SERVING

calories 124	**carbohydrates** 12 g
total fat 3.5 g	fiber 1 g
saturated fat 1.0 g	sugars 3 g
trans fat 0.0 g	**protein** 11 g
polyunsaturated fat 1.5 g	**DIETARY EXCHANGES**
monounsaturated fat 0.5 g	1 starch, 1 1/2 lean
cholesterol 19 mg	meat
sodium 361 mg	

SAUTÉED LEMON-GARLIC SARDINES AND FENNEL WITH FETTUCCINE

SERVES 4

Sardines are named after Sardinia, the Italian island where large schools of these fish were once found. Sardines are a very good source of omega-3s, important nutrients for good heart health. Serve this dish with a dark green, leafy salad with Zesty Tomato Dressing (page 105).

 4 ounces dried whole-grain fettuccine,
   linguine, or penne

 1 teaspoon olive oil and 2 teaspoons olive oil,
   divided use

 1/2 cup whole-wheat panko (Japanese-style
   bread crumbs)

 3 tablespoons shallots, finely chopped

 2 medium garlic cloves, finely chopped

 1 teaspoon grated lemon zest (optional)

 1 pound medium fennel bulbs, thinly sliced

 1/2 cup semi-dry white wine (Pinot Grigio or
   Pinot Blanc preferred), or 1/2 cup fat-
   free, low-sodium vegetable broth, such
   as on page 36

 1 teaspoon dried marjoram, crumbled

 12 ounces fresh or frozen sardine fillets, cut
   into 1/2-inch pieces

 1/2 cup chopped Italian (flat-leaf) parsley

 1/8 teaspoon crushed red pepper flakes or to
   taste (optional)

Prepare the pasta using the package directions, omitting the salt. Drain well in a colander, reserving 1/2 cup of the cooking liquid. Cover the pasta to keep warm. Set the pasta and cooking liquid aside.

Meanwhile, in a large nonstick skillet, heat 1 teaspoon oil over medium-high heat, swirling to coat the bottom. Cook the panko for about 3 to 5 minutes, or until golden brown, stirring constantly. Transfer to a small bowl. Wipe the skillet clean with paper towels.

In the same skillet, still over medium-high heat, heat the remaining 2 teaspoons oil, swirling to coat the bottom. Cook the shallots for 2 to

3 minutes, or until fragrant, stirring frequently. Stir in the garlic and lemon zest. Cook for 1 to 2 minutes, or until fragrant, stirring frequently.

Stir in the sliced fennel. Cook for 4 to 6 minutes, or until translucent and very tender, stirring occasionally.

Pour in the wine, stirring to combine. Reduce the heat to medium. Cook for 2 to 3 minutes, stirring frequently. Add the fish and marjoram. Cook for 3 to 4 minutes, or until the fish just turns opaque. Reduce the heat to medium low. Turn over the fish. Cook for 1 to 2 minutes, or until heated through. Stir in the pasta, parsley, panko, and 1/3 cup of the reserved cooking liquid. Cook for 1 to 2 minutes, stirring frequently to coat the pasta with the sauce. Stir in the remaining cooking liquid if needed. Just before serving, sprinkle with the red pepper flakes.

Cook's Tip: If you have trouble finding fresh sardine fillets for this recipe, you can substitute 12 ounces canned very low sodium albacore tuna that's packed in water. Try to avoid canned sardine fillets as they can be high in sodium, especially if the label says "smoked."

PER SERVING

calories 362	carbohydrates 39 g
total fat 12.5 g	fiber 8 g
saturated fat 2.0 g	sugars 2 g
trans fat 0.0 g	protein 25 g
polyunsaturated fat 3.0 g	DIETARY EXCHANGES
monounsaturated fat 6.0 g	2 starch, 2 vegetable,
cholesterol 55 mg	2 1/2 lean meat, 1/2 fat
sodium 179 mg	

YELLOWTAIL SNAPPER À L'ORANGE

SERVES 6

Cooking this one-dish entrée is as easy as 1-2-3 when all you need to do is (1) put the fish in a casserole dish, (2) pour the sauce over the fish, and (3) bake.

    Cooking spray
    1 1/2 pounds yellowtail snapper, branzino, or
       flounder fillets, rinsed and patted dry,
       cut into 6 pieces

    1 teaspoon grated orange zest
    2 tablespoons fresh orange juice
    1 teaspoon canola or corn oil
    Pepper to taste
    1/8 teaspoon ground nutmeg

Preheat the oven to 350°F. Lightly spray a 13 x 9 x 2-inch baking dish with cooking spray.

Arrange the fish in the baking dish.

In a small bowl, whisk together the orange zest, orange juice, oil, and pepper. Pour over the fish. Sprinkle the nutmeg over the fish.

Bake for 20 to 30 minutes, or until the fish flakes easily when tested with a fork.

PER SERVING

calories 119	sodium 49 mg
total fat 2.5 g	carbohydrates 1 g
saturated fat 0.5 g	fiber 0 g
trans fat 0.0 g	sugars 0 g
polyunsaturated fat 0.5 g	protein 22 g
monounsaturated fat 1.0 g	DIETARY EXCHANGES
cholesterol 40 mg	3 lean meat

CRISPY BAKED FILLET OF SOLE

SERVES 6

Fish fillets absorb Asian flavor from a soy-ginger marinade and then are coated with an aromatic panko coating and baked for crispness. Brown rice and Fresh Snow Peas with Water Chestnuts (page 403) complete the meal.

Marinade
    3/4 cup finely chopped onion
    2 teaspoons grated lime zest
    1/4 cup fresh lime juice
    1 tablespoon grated peeled gingerroot
    1 tablespoon canola or corn oil
    1 tablespoon soy sauce (lowest sodium
       available)
    1/4 teaspoon pepper
    1/8 teaspoon salt

■ ■ ■

(continued)

1 1/2 pounds thin fish fillets, such as sole, rinsed and patted dry

Cooking spray

1 1/4 cups whole-wheat panko (Japanese-style bread crumbs)

2 tablespoons chopped fresh parsley

2 tablespoons finely chopped green onions

In a large shallow glass dish, whisk together the marinade ingredients. Add the fish, turning to coat. Cover and refrigerate for 15 minutes to 1 hour, turning occasionally.

Preheat the oven to 450°F. Lightly spray a 13 x 9 x 2-inch glass baking dish with cooking spray.

In a large shallow dish, stir together the panko, parsley, and green onions. Drain the fish, discarding the marinade. Dip the fish into the panko mixture, turning to coat and gently shaking off any excess. Transfer to the baking dish.

Bake for 15 to 18 minutes, or until the fish flakes easily when tested with a fork.

PER SERVING

calories 165	**sodium** 226 mg
total fat 2.0 g	**carbohydrates** 12 g
saturated fat 0.5 g	fiber 2 g
trans fat 0.0 g	sugars 1 g
polyunsaturated fat 0.5 g	**protein** 24 g
monounsaturated fat 0.5 g	**DIETARY EXCHANGES**
cholesterol 54 mg	1 starch, 3 lean meat

SOLE WITH WALNUTS AND WHITE WINE

SERVES 4

White sauce, wine, and walnuts bring the wow factor to this dish. Serve with steamed broccoli and a whole grain such as bulgur or brown rice.

Cooking spray

4 thin fish fillets, such as sole, (about 4 ounces each), rinsed and patted dry

1/2 cup dry white wine and 1/2 cup dry white wine (regular or nonalcoholic), divided use

1/2 cup fat-free, low-sodium chicken broth and 1/2 cup fat-free, low-sodium chicken broth, such as on page 36, divided use

Dash of cayenne

2 tablespoons light tub margarine

2 tablespoons all-purpose flour

1/4 cup fat-free milk

Dash of pepper (white preferred)

2 tablespoons chopped walnuts, dry-roasted

Sprigs of fresh parsley (optional)

Preheat the oven to 325°F. Lightly spray a 9-inch square baking pan with cooking spray.

Put the fish in the pan. Pour in 1/2 cup wine and 1/2 cup broth. Sprinkle the cayenne over the fish.

Bake, covered, for 20 minutes, or until the fish flakes easily when tested with a fork.

Meanwhile, in a small saucepan, melt the margarine over low heat, swirling to coat the bottom. Whisk in the flour. Cook for 1 minute, whisking occasionally. (Don't let the flour brown.) Increase the heat to medium high.

Whisk in the milk, pepper, and the remaining 1/2 cup wine and 1/2 cup broth. Cook for 3 to 4 minutes, or until the sauce has thickened, whisking constantly.

Stir in the walnuts. Reduce the heat and simmer for 1 minute. Spoon over the fish. Garnish with the parsley.

PER SERVING

calories 188	**carbohydrates** 5 g
total fat 6.0 g	fiber 0 g
saturated fat 0.5 g	sugars 1 g
trans fat 0.0 g	**protein** 23 g
polyunsaturated fat 2.5 g	**DIETARY EXCHANGES**
monounsaturated fat 2.0 g	1/2 other
cholesterol 55 mg	carbohydrate, 3 lean
sodium 148 mg	meat

SOLE WITH PARSLEY AND MINT

SERVES 4

The herb rub on the fish pairs beautifully with french-cut green beans and Couscous with Dates and Walnuts *(page 417).*

Cooking spray

2 tablespoons finely chopped fresh parsley

1 tablespoon chopped fresh mint

2 teaspoons canola or corn oil

1 medium garlic clove, chopped

1/4 teaspoon salt

4 thin fish fillets, such as sole, (about
    4 ounces each), rinsed and patted dry

Sauce

1 teaspoon light tub margarine

1 medium green onion (green part only),
    chopped

1/2 cup dry white wine (regular or
    nonalcoholic)

1/4 cup water

1/4 teaspoon pepper (white preferred)

Preheat the broiler. Lightly spray the broiler pan and rack with cooking spray.

In a small bowl, stir together the parsley, mint, oil, garlic, and salt (the mixture will be pastelike). Rub the mixture over one side of the fish.

Broil the fish with the seasoned side up about 4 inches from the heat for 5 to 8 minutes, or until it flakes easily when tested with a fork.

Meanwhile, in a medium nonstick skillet, melt the margarine over medium-high heat, swirling to coat the bottom. Cook the green onion for 1 to 2 minutes, stirring frequently. Stir in the wine, water, and pepper. Cook for 2 to 3 minutes, or until heated through. Spoon over the fish.

Cook's Tip on White Pepper: Milder in flavor than black pepper, white pepper is often used because its color blends in with a white or light-colored sauce. You can buy whole white peppercorns or ground white pepper.

PER SERVING (WITH OPTIONAL SAUCE)

calories 153	**sodium** 250 mg
total fat 4.0 g	**carbohydrates** 1 g
saturated fat 0.5 g	fiber 0 g
trans fat 0.0 g	sugars 0 g
polyunsaturated fat 1.0 g	**protein** 22 g
monounsaturated fat 2.0 g	**DIETARY EXCHANGES**
cholesterol 54 mg	3 lean meat

PER SERVING (WITHOUT OPTIONAL SAUCE)

calories 126	**sodium** 239 mg
total fat 3.5 g	**carbohydrates** 1 g
saturated fat 0.5 g	fiber 0 g
trans fat 0.0 g	sugars 0 g
polyunsaturated fat 1.0 g	**protein** 22 g
monounsaturated fat 1.5 g	**DIETARY EXCHANGES**
cholesterol 54 mg	3 lean meat

SOLE PARMESAN

SERVES 4

Mild sole fillets are baked with an Italian-seasoned coating, then topped with cheese and a quick basil-scented tomato sauce. If your family likes chicken Parmesan, then they'll enjoy this dish. If you can't find farro, serve the sole with whole-grain pasta instead.

Cooking spray

1 cup uncooked farro

2 large egg whites, lightly beaten with a fork

3/4 cup plain dry bread crumbs (lowest
    sodium available)

1 teaspoon dried oregano, crumbled

1 teaspoon garlic powder

1/4 teaspoon pepper

4 sole fillets (about 4 ounces each), rinsed
    and patted dry

1/2 cup shredded low-fat mozzarella cheese

1/4 cup shredded or grated Parmesan cheese

1 teaspoon olive oil

1 small garlic clove, minced

1/2 cup no-salt-added tomato sauce

2 tablespoons chopped fresh basil

(continued)

Preheat the oven to 400°F. Line a baking sheet with aluminum foil. Lightly spray with cooking spray.

Prepare the farro using the package directions, omitting the salt. Fluff with a fork. Set aside.

Meanwhile, pour the egg whites into a shallow dish. In a separate shallow dish, stir together the bread crumbs, oregano, garlic powder, and pepper. Set the dishes and baking sheet in a row, assembly-line fashion. Dip the fish in the egg whites, then in the bread crumb mixture, turning to coat at each step and gently shaking off any excess. Transfer to the baking sheet. Lightly spray the top of the fish with cooking spray.

Bake for 10 minutes, or until the fish flakes easily when tested with a fork. Sprinkle the mozzarella and Parmesan over the fish. Bake for 2 minutes, or until the cheeses have melted.

Meanwhile, in a small saucepan, heat the oil over low heat, swirling to coat the bottom. Cook the garlic for 5 to 10 seconds, stirring occasionally.

Stir in the tomato sauce and basil. Increase the heat to medium high and bring to a simmer, stirring occasionally. Reduce the heat and simmer for about 5 minutes, stirring occasionally. Spoon over the fish. Serve with the farro.

Cook's Tip: Keep your pantry stocked with no-salt-added canned products such as tomato sauce, tomato paste, and diced and whole tomatoes. Tomato purée, however, is already so low in sodium that you won't find a no-salt-added version.

PER SERVING

calories 435	carbohydrates 52 g
total fat 6.5 g	fiber 5 g
saturated fat 2.0 g	sugars 3 g
trans fat 0.0 g	protein 39 g
polyunsaturated fat 1.0 g	DIETARY EXCHANGES
monounsaturated fat 2.0 g	3 starch, 1 vegetable,
cholesterol 63 mg	4 lean meat
sodium 487 mg	

TANDOORI-SPICED SWORDFISH-AND-VEGETABLE KEBABS
SERVES 4

Swordfish marinated in Tandoori spices, then threaded on skewers and grilled, makes a delicious complete meal. Serve with brown basmati rice and Raita (page 430).

Marinade
  1 cup fat-free plain Greek yogurt
  1/4 cup fresh lemon juice (about 1 large lemon)
  2 tablespoons minced fresh cilantro and 1 teaspoon chopped fresh cilantro, divided use
  1 small fresh jalapeño, seeds and ribs discarded, minced (optional; see Cook's Tip on Handling Hot Chiles, page 24)
  1 tablespoon chopped fresh mint
  1 tablespoon grated peeled gingerroot
  2 teaspoons garam marsala
  1/4 teaspoon ground turmeric

■ ■ ■

Cooking spray
  1 1-pound swordfish steak, rinsed and patted dry, cut into 12 1-inch cubes
  2 medium red or green bell peppers, or one of each, cut into 8 squares
  1 large zucchini, cut crosswise into 8 pieces
  8 medium button mushrooms
  8 cherry tomatoes
  2 medium lemons, each cut into 4 wedges

In a large bowl, whisk together the marinade ingredients. Add the fish, turning to coat. Cover and refrigerate for 25 to 30 minutes, turning occasionally.

Meanwhile, soak four 12-inch wooden skewers for at least 10 minutes in cold water to keep them from charring, or use metal skewers. Set aside.

Lightly spray the grill rack with cooking spray. Preheat the grill on high.

For each kebab, thread each skewer with 3 fish cubes, 2 bell pepper squares, 2 zucchini slices, 2 mushrooms, and 2 tomatoes.

Grill for 3 to 4 minutes on each side, or until the fish is the desired doneness. Serve the kebabs with the lemon wedges.

Cook's Tip: Substitute tuna, cod, or any firm white fish for the swordfish.

PER SERVING

calories 188	carbohydrates 9 g
total fat 7.0 g	fiber 3 g
saturated fat 1.5 g	sugars 6 g
trans fat 0.0 g	protein 22 g
polyunsaturated fat 1.5 g	DIETARY EXCHANGES
monounsaturated fat 3.0 g	2 vegetable, 3 lean
cholesterol 65 mg	meat
sodium 94 mg	

COCONUT-RUM BAKED FISH

SERVES 4

Take one bite of this sweet-and-crunchy macadamia-crusted fish and you'll want to make Hawaii your next destination. Stir-Fried Sugar Snap Peas (page 402) and slices of fresh pineapple make tasty accompaniments.

2 tablespoons rum or 1/2 teaspoon rum extract

1 teaspoon grated lime zest

1 tablespoon fresh lime juice

1/2 teaspoon coconut extract

4 tilapia fillets (about 4 ounces each), rinsed and patted dry

Cooking spray

1/2 cup egg substitute

1/4 cup all-purpose flour

1/3 cup whole-wheat panko (Japanese-style bread crumbs)

2 tablespoons shredded sweetened coconut

2 tablespoons chopped macadamia nuts

In a medium glass dish, whisk together the rum, lime zest, lime juice, and coconut extract. Add the fish, turning to coat. Cover and refrigerate for 10 minutes to 1 hour.

Preheat the oven to 400°F. Lightly spray a baking sheet with cooking spray.

Put the egg substitute and flour in separate shallow dishes. In a third shallow dish, stir together the panko, coconut, and macadamia nuts. Set the dishes and baking sheet in a row, assembly-line fashion. Drain the fish, discarding the marinade. Dip the fish in the egg substitute, then in the flour, and finally in the panko mixture, turning to coat at each step and gently shaking off any excess. Transfer to the baking sheet. Lightly spray the tops with cooking spray.

Bake for 10 to 12 minutes, or until the fish is light golden brown and flakes easily when tested with a fork.

PER SERVING

calories 218	sodium 137 mg
total fat 6.0 g	carbohydrates 13 g
saturated fat 2.0 g	fiber 2 g
trans fat 0.0 g	sugars 2 g
polyunsaturated fat 0.5 g	protein 28 g
monounsaturated fat 3.0 g	DIETARY EXCHANGES
cholesterol 57 mg	1 starch, 3 lean meat

BAKED TILAPIA WITH SAUSAGE-FLECKED RICE

SERVES 4

A small amount of low-fat sausage has a large impact on the flavor of this dish. The rice is similar to the New Orleans favorite, dirty rice.

1/3 cup uncooked brown rice

Cooking spray

4 tilapia fillets (about 4 ounces each), rinsed and patted dry

1/4 teaspoon dried thyme, crumbled

1/8 teaspoon salt and 1/4 teaspoon salt, divided use

Paprika to taste

3 ounces low-fat bulk breakfast sausage

1 medium red bell pepper, finely chopped

1/2 cup finely chopped green onions

1/4 cup finely chopped fresh parsley

1/8 teaspoon cayenne (optional)

(continued)

Prepare the rice using the package directions, omitting the salt and margarine.

Meanwhile, preheat the oven to 400°F. Line a baking sheet with aluminum foil. Lightly spray with cooking spray.

Put the fish on the baking sheet. In a small bowl, stir together the thyme, 1/8 teaspoon salt, and paprika. Sprinkle on top of the fish.

Bake for 12 minutes, or until the fish flakes easily when tested with a fork.

Meanwhile, in a medium nonstick skillet, cook the sausage over medium-high heat for 2 minutes, stirring to break up the larger pieces.

Stir in the bell pepper and green onions. Cook for 1 minute, or until the sausage begins to lightly brown, stirring constantly. Remove from the heat.

Stir in the rice, parsley, cayenne, and the remaining 1/4 teaspoon salt. Serve with the fish.

Cook's Tip on Buying Bulk Sausage: Bulk sausage is ground meat that hasn't been stuffed into a casing. Look for sausage that's packaged in a cylinder-shaped roll rather than in individual casings.

PER SERVING

calories 210	carbohydrates 16 g
total fat 3.0 g	fiber 2 g
saturated fat 1.0 g	sugars 2 g
trans fat 0.0 g	**protein** 28 g
polyunsaturated fat 0.5 g	**DIETARY EXCHANGES**
monounsaturated fat 0.5 g	1 starch, 3 1/2 lean
cholesterol 67 mg	meat
sodium 414 mg	

BAKED TILAPIA WITH TARRAGON BREAD CRUMBS

SERVES 4

Herbed panko provides a crispy coating for this mild fish, which is baked at a high temperature. Enjoy with Ratatouille *(page 414).*

Cooking spray
4 tilapia fillets (about 4 ounces each), rinsed and patted dry
1 tablespoon red wine vinegar
1 tablespoon olive oil and 1 tablespoon plus 1 teaspoon olive oil (extra-virgin preferred), divided use
1/4 teaspoon garlic powder
1/4 teaspoon dried basil, crumbled
1/4 teaspoon dried oregano, crumbled
1/2 cup whole-wheat panko (Japanese-style bread crumbs)
1/2 teaspoon dried tarragon, crumbled
Paprika to taste
1/8 teaspoon salt
1/8 teaspoon pepper

Preheat the oven to 400°F. Line a baking sheet with aluminum foil. Lightly spray with cooking spray.

Put the fish on the baking sheet. In a small bowl, whisk together the vinegar, 1 tablespoon oil, the garlic powder, basil, and oregano. Spoon over the fish.

In a separate small bowl, stir together the panko, tarragon, and paprika. Sprinkle over the fish.

Bake for 12 minutes, or until the fish flakes easily when tested with a fork.

Transfer the fish to plates. Drizzle with the remaining 1 tablespoon plus 1 teaspoon oil. Sprinkle with the salt and pepper.

PER SERVING

calories 216	sodium 144 mg
total fat 10.0 g	**carbohydrates** 7 g
saturated fat 2.0 g	fiber 1 g
trans fat 0.0 g	sugars 0 g
polyunsaturated fat 1.0 g	**protein** 24 g
monounsaturated fat 6.5 g	**DIETARY EXCHANGES**
cholesterol 57 mg	1/2 starch, 3 lean meat

TILAPIA AMANDINE

SERVES 4

Hints of tart, sweet, and nutty provide the flavor for this quick and easy dish. Try it with a whole grain and Pan-Roasted Broccoli (page 376) or Garlicky Broccolini with Charred Cherry Tomatoes (page 378).

1/4 cup all-purpose flour
1/2 teaspoon paprika
1/8 teaspoon pepper
4 tilapia fillets (about 4 ounces each), rinsed
   and patted dry
1/4 cup water
2 tablespoons fresh lemon juice
1 tablespoon light tub margarine
2 teaspoons Worcestershire sauce (lowest
   sodium available)
1/4 teaspoon salt
1/4 cup sliced almonds, dry-roasted

In a shallow dish, stir together the flour, paprika, and pepper. Dip the fish in the mixture, turning to coat and gently shaking off any excess. Transfer to a plate.

In a large nonstick skillet, cook the fish over medium heat for 5 minutes on each side, or until it flakes easily when tested with a fork. Transfer to plates.

Meanwhile, in a small bowl, whisk together the remaining ingredients except the almonds. Pour into the skillet, scraping the bottom and side with a rubber scraper to dislodge any browned bits. Cook for 2 minutes, or until the liquid is reduced by half (to about 1/4 cup). Spoon over the fish. Sprinkle with the almonds.

PER SERVING

calories 186	**sodium** 239 mg
total fat 6.0 g	**carbohydrates** 9 g
saturated fat 1.0 g	fiber 1 g
trans fat 0.0 g	sugars 1 g
polyunsaturated fat 1.5 g	**protein** 25 g
monounsaturated fat 3.0 g	**DIETARY EXCHANGES**
cholesterol 57 mg	1/2 starch, 3 lean meat

TILAPIA WITH LEMON-CAPER SAUCE

SERVES 4

One skillet is all you need to cook this fish, enveloped in a creamy lemon sauce. Serve with steamed asparagus and quinoa or whole-wheat couscous.

1/4 cup all-purpose flour
1 tablespoon grated lemon zest and
   1 teaspoon grated lemon zest, divided
   use
1 tablespoon fresh lemon juice
1 teaspoon dried parsley, crumbled
1/4 teaspoon pepper
4 tilapia fillets (about 4 ounces each), rinsed
   and patted dry
2 teaspoons olive oil
1/2 cup fat-free, low-sodium chicken broth,
   such as on page 36
1 tablespoon capers, drained

In a shallow dish, stir together the flour, 1 tablespoon lemon zest, the parsley, and pepper. Dip the fish in the flour mixture, turning to coat and gently shaking off any excess. Transfer to a plate.

In a large nonstick skillet, heat the oil over medium-high heat, swirling to coat the bottom. Cook the fish for 1 minute on each side, or until lightly browned.

Add the broth, capers, lemon juice, and the remaining 1 teaspoon lemon zest (don't stir). Bring to a simmer. Reduce the heat and simmer, covered, for 7 to 8 minutes, or until the fish flakes easily when tested with a fork. Transfer the fish to plates. Spoon the sauce over the fish.

PER SERVING

calories 162	**sodium** 128 mg
total fat 4.5 g	**carbohydrates** 7 g
saturated fat 1.0 g	fiber 1 g
trans fat 0.0 g	sugars 0 g
polyunsaturated fat 0.5 g	**protein** 24 g
monounsaturated fat 2.0 g	**DIETARY EXCHANGES**
cholesterol 57 mg	1/2 starch, 3 lean meat

TILAPIA WITH YELLOW TOMATOES AND CHARD

SERVES 6

The flavor of the wine sauce is heightened with fresh herb and citrus and is used in two ways—to infuse the fish as it bakes and as a finishing sauce for the whole dish. Serve with Brussels Sprouts and Pistachios *(page 379).*

Cooking spray
1 teaspoon olive oil
1 large onion, finely chopped
3 medium garlic cloves, minced
3 tablespoons water and (optional)
    2 tablespoons water, divided use
3 cups chopped peeled yellow tomatoes
1/2 cup dry white wine (regular or
    nonalcoholic)
10 ounces Swiss chard, stems discarded,
    coarsely torn
2 tablespoons finely chopped fresh dillweed
2 tablespoons chopped fresh parsley
2 tablespoons fresh lemon juice
6 tilapia fillets (about 4 ounces each), rinsed
    and patted dry
1/2 teaspoon pepper
2 tablespoons cornstarch (optional)

Preheat the oven to 400°F. Lightly spray a 13 x 9 x 2-inch glass baking dish with cooking spray.

In a large nonstick skillet, heat the oil over medium-high heat, swirling to coat the bottom. Cook the onion and garlic for 2 minutes, stirring frequently. Pour in 3 tablespoons water. Cook until all the water has evaporated, stirring constantly.

Stir in the tomatoes and wine. Using the back of a spoon, crush the tomatoes. Cook for 7 to 8 minutes, or until the liquid is reduced slightly.

Stir in the chard. Cook, covered, for 3 to 5 minutes, or until the chard is wilted. Remove from the heat. Stir in the dillweed, parsley, and lemon juice.

Pour half the sauce into the baking dish. Place the fish on the sauce. Sprinkle the pepper over the fish. Fold each fillet in half. Top with the remaining sauce.

Bake, covered, for 15 to 18 minutes, or until the fish flakes easily when tested with a fork. Transfer the fish to plates.

If the sauce is the consistency you like, spoon it over the fish. If you prefer a thicker sauce, cover the fish to keep warm. Pour the sauce into a large nonstick skillet. Put the cornstarch in a small bowl. Add the remaining 2 tablespoons water, whisking to dissolve. Stir into the sauce. Bring to a boil over medium-high heat. Cook until the desired consistency, stirring constantly. Spoon the sauce over the fish.

Cook's Tip on Cooking Wine: Avoid wine bottled and labeled as cooking wine. It's loaded with sodium. It won't do your dish—or your body—any good.

Cook's Tip on Peeling Tomatoes: To peel tomatoes easily, fill a medium saucepan with water and bring to a boil. Boil the tomatoes for 45 seconds to 1 minute, or until their skins start to wrinkle and split. Plunge the tomatoes in a bowl of ice water to stop the cooking process. The skins should slip off easily.

PER SERVING

calories 160	carbohydrates 8 g
total fat 3.0 g	fiber 2 g
saturated fat 1.0 g	sugars 3 g
trans fat 0.0 g	**protein** 25 g
polyunsaturated fat 0.5 g	**DIETARY EXCHANGES**
monounsaturated fat 1.0 g	2 vegetable, 3 lean
cholesterol 57 mg	meat
sodium 179 mg	

GRILLED FISH WITH MEDITERRANEAN SALSA

SERVES 4

Grill and chill with saucy tilapia fillets inspired by heart-healthy Mediterranean cuisine. Serve with some grilled zucchini spears and whole-grain pita wedges warmed on the grill.

Cooking spray
1 small Italian plum (Roma) tomato, diced

1 medium green onion, thinly sliced

2 tablespoons crumbled fat-free feta cheese

1 tablespoon sliced kalamata olives

2 teaspoons olive oil

1 teaspoon dried oregano, crumbled

1 teaspoon grated lemon zest

2 medium garlic cloves, minced

1/4 teaspoon pepper

4 tilapia fillets (about 4 ounces each), rinsed and patted dry

1 medium lemon, cut into 4 wedges

Lightly spray the grill rack with cooking spray. Preheat the grill on medium high.

Meanwhile, in a small bowl, stir together the tomato, green onion, feta, and olives. Cover and refrigerate until serving time.

In a separate small bowl, stir together the oil, oregano, lemon zest, garlic, and pepper. Spread the mixture over both sides of the fish. Using your fingertips, gently press the mixture so it adheres to the fish.

Grill the fish for 4 to 5 minutes. Turn over the fish. Put the lemon wedges on the grill. Grill the fish and lemon wedges for 4 to 5 minutes, or until the fish flakes easily when tested with a fork and the lemon wedges are slightly charred. Transfer to plates. Spoon the tomato mixture onto the fish.

Cook's Tip: If you grill fish frequently, you may want to buy a grilling basket designed for fish. It's especially useful for thin, delicate fish fillets, such as tilapia. A perforated flat grilling pan would work, too, and is useful for grilling other types of food as well.

PER SERVING

calories 152	sodium 177 mg
total fat 5.0 g	**carbohydrates** 3 g
saturated fat 1.0 g	fiber 1 g
trans fat 0.0 g	sugars 1 g
polyunsaturated fat 0.5 g	**protein** 24 g
monounsaturated fat 2.5 g	**DIETARY EXCHANGES**
cholesterol 57 mg	3 lean meat

ALMOND-TOPPED BAKED TROUT

SERVES 4

Dinner will be ready in minutes when you prepare this simple fish dish. While the fish is cooking, you can roast asparagus on another oven rack for a side dish that will be ready at the same time.

Cooking spray

4 trout fillets with skin (about 5 ounces each), rinsed and patted dry

1/4 cup whole-wheat panko (Japanese-style bread crumbs)

2 tablespoons shredded or grated Parmesan cheese

1/2 teaspoon dried basil, crumbled

1/2 teaspoon paprika

1/4 teaspoon garlic powder

1/4 teaspoon pepper

1/4 cup sliced almonds, dry-roasted

1 medium lemon, cut into 4 wedges

Preheat the oven to 400°F. Lightly spray a large baking sheet with cooking spray.

Place the fish with the skin side down on the baking sheet.

In a small bowl, stir together the panko, Parmesan, basil, paprika, garlic powder, and pepper. Spoon over the fish. Using your fingertips, gently press the mixture so it adheres to the fish.

Spoon the almonds over the panko mixture, lightly pressing so they adhere. Lightly spray with cooking spray.

Bake for 10 to 15 minutes, or until the fish flakes easily when tested with a fork. Remove the skin if desired (tongs work well for this).

Serve the fish with the lemon wedges.

PER SERVING

calories 218	**carbohydrates** 6 g
total fat 8.0 g	fiber 1 g
saturated fat 1.5 g	sugars 1 g
trans fat 0.0 g	**protein** 29 g
polyunsaturated fat 2.5 g	**DIETARY EXCHANGES**
monounsaturated fat 3.5 g	1/2 starch, 3 1/2 lean
cholesterol 77 mg	meat
sodium 88 mg	

BAKED TROUT WITH TARTAR SAUCE

SERVES 4

Panko and nutritious chia seeds give this trout a tasty, crisp coating, which is brightened by orange zest. Prepare Roasted Brussels Sprouts *(page 378) as a side dish.*

Olive oil cooking spray
1 teaspoon onion powder
1/4 teaspoon paprika
4 trout fillets with skin (about 5 ounces each), rinsed and patted dry
3 tablespoons all-purpose flour
1 large egg white, lightly beaten with a fork
1 teaspoon fresh orange juice

Coating

3/4 cup whole-wheat panko (Japanese-style bread crumbs)
3 tablespoons chia seeds (optional)
1 tablespoon chopped fresh dillweed
2 medium garlic cloves, minced
1 teaspoon grated orange zest
1/8 teaspoon salt
1/8 teaspoon cayenne

Tartar Sauce

1/4 cup light mayonnaise
1 tablespoon fat-free sour cream
1 tablespoon drained sweet pickle relish
1 tablespoon finely chopped red bell pepper
1 teaspoon fresh lemon juice
1/8 teaspoon paprika

■ ■ ■

1 small orange, cut into 4 wedges

Preheat the oven to 400°F. Line a baking sheet with aluminum foil. Lightly spray with cooking spray.

Sprinkle the onion powder and paprika over the fish.

Put the flour on a plate. In a shallow dish, whisk together the egg white and orange juice. Set the plate, dish, and baking sheet in a row, assembly-line fashion. Dip the flesh side of the fish in the flour, then in the egg white mixture, gently shaking off any excess. Transfer the fish with the skin side down to the baking sheet.

On a shallow plate, stir together the coating ingredients. Pat on the top of the fish. Lightly spray the top of the fish with cooking spray.

Bake for 10 minutes, or until the top is lightly browned and the fish flakes easily when tested with a fork.

Meanwhile, in a small bowl, stir together the tartar sauce ingredients.

Carefully place each piece of fish with the skin side up on a separate plate. Let cool for about 3 minutes. Remove the skin if desired (tongs work well for this). Turn over the fish. Serve with the tartar sauce and orange wedges.

Cook's Tip on Storing Fresh Dillweed: To store fresh dillweed, put it in a resealable plastic bag and refrigerate it in the crisper drawer. For longer storage, rinse the dillweed, pat it dry, and freeze it in an airtight container.

PER SERVING

calories 281	carbohydrates 20 g
total fat 8.5 g	fiber 2 g
saturated fat 1.0 g	sugars 2 g
trans fat 0.0 g	**protein** 30 g
polyunsaturated fat 4.0 g	**DIETARY EXCHANGES**
monounsaturated fat 2.0 g	1 1/2 starch, 3 1/2 lean
cholesterol 81 mg	meat
sodium 309 mg	

CRISP PAN-SEARED TROUT WITH GREEN ONIONS

SERVES 4

Rich in omega-3 fatty acids, trout gets dressed for dinner by putting on a crisp coat made of flour and Chinese five-spice powder. Serve with soba noodles tossed with a small amount of toasted sesame oil and steamed or Sweet Lemon Snow Peas *(page 402).*

3 tablespoons red wine vinegar
2 teaspoons soy sauce (lowest sodium available)
1 teaspoon toasted sesame oil

1/4 cup all-purpose flour

1 teaspoon five-spice powder

4 trout fillets with skin (about 5 ounces
each), rinsed and patted dry

2 teaspoons canola or corn oil

Cooking spray

8 medium green onions (green part only),
thinly sliced

In a small bowl, whisk together the vinegar, soy sauce, and sesame oil. Set aside.

In a shallow dish, stir together the flour and five-spice powder. Dip the fish in the flour mixture to coat the flesh side of the fish, gently shaking off any excess. Transfer to a plate.

In a large nonstick skillet, heat the canola oil over medium-high heat, swirling to coat the bottom. Cook the fish with the flesh side down for 3 to 4 minutes, or until browned. Remove from the heat.

Lightly spray the skin side of the fish with cooking spray. Cook with the skin side down for 3 to 4 minutes, or until the fish flakes easily when tested with a fork.

Transfer the fish with the skin side up to plates. Let cool for about 1 minute. Remove the skin if desired (tongs work well for this). Turn over the fish. Sprinkle with the green onions. Pour the vinegar mixture over the fish.

PER SERVING

calories 235	carbohydrates 11 g
total fat 8.0 g	fiber 2 g
saturated fat 1.5 g	sugars 2 g
trans fat 0.0 g	protein 27 g
polyunsaturated fat 2.5 g	DIETARY EXCHANGES
monounsaturated fat 3.5 g	1/2 starch, 1 vegetable,
cholesterol 75 mg	3 1/2 lean meat
sodium 115 mg	

TROUT WITH FRESH TOMATOES AND CAPERS

SERVES 4

You get maximum flavor for minimal effort when you prepare this trout. The brief amount of cooking integrates the fresh vegetables into a sauce that really makes a statement. Serve with a side of brown rice or whole-grain pasta and Minted Peas (page 397).

4 rainbow trout or tilapia fillets (about
4 ounces each), rinsed and patted dry

4 medium green onions, chopped

1/2 medium tomato, finely chopped

2 tablespoons capers, drained

1 teaspoon grated lemon zest

2 tablespoons fresh lemon juice

1 tablespoon olive oil (extra-virgin preferred)

3/4 teaspoon dried oregano, crumbled

1 medium garlic clove, minced

1/4 teaspoon salt

Heat a large nonstick skillet over medium-high heat. Cook the fish for 3 minutes. Turn over the fish.

In a small bowl, stir together the remaining ingredients. Spoon over the fish. Cook for 3 minutes, or until the fish flakes easily when tested with a fork.

PER SERVING

calories 183	sodium 314 mg
total fat 7.5 g	carbohydrates 4 g
saturated fat 1.5 g	fiber 2 g
trans fat 0.0 g	sugars 2 g
polyunsaturated fat 2.0 g	protein 24 g
monounsaturated fat 4.0 g	DIETARY EXCHANGES
cholesterol 67 mg	3 lean meat

BRAISED TUNA STEAKS WITH ORANGE-CRANBERRY GLAZE

SERVES 4

Simmering lightly browned tuna steaks keeps them moist, and the rosemary-infused glaze makes them delicious. The fall flavor of the glaze make this a great match for Sweet Potato–Apple Gratin with Walnuts (page 407) or Maple-Glazed Butternut Squash (page 377).

(continued)

1/2 teaspoon ground pink peppercorns or
   1/4 teaspoon pepper
4 tuna steaks (about 4 ounces each), rinsed
   and patted dry
1 teaspoon olive oil
1 teaspoon grated orange zest
1/2 cup fresh orange juice
1/2 cup 100% cranberry juice
2 tablespoons port (optional)
1 tablespoon coarsely chopped fresh rosemary
   or 1 teaspoon dried rosemary, crushed
2 teaspoons light brown sugar

Sprinkle the pepper over both sides of the fish.

In a large nonstick skillet, heat the oil over medium-high heat, swirling to coat the bottom. Cook the fish for 1 minute on each side, or until lightly browned.

Stir in the remaining ingredients. Bring to a simmer, covered, for 7 to 9 minutes, or until the fish is the desired doneness. Transfer to plates. Cover to keep warm.

Increase the heat to medium high. Cook the remaining liquid until reduced by half (to about 1/2 cup). Pour over the fish.

PER SERVING

calories 172	sodium 53 mg
total fat 2.0 g	**carbohydrates** 10 g
saturated fat 0.5 g	fiber 0 g
trans fat 0.0 g	sugars 9 g
polyunsaturated fat 0.5 g	**protein** 28 g
monounsaturated fat 1.0 g	**DIETARY EXCHANGES**
cholesterol 44 mg	1/2 fruit, 3 lean meat

GRILLED TUNA WITH SMOKY-SWEET FRUIT SALSA

SERVES 4

Citrus-marinated tuna sizzles on the grill, then is topped with a cool but smoky fruit salsa. This pairs perfectly with a summery side salad, such as Green Bean and Tomato Toss *(page 79) or* Confetti Coleslaw *(page 84).*

Marinade
   1 teaspoon grated lime zest
   2 tablespoons fresh lime juice
   2 tablespoons fresh orange juice
   1 tablespoon chopped fresh cilantro
   1 teaspoon canola or corn oil
   1/4 teaspoon salt
   1/8 teaspoon pepper

■ ■ ■

4 tuna steaks (about 4 ounces each), rinsed
   and patted dry
Salsa
   1 8-ounce can pineapple slices in their own
      juice, drained and patted dry
   1 medium nectarine, halved
   1 medium kiwifruit, peeled and halved
   2 tablespoons diced red onion
   1 tablespoon chopped fresh cilantro
   1 teaspoon fresh lemon juice

In a large shallow glass dish, whisk together the marinade ingredients. Add the fish, turning to coat. Cover and refrigerate for 15 minutes to 1 hour, turning occasionally.

Meanwhile, preheat the grill on medium high. Grill the pineapple for about 5 minutes, or until lightly browned on one side. Turn over the pineapple. Put the nectarine and kiwifruit on the grill with the cut side down. Grill for about 5 minutes, or until all the fruit is lightly browned. Transfer to a cutting board and let cool.

Dice the pineapple, nectarine, and kiwifruit. Transfer to a medium bowl. Stir in the remaining salsa ingredients. Cover and refrigerate until serving time.

Drain the fish, discarding the marinade. Grill the fish for 5 to 7 minutes on each side, or to the desired doneness. Transfer to plates. Top with the salsa.

calories 173

total fat 1.0 g

  saturated fat 0.0 g

  trans fat 0.0 g

  polyunsaturated fat 0.5 g

  monounsaturated fat 0.0 g

cholesterol 44 mg

sodium 201 mg

carbohydrates 12 g

  fiber 2 g

  sugars 9 g

protein 28 g

DIETARY EXCHANGES

  1 fruit, 3 lean meat

ALMOND-CRUSTED TUNA STEAKS WITH HORSERADISH SAUCE

SERVES 4

This pan-seared fish cooks in just minutes so it's a go-to dish on a busy night. The tuna sits on a bed of bok choy that cooks in the same skillet, so you'll have easy cleanup and veggies for everyone, too.

Sauce

    1/3 cup fat-free sour cream

    3 teaspoons fat-free milk

    1 tablespoon grated peeled horseradish

    1 tablespoon fresh chives or green onions, thinly sliced

    1 teaspoon fresh lemon juice

    1/4 teaspoon salt

    1/2 teaspoon pepper

■ ■ ■

    3 tablespoons almonds and 1 tablespoon almonds, dry-roasted, finely chopped, divided use

    2 teaspoons all-purpose flour

    1/4 teaspoon pepper

    1/8 teaspoon salt

    4 tuna steaks (about 4 ounces each), rinsed and patted dry

    1 teaspoon and 1 teaspoon canola or corn oil, divided use

    4 cups sliced bok choy

    1 medium garlic clove, minced

In a small bowl, whisk together the sauce ingredients. Set aside.

Meanwhile, in a shallow dish, stir together 3 tablespoons almonds, the flour, pepper, and salt.

Dip the fish in the mixture, turning to coat both sides. Don't shake off any excess. Transfer to a plate.

In a large skillet, heat 1 teaspoon oil over medium-high heat, swirling to coat the bottom. Cook the bok choy for 4 minutes, or until tender-crisp, stirring frequently. Stir in the garlic. Cook for 30 seconds, stirring constantly. Remove from the heat. Sprinkle the remaining 1 tablespoon almonds over the bok choy, tossing to combine.

Transfer the bok choy to a serving platter.

In the same skillet, heat the remaining 1 teaspoon oil, swirling to coat the bottom. Cook the fish for 1 to 2 minutes on each side, or the desired doneness.

Arrange the fish on the bok choy. Spoon the sauce over the fish and the bok choy.

calories 218

total fat 6.0 g

  saturated fat 0.5 g

  trans fat 0.0 g

  polyunsaturated fat 1.5 g

  monounsaturated fat 3.5 g

cholesterol 48 mg

sodium 334 mg

carbohydrates 9 g

  fiber 2 g

  sugars 3 g

protein 32 g

DIETARY EXCHANGES

  1/2 other carbohydrate,

  3 1/2 lean meat

CREOLE TUNA STEAK SANDWICH WITH CAPER TARTAR SAUCE

SERVES 4

The coarse, stone-ground mustard and the chili powder kicks up the flavor in this sauce. Serve with a cool, refreshing salad, such as Spiralized Cucumbers with Yogurt-Dill Dressing *(page 79) or* Confetti Coleslaw *(page 84).*

Sauce

    1/4 cup light mayonnaise

    1 tablespoon capers packed in balsamic vinegar, rinsed and drained

    1 tablespoon Creole mustard (lowest sodium available)

    1 teaspoon fresh lemon juice

    1/4 teaspoon chili powder

(continued)

■ ■ ■

1 pound tuna steaks (about 1 inch thick),
    rinsed and patted dry
Cooking spray
1 to 1 1/2 teaspoons chili powder
4 whole-grain round sandwich thins (lowest
    sodium available), split and toasted
2 medium Italian plum (Roma) tomatoes or
    2 small yellow tomatoes, thinly sliced
4 romaine lettuce leaves
1/2 cup thinly sliced cucumber

In a small bowl, whisk together the sauce ingredients. Set aside.

Preheat the grill on medium high.

Lightly spray both sides of the fish with cooking spray. Sprinkle the remaining 1 to 1 1/2 teaspoons chili powder on the fish. Grill for 4 to 5 minutes on each side, or until the desired doneness. Transfer to a cutting board. Let stand for 5 minutes. Cut into 12 strips.

To assemble, spread half the sauce on the bottom halves of the sandwich thins. Top with the tomatoes, lettuce, and cucumber. Place the fish on the cucumber, spreading the remaining sauce over the fish. Put the tops of the sandwich thins on the sandwiches.

Cook's Tip: You can make the sauce up to four days in advance. Cover and refrigerate it until needed.

PER SERVING

calories 271	carbohydrates 26 g
total fat 5.5 g	fiber 6 g
saturated fat 0.5 g	sugars 3 g
trans fat 0.0 g	**protein** 32 g
polyunsaturated fat 3.0 g	**DIETARY EXCHANGES**
monounsaturated fat 1.5 g	1 1/2 starch, 3 lean
cholesterol 49 mg	meat
sodium 492 mg	

TUNA QUICHE IN A BULGUR CRUST

SERVES 8

If you're a fan of classic tuna casserole, give this updated version a try. A whole grain takes the place of traditional egg noodles; mushrooms are used instead of cream of mushroom soup, and eggs make the dish lighter and fluffier.

Cooking spray
3/4 cup uncooked instant (fine-grain) bulgur
1 large egg, lightly beaten using a fork, and
    2 large eggs, divided use
1 teaspoon dried dillweed, crumbled
2 4.5-ounce cans very low sodium albacore
    tuna, packed in water, drained and
    flaked
1 medium onion, chopped
1 tablespoon chopped fresh parsley
1 tablespoon fresh lemon juice
1 cup fat-free milk
1/3 cup shredded low-fat sharp Cheddar
    cheese
10 medium button mushrooms, sliced
1/2 large green bell pepper, chopped

Preheat the oven to 350°F. Lightly spray a 9-inch pie pan with cooking spray.

Prepare the bulgur using the package directions, omitting the salt. Transfer to a medium bowl. Fluff with a fork.

Stir in the beaten egg and dillweed. Press the bulgur mixture on the bottom and up the side of the pie pan, forming a crust. Bake for 8 to 10 minutes. Remove from the oven. Increase the oven temperature to 425°F. Let the crust stand to cool.

In a medium bowl, stir together the tuna, onion, parsley, and lemon juice.

In a separate medium bowl, stir together the milk, Cheddar, and the remaining 2 eggs.

Spread the mushrooms on the crust. Spread the tuna mixture over the mushrooms. Sprinkle the bell pepper over the tuna mixture. Pour the milk mixture over all.

Bake for 10 minutes. Reduce the oven temperature to 350°F. Bake for 30 minutes, or until the top of the quiche is golden and the center is set (doesn't jiggle when the pan is gently shaken).

PER SERVING

calories 137	sodium 93 mg
total fat 3.0 g	carbohydrates 15 g
saturated fat 1.0 g	fiber 3 g
trans fat 0.0 g	sugars 4 g
polyunsaturated fat 0.5 g	protein 15 g
monounsaturated fat 1.0 g	DIETARY EXCHANGES
cholesterol 85 mg	1 starch, 2 lean meat

STUFFED SHELLS WITH ALBACORE TUNA AND VEGETABLES

SERVES 4

A tuna noodle casserole variation goes gourmet with individual stuffed shells and a first-class white sauce enhanced with Dijon mustard.

12 dried jumbo pasta shells (about 4 ounces)

1 cup fat-free, low-sodium chicken broth, such as on page 36

3 tablespoons all-purpose flour

1 cup fat-free half-and-half

2 teaspoons Dijon mustard (lowest sodium available)

1 teaspoon salt-free all-purpose seasoning blend

1/8 teaspoon salt

2 4.5-ounce cans very low sodium albacore tuna in water, drained and flaked

8 ounces finely chopped frozen broccoli florets, thawed

2 ounces diced roasted red bell pepper, drained if bottled

1/3 cup shredded low-fat sharp Cheddar cheese

Prepare the pasta using the package directions, omitting the salt. Drain well in a colander. Set aside.

Preheat the oven to 350°F.

In a medium saucepan, whisk together the broth and flour. Bring to a simmer over medium-high heat, whisking frequently. Reduce the heat and simmer for 1 to 2 minutes, or until thickened.

Whisk in the half-and-half, mustard, seasoning blend, and salt. Reduce the heat to medium low. Cook for 1 minute, or until the sauce is heated through, whisking occasionally. Remove from the heat.

In a medium bowl, stir together the tuna, broccoli, roasted peppers, and 1/4 cup sauce.

Gently spoon 1/4 cup tuna mixture into each pasta shell. Place the shells with the open side up in a nonstick 13 x 9 x 2-inch baking pan. Pour the remaining sauce over the shells. Sprinkle the Cheddar over all.

Bake, covered, for 25 to 30 minutes, or until heated through. Serve the stuffed shells topped with the sauce remaining in the pan.

PER SERVING

calories 277	carbohydrates 39 g
total fat 2.5 g	fiber 3 g
saturated fat 0.5 g	sugars 7 g
trans fat 0.0 g	protein 30 g
polyunsaturated fat 0.5 g	DIETARY EXCHANGES
monounsaturated fat 0.5 g	2 starch, 1 vegetable,
cholesterol 30 mg	3 lean meat
sodium 310 mg	

TUNA-ARTICHOKE CASSEROLE WITH BASIL AND DILL

SERVES 5

This riff on an established favorite adds artichokes, fresh basil, and dill for jazzed-up flavor. Cherry tomatoes and kale contribute bright color and texture. While this updated version dials up the flavor, it still retains the creaminess and crunchy topping found in the classic tuna casserole.

(continued)

Cooking spray

6 ounces dried whole-grain rotini

1 tablespoon olive oil

1/4 cup chopped shallots

2 medium garlic cloves, minced

2 tablespoons all-purpose flour

1 1/2 cups fat-free milk

9 ounces frozen artichoke hearts, thawed, drained, and chopped

1 cup coarsely chopped baby kale

3/4 cup halved cherry tomatoes

1 2.6-ounce vacuum-sealed pouch very low sodium chunk light tuna, packed in water, drained and flaked

2 tablespoons chopped fresh basil

2 tablespoons chopped fresh dillweed

1/2 cup coarsely crushed unsalted multigrain tortilla chips

Preheat the oven to 350°F. Lightly spray a 1 1/2-quart casserole dish with cooking spray.

Prepare the pasta using the package directions, omitting the salt. Drain well in a colander. Transfer to a large bowl.

Meanwhile, in a medium saucepan, heat the oil over medium heat, swirling to coat the bottom. Cook the shallots and garlic for 1 minute, or until fragrant, stirring constantly. Stir in the flour. Slowly pour in the milk, stirring to combine. Increase the heat to medium high and bring to a boil. Reduce the heat to low and simmer for 1 minute, stirring constantly. Stir the mixture into the pasta. Stir in the remaining ingredients except the tortilla chips. Spoon into the casserole dish. Sprinkle the chips over the casserole.

Bake for 35 to 45 minutes, or until the top is lightly browned and the casserole is hot. Let stand for 5 minutes before serving.

PER SERVING

calories 329	**carbohydrates** 44 g
total fat 6.0 g	fiber 9 g
saturated fat 0.5 g	sugars 7 g
trans fat 0.0 g	**protein** 26 g
polyunsaturated fat 1.5 g	**DIETARY EXCHANGES**
monounsaturated fat 3.0 g	2 starch, 3 vegetable,
cholesterol 38 mg	2 1/2 lean meat
sodium 372 mg	

SPICY TUNA PITAS
SERVES 4

The tang of lime juice combined with the distinctive flavor of cumin and the mildest kick from cayenne gives a unique twist to the classic tuna sandwich.

2 4.5-ounce cans very low sodium albacore tuna in water, drained and flaked

1/2 medium rib of celery, chopped

2 medium green onions, chopped

1/4 cup finely chopped fresh cilantro

1/3 cup light mayonnaise

1 tablespoon fresh lime juice

1 teaspoon ground cumin

1/8 teaspoon cayenne

2 7-inch whole-grain pita pockets, halved

4 medium lettuce leaves, such as red leaf

In a medium bowl, stir together the tuna, celery, green onions, and cilantro.

Stir in the mayonnaise, lime juice, cumin, and cayenne.

Line each pita half with lettuce. Spoon the tuna salad into the pitas.

PER SERVING

calories 211	**carbohydrates** 22 g
total fat 7.0 g	fiber 3 g
saturated fat 0.5 g	sugars 1 g
trans fat 0.0 g	**protein** 20 g
polyunsaturated fat 3.5 g	**DIETARY EXCHANGES**
monounsaturated fat 1.0 g	1 1/2 starch, 2 1/2 lean
cholesterol 34 mg	meat
sodium 400 mg	

LINGUINE WITH WHITE CLAM SAUCE
SERVES 4

You can't do better than this classic pasta dish, which has fresh spinach to add color, nutrients, and earthy flavor. Serve with Focaccia (page 443) or Parmesan-Herb Breadsticks (page 451). Caprese Salad with Grilled Zucchini (page 80) can start your meal off with panache.

2 6.5-ounce cans minced clams, drained, liquid reserved (about 1 cup)

1/2 cup dry white wine (regular or
nonalcoholic)
8 ounces dried whole-grain linguine
1 teaspoon olive oil
1/2 cup finely chopped onion
4 medium garlic cloves, minced
2 tablespoons all-purpose flour
2 cups baby spinach
2 tablespoons finely chopped fresh parsley
2 tablespoons shredded or grated Parmesan
cheese
Pepper to taste

In a small saucepan, whisk together the clam liquid and wine. Bring to a boil over high heat. Boil for about 5 minutes, or until the mixture is reduced to 1 1/4 cups. Set aside.

Prepare the pasta using the package directions, omitting the salt. Drain well in a colander. Cover to keep warm.

Meanwhile, in a small nonstick skillet, heat the oil over medium-high heat, swirling to coat the bottom. Cook the onion for about 3 minutes, or until soft, stirring frequently.

Stir in the garlic. Cook for 2 minutes, stirring frequently.

Stir in the flour. Cook for 1 minute, stirring frequently.

Pour in the clam liquid mixture. Cook for 2 to 3 minutes, or until the sauce has thickened, stirring constantly.

Stir in the clams, spinach, and parsley. Cook for 2 minutes, or until the spinach is wilted and the mixture is heated through, stirring constantly. Spoon over the pasta. Sprinkle with the Parmesan and pepper.

PER SERVING

calories 322	carbohydrates 54 g
total fat 3.5 g	fiber 7 g
saturated fat 0.5 g	sugars 3 g
trans fat 0.0 g	**protein** 17 g
polyunsaturated fat 0.5 g	**DIETARY EXCHANGES**
monounsaturated fat 1.5 g	3 1/2 starch, 1 1/2 lean
cholesterol 33 mg	meat
sodium 503 mg	

MINI CRAB CASSEROLES
SERVES 8

Try this twist on traditional crab cakes. Serve this divine crab dish in individual casseroles or ramekins for a special touch. Add a leafy green salad with Lemon Dressing (page 106) or steamed broccoli to complete the meal.

Cooking spray
1/2 teaspoon canola or corn oil
2 tablespoons minced onion
2 cups fat-free milk
3 tablespoons all-purpose flour
1 medium rib of celery, finely chopped, or
1/4 teaspoon celery seeds
1 2-ounce jar diced pimientos, drained
2 tablespoons minced green bell pepper
1 tablespoon chopped fresh parsley
Dash of red hot-pepper sauce
2 tablespoons dry sherry
1/4 cup egg substitute
3 cups flaked crabmeat, thawed if frozen or
rinsed and drained if canned, bits of
shell and cartilage discarded
1/4 teaspoon pepper, or to taste
2 slices whole-grain bread (lowest sodium
available), lightly toasted and crumbled

Preheat the oven to 350°F. Lightly spray eight ramekins or individual casserole dishes with cooking spray.

In a large nonstick skillet, heat the oil over medium-high heat, swirling to coat the bottom. Cook the onion for about 3 minutes, or until soft, stirring frequently.

In a medium bowl, whisk together the milk and flour. Stir into the onion. Cook for 3 to 5 minutes, or until thickened, stirring occasionally.

Stir in the celery, pimientos, bell pepper, parsley, and hot-pepper sauce. Remove from the heat. Stir in the sherry.

Pour the egg substitute into a small bowl. Whisk in a little of the onion mixture. Slowly pour the egg substitute mixture into the onion mixture in the skillet, whisking constantly.

(continued)

Stir in the crabmeat and pepper. Spoon into the casserole dishes. Sprinkle the bread crumbs over the casseroles. Lightly spray with cooking spray.

Bake for 15 to 20 minutes, or until lightly browned.

PER SERVING

calories 118	sodium 273 mg
total fat 1.0 g	carbohydrates 10 g
saturated fat 0.0 g	fiber 1 g
trans fat 0.0 g	sugars 4 g
polyunsaturated fat 0.5 g	protein 16 g
monounsaturated fat 0.0 g	DIETARY EXCHANGES
cholesterol 42 mg	1/2 starch, 2 lean meat

CRAB PRIMAVERA ALFREDO

SERVES 4

Lump crabmeat is a seafood lover's delight. Savor that delicacy combined with a creamy sauce and tender vegetables and served over fettuccine.

    4 ounces dried whole-grain fettuccine
    1 teaspoon olive oil
    2 medium shallots, coarsely chopped
    8 ounces broccoli florets, cut into bite-size pieces
    1/2 cup halved matchstick-size carrot strips
    1 medium yellow summer squash, thinly sliced
    1/2 cup fat-free, low-sodium chicken broth, such as on page 36
    1/2 cup fat-free half-and-half
    1 1/2 tablespoons all-purpose flour
    1/2 teaspoon dried dillweed, crumbled
    2 tablespoons shredded or grated Parmesan cheese
    1 6-ounce can lump crabmeat, rinsed and drained

Prepare the pasta using the package directions, omitting the salt. Drain well in a colander. Transfer to a medium bowl. Cover to keep warm.

Meanwhile, in a large skillet, heat the oil over medium-high heat, swirling to coat the bottom. Cook the shallots for about 3 minutes, or until soft, stirring frequently.

Stir in the broccoli and carrots. Cook for about 3 minutes, or until tender-crisp.

Stir in the squash. Cook for 2 to 3 minutes, or until the broccoli and carrots are tender.

In a small bowl, whisk together the broth, half-and-half, flour, and dillweed. Pour into the shallot mixture. Bring to a simmer. Reduce the heat and simmer for 1 to 2 minutes, or until thickened, stirring occasionally.

Stir in the Parmesan. Carefully fold in the crabmeat so the lumps don't break up too much. Cook for 2 to 3 minutes, or until heated through, gently stirring occasionally. Spoon over the pasta.

PER SERVING

calories 228	carbohydrates 35 g
total fat 3.5 g	fiber 6 g
saturated fat 0.5 g	sugars 6 g
trans fat 0.0 g	protein 17 g
polyunsaturated fat 0.5 g	DIETARY EXCHANGES
monounsaturated fat 1.5 g	2 starch, 1 vegetable,
cholesterol 43 mg	1 1/2 lean meat
sodium 271 mg	

OVEN-FRIED SCALLOPS WITH CILANTRO AND LIME

SERVES 4

Moist, tantalizing scallops soak in a cilantro-buttermilk marinade with the bright taste of lime before being coated in panko and baked. For a tasty side that bakes at the same temperature, try Roasted Chayote Squash (page 385).

    Cooking spray
    1/2 cup low-fat buttermilk
    2 tablespoons chopped fresh cilantro and 2 tablespoons chopped fresh cilantro, divided use
    2 tablespoons fresh lime juice
    1/4 teaspoon pepper
    1 pound sea scallops, rinsed and patted dry
    1/2 cup whole-wheat panko (Japanese-style bread crumbs)
    Dash of paprika
    1 medium lime, cut into 4 wedges (optional)

Preheat the oven to 400°F. Lightly spray a 9-inch round or square baking pan with cooking spray.

In a shallow glass bowl, whisk together the buttermilk, 2 tablespoons cilantro, lime juice, and pepper.

Stir the scallops into the buttermilk mixture, turning to coat. Let soak for 10 minutes. Drain, discarding the buttermilk mixture.

Put the panko on a plate. Roll the scallops in the panko to coat, gently shaking off any excess. Arrange the scallops in a single layer in the baking pan.

Sprinkle the paprika over the scallops. Lightly spray with cooking spray.

Bake for 10 to 13 minutes, or until opaque. Be careful not to overcook or the scallops will become rubbery. Just before serving, sprinkle with the remaining 2 tablespoons cilantro. Serve with the lime wedges.

PER SERVING

calories 132	sodium 210 mg
total fat 1.0 g	carbohydrates 9 g
saturated fat 0.0 g	fiber 0 g
trans fat 0.0 g	sugars 1 g
polyunsaturated fat 0.5 g	protein 20 g
monounsaturated fat 0.0 g	DIETARY EXCHANGES
cholesterol 38 mg	1/2 starch, 3 lean meat

LINGUINE WITH SCALLOPS AND ASPARAGUS

SERVES 4

A lemony sauce made with clam juice and tender asparagus complements the sweet flavor of scallops in this complete meal.

4 ounces dried whole-grain linguine
1 8-ounce bottle clam juice
1/2 cup dry white wine (regular or nonalcoholic)
3 tablespoons all-purpose flour
1/4 teaspoon pepper
6 ounces asparagus, trimmed, or 4 ounces frozen asparagus, thawed, sliced diagonally into 1-inch pieces

1 teaspoon light tub margarine
1/4 cup minced shallots (about 4 large)
1 pound sea or bay scallops, rinsed and patted dry, quartered if large
3 tablespoons finely chopped fresh parsley
1 tablespoon fresh lemon juice

Prepare the pasta using the package directions, omitting the salt. Drain well in a colander. Transfer to a medium bowl. Cover to keep warm.

Meanwhile, in a large saucepan, whisk together the clam juice, wine, flour, and pepper. Bring to a boil over medium-high heat. Boil for 4 to 5 minutes, or until thickened, stirring occasionally.

In a medium saucepan, steam the fresh asparagus for 2 minutes, or until tender-crisp. (Don't cook the asparagus if using thawed frozen.)

In a small nonstick skillet, melt the margarine over medium-high heat, swirling to coat the bottom. Cook the shallots for 2 to 3 minutes, or until soft, stirring frequently.

Stir the shallots and scallops into the clam juice mixture. Reduce the heat to medium and cook for 5 minutes, stirring frequently. Don't let the mixture come to a boil. Stir in the asparagus, parsley, and lemon juice. Cook for 2 to 3 minutes, or until the scallops are opaque and the mixture is heated through. Be careful not to overcook or the scallops will become rubbery. Serve over the pasta.

PER SERVING

calories 264	sodium 475 mg
total fat 2.0 g	carbohydrates 32 g
saturated fat 0.0 g	fiber 5 g
trans fat 0.0 g	sugars 3 g
polyunsaturated fat 0.5 g	protein 25 g
monounsaturated fat 0.5 g	DIETARY EXCHANGES
cholesterol 37 mg	2 starch, 3 lean meat

OVEN-FRIED OYSTERS

SERVES 4

If you love fried oysters, try these baked ones with a crunchy coating and a horseradish-spiked dipping sauce. Pair with Oven-Fried Onion Rings *(page 395) or* Baked Okra Bites *(page 394) for a healthy "fried" dinner.*

Cooking spray

1/4 cup low-fat buttermilk

1/2 teaspoon red hot-pepper sauce

24 shucked oysters, rinsed and drained

1/2 cup all-purpose flour

2 large egg whites, beaten until frothy

1 1/2 cups crushed cornflakes

1 tablespoon salt-free all-purpose seasoning
   blend

1/8 teaspoon cayenne

1/2 cup no-salt-added ketchup

1 tablespoon bottled white horseradish,
   drained

2 teaspoons fresh lemon juice

1 teaspoon Worcestershire sauce (lowest
   sodium available)

1 medium lemon, cut into 4 wedges

Preheat the oven to 400°F. Place a wire cooling rack on a large rimmed baking sheet. Lightly spray the rack and baking sheet with cooking spray.

In a medium bowl, whisk together the buttermilk and hot-pepper sauce. Add the oysters, stirring gently to coat. (For deeper flavor and additional tenderness, cover and refrigerate the oysters for up to 30 minutes at this point if desired.)

Put the flour in a medium shallow bowl. Put the egg whites in a separate medium shallow bowl. In a third medium shallow bowl, stir together the cornflakes, seasoning blend, and cayenne. Put the bowls and baking sheet in a row, assembly-line fashion.

Drain the oysters, discarding the buttermilk mixture. Dip the oysters in the flour, then in the egg whites, and finally in the cornflake mixture, turning to coat at each step and gently shaking off the excess. Using your fingertips, gently

press the coating so it adheres to the oysters. Place the oysters on the wire rack.

Bake for 7 to 8 minutes, or until the oysters are crisp on the outside and cooked on the inside (slightly firm when pressed with the back of a spoon).

Meanwhile, in a small bowl, whisk together the ketchup, horseradish, lemon juice, and Worcestershire sauce. Serve the oysters with the sauce and the lemon wedges.

PER SERVING

calories 171	**carbohydrates** 32 g
total fat 1.5 g	fiber 1 g
saturated fat 0.5 g	sugars 11 g
trans fat 0.0 g	**protein** 7 g
polyunsaturated fat 0.5 g	**DIETARY EXCHANGES**
monounsaturated fat 0.0 g	1 starch, 1 other
cholesterol 34 mg	carbohydrate, 1 lean
sodium 219 mg	meat

JAPANESE SHRIMP KEBABS

SERVES 4

Sake and mirin—popular ingredients used in Japanese cooking—provide the Asian flavor to the shrimp in this dish. Serve with Asian Linguine *(page 418) and* Asian Spinach and Mushrooms *(page 403).*

Marinade

2 tablespoons sake, dry sherry, or lemon juice
   (optional)

2 tablespoons soy sauce (lowest sodium
   available)

2 tablespoons mirin

2 teaspoons grated peeled gingerroot

1 medium green onion, finely chopped

2 to 3 drops toasted sesame oil or chili oil

■ ■ ■

32 medium shrimp, with shells and tails,
   rinsed and patted dry

In a medium glass bowl, whisk together the marinade ingredients. Add the shrimp, tossing to coat. Cover and refrigerate for up to 1 hour.

Meanwhile, soak eight 8-inch wooden skewers for at least 10 minutes in cold water to prevent charring, or use metal skewers.

Preheat the grill on medium high.

Drain the shrimp, reserving the marinade. In a small saucepan, bring the marinade to a boil over high heat. Boil for 5 minutes. Remove from the heat.

Meanwhile, thread 4 shrimp onto each skewer. Grill for 1 to 2 minutes on each side, or until pink on the outside. Brush the marinade onto the shrimp. Grill for about 1 minute, or until the shells look chalky with just a little char. Serve hot, at room temperature, or cold.

PER SERVING

calories 89	sodium 312 mg
total fat 0.5 g	carbohydrates 1 g
saturated fat 0.0 g	fiber 0 g
trans fat 0.0 g	sugars 1 g
polyunsaturated fat 0.0 g	protein 20 g
monounsaturated fat 0.0 g	DIETARY EXCHANGES
cholesterol 159 mg	3 lean meat

SCALLOPS IN WHITE WINE

SERVES 4

Scallops are very porous, so they absorb maximum flavor in a minimal amount of time and they cook quickly. To ensure their moistness, sweetness, and velvety texture, keep an eye on them as they cook so they don't get overdone. Basil Spinach (page 404) makes a colorful bed for the scallops.

> 1 pound scallops (sea scallops preferred), rinsed and patted dry
> 1 cup dry white wine (regular or nonalcoholic)
> 2 medium shallots, minced
> 3 sprigs of fresh parsley, chopped
> Pepper to taste (freshly ground preferred)
> 1 medium lemon, cut into 4 wedges

In a large skillet, arrange the scallops in a single layer. Pour in the wine. Sprinkle the shallots and parsley over the scallops. Cook over medium-high heat for 5 to 6 minutes, until opaque, turn-

ing once halfway through. Be careful not to overcook or the scallops will become rubbery.

Just before serving, sprinkle with the pepper. Serve with the lemon wedges.

PER SERVING

calories 106	sodium 185 mg
total fat 1.0 g	carbohydrates 4 g
saturated fat 0.0 g	fiber 0 g
trans fat 0.0 g	sugars 0 g
polyunsaturated fat 0.5 g	protein 19 g
monounsaturated fat 0.0 g	DIETARY EXCHANGES
cholesterol 37 mg	3 lean meat

SHRIMP AND OKRA ÉTOUFFÉE

SERVES 6

This heart-healthy version of étouffée (ay-too-FAY) is every bit as decadent tasting as the classic Creole dish popular in New Orleans cuisine. Serve with Creole Squash (page 406).

> 1 1/2 cups uncooked instant brown rice
> 1/4 cup all-purpose flour
> 1 teaspoon canola or corn oil
> 1 medium green bell pepper, finely chopped
> 1 medium onion, finely chopped
> 1 medium rib of celery, finely chopped
> 2 cups fresh or frozen sliced okra
> 2 cups fat-free, low-sodium chicken broth, such as on page 36
> 2 teaspoons salt-free Creole or Cajun seasoning blend
> 1 pound raw medium shrimp, peeled, rinsed, and patted dry

Prepare the rice using the package directions, omitting the salt and margarine. Cover to keep warm. Set aside.

Meanwhile, in a large nonstick skillet, cook the flour over medium heat for 8 to 10 minutes, or until browned, stirring occasionally. Transfer to a medium bowl. Let cool for 5 minutes. Wipe the skillet with paper towels.

(continued)

In the same skillet, heat the oil over medium heat, swirling to coat the bottom. Cook the bell pepper, onion, and celery for 2 to 3 minutes, or until the bell pepper and celery are tender-crisp and the onion is soft, stirring occasionally.

Stir in the okra. Cook for 2 to 3 minutes (4 to 5 minutes if using frozen), or until the okra is tender-crisp, stirring occasionally.

Whisk the broth into the flour (there may be a few lumps). Stir the broth mixture and seasoning blend into the bell pepper mixture. Increase the heat to medium high and bring to a simmer, stirring occasionally. Reduce the heat and simmer, covered, for 15 minutes.

Stir in the shrimp. Simmer, covered, for 2 to 3 minutes, or until the shrimp are pink on the outside. Serve over the rice.

PER SERVING

calories 206	carbohydrates 28 g
total fat 2.5 g	fiber 3 g
saturated fat 0.5 g	sugars 3 g
trans fat 0.0 g	protein 17 g
polyunsaturated fat 1.0 g	DIETARY EXCHANGES
monounsaturated fat 1.0 g	1 1/2 starch,
cholesterol 121 mg	1 vegetable, 2 lean
sodium 567 mg	meat

SEAFOOD JAMBALAYA

SERVES 4

This take on jambalaya uses shrimp, redfish, and the classic "holy trinity" of Cajun and Creole cooking: bell pepper, celery, and onion.

2 teaspoons olive oil

2 medium ribs of celery, finely diced

1 cup diced onion

1 medium green bell pepper, diced

3 medium garlic cloves, minced

3/4 cup uncooked brown rice (long-grain preferred)

2 teaspoons chopped fresh thyme or 1/2 teaspoon dried thyme, crumbled

1/8 teaspoon cayenne

1 14.5-ounce can no-salt-added diced tomatoes, undrained

1 1/2 cups water

1/4 teaspoon salt

1/8 teaspoon pepper

8 ounces raw medium shrimp, peeled, rinsed, and patted dry

8 ounces redfish, striped bass, tilapia, or cod, cut into 3/4-inch pieces, rinsed and patted dry

1 teaspoon salt-free Creole or Cajun seasoning blend

In a large saucepan or Dutch oven, heat the oil over medium heat, swirling to coat the bottom.

Cook the celery, onion, and bell pepper for 6 to 7 minutes, or until the celery and bell pepper are tender and the onion is soft, stirring occasionally. Stir in the garlic. Cook for 1 minute, or until fragrant, stirring frequently. Stir in the rice, thyme, and cayenne. Cook for 1 minute, stirring occasionally.

Increase the heat to medium high. Stir in the tomatoes with liquid, water, salt, and pepper. Bring to a simmer. Reduce the heat and simmer, covered, for 35 minutes.

Stir in the shrimp and fish. Sprinkle the seasoning blend over all (don't stir). Cook, covered, over low heat for 6 to 8 minutes, or until the rice is tender, the shrimp is pink on the outside, and the fish flakes easily when tested with a fork.

PER SERVING

calories 299	carbohydrates 38 g
total fat 4.5 g	fiber 4 g
saturated fat 1.0 g	sugars 6 g
trans fat 0.0 g	protein 26 g
polyunsaturated fat 1.0 g	DIETARY EXCHANGES
monounsaturated fat 2.5 g	2 starch, 2 vegetable,
cholesterol 108 mg	3 lean meat
sodium 273 mg	

FIERY SHRIMP DIJON

SERVES 4

The addition of fresh lime juice makes the other intense ingredients in this dish just explode with flavor. This entrée cooks so fast and with so little effort, you can have it on the table in just minutes.

2 tablespoons light tub margarine

2 tablespoons Dijon mustard (lowest sodium available)

1 1/2 teaspoons dried tarragon, crumbled

1/4 teaspoon cayenne

1/4 teaspoon pepper

1/16 teaspoon salt

Cooking spray

12 ounces raw medium shrimp, peeled, rinsed, and patted dry

2 medium limes, each cut into 4 wedges

In a small bowl, stir together the margarine, mustard, tarragon, cayenne, pepper, and salt.

Lightly spray a large skillet with cooking spray. Cook the shrimp over medium heat for 3 minutes, or until pink on the outside, stirring frequently.

Add the margarine mixture, stirring to coat. Serve the shrimp with the lime wedges.

PER SERVING

calories 106	sodium 336 mg
total fat 3.5 g	carbohydrates 2 g
saturated fat 0.0 g	fiber 1 g
trans fat 0.0 g	sugars 1 g
polyunsaturated fat 0.5 g	protein 18 g
monounsaturated fat 1.5 g	**DIETARY EXCHANGES**
cholesterol 137 mg	2 1/2 lean meat

CURRIED SHRIMP RISOTTO

SERVES 4

Plump shrimp, curry powder, veggies, and brown rice come together in this one-dish, no-stress risotto. A touch of fat-free half-and-half rounds out the curry flavor and adds the creaminess associated with risotto.

2 1/2 cups fat-free, low-sodium chicken broth, such as on page 36

1 teaspoon olive oil and 1 teaspoon olive oil, divided use

1 medium green bell pepper, chopped

1 pound raw medium shrimp, peeled, rinsed, and patted dry

1 tablespoon plus 1 teaspoon curry powder

1 cup chopped onion

3/4 cup thin carrot strips, coarsely chopped

1 cup uncooked instant brown rice

1 tablespoon grated peeled gingerroot

3 medium garlic cloves, minced

2 tablespoons fat-free half-and-half

1/2 teaspoon crushed red pepper flakes

1/8 teaspoon salt

3/4 cup frozen green peas, thawed

2 medium green onions, thinly sliced

In a small saucepan, bring the broth to a boil, covered, over low heat. Remove from the heat. Keep covered.

Meanwhile, pour 1 teaspoon oil into a Dutch oven, swirling to coat the bottom. Cook the bell pepper over medium-high heat for 3 minutes, or until tender-crisp, stirring occasionally.

Stir in the shrimp and curry powder. Cook for 3 minutes, or until the shrimp turn pink on the outside, stirring frequently. Transfer the mixture to a plate. Cover and set aside.

Decrease the heat to medium. Pour the remaining 1 teaspoon oil into the Dutch oven, swirling to coat the bottom. Add the onion and carrots. Stir in 2 tablespoons of the heated broth, continuing to keep the remaining broth covered. Cook for 2 minutes, or until the onion and carrots just begin to soften, stirring frequently.

Stir the rice, gingerroot, and garlic into the onion mixture. Cook for 2 minutes, stirring constantly.

Stir in the remaining broth. Bring to a simmer, still over medium heat. Reduce the heat and simmer, covered, for 10 minutes, or until the liquid is almost absorbed, stirring occasionally. Remove from the heat.

(continued)

In a small bowl, stir together the half-and-half, red pepper flakes, and salt. Add to the cooked rice mixture.

Stir in the green peas and shrimp mixture. Remove from the heat. Let stand, covered, for 2 minutes. Just before serving, sprinkle with the green onions.

PER SERVING

calories 278	carbohydrates 32 g
total fat 4.0 g	fiber 5 g
saturated fat 0.5 g	sugars 6 g
trans fat 0.0 g	**protein** 29 g
polyunsaturated fat 1.0 g	**DIETARY EXCHANGES**
monounsaturated fat 2.0 g	2 starch, 1 vegetable,
cholesterol 183 mg	3 lean meat
sodium 278 mg	

PECAN SHRIMP AND CRISP SAGE OVER PUMPKIN GRITS

SERVES 4

This seasonal variation of a southern favorite features shrimp sautéed with wine and served over cheesy, pumpkin-enriched cornmeal grits. Lightly crisped sage adds an autumnal flavor and is an attractive garnish for this dish. For the best flavor, look for coarse-ground cornmeal.

8 small sprigs of fresh sage

1 1/4 cups water

1/2 cup fat-free milk

1/2 cup coarse-ground cornmeal grits (yellow cornmeal preferred)

1/3 cup canned solid-pack pumpkin (not pie filling)

2 tablespoons shredded or grated Parmesan cheese

1/8 teaspoon ground nutmeg

1/8 teaspoon pepper

1 tablespoon olive oil

1/4 cup finely chopped shallots

10 ounces raw medium shrimp, peeled, but tails left on, rinsed, and patted dry (31 to 35 count)

2 tablespoons chopped pecans

1/4 cup white wine (regular or nonalcoholic)

Arrange the sprigs of sage on a double thickness of paper towels, keeping the leaves flat. Cover with a double thickness of paper towels. Microwave on 100 percent power (high) for 20 to 30 seconds, or until the sage is lightly dry and crisp (the leaves should still be light green). Gently crush half the sprigs. Reserve the remaining sprigs for garnish.

In a medium saucepan, bring the water and milk to a boil over medium-high heat. Slowly stir in the grits. Reduce the heat to low. Cook for 5 to 7 minutes, or until thickened, stirring occasionally. Stir in the pumpkin, Parmesan, nutmeg, and pepper. Cover to keep warm. Set aside.

In a large nonstick skillet, heat the oil over medium heat, swirling to coat the bottom. Cook the shallots for 30 seconds, or until fragrant, reducing the heat if necessary, stirring occasionally. Stir in the shrimp. Cook for 3 to 4 minutes, or until pink on the outside and slightly firm. Stir in the pecans. Cook for 30 seconds or until fragrant, stirring constantly. Increase the heat to medium-high. Stir in the wine. Bring to a boil and boil for 30 seconds to 1 minute, or until the mixture is reduced by half (to about 2 tablespoons).

Spoon the grits onto plates. Serve the shrimp mixture over the grits. Sprinkle with the crushed sprigs of sage. Garnish with the remaining sprigs of sage.

PER SERVING

calories 228	carbohydrates 22 g
total fat 7.5 g	fiber 3 g
saturated fat 1.0 g	sugars 3 g
trans fat 0.0 g	**protein** 18 g
polyunsaturated fat 1.5 g	**DIETARY EXCHANGES**
monounsaturated fat 4.0 g	1 1/2 starch, 2 lean
cholesterol 117 mg	meat
sodium 147 mg	

LITTLE SHRIMP CAKES

SERVES 4

Present these on a bed of dark green, leafy lettuce with Tartar Sauce (page 428) or Cocktail Sauce (page 429) on the side.

Cooking spray

12 ounces raw medium shrimp, peeled, rinsed, and patted dry

1 cup whole-wheat panko (Japanese-style bread crumbs)

3 large egg whites, lightly beaten with a fork

1/2 medium red bell pepper, finely chopped

1 medium green onion, finely chopped

2 tablespoons light mayonnaise

1 teaspoon lemongrass paste or powder, or to taste

1/2 teaspoon Worcestershire sauce (lowest sodium available)

1/2 teaspoon seafood seasoning blend (lowest sodium available)

1/8 to 1/4 teaspoon cayenne

2 teaspoons canola or corn oil and 2 teaspoons canola or corn oil, divided use

2 medium lemons, cut into 4 wedges

Lightly spray a large skillet with cooking spray. Cook the shrimp over medium heat for 3 minutes, or until pink on the outside, stirring frequently. Transfer to a baking sheet or sheet of aluminum foil, spreading in a single layer to cool quickly.

Meanwhile, in a medium bowl, stir together the panko, egg whites, bell pepper, green onion, mayonnaise, lemongrass paste, Worcestershire sauce, seasoning blend, and cayenne.

Finely chop the shrimp. Stir into the bread crumb mixture. Shape into 12 small patties.

In the same skillet, heat 2 teaspoons oil over medium heat, swirling to coat the bottom. Cook half the patties for 3 minutes. Turn over the patties. Cook for 2 to 3 minutes, or until golden. Transfer to a plate. Cover to keep warm. Repeat with the remaining 2 teaspoons oil and the remaining patties. Serve with the lemon wedges.

PER SERVING

calories 222
total fat 7.5 g
   saturated fat 0.5 g
   trans fat 0.0 g
   polyunsaturated fat 2.5 g
   monounsaturated fat 3.5 g
cholesterol 139 mg
sodium 310 mg

carbohydrates 16 g
   fiber 3 g
   sugars 2 g
protein 23 g
DIETARY EXCHANGES
   1 starch, 2 1/2 lean meat

Poultry

ROAST CHICKEN WITH GRAPES

SERVES 6

Juicy grapes impart flavor and moisture to chicken when they're roasted inside, and they make a sweet accompaniment when the bird is done. To complete the meal, serve this with baked sweet potatoes or Maple-Glazed Butternut Squash (page 377) and roasted green beans.

1 2 1/2- to 3-pound chicken, all visible fat, neck, and giblets discarded

2 teaspoons poultry seasoning

1 teaspoon pepper

1 cup seedless grapes, halved

1/2 medium onion, cut into wedges, and 1/2 medium onion, sliced, divided use

1 medium lemon, cut into wedges, and 1 medium lemon, cut into wedges, divided use

4 sprigs of fresh rosemary

1/2 cup dry white wine (regular or nonalcoholic)

2 tablespoons light tub margarine, melted

Preheat the oven to 425°F.

In a small bowl, stir together the poultry seasoning and pepper. Rub the mixture over the outside of the chicken and in the chicken cavity. Put the grapes, onion wedges, wedges of 1 lemon, and the rosemary in the cavity. Using kitchen twine, tie the legs together.

Put the sliced onion and the remaining lemon wedges in a nonstick roasting pan. Place the chicken with the breast side up on a rack in the pan (above the sliced onion and lemon wedges). Pour the wine and margarine over the chicken. Transfer the pan to the oven with the legs facing the back of the oven. Roast for 1 hour to 1 hour 15 minutes, or until the chicken registers 165°F on an instant-read thermometer, basting once halfway through. The chicken should be golden brown and its juices should run clear when the thigh is pierced with the tip of a sharp knife. Remove from the oven. Let stand, loosely covered, for 5 minutes.

Transfer the chicken to a serving platter. Discard the twine. Discard the onion wedges, lemon wedges, and rosemary. Remove the grapes from the chicken and arrange around the chicken. Arrange the sliced onion around the chicken. Discard the skin before carving the chicken.

To make gravy, skim and discard the fat from the cooking liquid in the roasting pan. Pour the remaining liquid into a small saucepan. Bring to a boil over medium-high heat. Boil for 5 minutes, stirring occasionally. Serve with the chicken.

Cook's Tip on Meat Thermometers: An instant-read thermometer is your best bet to ensure the safe preparation and cooking of meat, including poultry. Insert the thermometer into the center, or thickest part, of the meat, making sure the thermometer doesn't touch bone or fat.

PER SERVING

calories 146	sodium 88 mg
total fat 3.5 g	carbohydrates 6 g
saturated fat 0.5 g	fiber 1 g
trans fat 0.0 g	sugars 5 g
polyunsaturated fat 1.0 g	protein 22 g
monounsaturated fat 1.0 g	DIETARY EXCHANGES
cholesterol 69 mg	1/2 fruit, 3 lean meat

YEMENI LEMON CHICKEN

SERVES 4

Lots of lemon and garlic combine with warm and smoky spices to create this simple yet exotic dish from the Middle East. It's traditionally served with rice, such as Middle Eastern Rice (page 422). Or, roast some small red potatoes alongside the chicken.

Paste

2 tablespoons grated lemon zest

1/4 cup fresh lemon juice (about 1 large lemon)

3 to 4 garlic cloves, crushed or minced

1/2 teaspoon pepper

1/2 teaspoon ground cardamom

1/2 teaspoon ground cinnamon

1/2 teaspoon ground cumin

(continued)

■ ■ ■

2 medium lemons, cut into wedges
1 2 1/2- to 3-pound chicken, all visible fat,
   neck, and giblets discarded
Cooking spray

Preheat the oven to 425°F.

In a small bowl, whisk together all the paste ingredients.

Rub the lemon wedges over the outside of the chicken and in the chicken cavity. Put the lemon wedges in the cavity. Carefully loosen the skin from the breast and drumsticks by gently inserting your fingers between the skin and the meat, making a pocket for the paste. Don't break the skin. Discard any fat beneath the skin. Still working carefully, spread the paste under the loosened skin as well as possible. Using kitchen twine, tie the legs together.

Lightly spray a roasting pan with cooking spray. Put the chicken in the pan. Roast for 1 hour to 1 hour 15 minutes, or until the chicken registers 165°F on an instant-read thermometer. The chicken should be golden brown and its juices should run clear when the thigh is pierced with the tip of a sharp knife. Remove from the oven. Let stand, loosely covered, for 5 minutes.

Transfer the chicken to a serving platter. Discard the twine. Discard the lemon wedges. Discard the skin before carving the chicken. To make gravy, skim and discard the fat from the cooking liquid in the roasting pan. Pour the remaining liquid into a small saucepan. Bring to a boil over medium-high heat. Boil for 5 minutes, stirring occasionally. Serve the chicken with the gravy.

PER SERVING

calories 188	sodium 121 mg
total fat 4.5 g	carbohydrates 3 g
saturated fat 1.0 g	fiber 1 g
trans fat 0.0 g	sugars 1 g
polyunsaturated fat 1.0 g	protein 33 g
monounsaturated fat 1.5 g	DIETARY EXCHANGES
cholesterol 103 mg	4 1/2 lean meat

CHICKEN WITH ORANGE SAUCE
SERVES 4

Orange juice tenderizes and adds zip to this chicken, which is broiled until browned, then finished on the stovetop. Serve the chicken over couscous or egg noodles. Minted Peas (page 397) are a perfect complement as a side dish.

Cooking spray
1/2 teaspoon paprika
1 2 1/2-pound chicken, skin and all visible fat
   discarded, cut into serving pieces
1 medium onion, sliced

Sauce
1/2 cup 100% frozen orange juice concentrate
1/3 cup water
2 tablespoons light brown sugar
2 tablespoons chopped fresh parsley
1 teaspoon soy sauce (lowest sodium
   available)
1 teaspoon dry sherry (optional)
1/2 teaspoon ground ginger

Preheat the broiler. Lightly spray a heavy-duty baking sheet with cooking spray.

Sprinkle the paprika over the chicken. Put the chicken on the baking sheet.

Broil the chicken about 6 inches from the heat for about 2 minutes on each side, or until lightly browned. Transfer the chicken to a Dutch oven or large deep skillet.

Spread the onion over the chicken.

In a small bowl, whisk together the sauce ingredients. Pour over the chicken and onion.

Bring to a boil over medium-high heat. Reduce the heat and simmer, covered, for 55 minutes to 1 hour, or until the chicken is no longer pink in the center.

PER SERVING

calories 272	carbohydrates 24 g
total fat 7.0 g	fiber 1 g
saturated fat 2.0 g	sugars 22 g
trans fat 0.0 g	protein 28 g
polyunsaturated fat 1.5 g	DIETARY EXCHANGES
monounsaturated fat 2.5 g	1 fruit, 1/2 other
cholesterol 82 mg	carbohydrate,
sodium 118 mg	3 1/2 lean meat

OVEN-BARBECUED CHICKEN

SERVES 4

When it's too cold outside to fire up the grill, but you're in the mood for a barbequed meal, stay warm inside with this dish. The sauce is quick to put together and healthier than the bottled version with less sodium and added sugar. Serve with Baked Okra Bites (page 394) and Potato Salad with Pepper and Parsley (page 87).

Cooking spray
1/4 cup water
1/4 cup white or cider vinegar
3 tablespoons canola or corn oil
1/2 cup no-salt-added ketchup
3 tablespoons Worcestershire sauce (lowest
    sodium available)
1 tablespoon dry mustard
Red hot-pepper sauce to taste (optional)
Pepper to taste (freshly ground preferred)
2 tablespoons chopped onion (optional)
1 2 1/2- to 3-pound chicken, skin and all visible
    fat discarded, cut into serving pieces

Preheat the oven to 350°F. Lightly spray a large baking dish with cooking spray.

In a medium saucepan, whisk together the remaining ingredients except the chicken. Bring to a boil over medium-high heat. Reduce the heat and simmer for 10 minutes.

Put the chicken in the baking dish. Pour half the sauce over the chicken. Bake for 50 minutes to 1 hour, or until the chicken is no longer pink in the center, basting with the remaining sauce every 15 minutes.

PER SERVING

calories 347	**carbohydrates** 15 g
total fat 15.5 g	fiber 0 g
saturated fat 2.0 g	sugars 11 g
trans fat 0.0 g	**protein** 33 g
polyunsaturated fat 4.0 g	**DIETARY EXCHANGES**
monounsaturated fat 8.0 g	1 other carbohydrate,
cholesterol 103 mg	4 lean meat, 1 fat
sodium 171 mg	

LEMON BAKED CHICKEN

SERVES 4

A simple combination of citrus, herbs, and garlic infuses chicken with simple deliciousness. About halfway through the total cooking time for the chicken, add Italian Vegetable Bake (page 413) to the oven, so they'll be finished at the same time.

Cooking spray
2 tablespoons fresh lemon juice
2 tablespoons olive oil
1 medium garlic clove, minced
1/2 teaspoon dried thyme, crumbled
1/2 teaspoon dried parsley, crumbled
1/2 teaspoon pepper (freshly ground
    preferred)
1 2 1/2- to 3-pound chicken, skin and all visible
    fat discarded, cut into serving pieces

Preheat the oven to 350°F. Lightly spray a shallow casserole dish with cooking spray.

In a small bowl, whisk together the lemon juice, oil, garlic, thyme, parsley, and pepper.

Put the chicken in the dish. Pour the lemon juice mixture over the chicken. Bake, covered, for 40 minutes, or until the chicken is no longer pink in the center, basting occasionally. Uncover the dish. Bake for 10 minutes, or until the chicken is browned.

PER SERVING

calories 208	**sodium** 119 mg
total fat 7.5 g	**carbohydrates** 0 g
saturated fat 1.5 g	fiber 0 g
trans fat 0.0 g	sugars 0 g
polyunsaturated fat 1.5 g	**protein** 32 g
monounsaturated fat 4.0 g	**DIETARY EXCHANGES**
cholesterol 103 mg	4 lean meat

CHICKEN WITH SPANISH SAUCE

SERVES 4

Browning the chicken and vegetables before baking the casserole not only provides a rich color to the dish but also an extra layer of flavor. Pop the Orange Sweet Potatoes (page 408) in the oven, too; that recipe cooks at the same temperature as the main dish.

Cooking spray
2 tablespoons olive oil
1 2 1/2- to 3-pound chicken, skin and all visible fat discarded, cut into serving pieces
1/2 teaspoon pepper (freshly ground preferred)
1/2 cup minced onion
1/2 cup chopped green bell pepper
1 medium garlic clove, minced
1 28-ounce can no-salt-added diced tomatoes, drained
1/2 cup dry white wine (regular or nonalcoholic)
1/2 teaspoon dried thyme, crumbled
2 medium dried bay leaves

Preheat the oven to 350°F. Lightly spray a large casserole dish with cooking spray.

In a large, heavy skillet, heat the oil over medium-high heat, swirling to coat the bottom. Cook the chicken for 4 to 5 minutes, turning to brown on all sides. (The chicken won't be done at this point.) Transfer to the casserole dish. Sprinkle the pepper on the chicken. Set aside.

In the same skillet, still over medium-high heat, cook the onion and bell pepper for 4 to 6 minutes, or until the onion is lightly browned. Cook the garlic for 1 minute, or until lightly browned, stirring frequently. Transfer to the casserole dish. Add the tomatoes, wine, thyme, and bay leaves to the dish. Bake, covered, for 1 hour, or until the chicken is no longer pink in the center. Discard the bay leaves.

PER SERVING

calories 301	**carbohydrates** 12 g
total fat 11.0 g	fiber 2 g
saturated fat 2.0 g	sugars 7 g
trans fat 0.0 g	**protein** 34 g
polyunsaturated fat 2.0 g	**DIETARY EXCHANGES**
monounsaturated fat 6.5 g	2 vegetable, 4 lean
cholesterol 103 mg	meat
sodium 142 mg	

COUNTRY-TIME BAKED CHICKEN

SERVES 4 (PLUS 2 CHICKEN BREAST HALVES RESERVED)

As this nicely seasoned chicken bakes, it releases juices to reduce into a rich-tasting sauce. Reserve two of the cooked chicken breast halves. Use them later to top a side salad, in a side soup, or in a casserole, such as Chicken Curry in a Hurry (page 227) or Chicken and Broccoli in Mushroom Sauce (page 226).

Cooking spray
6 skinless chicken breast halves with bone (about 6 ounces each), all visible fat discarded
3/4 teaspoon poultry seasoning
1/2 teaspoon paprika
1/2 teaspoon onion powder
1/2 teaspoon garlic powder
1/4 teaspoon salt
1/4 teaspoon pepper
1 1/2 tablespoons olive oil
3 tablespoons chopped fresh parsley and 2 tablespoons chopped fresh parsley, divided use

Preheat the oven to 325°F. Lightly spray a 13 x 9 x 2-inch glass baking dish with cooking spray.

Put the chicken with the smooth side up in the dish.

In a small bowl, stir together the poultry seasoning, paprika, onion powder, garlic powder, salt, and pepper. Sprinkle over the top of the chicken.

Drizzle the oil over the chicken. Sprinkle 3 tablespoons parsley over the chicken.

Bake, covered, for 40 minutes, or until the chicken is no longer pink in the center, turning several times to coat the chicken with the drippings. Transfer 4 pieces of chicken to plates. Put the remaining chicken in an airtight storage container. Refrigerate for use within two or three days or freeze for later use.

Pour the drippings from the baking dish into a small saucepan. Bring to a boil over high heat. Boil for 2 minutes, or until reduced to 1/4 cup liquid. Spoon over the chicken. Sprinkle with the remaining 2 tablespoons parsley.

PER SERVING

calories 196	sodium 264 mg
total fat 7.0 g	carbohydrates 1 g
saturated fat 1.5 g	fiber 0 g
trans fat 0.0 g	sugars 0 g
polyunsaturated fat 1.0 g	protein 30 g
monounsaturated fat 3.5 g	DIETARY EXCHANGES
cholesterol 91 mg	4 lean meat

CHICKEN, BARLEY, AND BROCCOLI BAKE

SERVES 4

This creamy one-dish casserole has all you need in a meal. Once it's in the oven, you can prepare Baked Ginger Pears *(page 502) or* Apple-Cherry Drops *(page 484), both of which bake at the same temperature as the entrée, for dessert.*

> 2 cups fat-free, low-sodium chicken broth, such as on page 36
> 1 cup fat-free milk
> 2 tablespoons all-purpose flour
> 1 teaspoon dried basil, crumbled
> 1/4 teaspoon salt
> Dash of pepper
> 2/3 cup uncooked pearl barley
> 4 boneless, skinless chicken breast halves (about 4 ounces each), all visible fat discarded
> 10 ounces frozen chopped broccoli, partially thawed if needed to break into small pieces

Preheat the oven to 350°F.

In a medium saucepan, whisk together the broth, milk, flour, basil, salt, and pepper until smooth. Cook over medium heat for 7 to 10 minutes, or until the sauce just starts to boil, whisking frequently.

Meanwhile, spread the barley to cover the bottom of a 9-inch square metal pan. Top with the chicken. Pour the sauce over the chicken. Sprinkle the broccoli over the chicken.

Bake for 1 hour 20 minutes, or until the barley is cooked and has absorbed the sauce and the chicken is no longer pink in the center.

PER SERVING

calories 306	carbohydrates 36 g
total fat 3.5 g	fiber 8 g
saturated fat 1.0 g	sugars 5 g
trans fat 0.0 g	protein 33 g
polyunsaturated fat 1.0 g	DIETARY EXCHANGES
monounsaturated fat 1.0 g	2 starch, 1 vegetable,
cholesterol 74 mg	3 1/2 lean meat
sodium 335 mg	

CRISPY BAKED CHICKEN

SERVES 4

You can still treat yourself to the taste of fried chicken but in a much healthier way. This baked chicken has all the moistness and crunchiness you'd expect in its fried counterpart.

> Cooking spray
> 1 cup fat-free milk
> 1 cup cornflake crumbs
> 1 teaspoon dried rosemary, crushed
> 1/2 teaspoon pepper
> 4 boneless, skinless chicken breast halves (about 4 ounces each), all visible fat discarded

Preheat the oven to 400°F. Line a 13 x 9 x 2-inch baking pan with aluminum foil. Lightly spray with cooking spray.

(continued)

Pour the milk into a shallow dish. In a separate shallow dish, stir together the cornflake crumbs, rosemary, and pepper. Put the dishes and baking pan in a row, assembly-line fashion. Dip the chicken in the milk, then in the crumbs, turning to coat at each step and gently shaking off any excess. Place in the baking pan, arranging so the pieces don't touch. Let stand for 5 to 10 minutes so the coating will adhere.

Bake for 30 minutes, or until the chicken is no longer pink in the center and the crumbs form a crisp "skin."

PER SERVING

calories 216	carbohydrates 21 g
total fat 3.0 g	fiber 0 g
saturated fat 0.5 g	sugars 3 g
trans fat 0.0 g	protein 26 g
polyunsaturated fat 0.5 g	DIETARY EXCHANGES
monounsaturated fat 1.0 g	1 1/2 starch, 3 lean
cholesterol 73 mg	meat
sodium 298 mg	

LEMONGRASS-LIME BAKED CHICKEN

SERVES 4

Commonly used in Thai and Vietnamese cooking, lemongrass has a lemon-lime taste with just a hint of mint and ginger. In this recipe, it adds an exotic flavor to the triple dose of citrus. If you can't find the fresh stalks, look for lemongrass paste. Serve with a side of Thai-Style Lemon and Spinach Soup *(page 44).*

Cooking spray
1 tablespoon fresh lemon juice
1 tablespoon fresh lime juice
1 teaspoon canola or corn oil
1 medium garlic clove, minced
1/4 teaspoon pepper
2 stalks lemongrass, 1 tablespoon lemongrass paste, or 1 tablespoon grated lemon zest
4 boneless, skinless chicken breast halves (about 4 ounces each), all visible fat discarded

Preheat the oven to 350°F. Lightly spray a 9-inch square baking dish or 1-quart casserole dish with cooking spray.

In a medium bowl, whisk together the lemon juice, lime juice, oil, garlic, and pepper.

Remove the outer leaf of the lemongrass. Slice the bottom 6 to 8 inches of the stalk crosswise into 1/2-inch pieces. Stir into the lemon juice mixture.

Put the chicken in the baking dish. Pour the lemon juice mixture over the chicken.

Bake, covered, for 30 minutes, or until the chicken is no longer pink in the center, basting occasionally. Bake, uncovered, for 10 minutes, or until the chicken is lightly browned.

Discard the lemongrass pieces before serving.

PER SERVING

calories 143	sodium 132 mg
total fat 4.0 g	carbohydrates 1 g
saturated fat 0.5 g	fiber 0 g
trans fat 0.0 g	sugars 0 g
polyunsaturated fat 1.0 g	protein 24 g
monounsaturated fat 2.0 g	DIETARY EXCHANGES
cholesterol 73 mg	3 lean meat

BAKED PARMESAN CHICKEN

SERVES 6

Chicken takes a double dip—in buttermilk and in seasoned bread crumbs—then bakes on a rack at a high temperature to stay crisp all over. While the chicken bakes, prepare whole-grain spaghetti and Speedy Marinara Sauce *(page 435).*

Cooking spray
4 slices whole-grain bread (lowest sodium available), processed into fine crumbs
1/4 cup plus 2 tablespoons shredded or grated Parmesan cheese
1 1/2 tablespoons finely chopped fresh parsley
1 1/2 teaspoons paprika
3/4 teaspoon garlic powder
1/2 teaspoon dried thyme, crumbled

1/2 cup low-fat buttermilk

6 boneless, skinless chicken breast halves (about 4 ounces each), all visible fat discarded

Preheat the oven to 450°F. Lightly spray a baking sheet and slightly smaller cooling rack with cooking spray. Put the rack on the baking sheet.

Pour the buttermilk into a shallow dish. Put the bread crumbs in a separate shallow dish. Stir in the Parmesan, parsley, paprika, garlic powder, and thyme. Set the dishes and baking sheet in a row, assembly-line fashion. Dip the chicken in the buttermilk, then in the bread crumb mixture, turning to coat at each step and gently shaking off the excess. Using your fingertips, gently press the coating so it adheres to the chicken. Place the chicken on the rack.

Bake for 15 minutes. Turn over the chicken. Bake for 10 minutes, or until no longer pink in the center.

PER SERVING

calories 202	**carbohydrates** 9 g
total fat 5.0 g	fiber 2 g
saturated fat 1.5 g	sugars 1 g
trans fat 0.0 g	**protein** 29 g
polyunsaturated fat 0.5 g	**DIETARY EXCHANGES**
monounsaturated fat 1.5 g	1/2 starch, 3 1/2 lean
cholesterol 76 mg	meat
sodium 298 mg	

BAKED CHICKEN AND VEGETABLES

SERVES 4

This all-in-one meal cooks slowly in its own juices for a delectable flavor. Once the dish is in the oven, throw together Strawberry-Raspberry Ice (page 503) or Frozen Banana-Orange Push-Ups (page 504); either will have time to freeze and will be the perfect finish.

Cooking spray

1 medium potato, peeled and sliced

1 medium onion, cut into 8 wedges

1 large carrot, cut into sticks

4 skinless chicken breast halves with bone (about 6 ounces each), all visible fat discarded

1/4 cup dry sherry or orange juice

1/4 teaspoon pepper

1 tablespoon light tub margarine

1 1/2 tablespoons flour

2/3 cup fat-free, low-sodium chicken broth, such as on page 36

1 tablespoon finely chopped fresh parsley

1 tablespoon finely chopped green onions

Preheat the oven to 300°F. Lightly spray a deep baking dish with cooking spray.

Put the potato, onion, and carrot in the baking dish. Place the chicken on top of the vegetables. Pour the sherry over all. Sprinkle the pepper over all. Bake, covered, for 1 1/2 hours.

Transfer the chicken and vegetables to a warm serving platter, reserving 1/3 cup of the pan juices. Cover to keep warm.

In a small saucepan, melt the margarine over medium-high heat, swirling to coat the bottom. Cook the flour for 1 minute, whisking constantly. Whisk in the broth and the reserved pan juices. Bring to a boil, whisking constantly. Stir in the parsley and green onions. Pour over the chicken and vegetables.

PER SERVING

calories 242	**carbohydrates** 15 g
total fat 5.0 g	fiber 2 g
saturated fat 1.0 g	sugars 4 g
trans fat 0.0 g	**protein** 32 g
polyunsaturated fat 1.0 g	**DIETARY EXCHANGES**
monounsaturated fat 1.5 g	1/2 starch, 1 vegetable,
cholesterol 91 mg	4 lean meat
sodium 209 mg	

CHICKEN STEW WITH CORNMEAL DUMPLINGS

SERVES 6

Chicken and dumplings is a dish found on many southern dinner tables. This creamy healthier version is full of lean chicken and vegetables, topped with savory cornmeal dumplings.

2 teaspoons canola or corn oil and
    1 tablespoon canola or corn oil, divided
    use
1 medium onion, chopped
1 medium garlic clove, minced
4 boneless, skinless chicken breast halves
    (about 4 ounces each), all visible fat
    discarded
4 1/2 cups fat-free, low-sodium chicken broth,
    such as on page 36
2 medium ribs of celery, sliced
1 large carrot, sliced
1 medium dried bay leaf
1 1/2 teaspoons dried basil, crumbled
1 1/2 teaspoons dried oregano, crumbled
1/2 teaspoon pepper and 1/8 teaspoon
    pepper, divided use
1/4 teaspoon salt and 1/4 teaspoon salt,
    divided use
1/4 teaspoon dried sage
1 medium zucchini, halved lengthwise and
    sliced
1 medium yellow summer squash, halved
    lengthwise and sliced
1 cup fat-free milk and 1/4 cup fat-free milk,
    divided use
1/2 cup all-purpose flour and 1/2 cup all-
    purpose flour, divided use
1/3 cup cornmeal
1/4 cup chopped fresh parsley
1 1/2 teaspoons baking powder
1/4 cup egg substitute

In a Dutch oven, heat 2 teaspoons oil over medium-high heat, swirling to coat the bottom. Cook the onion and garlic for 3 minutes, or until the onion is soft, stirring frequently.

Add the chicken and cook for 2 to 3 minutes on each side, or until lightly browned (the chicken won't be done at this point).

Stir in the broth, celery, carrot, bay leaf, basil, oregano, 1/2 teaspoon pepper, 1/4 teaspoon salt, and the sage. Bring to a low boil, still over medium-high heat. Reduce the heat and simmer, covered, for 10 minutes, or until the chicken is no longer pink except in the center. Transfer the chicken to a cutting board. Discard the bay leaf.

Stir the zucchini and yellow squash into the stew.

In a medium bowl, whisk together 1 cup milk and 1/2 cup flour. Stir into the stew. Increase the heat to medium high and bring to a boil. Reduce the heat to medium and cook for 5 minutes, or until thickened and bubbly, stirring constantly.

When the chicken is cool enough to handle, cut into bite-size pieces. Stir into the stew. Bring to a simmer.

In a small bowl, stir together the cornmeal, parsley, baking powder, and the remaining 1/2 cup flour, 1/4 teaspoon salt, and 1/8 teaspoon pepper.

In a separate small bowl, whisk together the egg substitute and the remaining 1/4 cup milk and 1 tablespoon oil. Add to the cornmeal mixture, whisking just until moistened.

Using a spoon, drop the dumpling batter in 6 mounds on the simmering stew. Reduce the heat and simmer, covered, for 10 to 12 minutes, or until a wooden toothpick inserted in one of the dumplings comes out clean. (Don't peek at the dumplings while they cook.)

PER SERVING

calories 284	**carbohydrates** 32 g
total fat 6.5 g	fiber 3 g
saturated fat 1.0 g	sugars 7 g
trans fat 0.0 g	**protein** 24 g
polyunsaturated fat 1.5 g	**DIETARY EXCHANGES**
monounsaturated fat 3.0 g	1 1/2 starch,
cholesterol 49 mg	1 vegetable, 3 lean
sodium 468 mg	meat

CHICKEN CACCIATORE

SERVES 4

Cacciatore *means "hunter" in Italian, and this chicken is prepared "hunter-style," or with onion, tomato, and herbs. Serve this rustic stew with crusty, whole-grain bread or ladle it over whole-grain pasta.*

1 teaspoon dried oregano, crumbled

1 teaspoon dried basil, crumbled

1/2 teaspoon salt

1/4 teaspoon pepper

4 boneless, skinless chicken breasts (about 4 ounces each), all visible fat discarded

1/4 cup all-purpose flour

2 teaspoons olive oil

2 medium ribs of celery, chopped

2 medium leeks, cut into thin strips (white part only)

4 medium garlic cloves, minced

1 14.5-ounce can no-salt-added diced tomatoes, undrained

1 cup fat-free, low-sodium chicken broth, such as on page 36

1/2 cup dry white wine (regular or nonalcoholic), or 1/2 cup fat-free, low-sodium chicken broth, such as on page 36

In a small bowl, stir together the oregano, basil, salt, and pepper. Sprinkle all over the chicken. Using your fingertips, gently press the mixture so it adheres to the chicken. Put the flour in a shallow dish. Dip the chicken in the flour, turning to coat and gently shaking off any excess. Transfer the chicken to a large plate.

In a large skillet, heat the oil over medium-high heat, swirling to coat the bottom. Cook the chicken for 2 to 3 minutes on each side, or until browned. Transfer to a separate large plate (the chicken won't be done at this point).

Reduce the heat to medium. In the same skillet, cook the celery and leeks for 2 to 3 minutes, or until soft, stirring occasionally. Stir in the garlic. Cook for 1 minute, or until the garlic is fragrant, stirring frequently. Stir in the tomatoes with liquid, broth, and wine. Return the chicken to the skillet, spooning the vegetables over the chicken.

Bring to a simmer over medium-high heat. Reduce the heat and simmer, covered, for 20 minutes, or until the chicken is no longer pink in the center.

PER SERVING

calories 240	carbohydrates 15 g
total fat 5.5 g	fiber 2 g
saturated fat 1.0 g	sugars 5 g
trans fat 0.0 g	protein 27 g
polyunsaturated fat 1.0 g	DIETARY EXCHANGES
monounsaturated fat 2.5 g	1/2 starch, 1 vegetable,
cholesterol 73 mg	3 lean meat
sodium 468 mg	

ONE-POT CHICKEN DINNER

SERVES 4

This oven-braised entrée is a complete meal—cooked all in one pot. Although it takes next to no time to prepare, this dish cooks low and slow, so be sure to make it when you have a couple of hours at home.

4 boneless, skinless chicken breast halves (about 4 ounces each), all visible fat discarded

3 medium potatoes, peeled and cut into 1/2-inch slices

1 large onion, quartered

8 ounces green beans, trimmed, or 10 ounces frozen green beans, thawed

2 large carrots, peeled and quartered lengthwise, then cut crosswise into 2-inch slices

1 tablespoon chopped fresh parsley

Pepper to taste (freshly ground preferred)

1/2 cup dry sherry

Preheat the oven to 300°F.

Put the chicken in a large, heavy ovenproof pot.

(continued)

Place the potatoes on the chicken. Put the onion, green beans, and carrots in the pot. Sprinkle the parsley and pepper over the vegetables.

Pour the sherry over all.

Bake, tightly covered, for 2 hours, or until the vegetables are tender.

PER SERVING

calories 329	carbohydrates 42 g
total fat 3.5 g	fiber 6 g
saturated fat 0.5 g	sugars 8 g
trans fat 0.0 g	protein 30 g
polyunsaturated fat 0.5 g	DIETARY EXCHANGES
monounsaturated fat 1.0 g	2 starch, 2 vegetable,
cholesterol 73 mg	3 lean meat
sodium 172 mg	

CHICKEN JAMBALAYA

SERVES 4

Capture the flavors of Louisiana with this casserole. Your family will love the taste—and you'll love the simple preparation. Pair it with a side dish, such as Corn Bread Muffins *(page 464) or* Green Beans Oregano *(page 390), to complete your dinner.*

Cooking spray
1 cup fat-free, low-sodium chicken broth, such as on page 36
1 cup dry white wine (regular or nonalcoholic)
1 large onion, chopped
1 medium green bell pepper, chopped
2 medium ribs of celery, chopped
1/4 cup chopped fresh parsley
1/2 teaspoon dried basil, crumbled
1/2 teaspoon dried thyme, crumbled
1 large dried bay leaf
1/4 teaspoon red hot-pepper sauce
1 14.5-ounce can no-salt-added diced tomatoes, undrained
1 cup uncooked brown rice
1/2 cup cubed lower-sodium, low-fat ham
4 boneless, skinless chicken breast halves (about 4 ounces each), all visible fat discarded

Preheat the oven to 350°F. Lightly spray a 13 x 9 x 2-inch glass baking dish or 2-quart glass casserole dish with cooking spray.

In a medium saucepan, stir together the broth, wine, onion, bell pepper, celery, parsley, basil, thyme, bay leaf, and hot-pepper sauce. Bring to a boil over medium-high heat, stirring occasionally. Remove from the heat.

In the baking dish, stir together the tomatoes with liquid, rice, and ham. Place the chicken on top. Pour the hot broth mixture over all.

Bake, covered, for 45 to 55 minutes, or until the chicken is no longer pink in the center and the rice is tender. Discard the bay leaf.

PER SERVING

calories 414	carbohydrates 49 g
total fat 5.0 g	fiber 5 g
saturated fat 1.0 g	sugars 8 g
trans fat 0.0 g	protein 33 g
polyunsaturated fat 1.0 g	DIETARY EXCHANGES
monounsaturated fat 1.5 g	2 1/2 starch, 2 vegetable,
cholesterol 80 mg	3 1/2 lean meat
sodium 355 mg	

CHICKEN WITH PEACH GLAZE

SERVES 4

Sweet peaches and tart pineapple juice combine with a hint of heat to enhance the flavor of chicken breasts. Serve Rustic Potato Patties *(page 400) and a steamed bright green vegetable to complement this palate-pleaser.*

1/4 cup all-purpose flour
1/8 teaspoon pepper (white preferred)
4 boneless, skinless chicken breast halves (about 4 ounces each), all visible fat discarded
Cooking spray
1 tablespoon canola or corn oil
1/2 cup all-fruit peach spread
2/3 cup 100% pineapple juice
1 tablespoon dry sherry
2 teaspoons soy sauce (lowest sodium available)
1 teaspoon dried basil, crumbled

1 teaspoon grated peeled gingerroot

1 teaspoon grated lemon zest

1/8 teaspoon red hot-pepper sauce

16 ounces jarred peach slices in light syrup, drained with 2/3 of the liquid reserved, coarsely chopped

1 medium red bell pepper, diced

In a medium shallow dish, stir together the flour and pepper. Dip the chicken in the mixture, turning to coat and gently shaking off any excess. Transfer the chicken with the smooth side up to a plate. Lightly spray the top with cooking spray.

In a large nonstick skillet, heat the oil over medium-high heat, swirling to coat the bottom. Cook the chicken with the smooth side down for 5 to 6 minutes, or until lightly browned. Remove from the heat.

Lightly spray the unbrowned side of the chicken with cooking spray. Turn over the chicken. Cover the browned side of the chicken with the peach spread.

In a medium bowl, whisk together the pineapple juice, sherry, soy sauce, basil, gingerroot, lemon zest, hot-pepper sauce, and reserved peach liquid. Pour into the skillet. Bring to a simmer, still over medium-high heat. Reduce the heat and simmer, covered, for 10 minutes, or until the chicken is no longer pink in the center.

Stir in the bell pepper. Cook for 7 to 8 minutes. Serve the chicken topped with the peaches and sauce.

PER SERVING

calories 312	**carbohydrates** 36 g
total fat 6.5 g	fiber 1 g
saturated fat 1.0 g	sugars 23 g
trans fat 0.0 g	**protein** 26 g
polyunsaturated fat 1.5 g	**DIETARY EXCHANGES**
monounsaturated fat 3.0 g	1/2 starch, 2 fruit,
cholesterol 73 mg	3 lean meat
sodium 202 mg	

SHERRY CHICKEN AND VEGETABLES

SERVES 4

Everything you need for your dinner bakes together in just one pan, making cleanup super simple. Toss a dark green, leafy salad with Chunky Cucumber and Garlic Dressing *(page 106) to serve on the side.*

Cooking spray

2 medium potatoes, peeled and chopped into 1/2-inch cubes

2 large carrots, cut into 1-inch pieces

2 medium onions, each cut into 8 wedges

4 whole medium garlic cloves

1/4 teaspoon salt

4 boneless, skinless chicken breast halves (about 4 ounces each), all visible fat discarded

1/2 cup dry sherry

1/2 teaspoon pepper

1/2 teaspoon dried dillweed, crumbled

Preheat the oven to 350°F. Lightly spray a deep baking pan with cooking spray.

Put the potatoes, carrots, onions, and garlic in the pan. Sprinkle the salt over all. Arrange the chicken on top. Pour the sherry over all. Sprinkle the pepper and dillweed over all.

Bake, covered, for 30 minutes, or until the chicken is no longer pink in the center and the potatoes and carrots are tender and the onions are soft.

Cook's Tip: Be careful not to use cooking sherry, which contains added salt.

PER SERVING

calories 277	**carbohydrates** 30 g
total fat 3.0 g	fiber 4 g
saturated fat 0.5 g	sugars 7 g
trans fat 0.0 g	**protein** 28 g
polyunsaturated fat 0.5 g	**DIETARY EXCHANGES**
monounsaturated fat 1.0 g	1 1/2 starch,
cholesterol 73 mg	2 vegetable, 3 lean meat
sodium 313 mg	

ROSEMARY CHICKEN

SERVES 4

This delicately flavored dish needs just 30 minutes of baking time, so it's a great choice for a weeknight dinner. While the chicken is baking, steam some veggies and prepare Lemon-Basil Rice *(page 420).*

Cooking spray
4 boneless, skinless chicken breast halves (about 4 ounces each), all visible fat discarded
2 tablespoons chopped fresh rosemary, or 2 teaspoons dried rosemary, crushed
Cooking spray
2 ounces button mushrooms, thinly sliced
1/2 cup fat-free, low-sodium chicken broth, such as on page 36
1/4 cup dry white wine (regular or nonalcoholic)
1 tablespoon fresh lemon juice
Pepper to taste
1 medium lemon, cut into 4 wedges (optional)
4 sprigs of fresh parsley (optional)

Preheat the oven to 350°F. Lightly spray a 9-inch square baking dish with cooking spray.

Rub the chicken with the rosemary. Lightly spray with cooking spray. Place the chicken with the smooth side down in the dish.

Bake for 15 minutes.

Meanwhile, in a medium bowl, stir together the mushrooms, broth, wine, lemon juice, and pepper. Pour over the chicken.

Bake for 15 minutes, or until the chicken is no longer pink in the center. Garnish with the lemon wedges and parsley.

PER SERVING

calories 146	sodium 136 mg
total fat 3.0 g	**carbohydrates** 1 g
saturated fat 0.5 g	fiber 0 g
trans fat 0.0 g	sugars 0 g
polyunsaturated fat 0.5 g	**protein** 25 g
monounsaturated fat 1.0 g	**DIETARY EXCHANGES**
cholesterol 73 mg	3 lean meat

POACHED CHICKEN THREE WAYS

SERVES 4

Poaching is a tried-and-true cooking method that keeps chicken breasts moist and tender. With a few simple swaps in the poaching liquids and three different sauces, this recipe gives you three unique dinner options.

Use 4 boneless, skinless chicken breast halves (about 4 ounces each), all visible fat discarded, flattened to 3/4-inch thickness with each of these three combinations of poaching liquid and sauce:

CHICKEN À L'ORANGE

Poaching Liquid
1 1/2 cups fat-free, low-sodium chicken broth, such as on page 36
1/2 cup dry vermouth, dry white wine (regular or nonalcoholic), or water
1 small orange, thinly sliced
1 sprig of fresh rosemary, or 2 teaspoons dried rosemary, crushed

Marmalade Sauce
1/3 cup orange marmalade
1 tablespoon white wine vinegar
1 teaspoon chopped fresh rosemary, or 1/4 teaspoon dried rosemary, crushed

PER SERVING

calories 198	**carbohydrates** 18 g
total fat 3.0 g	fiber 0 g
saturated fat 0.5 g	sugars 16 g
trans fat 0.0 g	**protein** 24 g
polyunsaturated fat 0.5 g	**DIETARY EXCHANGES**
monounsaturated fat 1.0 g	1 other carbohydrate,
cholesterol 73 mg	3 lean meat
sodium 147 mg	

LEMON-DIJON CHICKEN

Poaching Liquid

> 1 1/2 cups fat-free, low-sodium chicken broth, such as on page 36
>
> 1 medium lemon, thinly sliced
>
> 2 tablespoons dry sherry
>
> 2 sprigs of fresh thyme

Dijon-Yogurt Sauce

> 1/2 cup fat-free plain Greek yogurt
>
> 1 tablespoon Dijon mustard (lowest sodium available)
>
> 1 tablespoon fresh lemon juice
>
> 1 teaspoon olive oil (extra-virgin preferred)
>
> 1/4 teaspoon pepper (freshly ground preferred)

PER SERVING

calories 162	sodium 219 mg
total fat 4.5 g	carbohydrates 2 g
saturated fat 1.0 g	fiber 0 g
trans fat 0.0 g	sugars 1 g
polyunsaturated fat 0.5 g	protein 27 g
monounsaturated fat 1.5 g	DIETARY EXCHANGES
cholesterol 74 mg	3 lean meat

SOUTHWESTERN LIME CHICKEN

Poaching Liquid

> 1 1/2 cups fat-free, low-sodium chicken broth, such as on page 36
>
> 1 medium lime, thinly sliced
>
> 1 tablespoon coriander seeds, crushed with a mortar and pestle
>
> 8 sprigs of fresh cilantro

Pico de Gallo

> 2 medium Italian plum (Roma) tomatoes, diced
>
> 2 tablespoons chopped onion
>
> 1 medium fresh serrano pepper, seeds and ribs discarded, diced, or 1/2 medium fresh jalapeño, seeds and ribs discarded, diced (see Cook's Tip on Handling Hot Chiles, page 24)
>
> 1 teaspoon fresh lime juice

For each variation, in a large shallow saucepan, stir together the poaching liquid ingredients.

Bring to a boil over high heat. Reduce the heat and simmer, covered, for 5 minutes.

Place the chicken in the poaching liquid. Increase the heat to medium high and return to a simmer. Reduce the heat and simmer, partially covered, for 8 minutes, or until the chicken is no longer pink in the center.

Meanwhile, in a small bowl, whisk together the sauce ingredients that correspond to the poaching liquid you're using. If making the Pico de Gallo, gently stir together the ingredients.

Using a slotted spoon or spatula, transfer the cooked chicken to a cutting board. Discard the poaching liquid. Cut the chicken diagonally across the grain into thick slices. Transfer to plates. Spoon the sauce over the chicken.

PER SERVING

calories 138	sodium 133 mg
total fat 3.0 g	carbohydrates 2 g
saturated fat 0.5 g	fiber 1 g
trans fat 0.0 g	sugars 1 g
polyunsaturated fat 0.5 g	protein 24 g
monounsaturated fat 1.0 g	DIETARY EXCHANGES
cholesterol 73 mg	3 lean meat

STUFFED CHICKEN WITH BLUE CHEESE

SERVES 4

Tangy blue cheese and earthy spinach are perfect partners to stuff chicken breasts in this dish. Serve with Roasted Beets (page 375).

> Cooking spray
>
> 10 ounces frozen chopped spinach, thawed and squeezed dry
>
> 1/2 cup finely chopped onion
>
> 2 teaspoons dried basil, crumbled
>
> 1/8 teaspoon crushed red pepper flakes
>
> 1 1/2 ounces low-fat blue cheese, crumbled
>
> 4 boneless, skinless chicken breast halves (about 4 ounces each), all visible fat discarded, flattened to 1/4-inch thickness
>
> Pepper to taste
>
> Paprika to taste

(continued)

Preheat the oven to 400°F. Line a baking sheet with aluminum foil. Lightly spray the foil with cooking spray.

In a small bowl, stir together the spinach, onion, basil, and red pepper flakes.

Gently stir the blue cheese into the spinach mixture.

Place the chicken with the smooth side down on the baking sheet. Spoon the spinach mixture down the center of each breast. Press down on the mixture to pack it. Roll up the breasts jelly-roll style. Place with the seam side down. Secure with wooden toothpicks. Lightly spray the chicken rolls with cooking spray. Sprinkle the pepper and paprika over the rolls.

Bake for 25 minutes, or until the chicken is no longer pink in the center.

PER SERVING

calories 190	carbohydrates 6 g
total fat 5.5 g	fiber 3 g
saturated fat 2.0 g	sugars 2 g
trans fat 0.0 g	protein 30 g
polyunsaturated fat 0.5 g	DIETARY EXCHANGES
monounsaturated fat 1.5 g	1 vegetable, 3 1/2 lean
cholesterol 78 mg	meat
sodium 329 mg	

SPICY CHICKEN AND GRITS

SERVES 4

This recipe uses a spice rub for lots of flavor, adds soothing grits, and keeps everything savory and moist with a chicken broth sauce. Add Southern-Style Greens (page 391) or "Fried" Green Tomatoes (page 409) to complete your meal.

1 cup uncooked quick-cooking grits
4 cups fat-free, low-sodium chicken broth
    and 2 cups fat-free, low-sodium chicken broth, such as on page 36, divided use
1 teaspoon paprika
1 teaspoon sugar
1/2 teaspoon pepper
1/2 teaspoon cayenne

1 pound boneless, skinless chicken breasts, all visible fat discarded
1 tablespoon olive oil
1 small onion, minced
1/2 medium green bell pepper, minced
1 medium garlic clove, minced

Prepare the grits using the package directions, substituting 4 cups broth for the water and omitting the salt and margarine. Cover to keep warm. Set aside.

Meanwhile, in a small bowl, stir together the paprika, sugar, pepper, and cayenne. Sprinkle the mixture all over the chicken. Using your fingertips, gently press the mixture so it adheres to the chicken. Transfer to a cutting board.

In a large nonstick skillet, heat the oil over medium heat, swirling to coat the bottom. Cook the onion, bell pepper, and garlic for 10 minutes, stirring occasionally.

Meanwhile, cut the chicken across the grain into thin slivers. Stir into the onion mixture. Increase the heat to high and cook for 3 minutes, stirring frequently and scraping to dislodge any browned bits. Transfer the chicken mixture to a large plate.

Pour the remaining 2 cups broth into the skillet. Boil rapidly for 5 minutes, or until the broth is reduced by two-thirds (to about 3/4 cup).

Stir the chicken mixture into the broth. Cook for 2 minutes, or until heated through. Transfer the grits to plates. Spoon the chicken mixture and broth over the grits.

PER SERVING

calories 341	carbohydrates 37 g
total fat 7.0 g	fiber 2 g
saturated fat 1.0 g	sugars 3 g
trans fat 0.0 g	protein 31 g
polyunsaturated fat 1.0 g	DIETARY EXCHANGES
monounsaturated fat 3.5 g	2 1/2 starch, 3 lean
cholesterol 73 mg	meat
sodium 172 mg	

SOUTHWESTERN CHICKEN

SERVES 6

Serve this spicy dish with warm corn tortillas to counter the heat of the dish. You can adjust the heat level by reducing or increasing the jalapeño and chili powder. Serve with Watermelon-Cilantro Sorbet *(page 504) for dessert.*

1 1/2 cups orange, red, or yellow bell pepper strips, or a combination

2 teaspoons seeded and minced fresh jalapeño (see Cook's Tip on Handling Hot Chiles, page 24)

1/2 cup diagonally sliced green onions

1/3 cup all-purpose flour

1 1/2 teaspoons chili powder and 1 teaspoon chili powder, divided use

1/4 teaspoon pepper and 1/4 teaspoon pepper, divided use

1/4 teaspoon salt

6 boneless, skinless chicken breast halves (about 4 ounces each), all visible fat discarded, flattened to 1/4-inch thickness

1 teaspoon canola or corn oil and 1 teaspoon canola or corn oil, divided use

1 28-ounce can no-salt-added whole tomatoes, undrained

1 teaspoon grated lime zest

In a large nonstick skillet, cook the bell peppers and jalapeño over medium-high heat for 4 to 5 minutes, stirring occasionally.

Stir in the green onions. Cook for 1 minute. Transfer the bell pepper mixture to a plate. Set aside.

In a medium shallow dish, stir together the flour, 1 1/2 teaspoons chili powder, 1/4 teaspoon pepper, and the salt. Dip the chicken in the mixture, turning to coat and gently shaking off any excess. Transfer to a separate plate.

In a large nonstick skillet, heat 1 teaspoon oil over medium-high heat, swirling to coat the bottom. Cook half the chicken for 3 to 4 minutes on each side, or until lightly browned on both sides (the chicken won't be done at this point). Transfer to

the plate with the bell pepper mixture. Repeat with the remaining 1 teaspoon oil and chicken.

Pour the tomatoes with liquid into the skillet, breaking up the tomatoes with a spoon.

Stir in the remaining 1 teaspoon chili powder and 1/4 teaspoon pepper. Reduce the heat and simmer for 3 to 4 minutes.

Stir in the lime zest, bell pepper mixture, and chicken. Increase the heat to medium. Cook for 5 to 6 minutes, or until the chicken is no longer pink in the center and the tomato mixture is heated through.

PER SERVING

calories 207	carbohydrates 14 g
total fat 5.0 g	fiber 3 g
saturated fat 1.0 g	sugars 5 g
trans fat 0.0 g	protein 26 g
polyunsaturated fat 1.0 g	DIETARY EXCHANGES
monounsaturated fat 2.0 g	1/2 starch, 1 vegetable,
cholesterol 73 mg	3 lean meat
sodium 265 mg	

SPICY GRILLED CHICKEN

SERVES 4 (PLUS 4 CHICKEN BREAST HALVES RESERVED)

Grill once, eat twice. Try these chicken breasts with Jícama Slaw *(page 83) and* Chile-Lime Grilled Corn *(page 386), and save the extras to use for* Chicken Fajita Bowls *(page 220).*

Marinade

1 small red onion, finely chopped

3 tablespoons fresh lime juice (about 2 medium limes)

2 tablespoons olive oil

2 tablespoons finely chopped fresh cilantro

1/2 teaspoon chili powder

1/2 teaspoon ground cumin

1/4 teaspoon salt

1 small garlic clove, minced

1/2 medium fresh jalapeño, seeds and ribs discarded, minced (see Cook's Tip on Handling Hot Chiles, page 24)

(continued)

■ ■ ■

8 boneless, skinless chicken breast halves
(about 4 ounces each), all visible fat
discarded
Cooking spray

In a large shallow glass dish, whisk together the marinade ingredients. Add the chicken, turning to coat. Cover and refrigerate for 2 to 3 hours, turning occasionally.

Lightly spray the grill rack with cooking spray. Preheat the grill on medium high.

Grill the chicken for 6 to 7 minutes on each side, or until no longer pink in the center.

PER SERVING

calories 129	**sodium** 204 mg
total fat 3.0 g	**carbohydrates** 0 g
saturated fat 0.5 g	fiber 0 g
trans fat 0.0 g	sugars 0 g
polyunsaturated fat 0.5 g	**protein** 24 g
monounsaturated fat 1.0 g	**DIETARY EXCHANGES**
cholesterol 73 mg	3 lean meat

CHIPOTLE CHICKEN WRAPS

SERVES 6

Smoky chicken saved from Mexican Chicken and Vegetables with Chipotle Peppers *is rolled in tortillas with classic fajita toppings. Serve with* Mexican Fried Rice *(page 421) or* Zesty Corn Relish *(page 78).*

4 cooked chicken breast halves from Mexican
    Chicken and Vegetables with Chipotle
    Peppers (page 213)
1 cup tomato mixture from Mexican Chicken
    and Vegetables with Chipotle Peppers
    (page 213)
6 8-inch whole-wheat tortillas (lowest
    sodium available)
1/2 cup fat-free sour cream
1/2 cup finely chopped red onion
1/4 cup chopped fresh cilantro (optional)
12 medium black olives, drained and
    quartered
Pepper to taste
Fresh lime juice to taste

In a small saucepan, warm the reserved chicken and the tomato sauce mixture over medium heat for 10 minutes, or until heated through, stirring occasionally.

Warm the tortillas using the package directions.

To assemble, layer as follows down the center of each tortilla: chicken mixture (use a slotted spoon), sour cream, onion, cilantro, olives, pepper, and lime juice. Roll the tortilla jelly-roll style over the filling, securing with a wooden toothpick if desired.

PER SERVING

calories 280	**carbohydrates** 37 g
total fat 5.0 g	fiber 5 g
saturated fat 0.5 g	sugars 9 g
trans fat 0.0 g	**protein** 23 g
polyunsaturated fat 1.5 g	**DIETARY EXCHANGES**
monounsaturated fat 2.0 g	2 starch, 1 vegetable,
cholesterol 52 mg	2 1/2 lean meat
sodium 519 mg	

JERK CHICKEN

SERVES 4

This spicy dish can be a welcome change to some of the more familiar chicken dishes in your cooking repertoire. Highlighted by the popular Jamaican "jerk" seasoning—a combination of cinnamon, nutmeg, onion, chiles, rum, and allspice—the chicken will need some time to soak it in so plan ahead. Enjoy with Calypso Rice *(page 421) and* Grilled Pineapple *(page 502).*

Marinade
  2 tablespoons fresh lime juice (about
    1 1/2 medium limes)
  1 medium fresh jalapeño pepper, seeds and
    ribs discarded, chopped (see Cook's Tip
    on Handling Hot Chiles, page 24)
  1 tablespoon red wine vinegar
  1 tablespoon rum, or 1/8 teaspoon rum
    extract
  1 tablespoon canola or corn oil
  1 medium shallot, peeled and chopped
  2 teaspoons ground allspice (freshly ground
    preferred), dry-roasted

1 1/2 to 2 teaspoons soy sauce (lowest sodium
available)
2 medium garlic cloves, minced
1/2 teaspoon ground gingerroot
1/4 teaspoon dried thyme, crumbled
1/4 teaspoon salt
1/4 teaspoon ground cinnamon
1/8 teaspoon ground nutmeg
1/8 teaspoon pepper

■ ■ ■

4 boneless, skinless chicken breast halves
(about 4 ounces each), all visible fat
discarded
Cooking spray

In a blender or food processor, process the marinade ingredients for 20 to 30 seconds. Pour into a shallow glass bowl.

Add the chicken, turning to coat. Cover and refrigerate for 2 to 10 hours, turning occasionally.

Preheat the grill on medium high.

Drain the chicken, discarding the marinade. Lightly spray both sides of the chicken with cooking spray. Grill for 6 to 8 minutes on each side, or until the chicken is no longer pink in the center.

PER SERVING

calories 131	sodium 334 mg
total fat 3.0 g	carbohydrates 0 g
saturated fat 0.5 g	fiber 0 g
trans fat 0.0 g	sugars 0 g
polyunsaturated fat 0.5 g	protein 24 g
monounsaturated fat 1.0 g	DIETARY EXCHANGES
cholesterol 73 mg	3 lean meat

POMEGRANATE CHICKEN WITH PISTACHIO RICE

SERVES 4

Pomegranate juice adds its sweet tang to the deep mahogany sauce in this truly delicious dish. Citrus and nuts transform basmati rice into a crunchy, tart side dish.

3/4 cup water
1 tablespoon grated orange zest
1/4 cup fresh orange juice
1/2 cup brown basmati rice
2 tablespoons chopped unsalted pistachios,
dry-roasted
2 teaspoons ground cumin
1 teaspoon poultry seasoning
1 teaspoon ground cinnamon
1/4 teaspoon ground turmeric
1/4 teaspoon ground nutmeg
4 boneless, skinless chicken breast halves
(about 4 ounces each), all visible fat
discarded
2 teaspoons olive oil and 1 teaspoon olive oil,
divided use
1 large onion, halved lengthwise, then each
half cut crosswise into 1/4-inch half-
circles
2 large garlic cloves, finely chopped
1/2 cup fat-free, low-sodium chicken broth,
such as on page 36
1 tablespoon no-salt-added tomato paste
1 cup 100% pomegranate juice
2 teaspoons frozen 100% orange juice
concentrate, thawed
2 teaspoons honey
1/4 teaspoon salt
1/8 teaspoon cayenne
1 tablespoon plus 1 teaspoon pomegranate
seeds (arils) (optional)

In a medium saucepan, bring the water and orange juice to a boil over high heat. Stir in the rice. Return to a boil. Reduce the heat and simmer, covered, for 22 minutes, or until the rice is tender and liquid is absorbed. Stir in the pistachios and orange zest. Set aside.

(continued)

Meanwhile, in a small bowl, stir together the cumin, poultry seasoning, cinnamon, turmeric, and nutmeg. Sprinkle all over the chicken. Using your fingertips, gently press the mixture so it adheres to the chicken.

In a large nonstick skillet, heat 2 teaspoons oil over medium-high heat, swirling to coat the bottom. Cook the chicken with the smooth side down for 4 minutes, or until lightly browned. Turn over the chicken. Cook for 2 minutes, or until crusty and lightly browned (the chicken won't be done at this point). Transfer the chicken to a large plate. Cover to keep warm. Set aside.

Reduce the heat to medium. In the same skillet, heat the remaining 1 teaspoon oil, swirling to coat the bottom. Add the onion. Reduce the heat to low. Cook for 8 minutes, or until the onion begins to turn light brown, stirring frequently.

Stir in the garlic. Cook for 1 minute, stirring constantly.

Stir in the broth and tomato paste. Bring to a simmer, still over low heat, and simmer for 3 minutes, or until most of the broth has cooked away, stirring frequently.

Stir in the pomegranate juice. Increase the heat to medium and bring to a boil. Reduce the heat and simmer for 5 minutes, or until the sauce thickens and becomes syrupy.

Stir in the juice concentrate, honey, salt, and cayenne. Add the chicken and any accumulated juices. Spoon the sauce over the chicken. Return to a simmer. Simmer, covered, for 5 minutes, or until the chicken is no longer pink in the center. Spoon the sauce over the chicken. Sprinkle with the pomegranate seeds. Serve with the rice mixture.

PER SERVING

calories 360	carbohydrates 43 g
total fat 8.5 g	fiber 3 g
saturated fat 1.5 g	sugars 18 g
trans fat 0.0 g	**protein** 28 g
polyunsaturated fat 1.5 g	**DIETARY EXCHANGES**
monounsaturated fat 4.5 g	1 1/2 starch, 1 fruit,
cholesterol 73 mg	1 vegetable, 3 lean
sodium 296 mg	meat

SUN-DRIED TOMATO AND KALAMATA OLIVE CHICKEN

SERVES 4

This Greek-inspired dish will transport you to the Greek Isles with its authentic flavors. Start the meal with Roasted-Pepper Hummus *(page 13) and raw veggie dippers or* Greek Egg and Lemon Soup (Avgolemono) *(page 35).*

> 1 cup uncooked whole-wheat couscous
> 10 dry-packed sun-dried tomato halves, chopped
> 1/4 cup boiling water
> 1/2 teaspoon dried oregano, crumbled, and 1/2 teaspoon dried oregano, crumbled, divided use
> 4 boneless, skinless chicken breast halves (about 4 ounces each), all visible fat discarded, flattened to 1/4-inch thickness
> 1/8 teaspoon salt
> 12 kalamata olives, finely chopped
> 1/4 cup finely chopped fresh parsley
> 1/8 teaspoon crushed red pepper flakes
> 1 ounce fat-free feta cheese, crumbled
> 2 teaspoons olive oil (extra-virgin preferred)

Prepare the couscous using the package directions, omitting the salt. Fluff with a fork. Cover to keep warm. Set aside.

In a small bowl, stir together the tomatoes and water. Let stand for 10 minutes. Drain in a colander. Transfer to a medium bowl.

Meanwhile, sprinkle 1/2 teaspoon oregano over the chicken, using 1/4 teaspoon on each side.

In a large nonstick skillet, cook the chicken over medium-high heat for 3 to 4 minutes on each side, or until no longer pink in the center. Remove from the heat. Sprinkle with the salt.

Stir the olives, parsley, red pepper flakes, and the remaining 1/2 teaspoon oregano into the drained tomatoes. Gently stir in the feta.

Spoon the couscous onto plates. Place the chicken on the couscous. Spoon the tomato mixture over the chicken. Drizzle with the oil.

calories 424
total fat 9.5 g
  saturated fat 1.5 g
  trans fat 0.0 g
  polyunsaturated fat 1.5 g
  monounsaturated fat 5.0 g
cholesterol 73 mg
sodium 502 mg

carbohydrates 51 g
  fiber 8 g
  sugars 2 g
protein 35 g
DIETARY EXCHANGES
  3 starch, 1 vegetable,
  3 lean meat

LEMON-CAYENNE CHICKEN

SERVES 4

Spicy cayenne and tart lemon provide the zip for these chicken breasts. Serve with Dilled Green Beans (page 388) and a whole grain, such as quinoa or bulgur.

1/2 cup all-purpose flour
3/4 teaspoon paprika
1/4 teaspoon salt
1/4 teaspoon cayenne
1/8 teaspoon pepper
4 boneless, skinless chicken breast halves (about 4 ounces each), all visible fat discarded, flattened to 1/4-inch thickness
1 tablespoon olive oil
3 tablespoons water
1 tablespoon light tub margarine
1 teaspoon fresh lemon juice
2 tablespoons finely chopped fresh parsley

In a shallow dish, stir together the flour, paprika, salt, cayenne, and pepper. Dip the chicken in the mixture, turning to coat and gently shaking off any excess. Transfer to a plate.

In a large nonstick skillet, heat the oil over medium-high heat for 1 minute, or until hot, swirling to coat the bottom. Cook the chicken for 3 to 4 minutes on each side, or until lightly browned on the outside and no longer pink in the center. Transfer to plates.

In the same skillet, stir together the water, margarine, and lemon juice, scraping to dislodge any browned bits. Bring the mixture to a boil. Boil for

about 30 seconds, or until the sauce is slightly thickened. Drizzle over the chicken. Sprinkle with the parsley.

PER SERVING

calories 229
total fat 7.5 g
  saturated fat 1.0 g
  trans fat 0.0 g
  polyunsaturated fat 1.0 g
  monounsaturated fat 4.0 g
cholesterol 73 mg

sodium 302 mg
carbohydrates 13 g
  fiber 1 g
  sugars 0 g
protein 26 g
DIETARY EXCHANGES
  1 starch, 3 lean meat

CHICKEN WITH BELL PEPPERS AND MUSHROOMS

SERVES 6

This chicken-and-veggie skillet one-dish meal becomes a super supper when it's served on a bed of Lemon-Basil Rice (page 420).

1/3 cup all-purpose flour
1/4 teaspoon pepper
1/4 teaspoon salt
6 boneless, skinless chicken breast halves (about 4 ounces each), all visible fat discarded, flattened to 1/4-inch thickness
1 teaspoon olive oil and 1 teaspoon olive oil, divided use
8 ounces medium button mushrooms, quartered
1 1/2 medium red bell peppers, cut into strips
3 medium garlic cloves, minced
1 1/2 cups fat-free, low-sodium chicken broth, such as on page 36
1/3 cup white wine (regular or nonalcoholic)
2 tablespoons fresh lemon juice
1/2 cup sliced green onions
Chopped fresh parsley (optional)

In a medium shallow dish, stir together the flour, pepper, and salt. Dip the chicken in the flour mixture, turning to coat and gently shaking off any excess. Transfer the chicken to a large plate.

(continued)

In a large nonstick skillet, heat 1 teaspoon oil over medium-high heat, swirling to coat the bottom. Cook half the chicken for 3 to 4 minutes on each side, or until lightly browned on both sides. Transfer to a separate large plate. Repeat with the remaining 1 teaspoon oil and chicken.

Put the mushrooms, bell peppers, and garlic in the skillet, stirring to combine. Reduce the heat to medium low. Cook, covered, for 7 to 9 minutes, stirring occasionally.

Pour in the broth, wine, and lemon juice. Add the chicken. Increase the heat to medium. Cook for 10 minutes, or until the sauce thickens slightly, stirring occasionally.

Stir in the green onions. Cook for 1 minute, or until the chicken is no longer pink in the center. Just before serving, sprinkle with the parsley.

PER SERVING

calories 204	**carbohydrates** 10 g
total fat 4.5 g	fiber 2 g
saturated fat 1.0 g	sugars 2 g
trans fat 0.0 g	**protein** 27 g
polyunsaturated fat 1.0 g	**DIETARY EXCHANGES**
monounsaturated fat 2.0 g	1/2 starch, 1 vegetable,
cholesterol 73 mg	3 lean meat
sodium 242 mg	

THREE-PEPPER CHICKEN WITH CARROTS

SERVES 4

The benefits of a stir-fried meal are that it cooks all in one pan and often includes lots of vegetables. This entrée is no exception; it offers a whole serving of colorful veggies for each diner. Showcase this visually appealing dish on a bed of brown rice or other whole grain and you have a complete meal.

> 4 boneless, skinless chicken breast halves (about 4 ounces each), all visible fat discarded, thinly sliced
> 1 tablespoon cornstarch and 1 1/2 teaspoons cornstarch, divided use

> 1 tablespoon soy sauce and 1 1/2 teaspoons soy sauce (lowest sodium available), divided use
> 1 1/2 tablespoons dry sherry
> 1 large egg white, slightly beaten
> 1 1/2 teaspoons canola or corn oil and 1 tablespoon canola or corn oil, divided use
> 1/2 teaspoon hot chili oil and 1/2 teaspoon hot chili oil, divided use
> 1/2 cup thinly sliced carrots
> 1/2 cup thinly sliced red bell pepper
> 1/2 cup thinly sliced yellow bell pepper
> 1/2 cup thinly sliced green bell pepper
> 2 tablespoons grated peeled gingerroot
> 2 medium garlic cloves, minced
> 1/2 cup fat-free, low-sodium chicken broth, such as on page 36
> 1/2 teaspoon pepper (coarsely ground preferred)

Put the chicken in a medium bowl.

Put 1 tablespoon cornstarch in a small bowl. Add 1 tablespoon soy sauce, the sherry, and egg white, whisking to dissolve. Pour over the chicken, stirring to coat. Cover and set aside for 30 minutes.

In a large skillet, heat 1 1/2 teaspoons canola oil and 1/2 teaspoon hot chili oil over high heat, swirling to coat the bottom. Cook the carrots and all the bell peppers for 1 to 2 minutes, stirring constantly. Transfer to a plate. Set aside.

In the same skillet, still over high heat, heat the remaining 1 tablespoon canola oil and 1/2 teaspoon hot chili oil, swirling to coat the bottom. Cook the gingerroot and garlic for 1 minute, stirring constantly. Stir in the chicken. Cook for 2 to 3 minutes.

Put the remaining 1 1/2 teaspoons cornstarch in a small bowl. Add the broth and the remaining 1 1/2 teaspoons soy sauce, whisking to dissolve. Stir the mixture into the chicken mixture. Cook for 1 to 2 minutes, or until the sauce is thickened and the chicken is no longer pink in the center.

Stir in the pepper and the carrot mixture. Cook for 30 seconds to 1 minute, or until heated through, stirring constantly.

Cook's Tip on _Mise en Place:_ _Mise en place (meez ahn plahs)_ is the French term for having all your ingredients ready (measured, sliced, melted, and so on) before you start cooking. This advance preparation is very important when stir-frying.

PER SERVING

calories 236	carbohydrates 9 g
total fat 9.5 g	fiber 2 g
saturated fat 1.0 g	sugars 3 g
trans fat 0.0 g	protein 27 g
polyunsaturated fat 2.5 g	DIETARY EXCHANGES
monounsaturated fat 5.0 g	2 vegetable, 3 lean
cholesterol 73 mg	meat
sodium 308 mg	

CHICKEN BREASTS WITH ZUCCHINI

SERVES 6

This Italian-style dish is superfast and easy, making it perfect for any busy night of the week. It includes vegetables, which cook right in the same pan. Serve over whole-wheat pasta or other whole grain for a well-rounded meal.

2 large egg whites, lightly beaten using a fork
2/3 cup whole-wheat panko (Japanese-style bread crumbs)
6 boneless, skinless chicken breasts, all visible fat discarded, pounded to 1/4-inch thickness
1 tablespoon canola or corn oil
2 cups canned no-salt-added diced tomatoes, undrained
1/4 teaspoon dried basil, crumbled
3 medium zucchini, each cut into slices 1/2 inch thick

Put the egg whites in a medium shallow dish. Put the panko in a separate medium shallow dish. Put the dishes and a large plate in a row, assembly-line fashion. Dip the chicken in the egg whites, then in the panko, turning to coat

at each step and gently shaking off any excess. Using your fingertips, gently press the coating so it adheres to the chicken. Place on the plate.

In a large skillet, heat the oil over medium-high heat, swirling to coat the bottom. Cook the chicken for 4 minutes, or until no longer pink in the center, turning once halfway through. Transfer to a separate large plate. Cover to keep warm.

In the same skillet, stir together the tomatoes and basil. Reduce the heat and simmer, tightly covered, for 10 minutes.

Stir in the zucchini. Cook, covered, for 5 minutes, or until the zucchini is tender-crisp.

Transfer the chicken to plates. Spoon the tomato mixture over the chicken.

PER SERVING

calories 208	carbohydrates 11 g
total fat 5.5 g	fiber 2 g
saturated fat 1.0 g	sugars 5 g
trans fat 0.0 g	protein 27 g
polyunsaturated fat 1.0 g	DIETARY EXCHANGES
monounsaturated fat 2.5 g	2 vegetable, 3 lean
cholesterol 73 mg	meat
sodium 171 mg	

SAFFRON-SCENTED GRILLED CHICKEN

SERVES 4

This super fast marinade packs a lot of punch with just three ingredients. If you don't feel like grilling, the chicken can just as easily be broiled, pan-seared, or even baked. Serve with grilled asparagus and a whole grain.

1/2 cup fresh lemon juice
1/2 teaspoon saffron threads, crumbled
1/2 teaspoon pepper, or to taste (freshly ground preferred)
4 boneless, skinless chicken breasts (about 4 ounces each), all visible fat discarded, pounded to 1/2-inch thickness
Cooking spray

(continued)

In a large glass baking dish, whisk together the lemon juice, saffron, and pepper. Add the chicken, turning to coat. Refrigerate, covered, for 30 minutes, turning occasionally.

Meanwhile, lightly spray the grill rack with cooking spray. Preheat the grill on medium high.

Drain the chicken, discarding the marinade. Grill the chicken for 5 to 7 minutes on each side, or until no longer pink in the center.

PER SERVING

calories 129	**sodium** 132 mg
total fat 3.0 g	**carbohydrates** 0 g
saturated fat 0.5 g	fiber 0 g
trans fat 0.0 g	sugars 0 g
polyunsaturated fat 0.5 g	**protein** 24 g
monounsaturated fat 1.0 g	**DIETARY EXCHANGES**
cholesterol 73 mg	3 lean meat

GRILLED LEMON-SAGE CHICKEN

SERVES 6

Fresh sage and rosemary impart a wonderfully earthy flavor to grilled chicken. Tomato halves and corn on the cob can grill along with the chicken.

Marinade
    1/4 cup chopped fresh sage
    1 teaspoon grated lemon zest
    1/4 cup fresh lemon juice
    1 tablespoon chopped fresh rosemary or
        1 teaspoon dried rosemary, crushed
    2 or 3 medium garlic cloves, minced
    1 teaspoon black peppercorns, cracked
    1 teaspoon olive oil
    1/2 teaspoon salt

■ ■ ■

6 boneless, skinless chicken breast halves
    (about 4 ounces each), all visible
    fat discarded, flattened to 1/4-inch
    thickness
6 lemon slices, halved (optional)
Fresh sage leaves (optional)

In a large shallow glass dish, stir together the marinade ingredients. Add the chicken, turning to coat. Cover and refrigerate for 30 minutes to 8 hours, turning occasionally.

Drain the chicken, discarding the marinade.

Preheat the grill on medium high.

Grill the chicken for 6 to 7 minutes on each side, or until no longer pink in the center. Garnish with the lemon slices and sage leaves.

PER SERVING

calories 129	**sodium** 325 mg
total fat 3.0 g	**carbohydrates** 1 g
saturated fat 0.5 g	fiber 0 g
trans fat 0.0 g	sugars 0 g
polyunsaturated fat 0.5 g	**protein** 24 g
monounsaturated fat 1.0 g	**DIETARY EXCHANGES**
cholesterol 73 mg	3 lean meat

CARIBBEAN GRILLED CHICKEN KEBABS

SERVES 4

An important part of this delicious blend of sweet and spicy island flavors, bananas are easier to handle on the grill if they're slightly under ripe. Serve on a bed of Calypso Rice *(page 421).*

Marinade
    2/3 cup 100% pineapple juice
    2 tablespoons minced onion
    2 tablespoons fresh lime juice
    1 tablespoon curry powder
    1 tablespoon honey
    1/4 teaspoon salt
    1/4 teaspoon pepper
    1/4 teaspoon red hot-pepper sauce

■ ■ ■

1 pound boneless, skinless chicken breasts,
    all visible fat discarded, cut into
    16 1 1/2-inch cubes
1 medium red onion, cut into 8 wedges
8 medium button mushrooms
8 cherry or grape tomatoes

1 large banana, slightly under ripe, cut crosswise into 8 pieces

In a large shallow glass dish, whisk together the marinade ingredients. Add the chicken, onion, mushrooms, and tomatoes, turning to coat. Cover and refrigerate for 1 hour, turning occasionally.

Meanwhile, soak eight 8-inch wooden skewers for at least 10 minutes in cold water to prevent charring, or use metal skewers.

Preheat the grill on medium.

Drain the chicken and vegetables. Pour the marinade into a small saucepan. Bring to a boil over high heat. Boil for at least 5 minutes (this destroys harmful bacteria).

Thread each skewer with 1 chicken cube, 1 onion wedge, 1 mushroom, 1 tomato, 1 piece of banana, and 1 chicken cube. Repeat. Grill the kebabs for 10 to 15 minutes, or until the chicken is no longer pink in the center, turning once halfway through. Just before serving, brush the kebabs with the marinade.

PER SERVING

calories 265	carbohydrates 33 g
total fat 3.5 g	fiber 4 g
saturated fat 1.0 g	sugars 19 g
trans fat 0.0 g	protein 27 g
polyunsaturated fat 0.5 g	DIETARY EXCHANGES
monounsaturated fat 1.0 g	1 1/2 fruit, 2 vegetable,
cholesterol 73 mg	3 lean meat
sodium 293 mg	

SESAME SOY CHICKEN

SERVES 6

This dish requires some time to absorb the flavors from this citrusy-ginger marinade, but it's well worth the wait. A short stay under the broiler makes a big difference in flavor; it brings out a rich caramelization in the chicken, so be sure not to skip this step. Serve with Edamame with Walnuts *(page 387) or* Stir-Fried Bok Choy with Green Onion Sauce *(page 375).*

1 cup finely chopped onion
1 teaspoon grated lime zest
1/2 cup fresh lime juice (about 4 large limes)
1/3 cup sherry or fresh orange juice
1/4 cup frozen 100% orange juice concentrate, thawed
3 tablespoons soy sauce (lowest sodium available)
2 tablespoons grated peeled gingerroot
1 tablespoon sugar
1 tablespoon hot chili oil
3 medium garlic cloves, minced
6 boneless, skinless chicken breast halves (about 4 ounces each), all visible fat discarded
1 tablespoon sesame seeds, dry-roasted

In a large broilerproof baking dish, stir together the onion, lime zest, lime juice, sherry, soy sauce, orange juice concentrate, gingerroot, sugar, hot chili oil, and garlic. Add the chicken, turning to coat. Cover and refrigerate for several hours or overnight, turning the chicken occasionally.

Preheat the oven to 400°F.

Bake the chicken with the marinade for 20 to 25 minutes, or until the chicken is no longer pink in the center. Remove from the oven. Preheat the broiler. Broil the chicken mixture for 5 minutes, turning the chicken halfway through. Just before serving, sprinkle with the sesame seeds.

PER SERVING

calories 215	carbohydrates 13 g
total fat 6.5 g	fiber 1 g
saturated fat 1.0 g	sugars 9 g
trans fat 0.0 g	protein 26 g
polyunsaturated fat 1.5 g	DIETARY EXCHANGES
monounsaturated fat 2.5 g	1 other carbohydrate,
cholesterol 73 mg	3 lean meat
sodium 330 mg	

CHICKEN AND SNOW PEA STIR-FRY

SERVES 6

This stir-fry offers crunch with its combination of water chestnuts, celery, and snow peas. Be sure to have all the ingredients prepped before you start cooking, because things move quickly when you're stir-frying.

1 cup uncooked instant brown rice
1/4 cup fat-free, low-sodium chicken broth, such as on page 36
1 tablespoon dry sherry or fresh orange juice
1 tablespoon soy sauce (lowest sodium available)
1 teaspoon grated peeled gingerroot
1 medium garlic clove, minced
1/8 teaspoon hot chili oil (optional)
2 teaspoons canola or corn oil
1 pound boneless, skinless chicken breasts, all visible fat discarded, thinly sliced
1 small onion, thinly sliced
1 medium rib of celery, thinly sliced
10 ounces frozen snow peas, thawed and patted dry
1 8-ounce can sliced water chestnuts, rinsed and drained
1 8-ounce can bamboo shoots, rinsed and drained
1 tablespoon cornstarch
1 teaspoon sugar
1/4 cup cold water
2 tablespoons slivered almonds, dry-roasted

Prepare the rice using the package directions, omitting the salt and margarine.

Meanwhile, in a small bowl, whisk together the broth, sherry, soy sauce, gingerroot, garlic, and hot chili oil. Set aside.

Heat a wok or large, heavy skillet over high heat. Pour in the canola oil, swirling to coat the wok. Cook the chicken for 3 to 4 minutes, or until no longer pink in the center, stirring constantly.

Stir in the onion and celery. Cook for 3 minutes, stirring constantly.

Stir in the snow peas, water chestnuts, bamboo shoots, and broth mixture. Reduce the heat to medium. Cook, covered, for 5 minutes.

Put the cornstarch and sugar in a small bowl. Add the water, whisking to dissolve. Stir into the chicken mixture. Increase the heat to medium high. Cook for 2 minutes, or until the sauce thickens, stirring frequently.

Transfer the rice to plates. Spoon the chicken mixture over the rice. Sprinkle with the almonds.

Cook's Tip on Cutting Chicken: Chicken is easier to slice if it's partially frozen. Put the chicken in the freezer for about 30 minutes before cutting. Make sure the chicken is thawed, though, before it goes into the hot oil in the wok or you'll have lots of oil splattering.

PER SERVING

calories 244	**carbohydrates** 26 g
total fat 5.5 g	fiber 5 g
saturated fat 0.5 g	sugars 5 g
trans fat 0.0 g	**protein** 22 g
polyunsaturated fat 1.5 g	**DIETARY EXCHANGES**
monounsaturated fat 2.5 g	1 1/2 starch,
cholesterol 48 mg	1 vegetable, 2 lean
sodium 219 mg	meat

CHICKEN MANDARIN

SERVES 4

Three types of citrus infuse the chicken as it simmers to brighten this Asian-style dish. Serve with Vegetable Stir-Fry (page 414) or Fresh Snow Peas with Water Chestnuts (page 403).

1/4 cup all-purpose flour
4 boneless, skinless chicken breast halves (about 4 ounces each), all visible fat discarded
2 teaspoons canola or corn oil
2 teaspoons light tub margarine
1/2 cup fresh orange juice
1/4 cup fresh lemon juice
1 11-ounce can mandarin oranges, packed in juice, drained, juice reserved
2 tablespoons honey

1 1/2 teaspoons soy sauce (lowest sodium available)
1/2 teaspoon ground ginger

Put the flour in a shallow dish. Dip the chicken in the flour, turning to coat and lightly shaking off any excess. Transfer to a plate.

In a large skillet, heat the oil and margarine over medium-high heat, swirling to coat the bottom. Cook the chicken for 1 minute on each side (the chicken won't be done at this point). Transfer to a large plate.

In a medium bowl, whisk together the orange juice, lemon juice, juice from the mandarin oranges, honey, soy sauce, and ginger.

Return the chicken to the skillet. Pour the sauce over the chicken. Reduce the heat to medium low. Simmer, covered, for 15 minutes, or until the chicken is no longer pink in the center. Add the mandarin oranges 5 to 10 minutes before the chicken is done.

PER SERVING

calories 259	carbohydrates 25 g
total fat 6.0 g	fiber 1 g
saturated fat 1.0 g	sugars 18 g
trans fat 0.0 g	protein 26 g
polyunsaturated fat 1.5 g	DIETARY EXCHANGES
monounsaturated fat 3.0 g	1 fruit, 1/2 other
cholesterol 73 mg	carbohydrate, 3 lean
sodium 199 mg	meat

SESAME CHICKEN

SERVES 4

Lemon juice and wine flavor this dish and keep the chicken moist as it bakes. Serve with Baked Cauliflower and Carrots with Nutmeg *(page 382), which bakes at the same temperature, and a whole grain.*

Cooking spray
1/3 cup all-purpose flour
1/4 teaspoon pepper
4 boneless, skinless chicken breast halves (about 4 ounces each), all visible fat discarded
1/4 cup sesame seeds
1 tablespoon fresh lemon juice

3 tablespoons minced green onions
1/2 cup dry white wine (regular or nonalcoholic) (plus more as needed)

Preheat the oven to 375°F. Lightly spray a 13 × 9 × 2-inch baking dish with cooking spray.

In a shallow dish, stir together the flour and pepper. Dip the chicken in the mixture, turning to coat and gently shaking off any excess. Lightly spray the smooth side with cooking spray. Transfer the chicken with the sprayed side down to the baking dish, arranging so the pieces don't touch. Lightly spray the top.

Sprinkle half the sesame seeds and the lemon juice over the chicken.

Bake for 30 minutes, or until lightly browned. Turn over the chicken. Sprinkle the green onions and the remaining sesame seeds over the chicken. Pour the wine around (not over) the chicken.

Bake for 30 to 45 minutes, or until the chicken is no longer pink in the center, basting occasionally with the liquid in the baking dish.

PER SERVING

calories 250	sodium 140 mg
total fat 9.0 g	carbohydrates 10 g
saturated fat 1.5 g	fiber 2 g
trans fat 0.0 g	sugars 0 g
polyunsaturated fat 3.0 g	protein 27 g
monounsaturated fat 3.0 g	DIETARY EXCHANGES
cholesterol 73 mg	1/2 starch, 3 lean meat

BROILED CHICKEN WITH HOISIN-BARBECUE SAUCE

SERVES 4

Ordinary barbecue sauce goes Asian in this one-dish meal. The sweet and savory kebabs are served with rice that's tinged bright yellow by turmeric and studded with green peas.

Cooking spray
1 cup uncooked instant brown rice
1/2 teaspoon ground turmeric

(continued)

Sauce

    1/4 cup hoisin sauce (lowest sodium
        available)

    2 tablespoons barbecue sauce (lowest
        sodium available)

    1 teaspoon sugar

    1 teaspoon cider vinegar

    3/4 teaspoon Worcestershire sauce (lowest
        sodium available)

    1/2 teaspoon grated peeled gingerroot

    1/8 teaspoon cayenne

■ ■ ■

    1 pound boneless, skinless chicken breasts,
        all visible fat discarded, cut into
        16 1 1/2-inch cubes

    16 medium button mushrooms

    12 medium green onions, each cut to 6 inches
        long and folded in half

    1 large red bell pepper, cut into 16 1-inch
        squares

    1 cup frozen green peas, thawed and patted
        dry

    1/4 cup finely chopped fresh cilantro or
        parsley

Soak four 12-inch wooden skewers for at least 10 minutes in cold water to prevent charring, or use metal skewers.

Preheat the broiler. Line the broiler pan with aluminum foil. Lightly spray the broiler rack with cooking spray.

Prepare the rice using the package directions, omitting the salt and margarine and adding the turmeric.

Meanwhile, in a small bowl, whisk together the sauce ingredients.

Thread each skewer with 4 chicken cubes, 4 mushrooms, 3 green onions, and 4 bell pepper squares. Put on the broiler rack.

Broil 2 to 3 inches from the heat for 3 minutes. Turn over the skewers. Spoon the sauce over all. Broil for 3 minutes, or until the chicken is no longer pink in the center.

Stir the peas into the rice. Spoon onto a platter. Arrange the skewers on the rice. Sprinkle with the cilantro.

PER SERVING

calories 341	fiber 7 g
total fat 4.0 g	sugars 16 g
saturated fat 0.5 g	**protein** 31 g
trans fat 0.0 g	**DIETARY EXCHANGES**
polyunsaturated fat 1.0 g	1 1/2 starch,
monounsaturated fat 1.0 g	2 vegetable, 1/2 other
cholesterol 73 mg	carbohydrate, 3 lean
sodium 330 mg	meat
carbohydrates 42 g	

CURRIED SWEET-AND-SOUR CHICKEN

Substitute 3/8 cup sweet-and-sour sauce for the hoisin and barbecue sauces, and substitute 1 teaspoon curry powder for the gingerroot.

Cook's Tip on Skewered Food: For a dramatic presentation, poke skewered items into a large, heavy vegetable. Try a butternut squash, an eggplant, or a red cabbage. Slice a thin piece off the bottom so it will sit flat. Surround the vegetable with sprigs of parsley or other fresh herbs. If you're serving fruit kebabs, stick them into a pineapple.

PER SERVING

calories 341	**carbohydrates** 42 g
total fat 4.5 g	fiber 7 g
saturated fat 0.5 g	sugars 16 g
trans fat 0.0 g	**protein** 31 g
polyunsaturated fat 1.0 g	**DIETARY EXCHANGES**
monounsaturated fat 1.0 g	1 1/2 starch, 2 vegetable,
cholesterol 73 mg	1/2 other carbohydrate, 3 lean
sodium 206 mg	meat

SPAGHETTI WITH GRILLED CHICKEN, MIXED BELL PEPPERS, AND ZUCCHINI

SERVES 4

A bit of apple juice gives a subtle sweetness to this all-in-one dish, providing a counterpoint to the heat of red pepper flakes and the tang of feta cheese.

8 ounces dried whole-grain spaghetti

1 cup 100% apple juice

3 or 4 medium garlic cloves, finely minced

1/4 teaspoon crushed red pepper flakes, or to taste

8 to 10 fresh basil leaves

2 boneless, skinless chicken breast halves (about 4 ounces each), all visible fat discarded

1 medium zucchini, quartered lengthwise

1 medium red bell pepper, quartered lengthwise

1 medium green bell pepper, quartered lengthwise

1 medium yellow bell pepper, quartered lengthwise

1 small red onion, cut into 1/4-inch wedges

Cooking spray

1 teaspoon dried Italian seasoning, crumbled

2 ounces crumbled fat-free feta cheese

1/4 teaspoon salt

Preheat the grill on medium high.

Prepare the pasta using the package directions, omitting the salt. Drain well in a colander. Set aside.

As soon as you put the water on to boil, put the apple juice, garlic, and red pepper flakes in a small saucepan and stir together. Cook over high heat for about 5 minutes, or until reduced by half (to about 1/2 cup). Remove from the heat. Set aside.

Meanwhile, stack the basil leaves into two piles, then roll up tightly from the tip end to the base. Cut crosswise into very thin strips. Transfer to a large serving bowl. Set aside.

Put the chicken, zucchini, and bell peppers on a large rimmed baking sheet. Tear off an 18-inch-long piece of aluminum foil. Fold in half crosswise, with the shiny side in, then roll up the edges to make a slightly raised rim. Put the onion on the foil. Spray the chicken, zucchini, bell peppers, and onion with cooking spray, turning to coat both sides. Sprinkle the Italian seasoning over all.

Transfer the chicken, zucchini, bell peppers, and foil with the onion to the grill. Grill, covered, for 10 minutes, or until the chicken is no longer pink in the center and the zucchini and bell peppers are just tender, turning or stirring once halfway through.

Transfer the zucchini and bell peppers to a cutting board. Slice them crosswise into 1/4-inch pieces. Stir into the basil. Stir in the onion. Cover the mixture to keep it warm. Transfer the chicken to the cutting board. Cut each piece in half lengthwise, then cut crosswise into 1/4-inch strips. Stir into the basil mixture. Stir in the feta, salt, and apple juice mixture. Toss gently with tongs. Serve over the pasta.

PER SERVING

calories 358	carbohydrates 60 g
total fat 3.5 g	fiber 9 g
saturated fat 0.5 g	sugars 14 g
trans fat 0.0 g	**protein** 24 g
polyunsaturated fat 1.0 g	**DIETARY EXCHANGES**
monounsaturated fat 1.0 g	3 starch, 2 vegetable,
cholesterol 36 mg	1/2 fruit, 2 lean meat
sodium 442 mg	

ITALIAN CHICKEN ROLL-UPS

SERVES 4

Serve these cheese-filled chicken rolls on a bed of Basil Spinach (page 404) and with Chocolate-Pistachio Biscotti (page 485) for dessert.

1 cup water

6 ounces no-salt-added tomato paste

1 medium garlic clove, minced

3/4 teaspoon dried oregano, crumbled

3/4 teaspoon dried basil, crumbled

1/2 teaspoon dried marjoram, crumbled

1/4 teaspoon pepper, or to taste

4 ounces fat-free ricotta cheese

4 boneless, skinless chicken breast halves (about 4 ounces each), all visible fat discarded, flattened to 1/4-inch thickness

2 ounces low-fat mozzarella cheese, shredded (about 1/2 cup)

(continued)

Preheat the oven to 350°F.

In a small saucepan, whisk together the water, tomato paste, and garlic.

In a small bowl, stir together the oregano, basil, marjoram, and pepper. Stir three-fourths of the mixture into the tomato paste mixture. Bring to a boil over medium-high heat. Reduce the heat and simmer for 10 minutes, stirring occasionally.

Meanwhile, stir the ricotta into the remaining oregano mixture. Leaving a 1/2-inch edge all around, spread over the chicken. Starting with a short side, roll up each breast jelly-roll style. Secure with wooden toothpicks.

Spoon half the tomato paste mixture into an 8-inch square glass baking dish. Arrange the chicken rolls with the seam side down on the sauce. Spoon the remaining sauce over the chicken rolls. Sprinkle the mozzarella over the rolls.

Bake for 45 minutes, or until the chicken is no longer pink in the center. If the chicken is getting too brown, cover it for the last 10 minutes of baking.

PER SERVING

calories 216	carbohydrates 10 g
total fat 4.5 g	fiber 2 g
saturated fat 1.0 g	sugars 6 g
trans fat 0.0 g	protein 33 g
polyunsaturated fat 0.5 g	DIETARY EXCHANGES
monounsaturated fat 1.5 g	2 vegetable, 4 lean
cholesterol 80 mg	meat
sodium 314 mg	

CHICKEN COLUMBO

SERVES 4

Seasoned wheat germ coats the chicken for a nutty flavor and a crunchy texture. A mushroom-wine sauce brings the dish together for a delicious meal. Serve with Baked Vegetable Casserole Italiano *(page 411).*

> 4 ounces dry whole-grain small or medium
>   pasta shells
> 1/2 cup fat-free milk

1/3 cup toasted wheat germ or plain dry
  bread crumbs (lowest sodium available)
1 teaspoon dried oregano, crumbled
1/4 teaspoon garlic powder
1/4 teaspoon onion powder
1/8 teaspoon salt
Pepper to taste
4 boneless, skinless chicken breast halves
  (about 4 ounces each), all visible fat
  discarded
1 tablespoon olive oil
8 ounces button mushrooms, sliced
1/4 cup dry marsala, dry sherry, or fat-free,
  low-sodium chicken broth, such as on
  page 36
1/4 cup water
3 tablespoons no-salt-added tomato paste
2 tablespoons chopped fresh parsley

Prepare the pasta using the package directions, omitting the salt. Set aside.

Meanwhile, pour the milk into a shallow dish. In a separate shallow dish, stir together the wheat germ, oregano, garlic powder, onion powder, salt, and pepper. Set the dishes and a plate in a row, assembly-line fashion. Dip the chicken in the milk, then in the wheat germ mixture, turning to coat at each step and gently shaking off any excess. Using your fingertips, gently press the coating so it adheres to the chicken. Place the chicken on the plate.

In a large nonstick skillet, heat the oil over medium-high heat, swirling to coat the bottom. Cook the chicken for 3 to 4 minutes on each side, or until lightly browned.

In a medium bowl, stir together the remaining ingredients except the parsley. Pour over the chicken. Reduce the heat and simmer for 10 minutes, or until the chicken is no longer pink in the center. Spoon the chicken and sauce over the pasta. Sprinkle with the parsley.

Cook's Tip on Wheat Germ: Wheat germ contains more nutrients per ounce than any other grain or vegetable and is very high in protein. Eat wheat germ as a cereal or sprinkle it over other cereals and other foods, such as casseroles, to add a nutty flavor, crunch, and nutrients. Store it in an airtight jar in the refrigerator.

PER SERVING

calories 329	carbohydrates 32 g
total fat 7.5 g	fiber 5 g
saturated fat 1.0 g	sugars 5 g
trans fat 0.0 g	protein 33 g
polyunsaturated fat 1.0 g	DIETARY EXCHANGES
monounsaturated fat 3.5 g	1 1/2 starch, 1 vegetable,
cholesterol 73 mg	3 lean meat
sodium 230 mg	

CHICKEN MARSALA

SERVES 4

Marsala, a type of fortified wine, is the key to this traditional Italian dish, which is generally prepared with veal. This version, prepared with chicken, offers an economical alternative.

1 tablespoon olive oil, 2 teaspoons olive oil, and 2 teaspoons olive oil, divided use

2 tablespoons minced shallot

10 ounces baby bella mushrooms, thinly sliced

1/2 teaspoon dried thyme, crumbled, and 1 1/2 teaspoons dried thyme, crumbled, divided use

1/4 teaspoon pepper and 1/4 teaspoon pepper, divided use

1/2 cup all-purpose flour

4 boneless, skinless chicken breast halves (about 4 ounces each), all visible fat discarded, flattened to 1/4-inch thickness

3/4 cup fat-free, low-sodium chicken broth, such as on page 36

1/4 cup marsala

2 tablespoons capers, drained

1 tablespoon balsamic vinegar

2 tablespoons chopped fresh parsley

In a large nonstick skillet, heat 1 tablespoon oil over medium-high heat, swirling to coat the bottom. Cook the shallot for 2 to 3 minutes, or until just soft, stirring constantly. Stir in the mushrooms, 1/2 teaspoon thyme, and 1/4 teaspoon

pepper. Cook for 7 to 10 minutes, or until the mushrooms are golden brown and the mushroom liquid has evaporated, stirring frequently. Transfer the mushroom mixture to a bowl. Set aside. Wipe the skillet clean with paper towels.

In a medium shallow dish, stir together the flour with the remaining 1 1/2 teaspoons thyme and 1/4 teaspoon pepper. Put the dish with the flour mixture and a large plate in a row, assembly-line fashion. Dip the chicken in the flour mixture, turning to coat and gently shaking off any excess. Using your fingertips, gently press the flour mixture so it adheres to the chicken. Place the chicken on the plate.

In the same skillet, still over medium-high heat, heat 2 teaspoons oil, swirling to coat the bottom. Cook 2 chicken breasts for 4 minutes. Turn over the chicken. Cook for 2 to 4 minutes, or until no longer pink in the center and golden brown on the outside. Transfer to a separate large plate. Wipe the skillet clean with paper towels. Repeat with the remaining 2 chicken breasts and the remaining 2 teaspoons oil.

Using a spatula or wooden spoon, stir together the broth and marsala in the skillet, scraping to dislodge any browned bits. Cook for 3 minutes, or until heated through, stirring constantly.

Stir in the capers, vinegar, and mushroom mixture. Cook for 2 to 3 minutes, or until the sauce has thickened, stirring constantly. Return the chicken to the skillet. Spoon the sauce over the chicken. Sprinkle with the parsley.

PER SERVING

calories 267	carbohydrates 12 g
total fat 11.0 g	fiber 2 g
saturated fat 2.0 g	sugars 3 g
trans fat 0.0 g	protein 28 g
polyunsaturated fat 1.5 g	DIETARY EXCHANGES
monounsaturated fat 6.5 g	1/2 starch, 1 vegetable,
cholesterol 73 mg	3 lean meat, 1/2 fat
sodium 271 mg	

ROSÉ CHICKEN WITH ARTICHOKE HEARTS AND MUSHROOMS

SERVES 4

Delicious as is, this one-skillet dish is also great over whole-grain couscous or steamed spinach. To start your meal, try a cup of Greek Egg and Lemon Soup (Avgolemono) (page 35).

1/4 cup all-purpose flour

4 boneless, skinless chicken breast halves (about 4 ounces each), all visible fat discarded

1/2 teaspoon olive oil and 1/2 teaspoon olive oil, divided use

8 ounces medium button mushrooms, quartered

2 medium garlic cloves, minced

9 ounces frozen artichoke hearts, thawed and halved

1 14.5-ounce can no-salt-added diced tomatoes, undrained

1/4 cup fat-free, low-sodium chicken broth, such as on page 36

1/4 cup rosé wine or dry white wine (regular or nonalcoholic)

1 tablespoon fresh lemon juice

1 teaspoon dried oregano, crumbled

1/4 teaspoon salt

1/2 cup thinly sliced green onions (green part only)

Put the flour in a shallow dish. Dip the chicken in the flour, turning to coat and gently shaking off any excess. Transfer to a large plate.

In a large nonstick skillet, heat 1/2 teaspoon oil over medium heat, swirling to coat the bottom. Cook the chicken for 4 minutes on each side. Transfer to a separate large plate.

Put the mushrooms, garlic, and the remaining 1/2 teaspoon oil in the skillet, stirring to combine. Cook, covered, for 7 minutes.

Stir in the artichoke hearts. Cook, uncovered, for 1 to 2 minutes, or until the liquid has evaporated.

Add the chicken and the remaining ingredients except the green onions. Cook for 10 minutes, or until the chicken is no longer pink in the center, stirring occasionally.

Stir in the green onions. Cook for 1 minute.

PER SERVING

calories 251	carbohydrates 21 g
total fat 4.5 g	fiber 8 g
saturated fat 1.0 g	sugars 5 g
trans fat 0.0 g	protein 29 g
polyunsaturated fat 0.5 g	DIETARY EXCHANGES
monounsaturated fat 1.5 g	1/2 starch, 3 vegetable,
cholesterol 73 mg	3 lean meat
sodium 363 mg	

CHICKEN VALENCIANA

SERVES 6

This recipe gets its name from Spain's citrus-growing region. While it's cooking, enjoy Gazpacho (page 49) or Watermelon Sangría (page 31).

6 boneless, skinless chicken breast halves (about 4 ounces each), all visible fat discarded

2 teaspoons pepper, or to taste

1/2 teaspoon salt

1 cup uncooked instant brown rice

1 cup 100% orange juice concentrate

2 medium ribs of celery, minced

1 medium onion

1 medium green bell pepper, diced

1 medium orange, diced

1 teaspoon dried oregano, crumbled

1 medium garlic clove, minced

1/2 teaspoon ground turmeric

Preheat the oven to 450°F.

Put the chicken in a large, heavy ovenproof pot. Sprinkle the pepper and salt over the chicken. Bake, uncovered, for 20 minutes.

Meanwhile, prepare the rice using the package directions, omitting the salt and margarine.

Stir the remaining ingredients into the cooked rice. Spoon the rice mixture into the pot.

Bake, covered, for 20 minutes.

calories 289
total fat 3.5 g
  saturated fat 0.5 g
  trans fat 0.0 g
  polyunsaturated fat 0.5 g
  monounsaturated fat 1.0 g
cholesterol 73 mg
sodium 343 mg

carbohydrates 36 g
  fiber 3 g
  sugars 22 g
protein 27 g
DIETARY EXCHANGES
  1 1/2 fruit, 1 starch,
  3 lean meat

CHICKEN CORDON BLEU

SERVES 4

The French words cordon bleu *translate to "blue ribbon." The term originally referred to prizes given for outstanding culinary creations. This first-class chicken entrée pairs winningly with* Mushrooms with White Wine and Shallots *(page 394) and* Peach Clafouti *(page 492) for dessert.*

> 4 boneless, skinless chicken breast halves (about 4 ounces each), all visible fat discarded, flattened to 1/4-inch thickness
> 2 slices low-fat Swiss cheese (about 2 ounces), halved
> 2 slices lower-sodium, low-fat ham (about 2 ounces), all visible fat discarded
> 1/2 cup chopped cooked spinach (about 8 to 10 ounces fresh)
> 4 teaspoons chopped fresh chives
> 3 tablespoons whole-wheat flour
> 1 teaspoon dry mustard
> 1/2 teaspoon paprika
> 2 teaspoons olive oil

Arrange the chicken on a work surface. Place half a slice of Swiss and a slice of ham on top of each breast. If the cheese or ham hangs over the edges of the chicken breast, cut it or fold it to fit it on top. Spread 2 tablespoons spinach on top of the ham. Sprinkle each breast with 1 teaspoon of chives. Starting with a short side, roll up jelly-roll style. Secure with wooden toothpicks.

In a medium shallow bowl, stir together the flour, mustard, and paprika. Dip the chicken in the flour mixture, turning lightly to coat and

gently shaking off any excess. Transfer to a large plate.

In a large nonstick skillet, heat the oil over medium-low heat, swirling to coat the bottom. Cook the chicken for about 15 minutes on each side, or until golden brown on the outside and no longer pink in the center. Cook each seam side for about 20 seconds to seal.

PER SERVING

calories 228
total fat 7.0 g
  saturated fat 1.5 g
  trans fat 0.0 g
  polyunsaturated fat 1.0 g
  monounsaturated fat 3.0 g
cholesterol 84 mg
sodium 337 mg

carbohydrates 8 g
  fiber 2 g
  sugars 1 g
protein 33 g
DIETARY EXCHANGES
  1/2 starch, 4 lean meat

CHICKEN IN WHITE WINE AND TARRAGON

SERVES 4

Make a double batch of this no-fuss chicken so you can serve it over angel hair pasta one night and still have enough for sandwiches or salads later in the week.

> 4 boneless, skinless chicken breast halves (about 4 ounces each), all visible fat discarded
> 1 cup dry white wine (regular or nonalcoholic)
> 1 tablespoon dried tarragon, crumbled
> 4 medium garlic cloves, minced
> 1 teaspoon dry mustard
> 1/4 teaspoon pepper

Preheat the oven to 350°F.

Put the chicken in a shallow broilerproof pan.

Pour the wine over the chicken.

In a small bowl, stir together the remaining ingredients. Sprinkle over the chicken. Using your fingertips, gently press the mixture so it adheres to the chicken.

(continued)

Bake, covered, for 35 minutes. Change the oven setting to broil. Broil the chicken, uncovered, about 5 inches from the heat for 2 to 3 minutes, or until lightly browned and no longer pink in the center.

PER SERVING

calories 164	sodium 134 mg
total fat 3.5 g	carbohydrates 2 g
saturated fat 0.5 g	fiber 1 g
trans fat 0.0 g	sugars 0 g
polyunsaturated fat 0.5 g	protein 25 g
monounsaturated fat 1.0 g	DIETARY EXCHANGES
cholesterol 73 mg	3 lean meat

ORANGE PECAN CHICKEN

SERVES 4

Sweet spices and tangy citrus hit high flavor notes in this French-inspired chicken dish, making diners sing for their supper. Serve over brown rice or with Whole-Wheat French Bread *(page 443) and* French Peas *(page 396).*

> 1/2 cup all-purpose flour
> 2 teaspoons grated orange zest
> 1 teaspoon paprika
> 1/2 teaspoon pepper (freshly ground preferred)
> 4 boneless, skinless chicken breast halves (about 4 ounces each), all visible fat discarded
> 1 teaspoon canola or corn oil
> 1/2 cup water
> 1 1/2 cups fresh orange juice
> 2 tablespoons brown sugar
> 1/4 teaspoon ground ginger
> 1/8 teaspoon ground cinnamon
> 1/4 cup finely chopped pecans

In a medium shallow bowl, stir together the flour, orange zest, paprika, and pepper. Dip the chicken in the flour mixture, turning to coat and shaking off any excess. Transfer the chicken to a large plate.

In a large, heavy nonstick skillet, heat the oil over medium-high heat, swirling to coat the bottom.

Cook the chicken for 2 minutes on each side, or until browned. Transfer to a large plate.

In the same skillet, add the water, orange juice, brown sugar, ginger, and cinnamon. Bring to a boil. Add the chicken, turning to coat. Reduce the heat and simmer, covered, for 10 to 12 minutes, or until the chicken is no longer pink in the center. Transfer chicken to a platter.

Increase the heat to medium high and bring to a boil. Boil for 2 minutes, or until the orange juice mixture is slightly thickened, stirring occasionally. Spoon over the chicken. Sprinkle with the pecans.

PER SERVING

calories 300	carbohydrates 27 g
total fat 9.5 g	fiber 2 g
saturated fat 1.0 g	sugars 15 g
trans fat 0.0 g	protein 27 g
polyunsaturated fat 2.5 g	DIETARY EXCHANGES
monounsaturated fat 4.5 g	1 fruit, 1 other
cholesterol 73 mg	carbohydrate, 3 lean
sodium 136 mg	meat

BURGUNDY CHICKEN WITH MUSHROOMS

SERVES 4

This delectable chicken dish is like a speedy version of coq au vin, *a classic French dish featuring chicken braised with red wine and mushrooms. Serve it with steamed red potatoes or* Potatoes with Leeks and Fresh Herbs *(page 398) and* Dilled Green Beans *(page 388).*

> 4 boneless, skinless chicken breast halves (about 4 ounces each), all visible fat discarded
> 8 ounces button mushrooms, sliced
> 1/4 cup finely chopped onion
> 2 tablespoons burgundy or other dry red wine (regular or nonalcoholic)
> 2 medium garlic cloves, minced
> 2 tablespoons finely chopped fresh parsley
> 1/4 teaspoon salt
> 2 teaspoons olive oil (extra-virgin preferred)

In a large nonstick skillet, cook the chicken over medium-high heat for 4 minutes. Turn over the chicken. Cook for 2 to 4 minutes, or until it begins to brown on the outside and is no longer pink in the center. Transfer to a plate.

Scrape the skillet to dislodge any browned bits. Put the mushrooms, onion, burgundy, and garlic in the skillet, stirring to combine. Cook for 2 minutes.

Add the chicken and any accumulated juices. Cook for 5 minutes, or until the mushrooms just begin to brown slightly. Spoon the mushroom mixture over the chicken. Sprinkle with the parsley and salt. Drizzle with the oil.

PER SERVING

calories 175	**sodium** 282 mg
total fat 5.5 g	**carbohydrates** 4 g
saturated fat 1.0 g	fiber 1 g
trans fat 0.0 g	sugars 2 g
polyunsaturated fat 1.0 g	**protein** 26 g
monounsaturated fat 2.5 g	**DIETARY EXCHANGES**
cholesterol 73 mg	3 lean meat

MEXICAN CHICKEN AND VEGETABLES WITH CHIPOTLE PEPPERS

SERVES 4 (PLUS 4 CHICKEN BREAST HALVES AND 1 CUP TOMATO MIXTURE RESERVED)

Chicken simmered with bell peppers and tomatoes, richly seasoned with chipotle peppers (smoked jalapeños), and served over yellow rice will satisfy the most demanding Mexican-food enthusiast. The extra chicken and sauce are ready for use in Chipotle Chicken Wraps (page 196) later in the week.

1 1/2 cups water

4 chipotle peppers (see Cook's Tip on Handling Hot Chiles, page 24)

Olive oil cooking spray

8 boneless, skinless chicken breast halves (about 4 ounces each), all visible fat discarded

2 large onions, chopped

4 medium garlic cloves, minced

1 cup uncooked instant brown rice

1/2 teaspoon ground turmeric

1 medium fresh jalapeño, seeds and ribs discarded, minced (optional; see Cook's Tip on Handling Hot Chiles, page 24)

1 14.5-ounce can no-salt-added diced tomatoes, undrained

1 medium green bell pepper, chopped

2 teaspoons ground cumin

1 1/2 teaspoons dried oregano, crumbled

1 teaspoon chili powder

1/2 teaspoon salt

1 to 2 teaspoons olive oil (extra-virgin preferred)

In a small saucepan, bring the water to a boil over high heat. Remove from the heat. Add the chipotle peppers. Let stand for 30 minutes.

Meanwhile, lightly spray a Dutch oven with cooking spray. Cook half the chicken with the smooth side down over medium-high heat for 4 minutes. Turn over the chicken. Cook for 2 to 4 minutes, or until no longer pink in the center. Transfer to a large plate. Repeat with the remaining chicken.

In the same pot, still over medium-high heat, cook the onions and garlic for 5 to 7 minutes, stirring frequently and scraping to dislodge any browned bits. Remove from the heat.

Drain the chipotle peppers, reserving the water. Discard the stems, seeds, and ribs from the peppers. In a food processor or blender, process the peppers and reserved water until smooth.

Prepare the rice using the package directions, omitting the salt and margarine and adding the turmeric. When the rice is done, stir in the jalapeño.

Meanwhile, chop or shred the chicken.

Stir the tomatoes with liquid, bell pepper, cumin, oregano, chili powder, chipotle pepper mixture, and chicken and any accumulated juices into the onion mixture. Bring to a boil over medium heat. Reduce the heat and simmer, covered, for 20 minutes. Remove from the heat.

(continued)

Transfer half the chicken and 1 cup tomato mixture to an airtight container. Refrigerate and reserve for use in Chipotle Chicken Wraps. Just before serving, stir the salt and oil into the remaining chicken mixture. Serve over the rice.

Cook's Tip: This stew is even better if refrigerated overnight. It's a good dish to make on the weekend for a quick dinner. Just reheat the stew, add the salt and oil, and prepare the rice.

PER SERVING

calories 225	**carbohydrates** 19 g
total fat 4.5 g	fiber 3 g
saturated fat 1.0 g	sugars 6 g
trans fat 0.0 g	**protein** 27 g
polyunsaturated fat 1.0 g	**DIETARY EXCHANGES**
monounsaturated fat 1.5 g	1/2 starch, 2 vegetable,
cholesterol 73 mg	3 lean meat
sodium 312 mg	

CHICKEN AND FENNEL STEW

SERVES 6

Fresh fennel is the star player in this dish, adding a unique taste reminiscent of licorice and anise. Its sweetness is a good complement to the pungent flavor of the onions. Serve with Easy Refrigerator Rolls (page 458).

1 tablespoon canola or corn oil

1 1/2 pounds boneless, skinless chicken breast, cut into 1-inch cubes, all visible fat discarded

1/2 teaspoon pepper, or to taste (freshly ground preferred)

1 large onion, chopped

1 small head of fennel, halved and sliced, feathery fronds reserved

1 large carrot, chopped

1/4 cup water

3 small green onions, chopped

1 1/2 pounds baby spinach

1 medium lemon, cut into 6 wedges

In a stockpot or large saucepan, heat the oil over medium-high heat, swirling to coat the bottom. Cook the chicken for 5 to 7 minutes, or until

browned on all sides, stirring frequently. (The chicken won't be done at this point.) Sprinkle the pepper over the chicken. Stir in the onion, fennel, and carrot. Cook for 2 to 3 minutes, or until the onion is soft and the carrot is tender-crisp, stirring occasionally.

Stir in the water and green onions. Reduce the heat and simmer, covered, for 10 to 12 minutes, or until the chicken is no longer pink in the center, adding more water if necessary during cooking. Stir in the spinach. Cook for 30 seconds to 1 minute, or until wilted.

Garnish with the lemon wedges and reserved fennel fronds.

PER SERVING

calories 212	**sodium** 254 mg
total fat 6.0 g	**carbohydrates** 12 g
saturated fat 1.0 g	fiber 5 g
trans fat 0.0 g	sugars 4 g
polyunsaturated fat 1.5 g	**protein** 28 g
monounsaturated fat 2.5 g	**DIETARY EXCHANGES**
cholesterol 73 mg	2 vegetable, 3 lean meat

SPICY CHICKEN SATAY WITH PEANUT DIPPING SAUCE

SERVES 4

A generous combination of sweet, savory, and acidic flavors makes this Thai-inspired dish a standout. Serve it with rice noodles or brown rice. The dipping sauce is too good to limit to just one recipe, so make extra and use it as a salad dressing on fresh spinach or kale or as a dipping sauce for spring rolls.

Marinade

1/3 cup sliced lemongrass

1/4 cup plus 1 tablespoon fresh lemon juice (about 2 medium lemons)

2 tablespoons light brown sugar

2 tablespoons mirin or sweet wine

2 1/2 teaspoons soy sauce (lowest sodium available)

2 medium garlic cloves, minced, or 1 teaspoon bottled minced garlic

1/8 teaspoon crushed red pepper flakes, or to taste

■ ■ ■

1 pound boneless, skinless chicken breast halves, all visible fat discarded, cut into 32 cubes

Sauce

2 tablespoons canola or corn oil

1/3 cup finely chopped green onions

1 tablespoon grated peeled gingerroot

1 medium garlic clove, finely chopped, or 1/2 teaspoon bottled minced garlic

1/2 cup water

1/4 cup plus 1 tablespoon creamy low sodium peanut butter

2 tablespoons tarragon wine vinegar or white vinegar

1 1/2 tablespoons light brown sugar

1 tablespoon soy sauce (lowest sodium available)

1/8 teaspoon crushed red pepper flakes

■ ■ ■

16 large button mushrooms, stems discarded, halved

In a large shallow glass dish, stir together the marinade ingredients. Add the chicken, turning to coat. Cover and refrigerate for 1 to 12 hours, turning occasionally.

In a small saucepan, heat the oil over medium-high heat, swirling to coat the bottom. Cook the green onions, gingerroot, and garlic for 1 minute, or until fragrant and glossy, stirring occasionally.

Stir in the remaining sauce ingredients. Reduce the heat and simmer until smooth, stirring occasionally. Remove from the heat. Let cool to room temperature.

Soak eight 8-inch wooden skewers for at least 10 minutes in cold water to keep them from charring, or use metal skewers.

Preheat the grill on medium high.

Drain the chicken, discarding the marinade. For each kebab, thread each skewer with 4 chicken cubes and 4 mushroom halves.

Grill the skewers for 5 minutes on each side, or until the chicken is no longer pink in the center. Serve the kebabs with the dipping sauce.

Cook's Tip: You can make the peanut dipping sauce several days in advance. Cover and refrigerate it until needed.

Cook's Tip on Lemongrass: Frequently used in Southeast Asian cuisines, lemongrass adds a lemon-like flavor to foods without the bitterness and acidity of lemons. Look for pale to medium-green stalks with a pale yellow to almost white root end. Discard the bulb and outer leaves, and use only the bottom 3 to 5 inches of the inner stalk. Lemongrass can be found in Asian markets and in the produce section of some grocery stores.

PER SERVING

calories 362	carbohydrates 15 g
total fat 20.0 g	fiber 3 g
saturated fat 3.0 g	sugars 10 g
trans fat 0.0 g	**protein** 32 g
polyunsaturated fat 5.0 g	**DIETARY EXCHANGES**
monounsaturated fat 10.0 g	1 other carbohydrate,
cholesterol 73 mg	4 lean meat, 2 fat
sodium 362 mg	

CHICKEN AND MUSHROOM STIR-FRY

SERVES 6

Stir-fries are an easy way to add more vegetables to your meals. Have all the ingredients ready before you start cooking, because things move fast once the heat is on. Serve over brown rice or for a change of pace try another whole grain such as quinoa or farro.

(continued)

1 tablespoon grated peeled gingerroot

1 tablespoon hot chili oil

3 medium garlic cloves, minced

1 teaspoon toasted sesame oil

1 pound boneless, skinless chicken breasts, all visible fat discarded, cut into 1-inch cubes

2 tablespoons light brown sugar

2 tablespoons fat-free, low-sodium chicken broth, such as on page 36

2 tablespoons dry sherry

1 tablespoon soy sauce (lowest sodium available)

1 tablespoon plain rice vinegar

1 teaspoon cornstarch

8 ounces button mushrooms, sliced

1 medium red bell pepper, diced

1 medium zucchini, diced

1/2 medium onion, sliced

9 cherry tomatoes, halved

In a large bowl, stir together the gingerroot, chili oil, garlic, and sesame oil. Add the chicken, stirring to coat. Cover and refrigerate for 15 minutes.

Meanwhile, in a small bowl, whisk together the brown sugar, broth, sherry, soy sauce, vinegar, and cornstarch until the brown sugar and cornstarch are dissolved. Set aside.

In a large nonstick skillet, cook the chicken with the marinade over medium-high heat for about 4 minutes, or until the chicken is lightly browned, stirring constantly.

Stir in the mushrooms, bell pepper, zucchini, and onion. Cook, covered, for 5 minutes, stirring occasionally.

Stir in the brown sugar mixture and tomatoes. Cook for 3 to 4 minutes, or until the sauce has thickened, stirring occasionally.

Cook's Tip: This stir-fry is also delicious with beef. Just substitute 1 pound thinly sliced sirloin or eye-of-round steak, all visible fat discarded, for the chicken.

PER SERVING

calories 169	**carbohydrates** 11 g
total fat 5.5 g	fiber 2 g
saturated fat 1.0 g	sugars 9 g
trans fat 0.0 g	**protein** 18 g
polyunsaturated fat 1.5 g	**DIETARY EXCHANGES**
monounsaturated fat 2.0 g	1 vegetable, 1/2 other
cholesterol 48 mg	carbohydrate,
sodium 163 mg	2 1/2 lean meat

CHINESE CHICKEN WITH PEPPERS AND ONIONS

SERVES 6

If you enjoy simple, classic Chinese cuisine with a little heat, then this dish will be one of your favorites when you're in the mood for takeout. Serve over brown rice and with Eggplant Hunan Style *(page 388).*

2 teaspoons canola or corn oil and 2 teaspoons canola or corn oil, divided use

12 ounces boneless, skinless chicken breasts, all visible fat discarded, cut into 1/2-inch cubes

4 pieces of peeled gingerroot (each about the size of a nickel)

3 small red chiles (see Cook's Tip on Handling Hot Chiles, page 24), or 1/8 teaspoon cayenne

3 medium green or red bell peppers (or a combination), cut into 1-inch squares

2 medium onions, quartered, then very thinly sliced

1 tablespoon sherry or orange juice

2 teaspoons soy sauce (lowest sodium available)

1 teaspoon toasted sesame oil

In a large skillet or wok, heat 2 teaspoons canola oil over high heat, swirling to coat the bottom.

Stir in the chicken, gingerroot, and chiles. Cook for 3 minutes, or until the chicken is no longer pink in the center, stirring constantly. Transfer the chicken to a plate.

Heat the remaining 2 teaspoons canola oil, still over high heat, swirling to coat the bottom. Stir in the bell peppers and onions. Cook for 2 minutes, or until the onions begin to soften, stirring frequently.

Return the chicken to the skillet. Pour in the sherry and soy sauce. Cook for 1 minute.

Just before serving, sprinkle with the sesame oil.

PER SERVING

calories 130	carbohydrates 7 g
total fat 5.5 g	fiber 2 g
saturated fat 0.5 g	sugars 5 g
trans fat 0.0 g	**protein** 13 g
polyunsaturated fat 1.5 g	**DIETARY EXCHANGES**
monounsaturated fat 2.5 g	1 vegetable, 2 lean
cholesterol 36 mg	meat
sodium 112 mg	

MEDITERRANEAN DOUBLE TOSS

SERVES 4

This one-dish meal combines the flavors of Greece and Italy for double the culinary enjoyment. It requires only two pots, one for the pasta and a skillet for the chicken and vegetables, so cleanup is a breeze.

4 ounces dried whole-grain penne
3/4 cup cherry tomatoes, quartered
5 kalamata olives, coarsely chopped
2 tablespoons chopped fresh basil
1 tablespoon plus 1 teaspoon capers, drained
8 ounces boneless, skinless chicken breasts,
    all visible fat discarded, cut into thin
    strips
1/2 medium red bell pepper, cut into thin
    strips
1 small zucchini, cut lengthwise into eighths,
    then cut crosswise into 2-inch pieces
1/4 medium onion, cut into 4 wedges
1 medium garlic clove, minced
Cooking spray
1/4 teaspoon salt
1 tablespoon olive oil (extra-virgin preferred)
2 ounces fat-free feta cheese, crumbled

Prepare the pasta using the package directions, omitting the salt. Drain well in a colander, reserving 1/4 cup pasta water. Set aside.

Meanwhile, in a small bowl, stir together the tomatoes, olives, basil, and capers. Set aside.

In a large nonstick skillet, cook the chicken over medium-high heat for 3 to 4 minutes, or until no longer pink in the center, stirring frequently. Transfer to a plate.

Put the bell pepper, zucchini, onion, and garlic in the skillet. Lightly spray the vegetables and garlic with cooking spray. Cook for 4 minutes, or until the bell pepper is just tender-crisp, stirring frequently.

Stir in the chicken, reserved pasta water, and salt.

Spoon the pasta onto a serving plate. Top with the chicken mixture. Drizzle with the oil. Spoon the tomato mixture over the chicken. Sprinkle with the feta.

PER SERVING

calories 247	carbohydrates 27 g
total fat 7.0 g	fiber 4 g
saturated fat 1.0 g	sugars 5 g
trans fat 0.0 g	**protein** 20 g
polyunsaturated fat 1.0 g	**DIETARY EXCHANGES**
monounsaturated fat 4.0 g	1 1/2 starch,
cholesterol 36 mg	1 vegetable, 2 1/2 lean
sodium 600 mg	meat

LINGUINE WITH CHICKEN AND ARTICHOKES

SERVES 4

A cheesy, creamy sauce blankets pasta and chicken in this comforting one-dish meal. Serve with a simple dark green, leafy salad with Chunky Cucumber and Garlic Dressing (page 106).

(continued)

4 ounces dried whole-grain linguine

12 ounces boneless, skinless chicken breasts, all visible fat discarded, cut into 1-inch cubes

1/4 teaspoon salt

2 teaspoons olive oil

2 medium garlic cloves, finely chopped

12 ounces frozen artichoke quarters (no thawing needed)

1 cup sliced onion

1/2 teaspoon crushed red pepper flakes

2 teaspoons cornstarch

3/4 cup fat-free, low-sodium chicken broth, such as on page 36

1/2 teaspoon dried rosemary, crushed

1/3 cup fat-free half-and-half

1/4 cup shredded or grated Parmesan cheese

Prepare the pasta using the package directions, omitting the salt and cooking for about 2 minutes less than instructed, just until almost tender. Drain well in a colander. Cover and set aside.

Put the chicken in a medium bowl. Sprinkle the salt over the chicken.

In a small bowl, stir together the oil and garlic. Using your fingertips, rub into the chicken.

In a large nonstick skillet, cook the chicken over medium-high heat for 3 minutes, or until lightly browned on the outside and no longer pink in the center, stirring constantly. Reduce the heat to medium.

Stir in the artichokes, onion, and red pepper flakes. Cook for 7 minutes, or until the onion begins to turn golden and the artichokes soften and turn light brown in spots, stirring frequently.

Meanwhile, put the cornstarch in a small bowl. Pour in the broth, whisking to dissolve. Stir in the rosemary. When the artichokes and onion have cooked, pour the broth mixture into the skillet. Bring to a simmer, still over medium heat, stirring frequently. Reduce the heat and simmer for 3 minutes, or until the sauce begins to thicken, stirring frequently.

Stir in the half-and-half. Return to a simmer.

Stir in the pasta. Return to a simmer and simmer for 1 to 2 minutes, or until heated through. Just before serving, sprinkle with the Parmesan.

PER SERVING

calories 314	carbohydrates 36 g
total fat 6.5 g	fiber 10 g
saturated fat 1.5 g	sugars 4 g
trans fat 0.0 g	protein 28 g
polyunsaturated fat 1.0 g	**DIETARY EXCHANGES**
monounsaturated fat 3.0 g	1 1/2 starch,
cholesterol 58 mg	2 vegetable, 3 lean
sodium 401 mg	meat

CHICKEN STUFINO

SERVES 6

The taste of chicken slowly oven-braised in a tomato-rich sauce with garden vegetables proves why homemade meals are worth the time.

1 tablespoon all-purpose flour

1/2 teaspoon salt

1/4 teaspoon pepper, or to taste

1 1/2 pounds boneless, skinless chicken breasts, all visible fat discarded, cut into large cubes

Olive oil cooking spray

1 teaspoon olive oil

1 cup dry white wine (regular or nonalcoholic)

2 medium carrots, finely chopped

2 medium ribs of celery, finely chopped

1 medium onion, finely chopped

1 to 2 medium garlic cloves, minced

1 14.5-ounce can no-salt-added stewed tomatoes, crushed, undrained

12 ounces dried whole-grain medium pasta shells

1 teaspoon dried Italian seasoning, crumbled

1/4 cup chopped fresh parsley (optional)

In a small bowl, stir together the flour, salt, and pepper.

Put the chicken on a plate. Sprinkle the flour mixture over the chicken. Gently shake off any excess.

Lightly spray a Dutch oven or heavy ovenproof skillet with cooking spray. Heat the oil over medium-high heat, swirling to coat the bottom. Cook the chicken for 2 to 3 minutes, stirring occasionally so it cooks evenly on all sides (the chicken won't be done at this point.)

Meanwhile, preheat the oven to 300°F.

Pour the wine into the Dutch oven, scraping to dislodge any browned bits. Stir in the carrots, celery, onion, and garlic. Cook for 2 to 3 minutes, stirring occasionally.

Stir in the tomatoes with liquid. Bring to a boil.

Bake, covered, for 1 hour, or until the chicken is no longer pink in the center.

Meanwhile, prepare the pasta using the package directions, omitting the salt and adding the Italian seasoning. Drain well in a colander. Transfer to plates. Top with the chicken. Sprinkle with the parsley.

PER SERVING

calories 410	**carbohydrates** 52 g
total fat 5.5 g	fiber 9 g
saturated fat 1.0 g	sugars 8 g
trans fat 0.0 g	**protein** 32 g
polyunsaturated fat 1.0 g	**DIETARY EXCHANGES**
monounsaturated fat 2.0 g	3 starch, 1 vegetable,
cholesterol 73 mg	3 lean meat
sodium 364 mg	

ONE-DISH ITALIAN CHICKEN AND RICE

SERVES 4

This one-dish meal combines classic Italian flavors in an easy-to-make casserole that fills the house with a tempting aroma that will have the family asking what's for dinner. While the casserole bakes, serve Spinach Salad with Chickpeas and Cider Vinaigrette (page 67).

Cooking spray

1 14.5-ounce can no-salt-added stewed tomatoes, undrained

1 pound boneless, skinless chicken breasts, all visible fat discarded, cut into bite-size pieces

3 ounces button or brown (cremini) mushrooms, sliced

2 ounces baby spinach, chopped

3/4 cup fat-free, low-sodium chicken broth, such as on page 36

3/4 cup uncooked instant brown rice

1/2 cup chopped onion

1/4 cup chopped fresh basil

2 medium garlic cloves, minced

1/2 teaspoon dried oregano, crumbled

1/2 teaspoon salt-free all-purpose seasoning blend

1/4 teaspoon pepper

1/8 teaspoon salt

2 tablespoons shredded or grated Parmesan cheese

Preheat the oven to 375°F. Lightly spray an 11 x 7 x 2-inch glass baking dish with cooking spray.

Pour the tomatoes with liquid into a large bowl. Break up any large pieces.

Stir in the remaining ingredients except the Parmesan. Pour into the baking dish.

Bake, covered, for 35 to 40 minutes, or until the chicken is no longer pink in the center and the rice is tender. Just before serving, sprinkle with the Parmesan.

Cook's Tip: Casseroles are the original one-dish meal. They are an easy way to include—or introduce veggies and whole grains into your family's meals. They also offer great variety and flexibility, so the next time you prepare this recipe try substituting kale or broccoli for the spinach.

PER SERVING

calories 254	**carbohydrates** 23 g
total fat 4.5 g	fiber 4 g
saturated fat 1.0 g	sugars 6 g
trans fat 0.0 g	**protein** 29 g
polyunsaturated fat 1.0 g	**DIETARY EXCHANGES**
monounsaturated fat 1.5 g	1 starch, 1 vegetable,
cholesterol 74 mg	3 lean meat
sodium 281 mg	

PAELLA

SERVES 4

Chicken or turkey andouille sausage packs plenty of heat and spice in this easy and delicious skillet dinner. Even the cold leftovers are tempting when tossed with lettuce for a light lunch.

- 1 1/4 cups fat-free, low-sodium chicken broth, such as on page 36
- 1/4 teaspoon saffron threads or 1/8 teaspoon crushed red pepper flakes
- 1 1/2 teaspoons olive oil and 1 1/2 teaspoons olive oil, divided use
- 8 ounces boneless, skinless chicken breasts, all visible fat discarded, cut crosswise into 1/2-inch strips
- 3 ounces cooked chicken or turkey andouille sausage link, cut crosswise into 1/4-inch pieces
- 1 cup uncooked brown rice
- 1 small red bell pepper, chopped
- 1 small onion or 1 large shallot, chopped
- 1 medium garlic clove, minced
- 8 large raw shrimp (about 4 ounces total), peeled, rinsed, and patted dry
- 8 cherry tomatoes, halved
- 1 cup cooked green peas
- 1/4 teaspoon salt
- 1/4 teaspoon pepper
- 1 teaspoon grated lemon zest
- 1 medium lemon, cut into 4 wedges

In a small saucepan, stir together the broth and saffron threads. Bring to a simmer over medium-high heat. Reduce the heat to low to keep the mixture heated until needed.

Meanwhile, in a large skillet or a Dutch oven, heat 1 1/2 teaspoons oil over medium-high heat, swirling to coat the bottom. Cook the chicken and sausage for 3 to 5 minutes (the chicken won't be done at this point), or until browned, stirring frequently. Transfer to a plate.

In the same skillet, heat the remaining 1 1/2 teaspoons oil, still over medium-high heat. Cook the rice, bell pepper, onion, and garlic for 3 minutes,

or until the bell pepper is almost tender, stirring frequently.

Stir in the hot broth mixture. Reduce the heat and simmer for 15 minutes. Add the chicken, sausage, and shrimp, tucking them into the rice. Cook for 8 to 10 minutes, or until the chicken is no longer pink in the center, the shrimp are pink on the outside, and the rice is tender (don't stir). Increase the heat to medium high and cook for 30 to 40 seconds, or until you can smell the rice toasting on the bottom. Remove from the heat. Sprinkle the tomatoes and peas on the rice. Let stand, covered, for 5 minutes.

Sprinkle with the salt, pepper, and lemon zest. Stir. Garnish with the lemon wedges.

Cook's Tip: The crunchy, toasted rice at the bottom of the pan is called a *socarrat* and is considered an integral part of a good paella.

PER SERVING

calories 366	**carbohydrates** 46 g
total fat 8.0 g	fiber 4 g
saturated fat 2.0 g	sugars 5 g
trans fat 0.0 g	**protein** 27 g
polyunsaturated fat 1.5 g	**DIETARY EXCHANGES**
monounsaturated fat 3.5 g	2 1/2 starch,
cholesterol 87 mg	1 vegetable, 3 lean
sodium 577 mg	meat

CHICKEN FAJITA BOWLS

SERVES 4

Spicy Grilled Chicken saved from another meal is the base for this super-speedy entrée. Serve with Tex-Mex Cucumber Salad (page 78) or Jícama Slaw (page 83).

- 1 cup uncooked instant brown rice
- 1 teaspoon canola or corn oil
- 1 large onion, thinly sliced
- 1 large green bell pepper, thinly sliced
- 4 cooked chicken breast halves from Spicy Grilled Chicken (page 195), thinly sliced
- 1 cup frozen or no-salt-added canned whole-kernel corn, thawed if frozen or rinsed and drained if canned

1 15.5-ounce can no-salt-added black beans, rinsed and drained
1 14.5-ounce can no-salt-added diced tomatoes, drained
1/2 cup salsa (lowest sodium available), such as Salsa Cruda (page 437)
1/2 small avocado, diced
1/4 cup chopped fresh cilantro
1 medium lime, cut into 4 wedges

Prepare the rice using the package directions, omitting the salt and margarine.

In a large nonstick skillet, heat the oil over medium-high heat, swirling to coat the bottom. Cook the onion and bell pepper for 5 minutes, or until the onion is slightly brown, stirring constantly.

Stir in the chicken. Cook for 2 to 3 minutes, or until heated through. Stir in the corn. Cook for 1 to 2 minutes, or until heated.

Put the rice in bowls. Place the chicken and vegetables on the rice. Top with the beans, tomatoes, salsa, and avocado. Sprinkle with the cilantro. Serve with the lime wedges.

PER SERVING

calories 458	carbohydrates 59 g
total fat 9.0 g	fiber 11 g
saturated fat 1.5 g	sugars 13 g
trans fat 0.0 g	**protein** 36 g
polyunsaturated fat 1.5 g	**DIETARY EXCHANGES**
monounsaturated fat 4.5 g	3 starch, 3 vegetable,
cholesterol 73 mg	4 lean meat
sodium 279 mg	

BONELESS BUFFALO WINGS

SERVES 4

These finger-lickin' "wings" are actually chicken tenders so you get more chicken and less bone to savor the sauce of your choice. Serve with Bourbon Barbecue Sauce *(page 431),* Sour Cream Sauce with Blue Cheese *(page 432), or* Ranch Dip *(page 14).*

Olive oil cooking spray
1/4 cup all-purpose flour

1 teaspoon salt-free all-purpose seasoning blend
8 chicken breast tenders (about 1 pound), all visible fat discarded, halved crosswise
1 tablespoon light tub margarine
1 teaspoon red hot-pepper sauce

Preheat the oven to 350°F. Lightly spray a baking sheet with cooking spray.

In a large shallow dish, stir together the flour and seasoning blend. Add the chicken tenders, turning to coat and gently shaking off any excess. Arrange the tenders in a single layer on the baking sheet. Lightly spray the chicken with cooking spray.

Bake for 20 to 25 minutes, or until lightly browned on the outside and no longer pink in the center.

Meanwhile, in a medium bowl, stir together the margarine and hot-pepper sauce. Add the cooked chicken, tossing to coat.

PER SERVING

calories 168	sodium 162 mg
total fat 4.0 g	**carbohydrates** 6 g
saturated fat 0.5 g	fiber 0 g
trans fat 0.0 g	sugars 0 g
polyunsaturated fat 0.5 g	**protein** 25 g
monounsaturated fat 1.5 g	**DIETARY EXCHANGES**
cholesterol 73 mg	1/2 starch, 3 lean meat

CHICKEN AND BARLEY CHILI

SERVES 4

Dig into a steaming bowl of this thick and hearty chili on a winter night and you'll feel like you've pulled on a cozy sweater. Complete your comfort food menu with a leafy green salad and Jalapeño Cheese Bread *(page 450).*

(continued)

Olive oil cooking spray

2 teaspoons olive oil

1 pound boneless, skinless chicken breasts, all visible fat discarded, cut into 1/2-inch cubes

1 small onion, chopped

1 small green bell pepper, chopped

1 medium fresh jalapeño, seeds and ribs discarded, minced (see Cook's Tip on Handling Hot Chiles, page 24)

3 medium garlic cloves, minced

2 tablespoons chili powder

2 teaspoons ground cumin

3 cups water

1 14.5-ounce can no-salt-added diced tomatoes, undrained

1 3/4 cups fat-free, low-sodium chicken broth, such as on page 36

1/2 cup uncooked pearl barley

2 tablespoons yellow cornmeal

1/4 cup chopped fresh cilantro

1 tablespoon fresh lime juice

Lightly spray a stockpot with cooking spray. In the same pot, heat the oil over medium-high heat, swirling to coat the bottom. Cook the chicken for 8 minutes, or until lightly browned on all sides, stirring frequently.

Stir in the onion, bell pepper, jalapeño, and garlic. Cook for 3 minutes, or until the onion is soft and the bell pepper is tender-crisp, stirring occasionally.

Stir in the chili powder and cumin. Stir in the water, tomatoes with liquid, broth, and barley. Increase the heat to high and bring to a boil. Reduce the heat and simmer, covered, for 30 minutes, or until the barley is tender yet firm to the bite.

Stir in the cornmeal. Increase the heat to medium high and cook, uncovered, for 3 to 5 minutes, or until the chili has thickened, stirring occasionally. Remove from the heat.

Stir in the cilantro and lime juice.

PER SERVING

calories 313	**carbohydrates** 35 g
total fat 6.5 g	fiber 8 g
saturated fat 1.0 g	sugars 7 g
trans fat 0.0 g	**protein** 30 g
polyunsaturated fat 1.0 g	**DIETARY EXCHANGES**
monounsaturated fat 2.5 g	1 1/2 starch,
cholesterol 73 mg	2 vegetable, 3 lean
sodium 262 mg	meat

BEAN AND BARLEY CHILI

To make a vegetarian version of the chili, omit the chicken and use fat-free, low-sodium vegetable broth, such as on page 36, in place of the chicken broth. Stir in one 15.5-ounce can no-salt-added black, pinto, or kidney beans, rinsed and drained, when you add the barley. Proceed as directed with the recipe.

PER SERVING

calories 275	**carbohydrates** 52 g
total fat 3.5 g	fiber 13 g
saturated fat 0.5 g	sugars 10 g
trans fat 0.0 g	**protein** 11 g
polyunsaturated fat 1.0 g	**DIETARY EXCHANGES**
monounsaturated fat 2.0 g	2 1/2 starch,
cholesterol 0 mg	2 vegetable, 1 lean
sodium 124 mg	meat

OVEN-FRIED PECAN CHICKEN FINGERS WITH ORANGE-YOGURT DIPPING SAUCE

SERVES 4

Chicken tenders are rolled in crunchy corn cereal crumbs that are seasoned with orange zest and southern pecans, and then baked to a crisp. Serve them with a cool and refreshing dip, featuring the bright flavor of orange all-fruit spread.

1 cup 100% orange juice concentrate, thawed

2 medium shallots, minced

1 tablespoon brown sugar (light or dark)

2 medium garlic cloves, minced

1/4 teaspoon pepper (freshly ground preferred)

8 boneless, skinless chicken tenders (about
1 pound), all visible fat discarded
Cooking spray
3 cups corn squares cereal, finely crushed
(about 1 1/2 cups of crumbs)
1/2 cup finely chopped pecans
1 tablespoon salt-free all-purpose seasoning
blend
1 tablespoon grated orange zest

Sauce
1/3 cup fat-free plain Greek yogurt
2 tablespoons orange juice concentrate,
thawed
1 tablespoon all-fruit orange spread
1 teaspoon orange zest
1/4 teaspoon light brown sugar

In a medium shallow glass dish, stir together
1 cup orange juice concentrate, the shallots,
brown sugar, garlic, and pepper until well combined. Add the chicken tenders, turning to coat.
Cover and refrigerate for 1 hour, turning once
halfway through. (For deeper flavor, marinate
the chicken overnight, turning occasionally.)

Drain the chicken, discarding the marinade.
Preheat the oven to 400°F. Line a large, heavy-
duty rimmed baking sheet with aluminum foil.
Place a slightly smaller cooling rack on the baking sheet. Lightly spray both the rack and the foil
with cooking spray.

In a medium shallow dish, stir together the cereal crumbs, pecans, seasoning blend, and orange zest. Arrange the dish with the chicken,
the dish with the cereal crumb mixture, and the
baking sheet in a row, assembly-line fashion.
Dip the chicken in the crumb mixture, turning
to coat and gently shaking off any excess. Using
your fingertips, gently press the crumbs so they
adhere to the chicken. Place the chicken on the
rack.

Bake the chicken for 15 to 20 minutes, or until no
longer pink in the center.

Meanwhile, in a small bowl, whisk together the
dipping sauce ingredients. Serve the chicken
with the dipping sauce.

PER SERVING

calories 301	**sodium** 272 mg
total fat 10.5 g	**carbohydrates** 24 g
saturated fat 1.5 g	fiber 2 g
trans fat 0.0 g	sugars 9 g
polyunsaturated fat 3.0 g	**protein** 28 g
monounsaturated fat 5.0 g	**DIETARY EXCHANGES**
cholesterol 73 mg	1 starch, 1/2 fruit,
	3 lean meat

CHICKEN GYROS WITH TZATZIKI SAUCE

SERVES 4

*Chicken tenders are anything but ordinary when
you season them with freshly squeezed citrus
juice, olive oil, and assertive spices. Greece's classic
yogurt-based sauce helps cool the palate.*

1 pound chicken tenders, all visible fat
discarded
1 teaspoon dried oregano, crumbled
1 teaspoon ground cumin
1 teaspoon onion powder
1/2 teaspoon paprika
1/8 teaspoon cayenne
1/8 teaspoon salt
3 tablespoons fresh lemon juice (about
1 medium lemon)
2 teaspoons olive oil
2 medium garlic cloves, minced
Cooking spray

Sauce
1/3 cup finely chopped peeled cucumber
1/3 cup fat-free plain yogurt
3 tablespoons fat-free sour cream
2 teaspoons chopped fresh dillweed
2 teaspoons fresh lemon juice
1 medium garlic clove, finely chopped
1/8 teaspoon pepper

Put the chicken in a medium glass bowl.

(continued)

In a small shallow glass dish, stir together the oregano, cumin, onion powder, paprika, cayenne, and salt. Sprinkle over the chicken. Using your fingertips, gently press the mixture so it adheres to the chicken.

In the same small dish, stir together 3 tablespoons lemon juice, the oil, and 2 minced garlic cloves. Pour over the chicken. Using your fingertips, rub into the chicken. Cover and refrigerate for 10 minutes.

Meanwhile, preheat the broiler. Line a baking sheet with aluminum foil. Lightly spray with cooking spray.

Drain the chicken, discarding the marinade. Transfer the chicken to the baking sheet.

Broil the chicken 4 to 5 inches from the heat for 8 minutes. Turn over the chicken. Broil for 3 minutes, or until no longer pink in the center.

Meanwhile, in a small bowl, stir together the sauce ingredients. Serve over the chicken.

Cook's Tip: If you prefer, you can serve the chicken in a sandwich. Fill six 6-inch whole-grain pita pockets (lowest sodium available) with chopped romaine and tomatoes. Top with thinly sliced red onion and the chicken. Spoon the sauce on top.

Cook's Tip on Tzatziki Sauce: This classic Greek sauce is also a great dip. Serve it with baked whole-grain pita triangles or raw veggie dippers.

PER SERVING

calories 161	carbohydrates 5 g
total fat 3.0 g	fiber 1 g
saturated fat 0.5 g	sugars 3 g
trans fat 0.0 g	**protein** 26 g
polyunsaturated fat 0.5 g	**DIETARY EXCHANGES**
monounsaturated fat 1.0 g	1/2 fat-free milk, 3 lean
cholesterol 75 mg	meat
sodium 231 mg	

SZECHUAN ORANGE CHICKEN
SERVES 4

When you want to give everyday ingredients an exotic touch, try this recipe. The spices, panko, and orange sauce add Asian flair without the high fat and sodium content of takeout. By using the high heat of the broiler and the speed of microwave cooking, you'll have this healthy version of fast food on the table in no time!

Cooking spray
1 teaspoon garlic powder
1 teaspoon onion powder
1 teaspoon ground ginger and 2 teaspoons
    ground ginger, divided use
1/2 teaspoon crushed red pepper flakes and
    1/2 teaspoon crushed red pepper flakes,
    divided use
1 pound chicken breast tenders, all visible fat
    discarded, cut into 1-inch cubes
1 teaspoon plain rice vinegar
1/4 cup egg substitute
1 cup panko (Japanese-style bread crumbs)
1/4 cup plus 2 tablespoons frozen 100%
    orange juice concentrate, thawed
1/4 cup plus 2 tablespoons water
1 tablespoon plus 1 teaspoon honey
2 teaspoons soy sauce (lowest sodium
    available)
2 medium garlic cloves, finely chopped
1 teaspoon toasted sesame oil

Preheat the broiler. Line a baking sheet with aluminum foil. Lightly spray with cooking spray.

In a medium bowl, stir together the garlic powder, onion powder, 1 teaspoon ginger, and 1/2 teaspoon red pepper flakes. Add the chicken, stirring to coat.

Drizzle with the vinegar, stirring to coat. Let stand for 5 minutes.

Meanwhile, pour the egg substitute into a shallow dish. Put the panko in a separate shallow dish. Set the dishes and baking sheet in a row, assembly-line fashion. Working in batches, dip the chicken cubes in the egg substitute, then in the panko, turning to coat at each step, and gently shaking off any excess. Place the chicken on the baking sheet in a single layer, arranging so the cubes don't touch. Lightly spray the top and sides of the chicken with cooking spray.

Broil about 6 inches from the heat for 8 minutes, or until the chicken is no longer pink in the center and the coating is golden brown and crisp.

Meanwhile, in a small microwaveable bowl, whisk together the orange juice concentrate, water, honey, soy sauce, garlic, and the remaining 2 teaspoons ginger. Microwave, covered, on 100 percent power (high) for 3 minutes, or until hot and bubbly.

Stir in the sesame oil and the remaining 1/2 teaspoon red pepper flakes. Drizzle over the chicken.

Cook's Tip on Plain Panko: Panko, or Japanese-style bread crumbs, is made from the soft centers of bread rather than the crust. It has a pleasant crunchiness, is lighter than traditional bread crumbs, and contains considerably less sodium and fewer calories.

PER SERVING

calories 274	carbohydrates 30 g
total fat 4.0 g	fiber 1 g
saturated fat 1.0 g	sugars 16 g
trans fat 0.0 g	protein 28 g
polyunsaturated fat 1.0 g	DIETARY EXCHANGES
monounsaturated fat 1.5 g	1 starch, 1 fruit, 3 lean
cholesterol 73 mg	meat
sodium 255 mg	

TANDOORI GINGER CHICKEN STRIPS

SERVES 4

This dish features the flavors of tandoori chicken, India's version of barbecued chicken, from the yogurt marinade and traditional spices. The recipe gets its name from the clay oven called a tandoor in which the chicken is cooked.

> 3/4 cup coarsely chopped onion
> 1 tablespoon coarsely chopped peeled gingerroot
> 2 medium garlic cloves
> 1 cup fat-free plain yogurt
> 2 tablespoons fresh lemon juice
> 1 tablespoon paprika
> 1 1/2 teaspoons curry powder
> 1/2 teaspoon ground cumin
> 1/4 teaspoon salt and 1/8 teaspoon salt, divided use
> 1/8 teaspoon cayenne
> 1 pound chicken tenders, all visible fat discarded
> Cooking spray

In a food processor or blender, process the onion, gingerroot, and garlic until smooth.

Add the yogurt, lemon juice, paprika, curry powder, cumin, 1/4 teaspoon salt, and the cayenne. Process until well blended.

Put the chicken in a large shallow glass dish. Pour the yogurt mixture over the chicken, turning to coat. Cover and refrigerate for 4 to 8 hours, turning occasionally.

After the chicken has marinated, preheat the broiler. Lightly spray a broiler pan and rack with cooking spray.

Remove the chicken from the marinade, leaving what clings to the chicken. Discard the marinade in the dish.

Broil the chicken about 4 inches from the heat for 6 minutes on each side, or until no longer pink in the center. Sprinkle with the remaining 1/8 teaspoon salt.

Cook's Tip: For peak flavor and texture, don't marinate the chicken any longer than the suggested time.

PER SERVING

calories 144	sodium 365 mg
total fat 3.0 g	carbohydrates 3 g
saturated fat 0.5 g	fiber 0 g
trans fat 0.0 g	sugars 2 g
polyunsaturated fat 0.5 g	protein 25 g
monounsaturated fat 1.0 g	DIETARY EXCHANGES
cholesterol 73 mg	3 lean meat

INDONESIAN CHICKEN CURRY

SERVES 4

Fragrant lemongrass, cinnamon, and kaffir lime perfume and flavor this dish, which owes its silky texture to a combination of chicken broth and coconut milk. If you can't find kaffir lime leaves, simply substitute freshly grated lime zest.

> 3/4 cup uncooked brown rice (jasmine preferred)
>
> 2 teaspoons canola or corn oil
>
> 4 boneless, skinless chicken thighs (about 4 ounces each), all visible fat discarded
>
> 1 cup fat-free, low-sodium chicken broth, such as on page 36
>
> 1/3 cup lite coconut milk
>
> 1 stalk lemongrass (use the bottom 8 inches of the stalk), cut in half lengthwise and slightly pounded with a meat mallet, or 1 teaspoon lemongrass paste
>
> 1 cinnamon stick (about 3 inches long)
>
> 2 medium garlic cloves, minced
>
> 2 medium kaffir lime leaves or 1 teaspoon grated lime zest
>
> 1 teaspoon minced peeled gingerroot
>
> 1/4 teaspoon salt
>
> 1/8 teaspoon pepper

Prepare the rice using the package directions, omitting the salt and margarine.

In a large skillet, heat the oil over medium-high heat, swirling to coat the bottom. Cook the chicken for 2 to 3 minutes on each side, or until browned. Stir in the remaining ingredients.

Bring to a simmer, still over medium-high heat. Reduce the heat and simmer, covered, for 30 minutes, or until the chicken is no longer pink in the center. Discard the lemongrass stalk, cinnamon stick, and lime leaves before serving the curry.

Cook's Tip on Kaffir Lime Leaves: These highly aromatic leaves have double leaf lobes and are emerald green in color. They are native to Indonesia, but are very popular in other Asian cuisines, such as Thai and Cambodian. Like bay leaves, kaffir lime leaves aren't eaten. They are usually sold in Asian grocery stores and some specialty markets.

PER SERVING

calories 302	**sodium** 263 mg
total fat 9.0 g	**carbohydrates** 28 g
saturated fat 2.0 g	fiber 1 g
trans fat 0.0 g	sugars 1 g
polyunsaturated fat 2.0 g	**protein** 25 g
monounsaturated fat 3.5 g	**DIETARY EXCHANGES**
cholesterol 108 mg	2 starch, 3 lean meat

CHICKEN AND BROCCOLI IN MUSHROOM SAUCE

SERVES 6

Earthy mushrooms, tender-crisp broccoli, and a cheesy creamy sauce team up to create a family favorite casserole.

> Cooking spray
>
> 10 ounces broccoli florets, or 10 ounces frozen broccoli florets, thawed
>
> 2 cups diced cooked skinless chicken breast, cooked without salt, all visible fat discarded

Sauce

> 1 teaspoon light tub margarine
>
> 8 ounces button mushrooms, sliced
>
> 1 1/3 cups fat-free, low-sodium chicken broth, such as on page 36
>
> 1 5-ounce can fat-free evaporated milk
>
> 1/4 cup all-purpose flour
>
> 1/4 cup sliced green onions
>
> 3 tablespoons shredded or grated Parmesan cheese
>
> Dash of ground nutmeg

Topping

> 1/4 cup whole-wheat panko (Japanese-style bread crumbs)
>
> 2 tablespoons finely chopped fresh parsley
>
> 1 teaspoon grated lemon zest

Lightly spray a 9-inch square baking dish with cooking spray.

In a medium saucepan, steam the broccoli for 5 to 6 minutes, or until tender-crisp. Plunge into a bowl of ice water to stop the cooking process. Drain well in a colander. Pat dry with paper towels. Arrange in a single layer in the baking dish.

Place the chicken on the broccoli. Set aside.

In a medium nonstick skillet, melt the margarine over medium heat, swirling to coat the bottom. Cook the mushrooms, covered, for 7 to 9 minutes, or until they have released their liquid. Increase the heat to high. Cook, uncovered, for 1 to 2 minutes, or until the liquid has evaporated.

Preheat the oven to 375°F.

Pour the broth and milk into a separate medium saucepan. Whisk in the flour. Bring to a boil over medium-high heat. Cook for 3 to 4 minutes, or until thickened, stirring occasionally.

Stir in the green onions, Parmesan, nutmeg, and mushrooms. Pour the sauce over the chicken and broccoli.

In a small bowl, stir together the topping ingredients. Sprinkle over the casserole.

Bake for 25 minutes.

PER SERVING

calories 168	carbohydrates 14 g
total fat 3.5 g	fiber 3 g
saturated fat 1.0 g	sugars 4 g
trans fat 0.0 g	protein 21 g
polyunsaturated fat 0.5 g	DIETARY EXCHANGES
monounsaturated fat 1.0 g	1 vegetable, 1/2 starch,
cholesterol 42 mg	2 1/2 lean meat
sodium 132 mg	

CHICKEN CURRY IN A HURRY

SERVES 4

Serve this quick and easy hit over steamed brown rice or rice pilaf. Add a splash of color by offering small bowls of toppings such as sliced green onions or Cranberry Chutney (page 424).

Cooking spray
1 teaspoon canola or corn oil
2 cups diced cooked skinless chicken or turkey breast, cooked without salt, all visible fat discarded

8 ounces button mushrooms, thinly sliced
1 small onion, chopped
3 tablespoons all-purpose flour
1 cup water
1 cup fat-free, low-sodium chicken broth, such as on page 36
1 medium Granny Smith apple, finely chopped
3/4 cup fat-free milk
1/4 cup chopped fresh parsley
1 1/2 teaspoons curry powder

Lightly spray a Dutch oven with cooking spray. Pour in the oil, swirling to coat the bottom. Heat over medium-high heat. Cook the chicken, mushrooms, and onion for 4 to 5 minutes, or until the chicken is warm, the mushrooms are tender, and the onion is very soft, stirring occasionally.

Put the flour in a small bowl. Add the water, whisking to dissolve. Pour into the pot.

Stir in the remaining ingredients. Bring to a boil over medium-high heat, stirring constantly. Reduce the heat and simmer for 3 minutes, or until the apple is tender-crisp, stirring constantly.

Cook's Tip on Curry Powder: If you feel like experimenting and making your own signature curry powder, combine 1/2 teaspoon each of the ground forms of cardamom, cinnamon, cloves, and turmeric (the last gives curry powder its characteristic yellow color). Then add small amounts to taste of any other spices commonly used in curry powder, such as chiles, coriander, cumin, fennel seed, fenugreek, mace, nutmeg, red and black pepper, poppy and sesame seeds, saffron, and tamarind.

PER SERVING

calories 222	carbohydrates 18 g
total fat 5.0 g	fiber 3 g
saturated fat 1.0 g	sugars 10 g
trans fat 0.0 g	protein 27 g
polyunsaturated fat 1.0 g	DIETARY EXCHANGES
monounsaturated fat 2.0 g	1/2 starch, 1/2 fruit,
cholesterol 60 mg	1 vegetable, 3 lean
sodium 88 mg	meat

CHICKEN POT PIE

SERVES 4

This healthy version of a family favorite eliminates a lot of sodium and saturated fat that is found in many of the frozen varieties. Enjoy this homemade classic with a dark green, leafy salad with Zesty Tomato Dressing (page 105).

Cooking spray

1 teaspoon canola or corn oil

1/2 cup chopped onion

1/2 cup chopped carrot

1/2 cup nonfat dry milk

3 tablespoons flour

1 1/2 cups fat free, low-sodium chicken broth, such as on page 36

1/2 teaspoon dried thyme, crumbled

1/2 teaspoon dried parsley, crumbled

1/2 teaspoon pepper (freshly ground preferred)

2 cups diced cooked skinless chicken breast, cooked without salt, all visible fat discarded

6 ounces frozen shelled edamame, thawed

6 ounces frozen whole-kernel corn, thawed

1/2 cup white whole-wheat flour

2 tablespoons canola or corn oil

1/8 teaspoon salt

Preheat oven to 400° F. Lightly spray a 1 1/2-quart casserole dish with cooking spray.

In a medium skillet, heat the oil over medium-high heat, swirling to coat the bottom. Cook the onion and carrot for 5 to 6 minutes, or until the onion is very soft and carrot is tender-crisp.

In a medium saucepan, stir together the dry milk and flour. Add the broth, whisking until smooth. Stir in the thyme, parsley, and pepper. Cook over medium heat for 5 minutes, or until thickened, stirring constantly. Remove from the heat. Stir in the chicken, edamame, corn, onions, and carrots.

Pour the mixture into a 1 1/2-quart casserole dish.

Put the flour in a small bowl. Stir in the oil and salt. Form into a ball. Put the ball on a sheet of wax paper, flattening the dough slightly. Place another sheet of wax paper on top of the dough. Roll out the dough. Place the dough over the casserole dish, pressing it firmly to the edge of the casserole. Using a sharp knife, cut a few slits (to release steam). Bake for 20 minutes, or until the crust is lightly browned.

PER SERVING

calories 410	carbohydrates 37 g
total fat 14.0 g	fiber 6 g
saturated fat 1.5 g	sugars 9 g
trans fat 0.0 g	protein 35 g
polyunsaturated fat 4.0 g	DIETARY EXCHANGES
monounsaturated fat 7.0 g	2 starch, 1 vegetable,
cholesterol 60 mg	4 lean meat
sodium 204 mg	

SESAME CHICKEN AND VEGETABLE STIR-FRY

SERVES 4

Goodbye, take-out! This Asian-influenced dish is loaded with vegetables and flavor. If you don't want to prepare that recipe, just use any leftover chicken that was cooked without added salt.

Sauce

1/3 cup fat-free, low-sodium chicken broth, such as on page 36

2 teaspoons cornstarch

2 teaspoons soy sauce (lowest sodium available)

1 teaspoon grated peeled gingerroot

1/2 teaspoon crushed red pepper flakes

1/2 teaspoon toasted sesame oil

1 small garlic clove, minced

■ ■ ■

1 teaspoon canola or corn oil

4 to 5 ounces broccoli florets, broken into bite-size pieces

2 medium carrots, cut diagonally into 1/8-inch slices

8 ounces sliced water chestnuts, drained

1 cup sliced green cabbage, slices 1/4 to 1/2 inch wide

3 ounces snow peas, trimmed

2 medium green onions, sliced

12 ounces cooked skinless chicken breast, cooked without salt, all visible fat discarded, cut into bite-size pieces

1/2 cup canned mandarin oranges in juice, drained

1/2 teaspoon toasted sesame oil

1 teaspoon sesame seeds

In a small bowl, whisk together all the sauce ingredients.

In a large nonstick skillet, heat the canola oil over medium-high heat, swirling to coat the bottom. Cook the broccoli and carrots for 3 minutes, stirring frequently.

Stir in the water chestnuts, cabbage, snow peas, and green onions. Cook for 3 minutes, stirring occasionally.

Stir in the chicken and sauce. Cook for 4 minutes, or until the chicken is heated through and the sauce has thickened, stirring frequently. Remove from the heat.

Stir in the mandarin oranges and sesame oil. Sprinkle with the sesame seeds.

PER SERVING

calories 240	carbohydrates 17 g
total fat 7.5 g	fiber 5 g
saturated fat 1.0 g	sugars 6 g
trans fat 0.0 g	**protein** 27 g
polyunsaturated fat 1.5 g	**DIETARY EXCHANGES**
monounsaturated fat 3.0 g	3 vegetable, 3 lean
cholesterol 73 mg	meat
sodium 242 mg	

CHICKEN-SPINACH MANICOTTI

SERVES 6

This twist on classic Italian stuffed shells is a great way to use leftover cooked chicken—and tuck in a vegetable. Serve with a dark green, leafy salad and Parmesan-Herb Breadsticks (page 451).

Cooking spray

12 dried manicotti shells

Filling

2 cups diced cooked skinless chicken breast, cooked without salt, all visible fat discarded

1 1/2 cups fat-free cottage cheese

10-ounces frozen chopped spinach, thawed and squeezed dry

3/4 cup egg substitute

1/3 cup shredded or grated Parmesan cheese

2 teaspoons dried basil, crumbled

Pepper to taste

Sauce

1 teaspoon olive oil

1 large onion, chopped

3 medium garlic cloves, minced

1 14.5-ounce can no-salt-added diced tomatoes, undrained

1 cup water

1 6-ounce can no-salt-added tomato paste

1 teaspoon dried Italian seasoning, crumbled

1 teaspoon dried basil, crumbled

∎ ∎ ∎

3 tablespoons shredded or grated Parmesan cheese

Lightly spray a 13 x 9 x 2-inch baking pan with cooking spray. Set aside.

Prepare the pasta using the package directions, omitting the salt. Drain well in a colander. Set aside.

Meanwhile, in a large bowl, stir together the filling ingredients. Set aside.

In a medium saucepan, heat the oil over medium-high heat, swirling to coat the bottom. Cook the onion for about 3 minutes, or until soft, stirring frequently.

Stir in the garlic. Cook for 1 minute, stirring occasionally.

Stir in the remaining sauce ingredients, including the tomatoes with liquid. Crush the tomatoes slightly. Bring to a simmer. Reduce the heat and simmer for 8 to 10 minutes. Spread 1 cup sauce in the pan.

(continued)

Meanwhile, preheat the oven to 375°F.

Gently stuff the shells with the filling. Place them on the sauce. Spoon the remaining sauce over the shells. Sprinkle with the remaining 3 tablespoons Parmesan.

Bake for 30 minutes, or until heated through.

MICROWAVE METHOD

Prepare the pasta as directed. In a large bowl, stir together the filling ingredients. In a 1-quart microwaveable bowl, stir together the oil, onion, and garlic. Microwave on 100 percent power (high) for 3 minutes. Stir in the remaining sauce ingredients. Microwave on 50 percent power (medium) for 10 minutes. Put half the sauce in a microwaveable baking dish. Fill the shells as directed. Place them on the sauce. Spoon the remaining sauce over the shells. Sprinkle 3 tablespoons Parmesan over all. Microwave, covered and vented, on 50 percent power (medium) for 25 minutes. Let stand, covered, for 5 minutes before serving.

PER SERVING

calories 359	carbohydrates 43 g
total fat 6.0 g	fiber 6 g
saturated fat 2.0 g	sugars 12 g
trans fat 0.0 g	protein 35 g
polyunsaturated fat 1.0 g	DIETARY EXCHANGES
monounsaturated fat 2.0 g	2 starch, 3 vegetable,
cholesterol 47 mg	3 1/2 lean meat
sodium 516 mg	

CHICKEN ENCHILADAS

SERVES 9

Need an easy dish for a fiesta? Try these individual rolled tortillas stuffed with a delicious veggie chicken filling. Serve with Mexican Fried Rice *(page 421).*

Cooking spray
8 ounces zucchini, chopped (about 1 cup)
8 ounces button mushrooms, sliced
18 6-inch corn tortillas
2 cups finely chopped cooked chicken, cooked without salt, all visible fat discarded

1 cup fat-free plain yogurt and 1 cup fat-free plain yogurt, divided use
1/4 cup chopped red onion
2 tablespoons chopped green onion
1 tablespoon chopped fresh cilantro and 1 tablespoon chopped fresh cilantro, divided use
1 cup chopped tomatoes

Preheat the oven to 350°F. Lightly spray a 13 x 9 x 2-inch baking dish with cooking spray.

In a medium saucepan, steam the zucchini and mushrooms, covered, for 3 to 4 minutes, or until the zucchini is tender and the mushrooms are soft. Drain well.

Wrap the tortillas in aluminum foil. Bake for 5 minutes to soften.

In a medium bowl, stir together the chicken, 1 cup yogurt, the red onion, green onion, and 1 tablespoon cilantro until combined. Gently stir in the zucchini and mushrooms.

Place the tortillas on a work surface. Spoon the filling down the center of each tortilla. Roll up jelly-roll style. Place with the seam side down in the baking dish.

Spoon the remaining 1 cup yogurt and the tomatoes over the enchiladas. Sprinkle the remaining 1 tablespoon cilantro over the yogurt.

Bake, covered, for 20 minutes.

PER SERVING

calories 147	carbohydrates 18 g
total fat 2.5 g	fiber 2 g
saturated fat 0.5 g	sugars 4 g
trans fat 0.0 g	protein 14 g
polyunsaturated fat 0.5 g	DIETARY EXCHANGES
monounsaturated fat 0.5 g	1 starch, 1 1/2 lean
cholesterol 27 mg	meat
sodium 95 mg	

SOUTHWESTERN ROASTED TURKEY

SERVES 12

For a southwestern-inspired version of a classic roasted turkey, try this lime-infused poultry rubbed with herbs and spices. If you like gravy, try Basic Gravy *(page 428) to drizzle over the turkey. Enjoy leftovers with sautéed onions and green bell peppers in warm corn tortillas topped with a dollop of fat-free sour cream and a squeeze of fresh lime.*

Cooking spray
3 medium limes, halved
1/2 cup chopped fresh cilantro or parsley
1 tablespoon dried oregano, crumbled
1 tablespoon Dijon mustard (lowest sodium available)
1 tablespoon olive oil
1 1/2 teaspoons ground cumin
2 teaspoons chili powder
1/2 teaspoon pepper (coarsely ground preferred)
2 medium garlic cloves, minced
1 5-pound turkey breast with skin

Preheat the oven to 325°F. Lightly spray a roasting pan and baking rack with cooking spray.

Squeeze the juice from the limes into a small bowl. Set aside the lime halves.

Whisk the cilantro, oregano, mustard, oil, cumin, chili powder, pepper, and garlic into the lime juice.

Using your fingers and keeping the skin attached, carefully lift the skin from the meat of the turkey so you can spread the lime juice mixture between the skin and meat. Cover as much area as possible, being careful not to tear the skin. Gently pull the skin over the top and sides. Put the turkey on the rack in the pan. Put the lime halves in the pan, directly under the turkey.

Roast the turkey for 1 hour and 30 minutes to 1 hour and 45 minutes, or until the thickest part of the breast registers about 165°F on an instant-read thermometer. Remove from the oven.

Transfer the turkey to a cutting board. Let stand, loosely covered, for 15 minutes. Discard the skin before slicing.

PER SERVING

calories 162	**sodium** 92 mg
total fat 2.5 g	**carbohydrates** 2 g
saturated fat 0.5 g	fiber 0 g
trans fat 0.0 g	sugars 0 g
polyunsaturated fat 0.5 g	**protein** 31 g
monounsaturated fat 1.0 g	**DIETARY EXCHANGES**
cholesterol 89 mg	4 lean meat

TURKEY BREAST WITH MOLE SAUCE

SERVES 8

If you enjoy a good "concoction," which is what the Nahuatl (language of the Aztecs) word molli *means, you'll enjoy this dish. Many traditional Mexican dishes use mole (MOH-lay), a rich, dark sauce that usually includes chocolate. To reduce the saturated fat, this recipe uses cocoa powder instead. For an interesting pairing, try this entrée with* Cocoa-Cayenne Kale Crisps *(page 392).*

1 teaspoon canola or corn oil and 1 teaspoon canola or corn oil, divided use
2 pounds boneless, skinless turkey breast, all visible fat discarded
1 cup water
1 medium onion, chopped
1 medium garlic clove, minced
1 cup fat-free, low-sodium chicken broth, such as on page 36
2 tablespoons unsweetened cocoa powder
2 tablespoons shelled unsalted sunflower seeds
2 tablespoons shelled unsalted pumpkin seeds
1 tablespoon chili powder
1/2 teaspoon sugar
1/4 teaspoon ground cumin
1/4 teaspoon salt
1/4 teaspoon ground cinnamon
1/8 teaspoon ground cloves

(continued)

In a large skillet, heat 1 teaspoon oil over medium heat, swirling to coat the bottom. Cook the turkey breast for 2 to 3 minutes on each side, or until browned. Pour in the water and bring to a boil. Reduce the heat and simmer, covered, for 1 hour, or until the turkey registers 165°F on an instant-read thermometer. Transfer the turkey to an ungreased 1-quart baking dish, discarding the cooking liquid. Set aside the turkey.

Preheat the oven to 350°F.

Meanwhile, in a small skillet, heat the remaining 1 teaspoon oil over medium-high heat, swirling to coat the bottom. Cook the onion and garlic for 3 minutes, or until the onion is soft, stirring occasionally.

In a food processor or blender, process the onion mixture and the remaining ingredients until smooth. Pour the mixture over the turkey. Bake for 30 minutes. Serve warm.

Cook's Tip on Grinding Dried Chiles, Herbs, and Spices: If you enjoy grinding your own dried chiles, an electric coffee grinder is the best tool for the job. If you choose this method, you will want to dedicate the coffee grinder to grinding only chiles—otherwise, "hot coffee" could take on a whole new meaning! Electric coffee grinders are also great for perking up your dried herbs or spices.

PER SERVING

calories 177	sodium 145 mg
total fat 4.5 g	carbohydrates 4 g
saturated fat 0.5 g	fiber 1 g
trans fat 0.0 g	sugars 2 g
polyunsaturated fat 1.5 g	protein 29 g
monounsaturated fat 1.5 g	DIETARY EXCHANGES
cholesterol 77 mg	3 lean meat

ONE-PAN CURRIED TURKEY WITH WATER CHESTNUTS

SERVES 6

Looking for an interesting way to use leftover turkey? Try this Asian-inspired one-dish meal. It offers crunch from water chestnuts and almonds, sweetness from pineapple and pimiento, and a sweet savory flavor balance from the blend of spices used in curry powder.

2 teaspoons canola or corn oil
8 medium green onions, sliced diagonally into 1/2-inch pieces
1 medium green bell pepper, sliced
1 small rib of celery, sliced diagonally into 1/2-inch pieces
2 cups diced cooked skinless turkey breast, cooked without salt, all visible fat discarded
2 cups canned sliced water chestnuts, drained, cut into thin strips
3 tablespoons white whole-wheat flour
2 tablespoons slivered almonds
1 teaspoon curry powder
1 teaspoon paprika
1/2 teaspoon dried basil, crumbled
1 1/2 cups fat-free, low-sodium chicken broth, such as on page 36
1 cup pineapple tidbits, canned in their own juice, drained
2 tablespoons chopped pimiento, drained
Pepper to taste (freshly ground preferred)

In a large skillet, heat the oil over medium-high heat, swirling to coat the bottom. Cook the green onions, bell pepper, and celery for 5 minutes, or until the onions are soft and slightly browned and the bell pepper and celery are tender, stirring frequently.

Reduce the heat to medium. Stir in the turkey, water chestnuts, flour, almonds, curry powder, paprika, and basil. Cook for 3 to 5 minutes, or until well blended, stirring constantly.

Stir in the broth, pineapple, and pimiento. Cook, covered, for 2 minutes.

Just before serving, sprinkle with the pepper.

calories 179
total fat 3.5 g
  saturated fat 0.5 g
  trans fat 0.0 g
  polyunsaturated fat 1.0 g
  monounsaturated fat 2.0 g
cholesterol 40 mg
sodium 57 mg

carbohydrates 20 g
  fiber 6 g
  sugars 7 g
protein 16 g
DIETARY EXCHANGES
  2 vegetable, 1/2 fruit,
  2 lean meat

ROASTED GARLIC–LEMON TURKEY BREAST

SERVES 14

A highly aromatic marinade of garlic, lemon, rosemary, thyme, and parsley flavors this roasted turkey breast. Use any leftover turkey in sandwiches, salads, or Turkey and Rice Soup *(page 109).*

Cooking spray
1 5 1/2- to 6-pound turkey breast with bone and skin, thawed if frozen
1/4 cup grated lemon zest
1/2 cup fresh lemon juice (about 4 large lemons)
1/4 cup olive oil
12 medium garlic cloves, minced
1 tablespoon Dijon mustard (lowest sodium available)
1 1/2 teaspoons dried rosemary, crushed
1 teaspoon dried thyme, crumbled
1 teaspoon salt
1 cup chopped fresh parsley

Lightly spray a large glass baking dish with cooking spray. Put the turkey in the baking dish.

In a small bowl, whisk together the remaining ingredients except the parsley. Stir in the parsley.

Using your fingers and keeping the skin attached, carefully lift the skin from the meat of the turkey so you can spread the lemon zest mixture between the skin and the meat. Cover as much area as possible, being careful not to tear the skin. Gently pull the skin back over the top and sides. Cover the turkey tightly with plastic wrap and refrigerate for 8 to 12 hours.

Preheat the oven to 325°F.

Remove the plastic wrap. Roast the turkey for about 1 hour 45 minutes to 2 hours, or until the thickest part of the breast registers 165°F on an instant-read thermometer. Remove from the oven.

Transfer the turkey to a cutting board. Let stand for 15 minutes, loosely covered. Discard the skin before slicing.

PER SERVING

calories 194
total fat 5.0 g
  saturated fat 1.0 g
  trans fat 0.0 g
  polyunsaturated fat 0.5 g
  monounsaturated fat 3.0 g
cholesterol 92 mg

sodium 249 mg
carbohydrates 2 g
  fiber 1 g
  sugars 1 g
protein 34 g
DIETARY EXCHANGES
  4 lean meat

CIDER-GLAZED TURKEY TENDERLOIN WITH HARVEST VEGETABLES

SERVES 4

Here's a turkey dinner with heart-healthy fixings that's easy to prepare and roasts while you're busy elsewhere. It's like Thanksgiving without the fuss—or all the extra calories! To make it even more reminiscent of the holidays, serve Pumpkin Pie Bites *(page 493) for dessert.*

Cooking spray
1 1-pound turkey tenderloin, all visible fat discarded
1 teaspoon olive oil and 2 teaspoons olive oil, divided use
1 medium carrot, cut into 1-inch pieces
1 medium parsnip, cut into 1-inch pieces
1/2 medium onion, cut into 1-inch wedges
1/4 small acorn squash, peeled, seeds and strings discarded, cut into 1 1/2-inch cubes
1/2 teaspoon dried thyme, crumbled
1/4 teaspoon salt
1/4 teaspoon pepper
1/4 teaspoon ground nutmeg
1 cup 100% apple cider

(continued)

Preheat the oven to 425°F.

Line a 13 x 9 x 2-inch baking pan with aluminum foil. Lightly spray the foil with cooking spray. Place the turkey in the pan. Brush the top of the turkey with 1 teaspoon oil.

In a large bowl, combine the carrot, parsnip, onion, and squash. Drizzle with the remaining 2 teaspoons oil. Stir to coat. Place around the turkey.

In a small bowl, stir together the remaining ingredients except the cider. Sprinkle over the turkey and vegetables.

Roast for 30 minutes.

Meanwhile, in a small saucepan, bring the cider to a boil over medium-high heat. Boil for 10 minutes, or until reduced by half (to about 1/2 cup). Remove from the heat.

Remove the baking pan from the oven after 30 minutes. Stir the vegetables. Pour the cider over the turkey and vegetables. Roast for 15 minutes, or until the turkey is no longer pink in the center and registers 165°F on an instant-read thermometer and the vegetables are tender. Remove from the oven.

Cover the turkey loosely with aluminum foil. Let stand for 10 minutes. Cut the turkey crosswise into slices about 3/4 inch thick. Serve with the vegetables.

Cook's Tip: Use the remaining acorn squash to make squash "fries" later. Preheat the oven to 425°F. Cut the squash into thick slices and arrange in a single layer on a large baking sheet. Lightly spray the squash with olive oil cooking spray, then bake for 35 to 40 minutes, or until lightly browned.

PER SERVING

calories 228	carbohydrates 19 g
total fat 4.0 g	fiber 3 g
saturated fat 0.5 g	sugars 11 g
trans fat 0.0 g	**protein** 28 g
polyunsaturated fat 0.5 g	**DIETARY EXCHANGES**
monounsaturated fat 2.5 g	1/2 starch, 1/2 fruit,
cholesterol 75 mg	1 vegetable, 3 lean
sodium 227 mg	meat

TURKEY SCHNITZEL

SERVES 4

Don't wait for Oktoberfest to try this healthy version of an Austrian and German classic, in which creamy mushroom gravy tops thyme-scented turkey. Pair it with potatoes, as Germans usually do, or try Spiced Red Cabbage (page 380).

Cooking spray
2 teaspoons chopped fresh thyme or
    1 teaspoon dried thyme, crumbled
1/4 teaspoon salt
1/8 teaspoon pepper and 1/8 to 1/4 teaspoon
    pepper (freshly ground preferred),
    divided use
1 pound turkey tenderloin, flattened to 1/2-inch
    thickness, cut into 3/4-inch slices
1/3 cup all-purpose flour and 2 teaspoons all-
    purpose flour, divided use
1 large egg
2 large egg whites
3/4 cup whole-wheat panko (Japanese-style
    bread crumbs)
1 tablespoon olive oil
1/2 cup chopped button mushrooms
1/2 cup chopped brown (cremini) mushrooms
1/4 cup fat-free, low-sodium chicken broth,
    such as on page 36
1/4 cup fat-free half-and-half

Preheat the oven to 375°F. Lightly spray a large rimmed baking sheet with cooking spray.

In a small bowl, stir together the thyme, salt, and 1/8 teaspoon pepper. Sprinkle over both sides of the turkey. Using your fingertips, gently press the mixture so it adheres to the turkey.

Put 1/3 cup flour in a shallow medium bowl. In a separate shallow medium bowl, whisk together the egg and egg whites for 1 minute, or until frothy. Put the panko in a third medium shallow bowl. Put the bowls and a large plate in a row, assembly-line fashion. Dip the turkey in the flour, then in the egg mixture, and finally in the panko, turning to coat at each step and gently shaking off any excess. Place the turkey on the plate.

In a large nonstick skillet, heat the oil over medium heat, swirling to coat the bottom. Cook the turkey for 2 minutes on each side, or until light golden brown. Transfer to the baking sheet.

Bake for 4 to 5 minutes, or until the turkey is no longer pink in the center. Remove from the oven. Cover to keep warm.

Meanwhile, in the same skillet, still over medium heat, cook both mushrooms for 3 to 4 minutes, or until soft, stirring occasionally.

In a medium bowl, whisk together the broth, half-and-half, and the remaining 2 teaspoons flour and 1/8 to 1/4 teaspoon pepper. Pour the broth mixture into the skillet. Increase the heat to medium high. Cook for 1 to 2 minutes, or until thickened, stirring frequently. Just before serving, spoon the gravy over the turkey.

PER SERVING

calories 231	sodium 238 mg
total fat 5.0 g	carbohydrates 14 g
saturated fat 1.0 g	fiber 1 g
trans fat 0.0 g	sugars 2 g
polyunsaturated fat 0.5 g	protein 32 g
monounsaturated fat 3.0 g	DIETARY EXCHANGES
cholesterol 89 mg	1 starch, 3 lean meat

TURKEY ROLLS WITH GARDEN PESTO

SERVES 4

Boldly colored pesto and a honey and soy sauce glaze are great complements to these turkey rolls. Prepare Risotto Milanese (page 423) while the turkey bakes.

Cooking spray

Pesto
1/2 cup tightly packed fresh basil
1 small tomato, peeled, seeded, and coarsely chopped
1 tablespoon pine nuts, dry-roasted
1 large garlic clove, minced
2 tablespoons shredded or grated Parmesan cheese

2 8-ounce turkey tenderloins, all visible fat discarded, halved lengthwise
1 tablespoon honey
1 tablespoon soy sauce (lowest sodium available)

Preheat the oven to 350°F. Lightly spray an 8-inch square baking dish with cooking spray.

In a food processor or blender, process the pesto ingredients except the Parmesan until nearly smooth. Stir in the Parmesan.

Spread 1 rounded tablespoon pesto mixture on a piece of turkey. Starting with a short side, roll up jelly-roll style. Secure with wooden toothpicks. Repeat with the remaining turkey and pesto mixture. Place the turkey rolls with the seam side down in the pan. Set aside any remaining pesto.

In a small bowl, whisk together the honey and soy sauce. Brush on the turkey rolls.

Bake for 40 to 45 minutes, or until the turkey is no longer pink in the center. Top the turkey rolls with the remaining pesto.

Cook's Tip on Peeling Tomatoes: Cut a small, shallow X in the bottom end of each tomato. Plunge the tomatoes into boiling water for 10 to 15 seconds, then into ice water for about 1 minute. Use a paring knife to peel off the skin easily.

PER SERVING

calories 166	carbohydrates 7 g
total fat 2.5 g	fiber 1 g
saturated fat 1.0 g	sugars 6 g
trans fat 0.0 g	protein 29 g
polyunsaturated fat 0.5 g	DIETARY EXCHANGES
monounsaturated fat 0.5 g	1/2 other
cholesterol 76 mg	carbohydrate, 3 lean
sodium 188 mg	meat

■ ■ ■

FIVE-SPICE TURKEY MEDALLIONS

SERVES 4

With its cinnamon, cloves, fennel, anise, and pepper blend, Chinese five-spice powder packs a pungent flavor punch.

PER SERVING

calories 185	carbohydrates 8 g
total fat 3.5 g	fiber 2 g
saturated fat 0.5 g	sugars 4 g
trans fat 0.0 g	protein 30 g
polyunsaturated fat 1.0 g	DIETARY EXCHANGES
monounsaturated fat 1.0 g	1 vegetable, 3 lean
cholesterol 70 mg	meat
sodium 124 mg	

2 teaspoons toasted sesame oil

1 teaspoon soy sauce and 1 teaspoon soy sauce (lowest sodium available), divided use

1 1/2 teaspoons five-spice powder

1 pound turkey tenderloins, cut crosswise into 1/4-inch slices

8 ounces snow peas, trimmed and halved

1/2 cup chopped red bell pepper

1/4 cup slivered red onion

3 tablespoons plain rice vinegar

1 tablespoon grated peeled gingerroot

1 medium garlic clove, minced

In a medium bowl, stir together the oil, 1 teaspoon soy sauce, and the five-spice powder. Add the turkey, stirring to coat.

In a large nonstick skillet, cook the turkey mixture over medium heat for about 5 minutes, or until the turkey is no longer pink in the center, stirring occasionally. Transfer to a plate. Cover to keep warm.

In the same skillet, still over medium heat, stir together the remaining ingredients. Cook for 4 to 5 minutes, or until the snow peas are tender-crisp, stirring occasionally.

Stir in the remaining 1 teaspoon soy sauce. Serve the turkey over the snow pea mixture.

Cook's Tip on Toasted Sesame Oil: Widely used in Asian and Indian cuisines, this polyunsaturated oil is also called Asian sesame oil and fragrant toasted sesame oil. Toasted sesame oil is darker and stronger in flavor than "plain" sesame oil.

TURKEY CUTLETS WITH FRESH HERBS

SERVES 6

No more dry turkey! The buttermilk tenderizes the cutlets and keeps them moist as they cook. Cranberry Chutney (page 424) pairs well with the cutlets. Refrigerate any leftovers and serve slices of chilled turkey over your favorite salad greens or in Southwestern Turkey Wraps (page 241).

Marinade

2 cups low-fat buttermilk

1 large onion, finely chopped

1 tablespoon finely chopped fresh dillweed

1 tablespoon finely chopped fresh tarragon

1 tablespoon finely chopped fresh cilantro

1 tablespoon finely chopped fresh rosemary

1 tablespoon canola or corn oil

1 teaspoon pepper

1/4 teaspoon salt

■ ■ ■

6 skinless turkey breast cutlets (about 4 ounces each), about 3/4 inch thick, all visible fat discarded

In a large shallow glass dish, stir together the marinade ingredients. Add the turkey, turning to coat. Cover and refrigerate for 1 to 12 hours, turning several times.

Preheat the grill on medium high or preheat the broiler.

Drain the turkey, discarding the marinade.

Grill for 4 to 5 minutes on each side or broil about 6 inches from the heat for 5 to 7 minutes on each side, or until no longer pink in the center.

Cook's Tip on Herbs: In most recipes, such as this one, you can substitute dried herbs for fresh, though the flavor won't be quite as good. Use about one-third as much as you would of the fresh herbs.

TURKEY, KALE, AND PORTOBELLO LASAGNA

SERVES 9

Here's the solution for what to take to potluck dinners, a lighter version of a family favorite. Serve with a dark green, leafy salad with Zesty Tomato Dressing (page 105) or Focaccia (page 443).

Cooking spray
8 ounces dried whole-grain lasagna noodles
1 pound ground skinless turkey breast
8 ounces portobello mushrooms, chopped
1/2 cup chopped onion
3 medium garlic cloves, minced
3 cups no-salt-added tomato sauce
2 teaspoons dried basil, crumbled
1/2 teaspoon dried oregano, crumbled
Pepper to taste
16 ounces fat-free ricotta cheese
10 ounces frozen chopped kale, thawed and squeezed dry
Dash of ground nutmeg
2 cups shredded or grated low-fat mozzarella cheese

Preheat the oven to 375°F. Lightly spray a 13 x 9 x 2-inch glass baking dish with cooking spray.

Prepare the noodles using the package directions, omitting the salt.

Meanwhile, in a large nonstick skillet over medium-high heat, stir together the turkey, mushrooms, onion, and garlic. Cook for 8 to 10 minutes, or until the turkey is no longer pink, stirring occasionally to turn and break up the turkey. Reduce the heat to low. Cook, covered, for 3 to 4 minutes, or until the mushrooms have released their liquid. Increase the heat to high. Cook, uncovered, for 2 to 3 minutes, or until the liquid evaporates.

Stir in the tomato sauce, basil, oregano, and pepper. Reduce the heat to low. Cook for 5 to 6 minutes, or until heated through.

In a large bowl, stir together the ricotta, kale, and nutmeg.

In the baking dish, layer one-third of the cooked noodles, one-half of the ricotta mixture, one-third of the turkey mixture, and one-third of the mozzarella. Repeat the layers. Finish in order with the remaining noodles, turkey, and mozzarella.

Bake, covered, for 35 to 40 minutes, or until the casserole is heated through and the mozzarella has melted.

THANKSGIVING MEAT LOAF WITH CRANBERRY GLAZE

SERVES 4

This meat loaf, packed with all the flavors of a holiday turkey dinner, is so moist—thanks to a mashed sweet potato—that you'll gobble it up! Serve with Creamy Pumpkin Soup (page 48).

(continued)

Cooking spray

Meat Loaf

1 pound lean ground skinless turkey breast

1 medium sweet potato, peeled, cooked, and mashed

2 teaspoons dried sage

2 teaspoons poultry seasoning

1 teaspoon dried thyme, crumbled

1/8 teaspoon salt

1/4 teaspoon pepper

1/2 cup grated or finely chopped onion

1/2 medium rib of celery, diced

1/4 cup chopped red bell pepper

1/4 cup egg substitute

■ ■ ■

1/2 cup cranberries, thawed if frozen

1/3 cup water

1 tablespoon no-salt-added ketchup

1 teaspoon honey

1 teaspoon hot chili sauce (sriracha preferred)

1/4 teaspoon dried rosemary, crushed

1/8 teaspoon salt

Preheat the oven to 350°F. Line a baking sheet with aluminum foil. Lightly spray the foil with cooking spray. Set aside.

Crumble the turkey into a large bowl. Add the remaining meat loaf ingredients. Using your hands or a spoon, combine the ingredients.

Transfer the turkey mixture to the baking sheet. Shape into a loaf about 8 x 5 inches. Bake for 30 minutes.

Meanwhile, in a small saucepan, stir together the cranberries, water, ketchup, honey, and chili sauce. Heat over medium-high heat until just beginning to boil. Reduce the heat and simmer for 10 minutes, or until the cranberries are soft. Using a potato masher or the back of a spoon, crush the cranberries until almost smooth. Stir in the rosemary and the remaining 1/8 teaspoon salt.

Spread the glaze over the top and sides of the meat loaf. Bake for 30 to 40 minutes, or until the

loaf registers 165°F on an instant-read thermometer. Let stand for 10 minutes before serving.

PER SERVING

calories 216	carbohydrates 20 g
total fat 1.0 g	fiber 3 g
saturated fat 0.5 g	sugars 7 g
trans fat 0.0 g	protein 31 g
polyunsaturated fat 0.0 g	DIETARY EXCHANGES
monounsaturated fat 0.0 g	1 1/2 starch, 3 lean
cholesterol 70 mg	meat
sodium 296 mg	

TURKEY CHILI

SERVES 8

Beans are high in protein and fiber, and they help stretch this chili to feed more people or provide extra for leftovers for later in the week. This recipe uses pinto and black beans, but you can substitute kidney beans, chickpeas, or your own favorites. Serve with Tex-Mex Cucumber Salad (page 78) and Corn Bread Muffins (page 464).

2 tablespoons canola or corn oil

1 large onion, chopped

1 1/4 pounds ground skinless turkey breast

2 large garlic cloves, minced

2 teaspoons chili powder

1/2 teaspoon pepper (freshly ground preferred)

1/2 teaspoon ground cumin

1 15.5-ounce can no-salt-added pinto beans, rinsed and drained

1 15.5-ounce can no-salt-added black beans, rinsed and drained

1 14.5-ounce can no-salt-added diced tomatoes, undrained

1 3/4 cups fat-free, low-sodium chicken broth, such as on page 36

1 cup frozen whole-kernel corn

1 6-ounce can no-salt-added tomato paste

4 to 5 medium green onions (green part only), chopped

In a Dutch oven or large saucepan, heat the oil over medium heat, swirling to coat the bottom.

Cook the onion for 5 minutes, or until soft, stirring frequently.

Stir in the turkey. Cook for 5 minutes, or until no longer pink, stirring to turn and break up the turkey. Stir in the garlic, chili powder, pepper, and cumin until well combined.

Stir in both beans, the tomatoes with liquid, broth, corn, and tomato paste. Cook for 5 to 7 minutes, or until the chili is heated through, stirring frequently.

Stir the green onions into the chili. Ladle the chili in bowls.

PER SERVING

calories 273	carbohydrates 32 g
total fat 4.5 g	fiber 7 g
saturated fat 0.5 g	sugars 10 g
trans fat 0.0 g	protein 26 g
polyunsaturated fat 1.5 g	**DIETARY EXCHANGES**
monounsaturated fat 2.5 g	2 starch, 1 vegetable,
cholesterol 48 mg	3 lean meat
sodium 71 mg	

SWEET AND SPICY TURKEY BURGERS

SERVES 4

These moist burgers pack a hint of heat from chipotle and a bit of sweet from mango. Serve with Grilled Tomato-Peach Salad (page 82) or Baked Sweet Potato Chips (page 407).

1 teaspoon canola or corn oil
1 medium Granny Smith apple, peeled and diced
1/4 cup chopped red onion
2 tablespoons chopped celery
1 pound ground skinless turkey breast
2 tablespoons whole-wheat panko (Japanese-style bread crumbs)
2 tablespoons coarsely chopped fresh cilantro
2 tablespoons fresh lemon juice
1/4 teaspoon pepper
1/4 teaspoon chipotle powder
1/8 teaspoon salt
Cooking spray

4 whole-grain hamburger buns (lowest sodium available), split
1/4 cup mango chutney (lowest sodium available)
1/2 medium fresh jalapeño, seeds and ribs discarded, minced (optional; see Cook's Tip on Handling Hot Chiles, page 24)

Preheat the grill on medium high.

In a small nonstick skillet, heat the oil over medium-high heat, swirling to coat the bottom. Cook the apple, onion, and celery for 6 to 8 minutes, or until the apple is tender and the onion is very soft, stirring frequently.

In a medium bowl, stir together the apple mixture, turkey, panko, cilantro, lemon juice, pepper, chipotle powder, and salt just until blended. Form into 4 patties, 1/4 to 1/2 inch thick. Lightly spray the top with cooking spray.

Grill the patties with the sprayed side down for 5 to 7 minutes on each side, or until no longer pink in the center. Grill the buns with the split side down for 30 seconds, or until lightly browned. Serve the patties on the buns, topping the patties with the chutney and jalapeño.

Cook's Tip on Sodium in Chutney: It is really important to compare Nutrition Facts labels on chutneys because the sodium varies drastically from one brand to another. The one used for this nutrition analysis has 55 milligrams of sodium in each tablespoon.

PER SERVING

calories 308	carbohydrates 37 g
total fat 4.0 g	fiber 4 g
saturated fat 0.5 g	sugars 14 g
trans fat 0.0 g	protein 32 g
polyunsaturated fat 1.5 g	**DIETARY EXCHANGES**
monounsaturated fat 1.5 g	1 1/2 starch, 1 fruit,
cholesterol 70 mg	3 lean meat
sodium 396 mg	

TURKEY MEATBALLS

SERVES 4

Ground turkey has less fat than ground beef, so this recipe uses milk to keep these meatballs moist. Serve with whole-grain pasta and Speedy Marinara Sauce *(page 435) or* Fresh Tomato and Roasted Red Bell Pepper Sauce *(page 434) and a simple dark green, leafy salad.*

Cooking spray

Meatballs

1 pound ground skinless turkey breast

1 small onion, grated

1/3 cup shredded or grated Parmesan cheese

1/4 cup whole-wheat bread crumbs (lowest sodium available)

1/4 cup fat-free milk

3 tablespoons chopped fresh parsley

1 large egg, well beaten

1 medium garlic clove, minced

1/4 teaspoon ground nutmeg

1/4 teaspoon pepper

■ ■ ■

1/4 cup all-purpose flour

Preheat the oven to 350°F. Lightly spray the broiler pan and rack with cooking spray.

In a medium bowl, using your hands or a spoon, combine the meatball ingredients. Shape into 35 balls, about 1 inch in diameter. Dust with the flour. Transfer to the broiler rack.

Broil the meatballs about 4 inches from the heat for 10 to 15 minutes, or until the tops are browned. Turn over the meatballs. Broil for 10 to 15 minutes, or until the meatballs are browned on the outside and no longer pink in the center.

PER SERVING

calories 242	sodium 245 mg
total fat 5.0 g	carbohydrates 15 g
saturated fat 1.5 g	fiber 1 g
trans fat 0.0 g	sugars 3 g
polyunsaturated fat .5 g	protein 35 g
monounsaturated fat 1.0 g	DIETARY EXCHANGES
cholesterol 98 mg	1 starch, 4 lean meat

SPAGHETTI BOLOGNESE

SERVES 8

A traditional Bolognese sauce is a thick meat sauce usually made of ground beef or pork, but this version uses ground poultry instead. While the dish simmers slowly for a couple of hours, prepare Kale Caesar Salad with Polenta Croutons *(page 69).*

Sauce

1 teaspoon olive oil

1 1/2 pounds ground skinless turkey breast

2 cups chopped onions

2 cups chopped celery

1 cup chopped green bell pepper

1 28-ounce can Italian plum (Roma) tomatoes, drained

1 6-ounce can no-salt-added tomato paste

1 tablespoon Worcestershire sauce (lowest sodium available)

2 medium dried bay leaves

1 teaspoon pepper

1 teaspoon dried oregano, crumbled

1 teaspoon garlic powder

■ ■ ■

16 ounces dried whole-wheat spaghetti

1/2 cup shredded or grated Parmesan cheese

In a large skillet, heat the oil over medium-low heat, swirling to coat the bottom. Cook the turkey for 3 minutes, stirring occasionally to turn and break up the turkey. Stir in the onions. Cook for 5 minutes, or until the onions are just beginning to brown. Stir in the celery and bell pepper. Cook for 2 to 3 minutes. Stir in the remaining sauce ingredients. Reduce the heat and simmer, covered, for 2 hours.

Right before the sauce finishes cooking, prepare the pasta using the package directions, omitting the salt. Drain well in a colander. Transfer to plates.

Discard the bay leaves from the sauce. Ladle the sauce onto the pasta. Sprinkle with the Parmesan.

calories 415
total fat 10.0 g
   saturated fat 3.0 g
   trans fat 0.0 g
   polyunsaturated fat 2.5 g
   monounsaturated fat 3.5 g
cholesterol 67 mg
sodium 384 mg

carbohydrates 57 g
   fiber 10 g
   sugars 10 g
protein 29 g
DIETARY EXCHANGES
   3 starch, 3 vegetable,
   2 1/2 lean meat

calories 190
total fat 5.0 g
   saturated fat 2.0 g
   trans fat 0.0 g
   polyunsaturated fat 1.0 g
   monounsaturated fat 1.5 g
cholesterol 49 mg

sodium 372 mg
carbohydrates 18 g
   fiber 2 g
   sugars 4 g
protein 17 g
DIETARY EXCHANGES
   1 starch, 2 lean meat

SOUTHWESTERN TURKEY WRAPS

SERVES 4

These wraps get their kick from salsa and Dijon mustard, and are an easy way to use leftover turkey. Because they're prepared ahead of time, they make a perfect halftime meal or snack during Thanksgiving weekend football games.

- 3 ounces light tub cream cheese
- 2 tablespoons salsa (lowest sodium available), such as Salsa Cruda (page 437)
- 2 tablespoons sliced green onion
- 1 teaspoon Dijon mustard (lowest sodium available)
- 4 6-inch whole-wheat tortillas (lowest sodium available)
- 1 cup shredded romaine
- 6 ounces very thinly sliced or finely chopped roasted turkey breast, cooked without salt, skin and all visible fat discarded
- 4 strips red bell pepper, about 1/4 inch wide

In a small bowl, stir together the cream cheese, salsa, green onion, and mustard.

To assemble, spread the cream cheese mixture over each tortilla. Top with the romaine, turkey, and bell pepper.

Roll the tortilla jelly-roll style over the filling, securing with a wooden toothpick if desired. Wrap tightly in plastic wrap. Refrigerate for several hours, or until serving time.

Cook's Tip: Cut each tortilla roll into fourths to serve as appetizers for eight.

Meats

FILET OF BEEF WITH *HERBES DE PROVENCE*

SERVES 6

You don't need much but garlic and a few seasonings to flavor this tender cut of beef. Serve with roasted red potatoes and Roasted Brussels Sprouts (page 378).

> Olive oil cooking spray
> 1 1 1/2-pound beef tenderloin, all visible fat and silver skin discarded
> 3 medium garlic cloves, minced
> 2 teaspoons dried *herbes de Provence* or mixed dried herbs, crumbled
> 1 teaspoon pepper, or to taste
> 2 medium carrots, finely diced
> 1 medium onion, sliced
> 1/4 teaspoon salt

Preheat the oven to 400°F. Lightly spray a roasting pan with cooking spray.

Tie the roast in three or four places with kitchen twine. Rub with the garlic. Sprinkle the *herbes de Provence* and pepper over the roast. Transfer to the pan. Lightly spray the roast with cooking spray. Scatter the carrots and onion on and around the roast.

Roast for 35 to 45 minutes for medium-rare, or until the roast registers 5 to 10 degrees below the desired doneness when tested with an instant-read thermometer. Transfer to a cutting board. Sprinkle with the salt. Cover with aluminum foil. Let stand for 10 to 15 minutes before slicing.

Cook's Tip on *Herbes de Provence*: *Herbes de Provence* is a combination of herbs used quite frequently in southern France: basil, thyme, rosemary, marjoram, sage, and lavender. If you don't have *herbes de Provence,* use a combination of at least two of these, blended in equal amounts.

PER SERVING

calories 182	carbohydrates 5 g
total fat 6.0 g	fiber 1 g
saturated fat 2.5 g	sugars 3 g
trans fat 0.0 g	**protein** 25 g
polyunsaturated fat 0.5 g	**DIETARY EXCHANGES**
monounsaturated fat 3.0 g	1 vegetable, 3 lean
cholesterol 61 mg	meat
sodium 185 mg	

POT ROAST RATATOUILLE AND PASTA

SERVES 8

This comforting dish slow-roasts, resulting in tender beef and melt-in-your-mouth vegetables to create the perfect meal on a cold winter's night. For variety, skip the pasta and serve the beef and vegetables over Mashed Potatoes with Parmesan and Green Onions (page 399).

> Olive oil cooking spray
> 1/2 teaspoon salt-free all-purpose seasoning blend
> 1/4 teaspoon pepper
> 1 1 1/2-pound eye-of-round roast, all visible fat discarded
> 1 10.75-ounce can tomato puree
> 10 ounces eggplant, chopped
> 2 medium zucchini, sliced
> 5 medium Italian plum (Roma) tomatoes, chopped
> 1 large onion, chopped
> 2 medium ribs of celery, sliced
> 1 teaspoon dried oregano or dried Italian seasoning, crumbled
> 1 medium garlic clove, minced
> 1 medium dried bay leaf
> 1/4 teaspoon dried basil, crumbled
> 8 ounces dried whole-grain pasta

Preheat the oven to 350°F. Lightly spray a Dutch oven with cooking spray.

Sprinkle the seasoning blend and pepper over the roast.

(continued)

Heat the Dutch oven over medium-high heat. Brown the roast for 2 to 3 minutes on each side.

Stir in the remaining ingredients except the pasta.

Roast, covered, for 2 hours, or until the beef is very tender when tested with a fork.

Shortly before the roast is done, prepare the pasta using the package directions, omitting the salt. Drain well in a colander.

Transfer the roast to a cutting board. Cover with aluminum foil. Let stand for 10 to 15 minutes before very thinly slicing diagonally across the grain, then slicing into thin strips. Discard the bay leaf from the sauce.

Spoon the pasta onto plates. Arrange the roast slices on the pasta. Top with the sauce.

Cook's Tip on Eye-of-Round Roast: For maximum tenderness, don't overcook an eye-of-round roast, and be sure to cut it into thin strips.

PER SERVING

calories 258	carbohydrates 32 g
total fat 3.0 g	fiber 6 g
saturated fat 1.0 g	sugars 8 g
trans fat 0.0 g	**protein** 26 g
polyunsaturated fat 0.5 g	**DIETARY EXCHANGES**
monounsaturated fat 1.5 g	1 1/2 starch,
cholesterol 40 mg	2 vegetable, 3 lean
sodium 76 mg	meat

BEEF ROAST WITH ROSEMARY AND HOISIN SAUCE

SERVES 8

Asian flavors infuse this braised eye-of-round roast. Serve thin slices of the roast and gravy on low-fat mashed potatoes spiked with wasabi or horseradish (see Cook's Tip in the next column).

Olive oil cooking spray
1 2-pound eye-of-round roast, all visible fat discarded
1 cup fat-free, low-sodium beef broth, such as on page 35
2 tablespoons dry vermouth or dry white wine (regular or nonalcoholic)

2 tablespoons hoisin sauce (lowest sodium available)
1 tablespoon balsamic vinegar
2 teaspoons soy sauce (lowest sodium available)
1 teaspoon dried rosemary, crushed
2 medium garlic cloves, minced
1 1/2 tablespoons cornstarch
1/4 cup water

Preheat the oven to 350°F. Lightly spray a Dutch oven with cooking spray.

Heat the Dutch oven over medium-high heat. Brown the roast for 2 to 3 minutes on each side.

Stir in the broth, vermouth, hoisin sauce, vinegar, soy sauce, rosemary, and garlic. Bring to a simmer.

Roast, covered, for about 2 hours, or until the beef is very tender when tested with a fork. Transfer to a cutting board, leaving the liquid in the pot. Cover the roast with aluminum foil. Let stand for 10 to 15 minutes before slicing diagonally across the grain into very thin pieces. Transfer to plates.

Put the cornstarch in a small bowl. Add the water, whisking to dissolve. Whisk into the cooking liquid. Bring to a simmer over medium-high heat. Reduce the heat and simmer for 1 to 2 minutes, or until the mixture has thickened, whisking occasionally. Spoon over the beef.

Cook's Tip on Wasabi or Horseradish Mashed Potatoes: For mashed potatoes with some firepower, just stir 1 to 2 teaspoons of wasabi paste or wasabi powder, or 1 tablespoon bottled white horseradish, into 4 cups mashed potatoes (mashed with fat-free milk and 1 tablespoon olive oil instead of butter).

PER SERVING

calories 157	sodium 125 mg
total fat 2.5 g	**carbohydrates** 4 g
saturated fat 1.0 g	fiber 0 g
trans fat 0.0 g	sugars 2 g
polyunsaturated fat 0.0 g	**protein** 27 g
monounsaturated fat 1.5 g	**DIETARY EXCHANGES**
cholesterol 54 mg	3 lean meat

SIMPLE SAUERBRATEN

SERVES 8

German for "sour roast," sauerbraten usually calls for the meat to marinate for days and simmer for hours. In this version, the roast cooks for just a bit over 2 hours, but tastes just as delicious as the classic recipe. Sauerbraten is traditionally served with dumplings, boiled potatoes, or noodles.

> Cooking spray
> Pepper to taste (freshly ground preferred)
> 3 pounds boneless lean chuck shoulder roast, all visible fat discarded
> 1 cup white wine vinegar
> 1 cup water
> 1 medium onion, sliced
> 2 medium dried bay leaves
> 16 low-fat gingersnaps, crushed to fine crumbs

Preheat the oven to 475°F. Lightly spray a Dutch oven with cooking spray.

Sprinkle the pepper over the roast. Transfer to the Dutch oven. Roast for 8 to 10 minutes, or until browned, turning once halfway through. Remove from the oven.

Pour the vinegar and water over the beef. Arrange the onion slices on the beef. Put the bay leaves in the pot liquid.

Reduce the heat to 350°F. Roast, covered, for 1 1/2 hours. Remove from the oven.

Sprinkle the gingersnap crumbs over the beef and gravy. Roast, covered, for 30 minutes, or to the desired doneness. Add water as needed to thin the gravy. Transfer the beef to a cutting board. Very thinly slice the beef diagonally across the grain. Discard the bay leaves. Serve with the gravy.

PER SERVING

calories 263	carbohydrates 13 g
total fat 9.0 g	fiber 0 g
saturated fat 3.0 g	sugars 6 g
trans fat 0.0 g	**protein** 32 g
polyunsaturated fat 0.5 g	**DIETARY EXCHANGES**
monounsaturated fat 4.0 g	1 other carbohydrate,
cholesterol 98 mg	4 lean meat
sodium 114 mg	

CHICKEN-"FRIED" STEAK

SERVES 4

This southern-accented comfort food with creamy gravy doesn't have to be off-limits. Cube steak stays tender and whole-grain crackers provide crunch with an extra helping of fiber.

> 1/4 cup white whole-wheat or whole-wheat pastry flour
> 1/2 teaspoon dried thyme, crumbled
> 1/2 teaspoon onion powder
> 1/2 teaspoon garlic powder
> 1/4 teaspoon pepper (freshly ground preferred)
> 1/2 cup low-fat buttermilk
> 3/4 cup finely crushed whole-grain crackers (lowest sodium available)
> 4 cube steaks (about 4 ounces each), all visible fat discarded
> 2 teaspoons olive oil
> Cooking spray
> 1/2 cup fat-free, low-sodium chicken broth, such as on page 36
> 1/2 cup fat-free half-and-half
> 1/4 teaspoon salt

In a shallow dish, stir together the flour, thyme, onion powder, garlic powder, and pepper. Set aside 1 tablespoon of the mixture. Pour the buttermilk into a separate shallow dish. Put the cracker crumbs in a third shallow dish. Put the dishes and a large plate in a row, assembly-line fashion. Dip the beef in the flour mixture, then in the buttermilk, and finally in the cracker crumbs, turning to coat at each step and gently shaking off any excess. Using your fingertips, gently press the coating so it adheres to the beef. Place the beef on the plate. Cover and refrigerate for 30 minutes to 4 hours.

In a large nonstick skillet, heat the oil over medium-high heat, swirling to coat the bottom. Cook the beef for 4 to 5 minutes, or until golden brown on the bottom. Remove the skillet from the heat. Lightly spray the top of the beef twice with cooking spray. Turn over the beef. Cook for 4 to 5 minutes, or until golden brown. Transfer

(continued)

the steaks to a platter. Cover to keep warm. Remove the skillet from the heat and let cool slightly.

In a small bowl, whisk together the broth, half-and-half, 1/4 teaspoon salt, and the reserved 1 tablespoon flour mixture. Pour into the skillet. Cook over medium heat for 2 to 3 minutes, or until the mixture comes to a simmer and thickens, stirring occasionally.

Just before serving, spoon the gravy over the beef or serve it on the side.

PER SERVING

calories 255	**sodium** 280 mg
total fat 7.0 g	**carbohydrates** 17 g
saturated fat 2.0 g	fiber 2 g
trans fat 0.0 g	sugars 3 g
polyunsaturated fat 1.5 g	**protein** 31 g
monounsaturated fat 3.5 g	**DIETARY EXCHANGES**
cholesterol 54 mg	1 starch, 3 lean meat

CUBE STEAK WITH MUSHROOM SAUCE

SERVES 4

Shallots impart a subtle onion flavor that doesn't overpower this quick-to-prepare steak and mushroom dish. Serve with French Peas *(page 396) and* Garlic Potatoes *(page 401).*

> 1/2 teaspoon salt-free onion and herb seasoning blend
> 1/2 teaspoon garlic powder
> 1/2 teaspoon pepper
> 4 cube steaks (about 4 ounces each), all visible fat discarded
> 2 teaspoons olive oil
> 8 ounces button mushrooms, sliced
> 2 medium shallots, finely chopped
> 1 1/2 tablespoons all-purpose flour
> 1 cup fat-free, low-sodium beef broth, such as on page 35
> 3 tablespoons all-fruit grape spread

In a small bowl, stir together the seasoning blend, garlic powder, and pepper. Sprinkle over both sides of the beef. Using your fingertips,

gently press the mixture so it adheres to the beef.

In a large nonstick skillet, heat the oil over medium-high heat, swirling to coat the bottom. Cook the beef for 4 to 5 minutes on each side, or until browned. Transfer to a large plate. Cover to keep warm.

In the same skillet, still over medium-high heat, cook the mushrooms and shallots for 4 to 5 minutes, or until soft, stirring frequently.

Stir in the flour. Stir in the broth and grape spread. Bring to a boil. Reduce the heat and simmer for 1 to 2 minutes, or until thickened, stirring constantly.

Add the beef, spooning the sauce over it. Simmer for 1 to 2 minutes, or until heated through.

Cook's Tip on Shallots: Shallots resemble garlic bulbs, but are actually part of the onion family. A staple of French cooking, they offer a more delicate flavor than other onions.

PER SERVING

calories 217	**carbohydrates** 13 g
total fat 5.0 g	fiber 1 g
saturated fat 1.5 g	sugars 9 g
trans fat 0.0 g	**protein** 29 g
polyunsaturated fat 0.5 g	**DIETARY EXCHANGES**
monounsaturated fat 3.0 g	1 other carbohydrate,
cholesterol 58 mg	3 lean meat
sodium 81 mg	

GREEK-STYLE EYE-OF-ROUND STEAKS

SERVES 4

Lean eye-of-round steaks are braised until fork-tender with popular ingredients used in Greek cooking. This dish is even more delicious the day after you make it. Serve with Bulgur Pilaf with Lemon and Spinach *(page 416).*

> Olive oil cooking spray
> 4 eye-of-round steaks (about 4 ounces each), all visible fat discarded
> 1 large green bell pepper, cut into 1-inch squares

1 cup frozen pearl onions, thawed

1 14.5-ounce can no-salt-added diced tomatoes, undrained

1/2 cup dry red wine (regular or nonalcoholic)

2 tablespoons chopped kalamata olives

1 teaspoon grated lemon zest

1 tablespoon fresh lemon juice

1 teaspoon dried oregano, crumbled

1/8 teaspoon ground cinnamon

Lightly spray a medium skillet with cooking spray. Cook the beef over medium-high heat for 3 minutes on each side, or until browned.

Stir in the bell pepper and onions. Cook for 1 to 2 minutes, or until the pepper is tender-crisp.

Stir in the remaining ingredients. Bring to a simmer. Reduce the heat and simmer, covered, for 1 hour 30 minutes, or until the beef is tender, stirring occasionally.

PER SERVING

calories 238	carbohydrates 16 g
total fat 4.0 g	fiber 3 g
saturated fat 1.5 g	sugars 7 g
trans fat 0.0 g	protein 28 g
polyunsaturated fat 0.5 g	**DIETARY EXCHANGES**
monounsaturated fat 2.0 g	3 vegetable, 3 lean
cholesterol 54 mg	meat
sodium 174 mg	

GRILLED LEMONGRASS FLANK STEAK

SERVES 4 (PLUS 6 OUNCES RESERVED)

Flank steak is marinated in a fragrant lemongrass mixture that also spotlights delicate rice vinegar and zesty chili garlic sauce. Serve four people tonight and refrigerate the extra two servings to use in sandwiches or Grilled Flank Steak Salad with Sweet-and-Sour Sesame Dressing *(page 97) later in the week.*

Marinade

3 stalks of lemongrass, 3 teaspoons lemongrass paste, 3 teaspoons ground dried lemongrass, or 3 teaspoons grated lemon zest

1/3 cup plain rice vinegar

3 medium garlic cloves, minced

1 teaspoon chili garlic sauce or chili garlic paste

1 teaspoon soy sauce (lowest sodium available)

1 teaspoon canola or corn oil

■ ■ ■

1 1 1/2-pound flank steak, all visible fat and silver skin discarded

Trim about 6 inches off the slender green end of the lemongrass stalks and discard. Remove the outer layer of leaves from the roots of the stalks. Halve the stalks lengthwise. (Lemongrass stalks are slightly tough, so be careful as you slice.)

In a large glass dish, stir together the marinade ingredients. Add the beef, turning to coat. Cover and refrigerate for 2 to 12 hours, turning occasionally.

Preheat the grill on medium high.

Drain the beef, discarding the marinade. Grill the beef for 8 to 9 minutes on each side, or to the desired doneness. Transfer to a cutting board. Let stand for 5 minutes before thinly slicing diagonally across the grain. Serve 12 ounces (about two-thirds) of the cooked beef. Cover and refrigerate the remaining beef (about 6 ounces) for use in Grilled Flank Steak Salad.

PER SERVING

calories 158	sodium 102 mg
total fat 6.5 g	carbohydrates 0 g
saturated fat 3.0 g	fiber 0 g
trans fat 0.0 g	sugars 0 g
polyunsaturated fat 0.5 g	protein 23 g
monounsaturated fat 2.5 g	**DIETARY EXCHANGES**
cholesterol 65 mg	3 lean meat

SIZZLING FLANK STEAK

SERVES 4

It sizzles onto your table from the grill during the summer, but you can also broil it when the weather turns much colder. Just be sure to plan ahead—the beef needs a half to full day to marinate. Serve it with Chile-Lime Grilled Corn *(page 386) or grilled or broiled zucchini spears.*

Marinade
- 1 medium onion, grated
- 1/4 cup plus 1 tablespoon fresh lemon juice (about 2 large lemons)
- 2 tablespoons chopped fresh parsley
- 2 tablespoons grated peeled gingerroot
- 2 tablespoons soy sauce (lowest sodium available)
- 1 tablespoon ground cumin
- 1 tablespoon chili powder
- 2 teaspoons olive oil
- 2 teaspoons dry sherry (optional)
- 2 large garlic cloves, crushed or minced
- 1 teaspoon ground turmeric
- 1 teaspoon dried oregano, crumbled
- 1 teaspoon pepper

■ ■ ■

- 1 1-pound flank steak, all visible fat and silver skin discarded
- Cooking spray
- Sprigs of fresh cilantro

In a shallow glass baking dish, stir together all the marinade ingredients. Add the beef, turning to coat. Cover and refrigerate for 12 to 24 hours, turning occasionally.

Lightly spray the grill rack or broiler pan and rack with cooking spray. Preheat the grill on medium high or preheat the broiler.

Drain the beef, reserving the marinade. Grill the beef or broil it about 4 inches from the heat for about 5 minutes on each side for medium, or to the desired doneness. Transfer to a cutting board. Let stand for about 5 minutes. Cut the beef diagonally across the grain into thin slices. Arrange on a platter.

Meanwhile, strain the marinade into a small saucepan, discarding the solids. Bring to a boil over high heat. Pour the desired amount of sauce over the beef, discarding any extra. Garnish with the cilantro.

PER SERVING

calories 202	**carbohydrates** 5 g
total fat 9.5 g	fiber 1 g
saturated fat 3.0 g	sugars 2 g
trans fat 0.0 g	**protein** 24 g
polyunsaturated fat 0.5 g	**DIETARY EXCHANGES**
monounsaturated fat 4.5 g	1/2 other carbohydrate,
cholesterol 65 mg	3 lean meat
sodium 277 mg	

MARINATED STEAK

SERVES 6

Classic Asian and Italian ingredients combine in this marinade to create a fusion of flavors. Plan ahead for this dish, since the beef needs at least a half day to marinate. Serve with Ratatouille *(page 414) or* Vegetable Stir-Fry *(page 414).*

Marinade
- 2/3 cup dry red wine (regular or nonalcoholic)
- 2 teaspoons dry sherry
- 1 teaspoon soy sauce (lowest sodium available)
- 1/8 teaspoon dried oregano, crumbled
- 1/8 teaspoon dried marjoram, crumbled
- 1/8 teaspoon grated peeled gingerroot
- 1/8 teaspoon toasted sesame oil
- Pepper to taste (freshly ground preferred)

■ ■ ■

- 1 1/2 pounds flank steak, all visible fat and silver skin discarded

In a large shallow glass dish, whisk together the marinade ingredients. Add the beef, turning to coat. Cover and refrigerate for at least 12 to 18 hours, turning occasionally.

Preheat the broiler. Drain the beef, discarding the marinade.

Broil 4 to 6 inches from the heat for 5 minutes on each side. Transfer to a cutting board. Thinly slice the beef diagonally across the grain.

PER SERVING

calories 158	**sodium** 67 mg
total fat 6.5 g	**carbohydrates** 0 g
saturated fat 3.0 g	fiber 0 g
trans fat 0.0 g	sugars 0 g
polyunsaturated fat 0.5 g	**protein** 23 g
monounsaturated fat 2.5 g	**DIETARY EXCHANGES**
cholesterol 65 mg	3 lean meat

ROPA VIEJA

SERVES 6

This stew has Cuban and Caribbean origins, and its name translates to "old clothes." It's made with an inexpensive piece of meat that's tenderized by long cooking and then shredded, causing it to resemble strips of cloth or rags. Prepare this dish when you have some time at home, since it'll take a few hours to cook. Serve it wrapped in whole-grain tortillas or with a side portion of Cuban Black Beans *(page 332).*

1 1/2 teaspoons canola or corn oil,

    1 1/2 teaspoons canola or corn oil, and

    1 teaspoon canola or corn oil, divided use

1 1/2-pounds boneless round steak, all visible fat discarded

1 cup water

1 medium dried bay leaf

1/4 teaspoon salt

1/8 teaspoon pepper

1 medium onion, sliced

1 medium green bell pepper, sliced

2 medium garlic cloves, minced

1 14.5-ounce can no-salt-added diced tomatoes, undrained

1/8 teaspoon ground cinnamon

In a Dutch oven, heat 1 1/2 teaspoons oil over medium heat, swirling to coat the bottom. Cook the beef on one side for about 4 minutes, or until browned on the bottom. Transfer to a plate. Pour in 1 1/2 teaspoons oil, swirling to coat the bottom. Return the beef to the pot with the uncooked side down. Cook for about 4 minutes, or until browned on the bottom.

Pour in the water and add the bay leaf, salt, and pepper. Reduce the heat and simmer, covered, for 2 to 3 hours, or until the beef is very tender. Discard the bay leaf.

Transfer the beef to a cutting board, leaving the juices in the pot. Set aside.

In a medium skillet, heat the remaining 1 teaspoon oil over medium-high heat, swirling to coat the bottom. Cook the onion, bell pepper, and garlic for about 3 minutes, or until the onion is soft and the bell pepper is tender, stirring frequently.

Stir the onion mixture, tomatoes with liquid, and cinnamon into the juices in the Dutch oven.

Using two forks, shred the beef, discarding any visible fat or gristle. Stir the shredded beef into the stew. Cook for 10 to 15 minutes, or until heated through.

PER SERVING

calories 193	**carbohydrates** 7 g
total fat 5.5 g	fiber 1 g
saturated fat 1.5 g	sugars 4 g
trans fat 0.0 g	**protein** 27 g
polyunsaturated fat 1.0 g	**DIETARY EXCHANGES**
monounsaturated fat 3.0 g	1 vegetable, 3 lean
cholesterol 53 mg	meat
sodium 176 mg	

YOGURT-MARINATED GRILLED ROUND STEAK

SERVES 4

Round steak usually needs long, slow cooking to become tender. In this recipe the acidity of the yogurt and lemon does the job instead. Let the steak marinate while you're at work or out for the day, and then come home and fire up the grill. Serve with Caprese Salad with Grilled Zucchini *(page 80).*

(continued)

Marinade

        6 ounces fat-free plain yogurt
        1/4 cup thinly sliced green onions
        2 tablespoons chopped fresh parsley (Italian,
            or flat-leaf, preferred)
        2 teaspoons grated lemon zest
        1 tablespoon fresh lemon juice
        1 medium garlic clove, minced

                    ■ ■ ■

        1 1-pound boneless round steak, all visible fat
            discarded
        1/4 cup fat-free sour cream
        1/4 teaspoon salt

In a large shallow glass dish, stir together the marinade ingredients. Pour 1/4 cup marinade into a small bowl. Add the beef to the remaining marinade, turning to coat. Cover and refrigerate the beef for 8 hours, turning occasionally.

Stir the sour cream into the marinade in the small bowl. Cover and refrigerate until ready to serve.

Preheat the grill on medium high.

Scrape the marinade off the beef, discarding the marinade. Sprinkle the salt over the beef.

Grill the beef for 6 to 8 minutes on each side, or to the desired doneness. Transfer to a cutting board and let stand for 3 to 5 minutes. Thinly slice the beef diagonally across the grain. Serve with the sauce.

PER SERVING

calories 158	**sodium** 237 mg
total fat 3.0 g	**carbohydrates** 4 g
saturated fat 1.0 g	fiber 0 g
trans fat 0.0 g	sugars 2 g
polyunsaturated fat 0.0 g	**protein** 28 g
monounsaturated fat 1.5 g	**DIETARY EXCHANGES**
cholesterol 61 mg	3 lean meat

SWISS STEAK
SERVES 4

Baking lean round steak makes it fork-tender. Try this classic dish with steamed green beans and fluffy low-fat mashed potatoes, such as Mashed Potatoes with Parmesan and Green Onions *(page 399).*

        Cooking spray
        1 1-pound boneless top round steak, about
            3/4 inch thick, all visible fat discarded,
            quartered
        1/4 teaspoon pepper
        1/8 teaspoon salt
        1 cup chopped onion
        1 medium carrot, chopped
        1 medium rib of celery, chopped
        1/4 small green bell pepper, chopped
        3 medium button mushrooms, chopped
        1 14.5-ounce can no-salt-added diced
            tomatoes, drained
        1/2 cup fat-free, low-sodium beef broth, such
            as on page 35
        1/2 teaspoon dried thyme, crumbled
        1/2 teaspoon Worcestershire sauce (lowest
            sodium available)

Preheat the oven to 350°F. Lightly spray a Dutch oven with cooking spray.

Cook the beef over medium-high heat for about 3 minutes on each side, or until well browned. Pour off any liquid.

Sprinkle the pepper and salt over both sides of the beef. Place the onion, carrot, celery, bell pepper, and mushrooms around the beef. Cook for 2 to 3 minutes, stirring frequently.

Stir in the remaining ingredients.

Bake, covered, for 45 to 50 minutes, or until the beef is tender.

PER SERVING

calories 187	**carbohydrates** 10 g
total fat 3.0 g	fiber 3 g
saturated fat 1.0 g	sugars 6 g
trans fat 0.0 g	**protein** 30 g
polyunsaturated fat 0.5 g	**DIETARY EXCHANGES**
monounsaturated fat 1.5 g	2 vegetable, 3 lean
cholesterol 54 mg	meat
sodium 248 mg	

POT ROAST–STYLE STEAK WITH TOMATOES

SERVES 4

Since this dish cooks quickly, the flavors of the meat and seasonings remain distinct. You can also stew the meat for a much longer time, melding the flavors to create a melt-in-your-mouth feast.

1 1/2 teaspoons olive oil
4 boneless sirloin steaks (about 4 ounces each), all visible fat discarded
2 medium garlic cloves, crushed or minced
2 medium Italian plum (Roma) tomatoes, chopped
1 teaspoon fresh lemon juice
1/4 teaspoon dried oregano, crumbled
1/8 teaspoon salt
Pepper to taste

In a large skillet, heat the oil over medium heat, swirling to coat the bottom. Cook the beef for 4 to 5 minutes on each side (for rare), or until the desired doneness. Transfer to a serving platter. Cover to keep warm.

Reduce the heat to low. Cook the garlic for 2 minutes, or until golden, stirring constantly. Watch carefully so it doesn't burn. Stir in the remaining ingredients. Increase the heat to medium. Cook for 5 minutes, or until the tomatoes are tender but still have some texture, stirring occasionally. Return the beef along with any accumulated juices to the skillet. Cook for 2 to 3 minutes to allow the flavors to combine, stirring gently.

Transfer the beef and sauce to the platter. Serve immediately.

Cook's Tip: Keep in mind that the beef will continue to cook slightly both when covered on the platter and when returned to the sauce. If you like your beef on the pink side, you might want to undercook it a bit to ensure desired doneness.

PER SERVING

calories 173	sodium 142 mg
total fat 6.0 g	carbohydrates 2 g
saturated fat 2.0 g	fiber 0 g
trans fat 0.0 g	sugars 1 g
polyunsaturated fat 0.5 g	protein 26 g
monounsaturated fat 3.5 g	**DIETARY EXCHANGES**
cholesterol 60 mg	3 lean meat

ROSEMARY-DIJON SIRLOIN

SERVES 6

Citrus needs at least several hours to tenderize the meat, so be sure to plan ahead for this recipe. Once the steak is done marinating, however, grilling it will go quickly. Serve with Grilled Pineapple (page 502) or Grilled Tomato-Peach Salad (page 82).

3/4 cup canola or corn oil
1/2 cup chopped onion
1/4 cup fresh lemon juice (about 1 large lemon)
3 tablespoons dry white wine (regular or nonalcoholic)
2 tablespoons finely chopped fresh rosemary
2 tablespoons finely chopped fresh sage
1 tablespoon Dijon mustard (lowest sodium available)
3 medium garlic cloves, minced
1/2 teaspoon salt
6 top sirloin steaks (about 4 ounces each), about 1 inch thick, all visible fat discarded
Cooking spray

In a large glass baking dish, whisk together all the ingredients except the beef. Add the beef, turning to coat. Cover and refrigerate for several hours or overnight, turning occasionally.

Lightly spray the grill rack with cooking spray. Preheat the grill on medium high.

Drain the beef, discarding the marinade.

Grill the beef for 5 to 7 minutes on each side, or until the desired doneness.

PER SERVING

calories 141	sodium 312 mg
total fat 3.5 g	carbohydrates 0 g
saturated fat 1.5 g	fiber 0 g
trans fat 0.0 g	sugars 0 g
polyunsaturated fat 0.5 g	protein 25 g
monounsaturated fat 1.5 g	**DIETARY EXCHANGES**
cholesterol 58 mg	3 lean meat

SIRLOIN STEAKS WITH CREAMY SPINACH

SERVES 4

Beef, baked potato, and creamed spinach are a classic steakhouse meal. Enjoy this healthier version at home. Try the spinach spooned over Twice-Baked Potatoes *(page 398).*

2 teaspoons no-salt-added steak grilling blend
1 1-pound boneless sirloin steak, all visible fat discarded
1 teaspoon canola or corn oil
Cooking spray
1 large onion, chopped
10 ounces frozen chopped spinach, thawed and squeezed dry
3/4 cup fat-free half-and-half
1 1/2 ounces light tub cream cheese, cut into small pieces
1 medium garlic clove, minced
1/4 teaspoon salt
1 tablespoon shredded or grated Parmesan cheese

Sprinkle the grilling blend over both sides of the beef.

In a large skillet, heat the oil over medium-high heat, swirling to coat the bottom. Cook the beef for 4 minutes on each side for medium-rare, or until the desired doneness. Transfer to a cutting board. Let stand for 5 minutes. Thinly slice the beef diagonally across the grain.

Meanwhile, lightly spray a medium skillet with cooking spray. Heat over medium heat. Cook the onion for 3 minutes, or until almost soft, stirring occasionally.

Stir in the spinach, half-and-half, cream cheese, and garlic until well blended. Reduce the heat and simmer, covered, for 5 minutes. Remove from the heat.

Stir in the salt. Sprinkle with the Parmesan. Serve with the beef.

PER SERVING

calories 239	carbohydrates 14 g
total fat 8.0 g	fiber 3 g
saturated fat 3.5 g	sugars 7 g
trans fat 0.0 g	**protein** 29 g
polyunsaturated fat 0.5 g	**DIETARY EXCHANGES**
monounsaturated fat 2.5 g	1/2 starch, 2 vegetable,
cholesterol 64 mg	3 lean meat
sodium 355 mg	

ZESTY HOT-OVEN SIRLOIN

SERVES 4

The marinade in this dish is transformed into an intense sauce that packs a palatable punch. A little sauce goes a long way! Serve with Pecan Broccoli *(page 376) and a whole grain. You'll need to marinate the sirloin for 8 hours, so get this prepped before work and dinner will be quick and easy when you get home.*

Marinade
2 tablespoons soy sauce (lowest sodium available)
2 tablespoons balsamic vinegar
2 tablespoons fresh lemon juice
1 tablespoon Worcestershire sauce (lowest sodium available)
2 teaspoons dried oregano, crumbled
2 medium garlic cloves, minced

■ ■ ■

1 1-pound boneless sirloin steak, about 1 inch thick, all visible fat discarded
Cooking spray
1/4 cup water
1 1/2 teaspoons light tub margarine
1/4 teaspoon pepper
2 tablespoons finely chopped fresh parsley

In a medium glass dish, whisk together the marinade ingredients. Add the beef, turning to coat. Cover and refrigerate for 8 hours, turning occasionally.

Preheat the oven to 500°F. Lightly spray a rimmed baking sheet with cooking spray.

Drain the beef, reserving the marinade. Transfer the beef to the baking sheet.

Roast the beef on the top oven rack for 12 to 14 minutes, or to the desired doneness. Cut into 4 pieces.

Meanwhile, in a small saucepan, bring the marinade and water to a boil over high heat. Reduce the heat and simmer for 3 minutes, or until reduced by two-thirds (to about 1/4 cup). Remove from the heat.

Add the margarine and pepper to the marinade mixture, stirring until the margarine has melted. Spoon over the beef. Sprinkle with the parsley.

Cook's Tip: To reduce smoke, be sure your oven is clean before roasting at a high temperature.

PER SERVING

calories 178	**carbohydrates** 5 g
total fat 5.0 g	fiber 0 g
saturated fat 2.0 g	sugars 4 g
trans fat 0.0 g	**protein** 26 g
polyunsaturated fat 0.5 g	**DIETARY EXCHANGES**
monounsaturated fat 2.5 g	1/2 other
cholesterol 60 mg	carbohydrate, 3 lean
sodium 295 mg	meat

ROSEMARY-SAGE STEAK

SERVES 4

Have a meat-and-potatoes dinner with this herb-enhanced steak and Rustic Potato Patties *(page 400), but add a side salad, such as* Dijon-Marinated Vegetable Medley *(page 82).*

Marinade
- 1/4 cup chopped onion
- 2 tablespoons fresh lemon juice
- 1 1/2 tablespoons dry white wine (regular or nonalcoholic)
- 1 tablespoon finely chopped fresh rosemary or 2 teaspoons dried rosemary, crushed
- 1 tablespoon finely chopped fresh sage or 2 teaspoons dried sage
- 1 1/2 teaspoons Dijon mustard (lowest sodium available)
- 2 medium garlic cloves, minced

- 1 teaspoon olive oil
- 1/4 teaspoon pepper
- 1/4 teaspoon salt

■ ■ ■

- 1 pound boneless top sirloin steak, all visible fat discarded

In a large baking dish, whisk together the marinade ingredients. Add the beef, turning to coat. Cover and refrigerate for 1 to 24 hours, turning occasionally.

Preheat the grill on medium high.

Drain the beef, discarding the marinade.

Grill for 8 to 12 minutes on each side, or until the desired doneness. Transfer the beef to a cutting board. Let stand for 3 minutes before thinly slicing diagonally across the grain.

Cook's Tip on Fresh Rosemary: For a real taste treat, save woody, more mature rosemary stems to use as skewers. Strip the leaves to use in recipes such as this one. With a sharp object—a wooden or thin metal skewer works well—poke a hole through the foods you'll use for your kebabs. Thread the rosemary stem through the hole and grill or broil those foods as usual.

PER SERVING

calories 127	**sodium** 227 mg
total fat 4.0 g	**carbohydrates** 0 g
saturated fat 1.5 g	fiber 0 g
trans fat 0.0 g	sugars 0 g
polyunsaturated fat 0.0 g	**protein** 21 g
monounsaturated fat 1.5 g	**DIETARY EXCHANGES**
cholesterol 56 mg	3 lean meat

GINGER-LIME SIRLOIN

SERVES 4

The same tasty combination serves as both marinade and sauce for the broiled steak in this Asian-inspired recipe. Serve with Edamame with Walnuts (page 387) and brown rice. This dish needs to be prepped early in the day—the sirloin needs 8 hours to marinate in the fridge.

Marinade
> 3 tablespoons soy sauce (lowest sodium available)
> 2 tablespoons plus 2 teaspoons sugar
> 2 tablespoons cider vinegar
> 1 tablespoon fresh lime juice
> 1 teaspoon grated peeled gingerroot
> 1 medium garlic clove, minced
> 1/2 teaspoon crushed red pepper flakes

■ ■ ■

> 1 1-pound boneless sirloin steak, about 1 inch thick, all visible fat discarded
> Cooking spray

In a small glass bowl, whisk together the marinade ingredients until the sugar is dissolved.

Pour half the marinade into a medium glass dish. Add the beef, turning to coat. Cover and refrigerate for 8 hours, turning occasionally. Cover and refrigerate the remaining marinade.

Preheat the broiler. Lightly spray a broiler pan and rack with cooking spray.

Drain the beef, discarding the marinade in the glass dish.

Broil the beef about 4 inches from the heat for 5 minutes. Turn over the beef. Broil for 8 minutes, or to the desired doneness. Transfer to a cutting board. Let stand for 5 minutes before cutting diagonally across the grain into thin slices. Transfer to plates.

Meanwhile, in a small saucepan, bring the reserved marinade to a boil over high heat. Boil for 1 to 2 minutes, or until reduced to about 2 tablespoons, stirring frequently. Spoon over the beef.

Cook's Tip: The beef is cooked longer on one side to allow it to blacken slightly.

PER SERVING

calories 176	**carbohydrates** 6 g
total fat 4.5 g	fiber 0 g
saturated fat 2.0 g	sugars 6 g
trans fat 0.0 g	**protein** 26 g
polyunsaturated fat 0.5 g	**DIETARY EXCHANGES**
monounsaturated fat 2.0 g	1/2 other
cholesterol 60 mg	carbohydrate, 3 lean
sodium 361 mg	meat

STEAK MARINATED IN BEER AND GREEN ONIONS

SERVES 8

Many Asian hosts serve beer rather than wine for special meals. It makes sense, then, that beer is also used in many Asian recipes, including this one.

Marinade
> 12 ounces light beer (regular or nonalcoholic)
> 4 medium green onions, minced
> 2 tablespoons light brown sugar
> 2 tablespoons dry sherry
> 1 tablespoon grated peeled gingerroot
> 1 tablespoon soy sauce (lowest sodium available)
> 2 medium garlic cloves, minced
> 1 teaspoon crushed red pepper flakes
> 1 teaspoon canola or corn oil
> Dash of red hot-pepper sauce

■ ■ ■

> 2 pounds boneless top sirloin steak, all visible fat discarded

In a large glass dish, stir together the marinade ingredients until the brown sugar is dissolved. Add the beef, turning to coat. Cover and refrigerate for 1 to 24 hours, turning occasionally.

Preheat the grill on medium high.

Drain the beef, discarding the marinade.

Grill the beef for 8 to 12 minutes on each side, or to the desired doneness.

Cook's Tip on Marinating: The purpose of a marinade is for food to absorb the flavors of the marinade and also to tenderize meat. In some recipes, you'll see a range of marinating times; use the amount of time within the range that best suits your schedule. Whether you marinate the meat for the minimum or maximum time, it'll still be delicious.

PER SERVING

calories 135	sodium 95 mg
total fat 4.5 g	carbohydrates 0 g
saturated fat 1.5 g	fiber 0 g
trans fat 0.0 g	sugars 0 g
polyunsaturated fat 0.0 g	protein 22 g
monounsaturated fat 1.5 g	DIETARY EXCHANGES
cholesterol 59 mg	3 lean meat

SIRLOIN WITH CREAMY HORSERADISH SAUCE

SERVES 4

Season, sear, and serve—that's all it takes to put this family favorite on the table. The pungent sauce also makes a great topping for baked potatoes or dip for fresh vegetables.

> 1 medium garlic clove, halved crosswise
> 1 1-pound boneless sirloin steak, all visible fat discarded
> 1/2 teaspoon chili powder
> 1/2 teaspoon onion powder
> 1 teaspoon olive oil
> 1/8 teaspoon salt

Sauce
> 1/2 cup fat-free sour cream
> 2 teaspoons bottled white horseradish, drained
> 2 teaspoons olive oil
> 1 teaspoon Dijon mustard (coarse-ground preferred) (lowest sodium available)
> 1/2 medium garlic clove, minced
> 1/2 teaspoon Worcestershire sauce (lowest sodium available)
> 1/8 teaspoon salt

1/4 cup water
Pepper, to taste (coarsely ground preferred)

Rub the halved garlic over both sides of the beef.

Sprinkle the chili powder and onion powder over both sides of the beef. Using your fingertips, gently press the mixture so it adheres to the beef.

In a large nonstick skillet, heat 1 teaspoon oil over medium-high heat, swirling to coat the bottom. Cook the beef for 5 minutes. Turn over the beef. Reduce the heat to medium and cook for 5 minutes, or to the desired doneness. Transfer the beef to a cutting board, leaving any browned bits in the skillet.

Sprinkle the beef with 1/8 teaspoon salt. Let stand for 3 minutes before slicing diagonally across the grain.

Meanwhile, in a small bowl, whisk together the sauce ingredients. Set aside.

Add the water to the skillet, scraping to dislodge any browned bits. Increase the heat to medium high and bring to a boil. Boil for 1 to 1 1/2 minutes, or until the liquid is reduced by half (to about 2 tablespoons).

Transfer the beef to plates. Top with the pan juices and pepper. Serve the sauce on the side.

PER SERVING

calories 201	carbohydrates 6 g
total fat 8.0 g	fiber 0 g
saturated fat 2.0 g	sugars 3 g
trans fat 0.0 g	protein 24 g
polyunsaturated fat 0.5 g	DIETARY EXCHANGES
monounsaturated fat 4.0 g	1/2 other
cholesterol 64 mg	carbohydrate, 3 lean
sodium 262 mg	meat

■ ■ ■

SMOTHERED STEAK WITH SANGRÍA SAUCE

SERVES 4

Different and easy, this dish turns simple steak into something special, with a sweet and herb-filled sauce that brings out the beefy flavor of the sirloin. Serve it over brown rice or whole-grain pasta.

Sauce

1 cup sangría (white preferred)
1 medium tomato, chopped
1 small green bell pepper, chopped
1/4 cup golden raisins
1/4 cup dried apricots, coarsely chopped
1 large dried bay leaf
1 teaspoon dried basil, crumbled
1/2 teaspoon dried thyme, crumbled
1/4 teaspoon pepper, or to taste

■ ■ ■

Cooking spray
4 thin boneless sirloin steaks (about 4 ounces each), all visible fat discarded

In a medium bowl, stir together the sauce ingredients.

Lightly spray a large skillet with cooking spray. Cook the beef over medium-high heat for 2 to 3 minutes on each side.

Pour the sauce into the skillet. Reduce the heat and simmer, covered, for 30 to 40 minutes, or until the beef is tender. Discard the bay leaf.

Time-Saver: Use cube steaks instead of sirloin steaks and reduce the simmering time to 20 to 25 minutes.

PER SERVING

calories 235	carbohydrates 21 g
total fat 4.5 g	fiber 2 g
saturated fat 1.5 g	sugars 14 g
trans fat 0.0 g	**protein** 23 g
polyunsaturated fat 0.0 g	**DIETARY EXCHANGES**
monounsaturated fat 2.0 g	1 fruit, 1/2 other
cholesterol 59 mg	carbohydrate, 3 lean
sodium 54 mg	meat

PEPPER-COATED STEAK

SERVES 4

In France, where it's called boeuf au poivre, *this steak is typically served with skillet-fried potatoes. For a more healthful option, choose* Potatoes with Leeks and Fresh Herbs *(page 398) and* Hot and Spicy Arugula and Romaine Salad *(page 71).*

2 teaspoons coarsely cracked black pepper
4 beef tenderloin steaks (about 4 ounces each), all visible fat discarded
Cooking spray
1/4 cup brandy or 100% apple juice
1 5-ounce can fat-free evaporated milk

Sprinkle the pepper over both sides of the beef. Using your fingertips, gently press the pepper so it adheres to the beef.

Lightly spray a large skillet with cooking spray. Heat over medium-high heat. Cook the beef for 5 minutes. Turn over the beef. Cook for 3 to 5 minutes, or until the desired doneness.

Transfer the beef to a plate. Cover to keep warm. Remove the skillet from the heat. Let cool for 1 minute.

Reduce the heat to low. Return the skillet to the heat. Gradually pour the brandy into the skillet. Cook for 1 minute, scraping to dislodge any browned bits.

Stir in the milk. Increase the heat to high and bring to a boil. Reduce the heat and simmer for 2 to 3 minutes, or until the sauce has thickened, stirring frequently.

Just before serving, pour the sauce over the beef.

Cook's Tip on Peppercorns: If you don't have a pepper mill, you can buy pepper that's already coarsely ground or use a mortar and pestle to crack whole peppercorns.

calories 188	sodium 84 mg
total fat 6.0 g	carbohydrates 5 g
saturated fat 2.0 g	fiber 0 g
trans fat 0.0 g	sugars 4 g
polyunsaturated fat 0.0 g	protein 24 g
monounsaturated fat 2.5 g	DIETARY EXCHANGES
cholesterol 61 mg	1/2 fat-free milk, 3 lean meat

PHILADELPHIA-STYLE CHEESE STEAK WRAP

SERVES 6

What do you get when you cross seasoned slices of tender beef, sautéed onions, and melted Cheddar cheese with a tortilla? Try this recipe based on the Philly classic (but much healthier) and you'll find out it's utterly delicious! Set aside time for the steak to marinate.

Marinade
  1 tablespoon balsamic vinegar or red wine vinegar
  2 teaspoons Worcestershire sauce (lowest sodium available)
  1 teaspoon sugar
  1 teaspoon dried oregano, crumbled
  1 teaspoon olive oil
  2 medium garlic cloves, minced
  1/4 teaspoon pepper

■ ■ ■

  12 ounces eye-of-round roast, all visible fat discarded, cut diagonally across the grain into 1/8-inch slices
  1 small onion, thinly sliced
  1 medium green bell pepper, thinly sliced
  6 6-inch whole-wheat tortillas (lowest sodium available)
  2 1-ounce slices fat-free sharp Cheddar cheese, each cut into thirds

In a medium glass dish, stir together the marinade ingredients until the sugar is dissolved. Add the beef, turning to coat. Cover and refrigerate for 10 minutes to 8 hours, turning occasionally.

Preheat the oven to 350°F.

Heat a nonstick griddle or large nonstick skillet over medium-high heat. Drain the beef, discarding the marinade. Cook for 3 to 5 minutes, or until no longer pink, stirring occasionally. Transfer to a bowl. Cover to keep warm.

Wipe the griddle with paper towels. Cook the onion and bell pepper for about 5 minutes, or until soft, stirring occasionally.

Place the tortillas in a large shallow baking pan. Spoon the beef down the center of each tortilla. Top with the onion mixture and Cheddar. Cover with aluminum foil. Heat in the oven for 4 to 5 minutes. Roll the tortillas jelly-roll style over the filling, securing with wooden toothpicks if desired.

MICROWAVE METHOD
Place the tortillas on a microwaveable plate. Add the filling as directed. Microwave on 100 percent power (high) for 30 seconds. Roll up the tortillas as directed.

PER SERVING

calories 173	sodium 334 mg
total fat 2.5 g	carbohydrates 18 g
saturated fat 0.5 g	fiber 3 g
trans fat 0.0 g	sugars 4 g
polyunsaturated fat 0.5 g	protein 19 g
monounsaturated fat 1.5 g	DIETARY EXCHANGES
cholesterol 29 mg	1 starch, 2 lean meat

SAVORY BEEF STEW

SERVES 12

This classic stew is everything you'd expect and more thanks to mushrooms and bell pepper. Serve with Whole-Wheat French Bread (page 443) to soak up the stew's delicious juices.

  Cooking spray
  2 1/2 pounds eye-of-round roast, all visible fat discarded, cut into bite-size pieces
  1 teaspoon olive oil
  1 large onion, finely chopped

(continued)

5 1/2 cups fat-free, low-sodium beef broth and 2 cups fat-free, low-sodium beef broth, such as on page 35, divided use
1 teaspoon dried thyme, crumbled, and 1 teaspoon dried thyme, crumbled, divided use
1 teaspoon dried marjoram, crumbled
1 medium dried bay leaf
1 pound red potatoes, cut into chunks
2 large carrots, sliced
8 ounces button mushrooms, quartered
1 medium red bell pepper, diced
4 medium green onions, thinly sliced
1/4 cup plus 2 tablespoons cornstarch
1/4 cup no-salt-added tomato paste
1 teaspoon dried Italian seasoning, crumbled
3/4 teaspoon pepper
1/4 teaspoon salt

PER SERVING

calories 194
total fat 3.0 g
    saturated fat 1.0 g
    trans fat 0.0 g
    polyunsaturated fat 0.5 g
    monounsaturated fat 1.5 g
cholesterol 45 mg
sodium 146 mg

carbohydrates 16 g
    fiber 2 g
    sugars 4 g
protein 25 g
DIETARY EXCHANGES
    1/2 starch, 1 vegetable,
    3 lean meat

Lightly spray a stockpot with cooking spray. Heat over medium-high heat. Cook the beef for 2 to 3 minutes on each side, or until browned. Transfer to a large plate.

In the same pot, heat the oil, swirling to coat the bottom. Cook the onion for 3 minutes, or until soft, stirring frequently.

Stir in the beef and any accumulated juices, 5 1/2 cups broth, 1 teaspoon thyme, the marjoram, and bay leaf. Increase the heat to high and bring to a boil. Reduce the heat and simmer, covered, for 1 hour 30 minutes, or until the beef is tender.

Stir in the potatoes, carrots, and mushrooms. Simmer, covered, for 30 minutes.

Stir in the bell pepper and green onions.

In a medium bowl, whisk together the cornstarch, tomato paste, Italian seasoning, pepper, salt, and the remaining 2 cups broth and 1 teaspoon thyme until the cornstarch is dissolved. Pour into the stew. Increase the heat to high and bring to a boil, stirring constantly. Reduce the heat to low. Cook for 5 minutes, or until the sauce has thickened, stirring constantly. Discard the bay leaf.

BEEF BOURGUIGNON

SERVES 8

Like other stews, Beef Bourguignon tastes best when made ahead so the flavors have time to blend, therefore you should plan about 3 hours to get this dish completed. Serve it over brown rice or whole-grain noodles.

Cooking spray
1 tablespoon olive oil
5 medium onions, sliced
2 pounds boneless top sirloin roast, all visible fat discarded, cut into 1-inch cubes
1 1/2 tablespoons all-purpose flour
1/2 teaspoon pepper, or to taste
1/4 teaspoon dried marjoram, crumbled
1/4 teaspoon dried thyme, crumbled
1 cup dry red wine (regular or nonalcoholic) (plus more as needed)
1/2 cup fat-free, low-sodium beef broth, such as on page 35 (plus more as needed)
8 ounces sliced button mushrooms
1/2 teaspoon salt

Lightly spray a Dutch oven with cooking spray. Pour in the oil, swirling to coat the bottom. Heat over medium-high heat. Cook the onions for 5 minutes, or until soft, stirring frequently. Transfer to a large plate.

In the same pot, cook the beef for 10 to 12 minutes, or until browned on all sides.

Sprinkle the beef with the flour, pepper, marjoram, and thyme. Stir well. Stir in the wine and broth. Reduce the heat and simmer, covered, for 1 hour 30 minutes to 2 hours, or until the beef is almost tender. Add more wine and broth (2 parts wine to 1 part broth) as needed to keep the beef barely covered.

Return the onions to the pot. Stir in the mushrooms and salt. Cook, covered, for 30 minutes, stirring occasionally and adding more wine and broth if necessary. The sauce should be thick and dark brown.

Cook's Tip on Marjoram: Available fresh as well as dried, marjoram tastes much like oregano, but is a bit milder. It's especially good with meats and vegetables.

Time-Saver: Reduce the simmering time of the beef in the wine and broth mixture to 30 minutes if you're in a hurry. The flavor won't be as full, but it will still be good.

PER SERVING

calories 230	sodium 220 mg
total fat 6.5 g	carbohydrates 11 g
saturated fat 2.0 g	fiber 2 g
trans fat 0.0 g	sugars 6 g
polyunsaturated fat 0.5 g	protein 27 g
monounsaturated fat 3.5 g	DIETARY EXCHANGES
cholesterol 60 mg	2 vegetable, 3 lean meat

BEEF AND MUSHROOM CASSEROLE

SERVES 4

This is a perfect dish for a day you're planning to be at home because it needs a few hours to bake for maximum flavor. Once you spend a few minutes watching the meat brown under the broiler, you can let the oven do the rest.

Cooking spray

1 pound beef chuck roast, cut into cubes, all visible fat discarded

1 1/4 cups fat-free, low-sodium beef broth, such as on page 35

1/2 cup dry red wine (regular or nonalcoholic)

1/4 cup flour

3 tablespoons no-salt-added tomato paste

1/4 teaspoon garlic powder

1/4 teaspoon dried rosemary, crushed

8 ounces sliced mushrooms

1 cup chopped onion

Preheat the broiler. Lightly spray the broiler pan with cooking spray.

Broil the beef about 6 inches from the heat for 10 to 15 minutes, turning to brown on all sides. Remove from the oven. Preheat the oven to 300°F.

In a 1 1/2-quart casserole, stir together the broth, wine, flour, tomato paste, garlic powder, and rosemary. Stir in the beef, mushrooms, and onion. Bake, covered, for 2 1/2 to 3 hours, or until the beef is tender.

PER SERVING

calories 215	carbohydrates 15 g
total fat 4.5 g	fiber 2 g
saturated fat 1.5 g	sugars 4 g
trans fat 0.0 g	protein 26 g
polyunsaturated fat 0.5 g	DIETARY EXCHANGES
monounsaturated fat 2.0 g	1/2 starch, 1 vegetable,
cholesterol 44 mg	3 lean meat
sodium 57 mg	

JAMAICAN BEEF AND OKRA STEW

SERVES 4

Traditionally, Jamaican stews are cooked in a "Dutch Pot" (Dutch oven) to develop flavors and tenderize tougher meats. Nutmeg, sweet potatoes, thyme, and allspice are all distinctive Jamaican ingredients in this stew, but there's one notable omission: the Scotch Bonnet pepper. Because it's one of the world's hottest peppers, it was purposely omitted, but add one, or even two, if you're feeling adventurous

1 tablespoon canola or corn oil, 1 tablespoon canola or corn oil, and 1 teaspoon canola or corn oil, divided use

1 pound boneless top round steak, all visible fat discarded, cut into 3/4-inch cubes

1 large onion, chopped

1 large sweet potato (yam), peeled and chopped into 1-inch cubes

4 medium garlic cloves, minced

1 teaspoon dried thyme, crumbled

1/2 teaspoon ground allspice

(continued)

1/2 teaspoon ground cinnamon

1/4 teaspoon ground nutmeg (freshly grated preferred)

1/4 teaspoon pepper (freshly ground preferred)

1/8 teaspoon cayenne (optional)

3 cups fat-free, low sodium beef broth, such as on page 35

1 14.5-ounce can diced fire-roasted tomatoes (lowest sodium available), or 1 14.5 ounce can diced no-salt-added tomatoes, undrained

1 tablespoon no-salt-added tomato paste

1 tablespoon Jamaican-style hot sauce (with tamarind preferred) (optional)

2 cups small fresh okra pods, thinly sliced and stem ends discarded, or 2 cups frozen petite okra (about half a 15-ounce package)

1/4 cup chopped fresh cilantro (optional)

2 medium lemons, cut into 8 wedges

In a Dutch oven, heat 1 tablespoon oil over medium-high heat, swirling to coat the bottom. Cook half the beef for 4 to 5 minutes, or until browned on all sides, stirring occasionally, Transfer to a medium bowl. Repeat with 1 tablespoon oil and the remaining beef.

In the same Dutch oven, still over medium-high heat, heat the remaining 1 teaspoon oil, swirling to coat the bottom. Cook the onion for 3 minutes, or until soft, stirring frequently. Stir in the sweet potato, garlic, thyme, allspice, cinnamon, nutmeg, pepper, and cayenne. Cook for 3 to 4 minutes, or until fragrant, stirring constantly.

Stir in the broth, tomatoes with liquid, tomato paste, and hot sauce. Increase the heat to high and bring just to a boil. Boil for about 4 to 5 minutes, stirring frequently.

Return the beef and any accumulated juices to the pot. Reduce the heat and simmer, partially covered, for 1 1/2 hours, or until the beef is just tender. Increase the heat to medium-high and bring just to a boil. Stir in the okra. Immediately reduce the heat and simmer for 10 to 12 minutes, or until the okra is tender, but not mushy. Stir in

the cilantro. Just before serving, garnish with the lemon wedges.

PER SERVING

calories 360	carbohydrates 33 g
total fat 11.0 g	fiber 7 g
saturated fat 2.0 g	sugars 11 g
trans fat 0.0 g	protein 32 g
polyunsaturated fat 2.5 g	DIETARY EXCHANGES
monounsaturated fat 6.5 g	1 starch, 3 vegetable,
cholesterol 58 mg	3 lean meat
sodium 377 mg	

BOWL OF RED

SERVES 4

Texans love to eat chili almost as much as they love to argue over which version is the best. This one has cubed beef and, as is the custom, skips the beans.

Cooking spray

Chili

1 pound boneless top round steak, all visible fat discarded, cut into 1/2-inch cubes

1 cup water

1 cup dark or regular beer (regular or nonalcoholic)

1/2 medium onion, chopped

1/2 8-ounce can no-salt-added tomato sauce

3 ancho chiles, seeds and ribs discarded, chopped (see Cook's Tip on Handling Hot Chiles, page 24)

1 medium fresh jalapeño or serrano pepper, seeds and ribs discarded, chopped (see Cook's Tip on Handling Hot Chiles, page 24)

1 tablespoon chili powder

1 tablespoon ground cumin

2 medium garlic cloves, minced

1/2 teaspoon ground coriander

1/2 teaspoon dried oregano, crumbled

1/4 teaspoon salt

1/8 teaspoon pepper

1/8 teaspoon cayenne, or to taste

■ ■ ■

1/4 cup fat-free sour cream (optional)

Fresh cilantro, chopped (optional)

Lightly spray a Dutch oven with cooking spray. Heat over medium-high heat. Cook the beef for 3 to 5 minutes, or until browned on the outside and no longer pink in the center, stirring occasionally.

Stir in the remaining chili ingredients. Bring to a boil. Reduce the heat and simmer, covered, for 1 hour, stirring occasionally. Simmer, uncovered, for 15 to 30 minutes, or until the desired consistency, stirring occasionally.

Ladle the chili into bowls. Top each serving with the sour cream. Sprinkle with the cilantro.

PER SERVING

calories 225	carbohydrates 15 g
total fat 4.5 g	fiber 5 g
saturated fat 1.5 g	sugars 3 g
trans fat 0.0 g	protein 29 g
polyunsaturated fat 1.0 g	**DIETARY EXCHANGES**
monounsaturated fat 1.5 g	3 vegetable, 3 lean
cholesterol 58 mg	meat
sodium 263 mg	

GINGER-BEEF KOREAN BARBECUE (BULGOGI)

SERVES 4

This sweet-and-spicy dish, called bulgogi *in Korean, is traditionally cooked on a tabletop grill. Serve it with* Asian Coleslaw *(page 84) and* Baked Sweet Potato Chips *(page 407). Sweet potatoes are very popular in Korean cuisine.*

Marinade

- 1 medium green onion, finely chopped
- 1 1/2 tablespoons dry sherry (optional)
- 1 tablespoon oyster sauce (lowest sodium available)
- 1 1/2 teaspoons hoisin sauce (lowest sodium available)
- 1 1/2 teaspoons toasted sesame oil
- 2 medium garlic cloves, minced
- 1/2 teaspoon grated peeled gingerroot
- 1/2 teaspoon no-salt-added liquid smoke
- 1/4 teaspoon sugar
- Pepper to taste
- Dash of red hot-pepper sauce, or to taste

■ ■ ■

1 pound boneless sirloin steak, all visible fat discarded, cut across the grain into strips about 1/8 inch wide

In a large glass dish, stir together the marinade ingredients until the sugar is dissolved. Add the beef, turning to coat. Cover and refrigerate for about 1 hour, turning several times. Drain the beef, discarding the marinade.

Heat a large skillet over medium-high heat until hot. Quickly arrange the beef in a single layer. Cook for about 1 minute on each side, or until the desired doneness. Turn over the beef only once or it will become dry and tough.

PER SERVING

calories 157	sodium 245 mg
total fat 4.5 g	carbohydrates 1 g
saturated fat 2.0 g	fiber 0 g
trans fat 0.0 g	sugars 1 g
polyunsaturated fat 0.5 g	protein 26 g
monounsaturated fat 2.0 g	**DIETARY EXCHANGES**
cholesterol 60 mg	3 lean meat

PORTOBELLO MUSHROOMS AND SIRLOIN STRIPS OVER SPINACH PASTA

SERVES 4

Beef and robust portobello mushrooms, both marinated in red wine and seasonings, make a hearty combination in this one-dish meal. If you prefer, you can serve the beef and mushrooms over steamed spinach instead of pasta.

Marinade

- 1/3 cup burgundy or other dry red wine (regular or nonalcoholic)
- 3 tablespoons soy sauce (lowest sodium available)
- 3 tablespoons Worcestershire sauce (lowest sodium available)
- 6 medium garlic cloves, minced
- 2 teaspoons olive oil
- 1 1/2 teaspoons dried oregano, crumbled

(continued)

12 ounces boneless top sirloin steak, all visible fat discarded, cut into thin strips
12 ounces portobello mushrooms, sliced
8 ounces dried spinach fettuccine

In a medium glass dish, stir together the marinade ingredients. Add the beef and mushrooms, turning to coat. Cover and refrigerate for 30 minutes, turning frequently.

Meanwhile, prepare the pasta using the package directions, omitting the salt. Drain well in a colander.

Drain the beef mixture, discarding the marinade. In a large nonstick skillet, cook half the beef over medium-high heat for 4 minutes, or until no longer pink, stirring frequently. Transfer to a plate. Repeat with the remaining beef mixture, leaving it in the skillet. Return the other half of the beef mixture and any accumulated juices to the skillet. Increase the heat to high and bring to a boil. Cook for 5 minutes, stirring frequently. Remove from the heat.

Transfer the pasta to plates. Spoon the beef mixture over the pasta.

PER SERVING

calories 349	sodium 416 mg
total fat 5.0 g	**carbohydrates** 48 g
saturated fat 1.5 g	fiber 3 g
trans fat 0.0 g	sugars 7 g
polyunsaturated fat 1.0 g	**protein** 30 g
monounsaturated fat 2.0 g	**DIETARY EXCHANGES**
cholesterol 45 mg	3 starch, 3 lean meat

ASIAN BEEF STIR-FRY

SERVES 4

Cauliflower isn't commonly found in Chinese dishes, but the mild vegetable is ideal for absorbing the pungent flavors of the sauce. Red bell peppers and snow peas add a crisp texture contrast. Try this stir-fry over a bed of brown rice or quinoa.

2 tablespoons dry sherry
2 tablespoons water
1 tablespoon cornstarch
1 tablespoon soy sauce (lowest sodium available)
1 1/2 teaspoons grated peeled gingerroot
1/8 teaspoon red hot-pepper sauce
8 ounces flank steak, all visible fat and silver skin discarded, cut against the grain into strips 2 to 3 inches long and 1/2 to 1 inch wide
2 teaspoons canola or corn oil
1/4 cup chopped onion
1 to 2 medium garlic cloves, minced
2 cups small cauliflower florets (about 1/2 medium head)
1 cup fat-free, low-sodium beef broth, such as on page 35
1 small or medium red bell pepper, diced
3 ounces snow peas, trimmed

In a small bowl, whisk together the sherry, water, cornstarch, soy sauce, gingerroot, and hot-pepper sauce until the cornstarch is dissolved. Set aside.

In a wok or large nonstick skillet, cook half the beef over medium-high heat for 3 to 4 minutes, or just until browned, stirring constantly. Transfer to a bowl. Repeat with the remaining beef.

In the same wok or skillet, still over medium-high heat, heat the oil, swirling to coat the bottom. Cook the onion and garlic for 3 minutes, or until the onion is soft, stirring frequently.

Stir in the cauliflower and broth. Cook for 2 minutes.

Stir in the bell pepper and snow peas. Cook for 1 minute.

Stir the sherry mixture and beef into the cauliflower mixture. Cook for 2 to 3 minutes, or until the sauce has thickened.

PER SERVING

calories 155	**carbohydrates** 10 g
total fat 6.0 g	fiber 2 g
saturated fat 1.5 g	sugars 4 g
trans fat 0.0 g	**protein** 14 g
polyunsaturated fat 1.0 g	**DIETARY EXCHANGES**
monounsaturated fat 3.0 g	2 vegetable, 1 1/2 lean
cholesterol 32 mg	meat
sodium 148 mg	

CLASSIC CHINESE BEEF STIR-FRY

SERVES 4

Put away the Chinese takeout menu and instead serve this lean beef and crisp vegetables in a soy-hoisin sauce over brown rice. Finish your meal with Sunny Mango Sorbet (page 506).

1 cup uncooked instant brown rice
1/2 cup fat-free, low-sodium beef broth, such as on page 35
1 tablespoon soy sauce (lowest sodium available)
2 teaspoons cornstarch
1 teaspoon toasted sesame oil
1 pound boneless sirloin steak, all visible fat discarded, cut into thin strips
1/2 cup matchstick-size carrot strips
1 cup frozen shelled edamame, thawed
4 ounces broccoli florets, cut into bite-size pieces
1/4 cup canned sliced water chestnuts, drained
2 medium green onions, cut into 1-inch pieces
2 tablespoons sesame seeds, dry-roasted

Prepare the rice using the package directions, omitting the salt and margarine.

Meanwhile, in a small bowl, whisk together the broth, soy sauce, cornstarch, and oil until the cornstarch is dissolved. Set aside.

In a wok or large nonstick skillet, cook the beef over medium-high heat for 5 minutes, or until the desired doneness, stirring constantly. Transfer to a bowl.

In the same wok or skillet, cook the carrots for 3 to 4 minutes, or until tender-crisp, stirring constantly.

Stir in the edamame, broccoli, water chestnuts, and green onions. Cook for 2 to 3 minutes, or until the edamame and broccoli are tender-crisp, stirring constantly.

Stir in the broth mixture and beef. Cook for 2 to 3 minutes, or until the sauce has thickened and the mixture is heated through, stirring con-

stantly. Spoon the beef and vegetables over the rice. Garnish with the sesame seeds.

PER SERVING

calories 360	carbohydrates 29 g
total fat 11.0 g	fiber 6 g
saturated fat 2.5 g	sugars 4 g
trans fat 0.0 g	protein 35 g
polyunsaturated fat 3.0 g	DIETARY EXCHANGES
monounsaturated fat 5.0 g	1 1/2 starch,
cholesterol 60 mg	1 vegetable, 4 lean
sodium 202 mg	meat

SOUTHWESTERN BEEF STIR-FRY

SERVES 4

Try this dish with some classic Latin American ingredients—chayote and tomatillos (Mexican green tomatoes) for an authentic-tasting meal.

1 cup uncooked instant brown rice
1 pound boneless sirloin steak, all visible fat discarded, cut into thin strips
1 medium chayote, peeled, sliced, and pitted, or 1 medium yellow summer squash, peeled and sliced
1 medium zucchini, thinly sliced
5 medium tomatillos (about 4 ounces total), papery husks discarded, rinsed, and quartered
1 14.5-ounce can no-salt-added diced tomatoes, undrained
2 tablespoons canned green chiles, drained
1/2 teaspoon ground cumin
1/4 teaspoon salt

Prepare the rice using the package directions, omitting the salt and margarine.

Meanwhile, in a wok or large nonstick skillet, cook the beef over medium-high heat for 4 to 5 minutes, or until the desired doneness, stirring constantly. Transfer to a bowl.

In the same wok or skillet, cook the chayote, zucchini, and tomatillos for 3 to 4 minutes, or until the chayote and zucchini are tender-crisp, stirring constantly.

(continued)

Stir in the tomatoes with liquid, chiles, cumin, and salt. Cook for 3 to 4 minutes, or until the chayote and zucchini are tender, stirring constantly.

Stir in the beef. Cook for 2 minutes, or until heated through, stirring constantly. Spoon over the rice.

PER SERVING

calories 284	carbohydrates 28 g
total fat 6.0 g	fiber 5 g
saturated fat 2.0 g	sugars 6 g
trans fat 0.0 g	protein 30 g
polyunsaturated fat 1.0 g	DIETARY EXCHANGES
monounsaturated fat 2.5 g	1 starch, 2 vegetable,
cholesterol 60 mg	3 lean meat
sodium 293 mg	

MEDITERRANEAN BEEF AND VEGETABLE STIR-FRY

SERVES 4

Stir-fries aren't just for Asian cuisine. Enjoy this Mediterranean-style stir-fry on a bed of Lemon-Basil Rice *(page 420).*

> 2 teaspoons canola or corn oil
> 1 pound boneless sirloin steak, all visible fat discarded, cut into thin strips
> 2 medium shallots, coarsely chopped
> 1 small eggplant (about 1 pound), cut into 1/2-inch cubes
> 2 tablespoons fat-free, low-sodium chicken broth, such as on page 36
> 1 14.5-ounce can artichoke hearts, drained and coarsely chopped
> 1 small yellow summer squash, cut into thin slices
> 1 14.5-ounce can no-salt-added diced tomatoes, undrained
> 1/4 cup coarsely chopped fresh basil
> 2 tablespoons chopped kalamata olives
> 1/4 teaspoon salt
> 1/4 teaspoon pepper

In a wok or large nonstick skillet, heat the oil over medium-high heat, swirling to coat the bottom. Cook the beef for 4 to 5 minutes, or to the de-sired doneness, stirring constantly. Transfer to a bowl. Set aside.

In the same wok or skillet, cook the shallots for 1 minute, or until tender-crisp, stirring constantly.

Stir in the eggplant and broth. Cook for 4 to 5 minutes, or until the eggplant is tender, stirring constantly.

Stir in the artichoke hearts and squash. Cook for 2 to 3 minutes, or until the squash is tender-crisp, stirring constantly.

Stir in the tomatoes with liquid, basil, olives, salt, and pepper. Cook for 2 to 3 minutes, or until the mixture is almost heated through, stirring constantly.

Stir in the beef. Cook for 1 to 2 minutes, or until heated through, stirring constantly.

Cook's Tip: For easier slicing, first put the raw beef in the freezer for about 30 minutes.

PER SERVING

calories 263	carbohydrates 19 g
total fat 8.0 g	fiber 6 g
saturated fat 2.0 g	sugars 9 g
trans fat 0.0 g	protein 30 g
polyunsaturated fat 1.0 g	DIETARY EXCHANGES
monounsaturated fat 4.5 g	4 vegetable, 3 lean
cholesterol 60 mg	meat
sodium 492 mg	

CARIBBEAN KEBABS

SERVES 4

This recipe makes a complete island dinner, with meat, vegetables, fruit, and rice. You'll need to set aside some time for the beef to soak in the citrus-sweet marinade. For a finishing touch, serve Watermelon-Cilantro Sorbet (page 504).

> 1 20-ounce can pineapple chunks in their own juice, drained, 1/4 cup juice reserved
> 1 teaspoon grated lemon zest
> 2 tablespoons fresh lemon juice
> 1 teaspoon light molasses
> 1/8 teaspoon pepper
> 1 pound boneless sirloin steak, all visible fat discarded, cut into 16 1-inch cubes

1 medium mango, cut into 8 cubes, or
    1 medium star fruit (carambola), cut
    crosswise into 8 slices, seeds discarded
2/3 cup uncooked instant brown rice
Cooking spray
1 medium zucchini, cut into 8 slices
12 pearl onions, thawed if frozen
1 medium red bell pepper, cut into 12 1-inch
    squares
1 tablespoon plus 1 teaspoon shredded
    unsweetened coconut, toasted

Set the pineapple chunks aside. Pour the reserved pineapple juice into a shallow glass bowl or casserole dish. Stir the lemon zest, lemon juice, molasses, and pepper into the pineapple juice. Add the beef cubes, turning to coat. Cover and refrigerate for 2 to 12 hours, stirring occasionally. Drain the beef, discarding the marinade.

Soak four 10-inch wooden skewers for at least 10 minutes in cold water to keep them from charring (these will be for skewering the beef), or use metal skewers. On four unsoaked 10-inch wooden or metal skewers, thread the pineapple chunks and mango cubes so they're evenly distributed among the skewers. Cover and refrigerate.

Prepare the rice using the package directions, omitting the salt and margarine. Set aside.

Meanwhile, preheat the broiler. Lightly spray a broiler pan with cooking spray. For each kebab, thread each skewer with 4 beef cubes, 2 zucchini slices, 3 onions, and 3 bell pepper squares. Transfer the beef skewers to the broiler pan.

Broil 4 to 6 inches from the heat for 3 to 4 minutes on each side, or until the desired doneness. You can also grill these skewers over medium-high heat for 3 to 4 minutes on each side, or until the desired doneness.

Spoon the rice down the center of each plate. Place a beef skewer on one side of the plate and a chilled fruit skewer on the other. Sprinkle the coconut over the rice.

Cook's Tip on Toasting Coconut: To toast coconut, preheat the oven to 350°F. Spread the coconut on a small rimmed baking sheet. Bake for about 10 minutes, or until beginning to brown, stirring occasionally. Watch carefully so it doesn't burn.

PER SERVING

calories 361	carbohydrates 47 g
total fat 7.0 g	fiber 5 g
saturated fat 3.0 g	sugars 31 g
trans fat 0.0 g	protein 29 g
polyunsaturated fat 0.5 g	DIETARY EXCHANGES
monounsaturated fat 2.5 g	2 fruit, 1 starch,
cholesterol 60 mg	1 vegetable, 3 lean
sodium 79 mg	meat

STEAK AND VEGETABLE KEBABS
SERVES 4

The beef marinates for several hours so it can absorb the hearty flavors. For a refreshing dessert, prepare Strawberry-Raspberry Ice *(page 503); it'll have plenty of time to freeze during the marinating time. Serve the kebabs over* Brown Rice Pilaf with Summer Squash *(page 404).*

Marinade
    1 small onion, chopped
    1/2 cup dry red wine (regular or nonalcoholic)
    2 tablespoons red wine vinegar
    1 tablespoon brown sugar
    4 medium garlic cloves, minced
    1 teaspoon paprika
    1/2 teaspoon pepper

■ ■ ■

    1 pound sirloin tip steak, all visible fat
        discarded, cut into 16 cubes
Cooking spray
    1 large red onion, cut into 16 wedges
    1 small red bell pepper, cut into 16 squares
    16 cherry tomatoes
    1 small yellow bell pepper, cut into 16 squares
    1/4 teaspoon salt

In a large glass dish, stir together the marinade ingredients until the sugar is dissolved. Add the beef, turning to coat. Cover and refrigerate for 8 hours, turning occasionally. Drain the beef, discarding the marinade.

(continued)

Soak eight 12-inch wooden skewers for at least 10 minutes in cold water to keep them from charring, or use metal skewers.

Lightly spray the grill rack with cooking spray. Preheat the grill on medium high.

For each kebab, thread each skewer with 4 beef cubes, 4 onion wedges, 4 red bell pepper squares, 4 cherry tomatoes, and 4 yellow bell pepper squares. Sprinkle the salt over the kebabs.

Grill the kebabs for 12 to 15 minutes, or until the desired doneness, turning frequently.

PER SERVING

calories 173	carbohydrates 8 g
total fat 3.0 g	fiber 2 g
saturated fat 1.0 g	sugars 5 g
trans fat 0.0 g	**protein** 26 g
polyunsaturated fat 0.5 g	**DIETARY EXCHANGES**
monounsaturated fat 1.5 g	2 vegetable, 3 lean
cholesterol 58 mg	meat
sodium 221 mg	

Stir in the onion and garlic. Cook for 3 minutes, or until the onion is soft, stirring frequently.

Stir in the broth, wine, and soy sauce. Bring to a boil. Reduce the heat and simmer, covered, for 1 hour 30 minutes, or until the beef is tender. Transfer the beef to a platter.

Put the cornstarch in a small bowl. Add the water, whisking to dissolve. Slowly pour into the skillet, stirring constantly. Increase the heat to medium high. Cook for 2 to 3 minutes, or until the sauce has thickened, stirring constantly. Serve with the beef. Sprinkle with the parsley.

PER SERVING

calories 162	**sodium** 124 mg
total fat 3.0 g	**carbohydrates** 4 g
saturated fat 1.0 g	fiber 1 g
trans fat 0.0 g	sugars 2 g
polyunsaturated fat 0.5 g	**protein** 26 g
monounsaturated fat 1.5 g	**DIETARY EXCHANGES**
cholesterol 58 mg	3 lean meat

BRAISED SIRLOIN TIPS

SERVES 8

Beef cooks in a wine and broth bath, which becomes the base for a sauce. Sweet Lemon Snow Peas *(page 402)* and Scalloped Potatoes *(page 399) are tasty accompaniments.*

1/4 teaspoon pepper
2 pounds sirloin tip, all visible fat discarded, cut into 1-inch cubes
1 small to medium onion, finely chopped
2 medium garlic cloves, minced
1 1/4 cups fat-free, low-sodium beef broth, such as on page 35
1/3 cup dry red wine (regular or nonalcoholic)
1 tablespoon soy sauce (lowest sodium available)
2 tablespoons cornstarch
1/4 cup cold water
1/4 cup chopped fresh parsley

Sprinkle the pepper over the beef.

In a large, heavy nonstick skillet, cook the beef over medium-high heat for 8 to 10 minutes, or until well browned on all sides, stirring frequently.

NIGERIAN BEEF-SPINACH STEW

SERVES 8

This recipe is a take on a Nigerian stew, which is tomato-based and traditionally combines onion and red hot peppers with meat, fish, or a combination of both, with seasonings. Serve with yams or plantains for an authentic side dish.

1 28-ounce can no-salt-added fire-roasted diced tomatoes, undrained
3 medium onions, quartered, and quarters halved
2 pounds boneless top sirloin, all visible fat discarded, cut into cubes
1 cup fat-free, low-sodium beef broth, such as on page 35
1/2 teaspoon curry powder
1/2 teaspoon crushed red pepper flakes
1/4 teaspoon salt
1/4 teaspoon pepper
Pinch of thyme
1 1/3 cups uncooked instant brown rice
2 teaspoons cornstarch
1 tablespoon cold water

10 ounces spinach, leaves torn into small
    pieces

In a food processor or blender, process the tomatoes with liquid and onions until smooth. Set aside.

In a Dutch oven, cook the beef cubes over medium-high heat for 5 minutes, or until browned, stirring occasionally. Stir in the tomato mixture, broth, curry powder, red pepper flakes, salt, pepper, and thyme. Reduce the heat and simmer, covered, for 1 hour, or until the beef is tender.

Meanwhile, prepare the rice using the package directions, omitting the salt and margarine. Set aside.

Put the cornstarch in a small bowl. Add the water, stirring to dissolve. Stir into the stew. Cook for 1 to 2 minutes, or until slightly thickened, stirring occasionally.

Stir in the spinach. Return to a simmer. Simmer, covered, for 5 minutes, or until the spinach is just tender.

Spoon the stew over the rice.

PER SERVING

calories 259	**carbohydrates** 23 g
total fat 5.0 g	fiber 3 g
saturated fat 2.0 g	sugars 7 g
trans fat 0.0 g	**protein** 29 g
polyunsaturated fat 0.5 g	**DIETARY EXCHANGES**
monounsaturated fat 2.5 g	1 starch, 2 vegetable,
cholesterol 60 mg	3 lean meat
sodium 189 mg	

BEEF AND BROCCOLI

SERVES 4; 1 CUP PER SERVING

Savory lean beef is teamed with tender-crisp broccoli and served on nutty brown rice in this popular one-dish stir-fry. Use the wok or skillet to cook Spiced Skillet Apples (page 503) or Spiced Skillet Bananas (page 503) for dessert.

3/4 cup uncooked brown rice (jasmine
    preferred)

1 tablespoon cornstarch and 2 teaspoons
    cornstarch, divided use
1 tablespoon water
2 medium garlic cloves, minced
1 teaspoon grated peeled gingerroot
1 pound boneless sirloin steak, all visible fat
    discarded, cut across the grain into thin
    strips
1/2 cup fat-free, low-sodium beef broth, such
    as on page 35
1 tablespoon soy sauce (lowest sodium
    available)
1 tablespoon hoisin sauce (lowest sodium
    available)
2 teaspoons toasted sesame oil
1 teaspoon canola or corn oil
2 cups broccoli florets
4 medium green onions, cut into 1-inch pieces

Prepare the rice using the package directions, omitting the salt and margarine. Set aside.

In a medium shallow dish, whisk together 1 tablespoon cornstarch, the water, garlic, and gingerroot until the cornstarch is dissolved. Add the beef, turning to coat. Cover and refrigerate for 15 minutes to 8 hours, turning occasionally.

In a small bowl, whisk together the broth, soy sauce, hoisin sauce, sesame oil, and the remaining 2 teaspoons cornstarch until the cornstarch is dissolved. Set aside.

In a wok or large skillet, heat the canola oil over medium-high heat, swirling to coat the bottom. Cook the broccoli and green onions for 2 to 3 minutes, or until tender-crisp, stirring constantly. Transfer to a bowl. Set aside.

In the same wok or skillet, still over medium-high heat, cook the beef with the marinade for 4 to 5 minutes, or until the beef is almost cooked through, stirring frequently. Stir in the broth mixture. Bring to a simmer over medium-high heat. Stir in the broccoli mixture. Cook for 1 to 2 minutes, or until the sauce is thickened, stirring constantly.

(continued)

Spoon the rice onto plates. Spoon the beef mixture over the rice.

PER SERVING

calories 337	carbohydrates 37 g
total fat 7.5 g	fiber 4 g
saturated fat 1.5 g	sugars 3 g
trans fat 0.0 g	protein 29 g
polyunsaturated fat 1.5 g	DIETARY EXCHANGES
monounsaturated fat 3.0 g	2 starch, 1 vegetable,
cholesterol 58 mg	3 lean meat
sodium 209 mg	

STIR-FRIED STROGANOFF

SERVES 4

Lighten up classic beef stroganoff by stir-frying the components and then topping them with a dollop of fat-free sour cream instead of drenching them in a heavy sauce laden with saturated fat. Dilled Green Beans *(page 388) or* Minted Peas *(page 397) complete the meal.*

6 ounces dried egg noodles

1/2 teaspoon pepper, or to taste

1 pound boneless sirloin steak, all visible fat discarded, cut into 1-inch cubes

1 teaspoon canola or corn oil

1 pound brown (cremini) mushrooms, sliced

1 medium red onion, thinly sliced

1/4 cup chopped fresh parsley

1/4 cup fat-free sour cream

1 tablespoon plus 1 teaspoon chopped fresh dillweed

Prepare the noodles using the package directions, omitting the salt. Drain well in a colander. Set aside.

Meanwhile, sprinkle the pepper over the beef.

In a wok or large skillet, heat the oil over medium-high heat, swirling to coat the bottom. Cook the beef for 4 to 6 minutes, or until the desired doneness, stirring frequently. Transfer to a bowl.

In the same wok, cook the mushrooms and onion for 8 minutes, or until the mushrooms are browned and their liquid has evaporated, stir-

ring frequently. Return the beef to the wok. Stir in the parsley.

Transfer the noodles to plates. Spoon the beef mixture over the noodles. Top with the sour cream. Sprinkle with the dillweed.

Cook's Tip: If you prefer, you can prepare this dish with ground beef instead. In a wok or large skillet, cook 1 pound extra-lean ground beef over medium-high heat for 4 to 5 minutes, or until no longer pink, stirring frequently to turn and break up the beef. Proceed as directed.

PER SERVING

calories 346	carbohydrates 41 g
total fat 6.0 g	fiber 4 g
saturated fat 1.5 g	sugars 7 g
trans fat 0.0 g	protein 31 g
polyunsaturated fat 0.5 g	DIETARY EXCHANGES
monounsaturated fat 2.5 g	2 1/2 starch,
cholesterol 58 mg	1 vegetable, 3 lean
sodium 87 mg	meat

ASIAN BEEF LETTUCE WRAPS WITH VIETNAMESE DIPPING SAUCE

SERVES 4

Seasoned ground beef and crunchy vegetables are tucked into soft lettuce leaves, creating a meal wrapped up in deliciousness. You might want to make extra sauce and serve with Sweet-and-Sour Spring Rolls *(page 23).*

Sauce

2 tablespoons plain rice vinegar

2 tablespoons fresh lime juice

2 tablespoons water

1 tablespoon chopped fresh cilantro

2 teaspoons fish sauce (lowest sodium available)

1/2 teaspoon finely chopped serrano pepper, seeds and ribs discarded

1/2 teaspoon honey

∎ ∎ ∎

12 ounces extra-lean ground beef

1 tablespoon dark molasses

1 tablespoon water

2 teaspoons white wine vinegar

1 teaspoon soy sauce (lowest sodium available)

1/2 teaspoon toasted sesame oil

1/4 cup sliced green onions

1/4 cup chopped fresh cilantro

12 large Boston or butter lettuce leaves

1/2 cup matchstick-size carrot strips

1/2 cup chopped zucchini

1/2 cup chopped red bell pepper

In a small glass bowl, whisk together all the sauce ingredients.

In a large nonstick skillet, cook the beef over medium-high heat for 5 to 7 minutes, or until browned on the outside and no longer pink in the center, stirring frequently to turn and break up the beef.

Meanwhile, in a small cup, whisk together the molasses, the remaining 1 tablespoon water, the white wine vinegar, soy sauce, and oil. Stir the mixture into the beef. Bring to a boil. Stir in the green onions and cilantro.

Place the lettuce leaves on a serving platter. Spoon the beef mixture onto the leaves. Top with the carrots, zucchini, and bell pepper. Serve the wraps with the dipping sauce.

PER SERVING

calories 156	carbohydrates 10 g
total fat 5.0 g	fiber 2 g
saturated fat 2.0 g	sugars 7 g
trans fat 0.0 g	**protein** 17 g
polyunsaturated fat 0.5 g	**DIETARY EXCHANGES**
monounsaturated fat 2.0 g	1 vegetable, 1/2 other
cholesterol 47 mg	carbohydrate,
sodium 283 mg	2 1/2 lean meat

SALISBURY STEAKS WITH MUSHROOM SAUCE

SERVES 4

Salisbury steak is actually not a steak at all, but a ground beef patty that's been flavored with onion and seasonings before being cooked and is often served with a gravy.

1/2 to 3/4 ounce dried mushrooms, any variety or combination

1 cup warm water

Patties

12 ounces extra-lean ground beef

1/2 medium onion, grated or minced

1 1/2 tablespoons all-purpose flour

1 1/2 teaspoons Worcestershire sauce (lowest sodium available)

1/2 teaspoon salt-free all-purpose seasoning blend

1/4 teaspoon dried thyme, crumbled

1/4 teaspoon salt

1/8 teaspoon pepper

2 tablespoons fat-free milk

■ ■ ■

1/2 cup fat-free, low-sodium beef broth, such as on page 35

1/2 cup dry red wine (regular or nonalcoholic)

1/2 medium carrot, grated

2 to 3 tablespoons chopped fresh parsley

In a small bowl, soak the mushrooms in the water for 20 to 30 minutes.

Meanwhile, in a large bowl, using your hands or a spoon, combine all the patty ingredients except the milk. Pour in the milk and combine. Shape into 4 patties.

Using a small sieve, scoop up the mushrooms, reserving the liquid. Rinse the mushrooms, then chop. Strain the liquid through a damp coffee filter, paper towel, or cheesecloth into a 2-cup liquid measuring cup to remove any dirt. Add enough broth to the strained liquid to make 1 cup.

Stir the wine into the broth mixture.

In a heavy nonstick skillet, cook the patties over medium-high heat for 5 to 6 minutes on each side, or until they are browned and register 160°F on an instant-read thermometer. Reduce the heat to medium if the patties are browning too quickly. Drain on paper towels. Discard any liquid left in the skillet.

(continued)

In the same skillet, bring the mushrooms, broth mixture, and carrot to a boil over high heat. Boil for 4 to 5 minutes, or until the liquid is reduced by one-third (to about one-half cup).

Add the patties. Reduce the heat and simmer for 10 minutes. Serve sprinkled with the parsley.

PER SERVING

calories 173	carbohydrates 9 g
total fat 4.5 g	fiber 2 g
saturated fat 2.0 g	sugars 3 g
trans fat 0.0 g	protein 19 g
polyunsaturated fat 0.5 g	DIETARY EXCHANGES
monounsaturated fat 2.0 g	1/2 other
cholesterol 47 mg	carbohydrate,
sodium 214 mg	2 1/2 lean meat

GRILLED HAMBURGERS WITH VEGETABLES AND FETA

SERVES 6

The vegetables in this meal are built right into the hamburger. Serve with Garden Vegetable Salad in Garlicky Vinaigrette *(page 85) or* Spiralized Cucumbers with Yogurt-Dill Dressing *(page 79).*

Cooking spray

Hamburgers
- 1 pound extra-lean ground beef
- 2 cups shredded broccoli (packaged broccoli slaw)
- 1 medium portobello mushroom, stem discarded, finely chopped
- 1/4 cup low-fat feta cheese
- 1/2 teaspoon salt-free lemon pepper

■ ■ ■

- 6 whole-grain hamburger buns (lowest sodium available), split

Lightly spray the grill rack with cooking spray. Preheat the grill on medium high.

In a medium bowl, using your hands or a spoon, combine the hamburger ingredients. Shape into 6 patties.

Grill the patties for 4 to 5 minutes on each side, or until they register 160°F on an instant-read

thermometer. Grill the buns with the split side down for 30 seconds, or until lightly browned. Serve the patties on the buns.

Cook's Tip: Rather than using traditional burger condiments, try Mustard and Green Onion Sauce (page 433), Fresh Herb Chimichurri Sauce (page 437), or Cranberry Chutney (page 424).

PER SERVING

calories 234	carbohydrates 24 g
total fat 6.5 g	fiber 4 g
saturated fat 2.5 g	sugars 4 g
trans fat 0.0 g	protein 22 g
polyunsaturated fat 1.5 g	DIETARY EXCHANGES
monounsaturated fat 2.0 g	1 1/2 starch, 2 lean
cholesterol 44 mg	meat
sodium 371 mg	

BEEF, KALE, AND MUSHROOM LASAGNA

SERVES 6

This healthier version of the traditional Italian dish is just as satisfying and includes two vegetables as an added benefit. Enjoy with Focaccia *(page 443) or* Parmesan-Herb Breadsticks *(page 451) and* Marinated Tomato Salad *(page 81).*

- Cooking spray
- 8 dried whole-grain lasagna noodles
- 10 ounces frozen chopped kale or spinach, thawed and squeezed dry
- 8 ounces fat-free cottage cheese
- 1 pound extra-lean ground beef
- 1/4 cup minced onion
- 3 cups no-salt-added tomato sauce
- 4 ounces button mushrooms, chopped
- 1 teaspoon dried basil, crumbled
- 1 teaspoon chopped fresh parsley
- 1/2 teaspoon dried oregano, crumbled
- 1 medium garlic clove, minced
- Pepper to taste (freshly ground preferred)
- 4 ounces low-fat mozzarella cheese, shredded (about 1 cup)

Preheat the oven to 375°F. Lightly spray a 13 x 9 x 2-inch baking dish with cooking spray.

Prepare the noodles using the package directions, omitting the salt. Drain well in a colander. Carefully arrange the noodles in a single layer on a large piece of wax paper and pat dry with paper towels.

In a medium bowl, stir together the kale and cottage cheese.

In a medium nonstick skillet, cook the beef and onion over medium-high heat for 8 to 10 minutes, or until the beef is browned on the outside and no longer pink in the center, stirring occasionally to turn and break up the beef.

Stir in the tomato sauce, mushrooms, basil, parsley, oregano, garlic, and pepper.

In the baking dish, layer as follows: half the noodles, half the kale mixture, half the beef mixture, and half the mozzarella. Repeat the layers.

Bake for 15 to 20 minutes, or until hot and bubbly.

PER SERVING

calories 338	carbohydrates 38 g
total fat 7.0 g	fiber 8 g
saturated fat 2.5 g	sugars 8 g
trans fat 0.0 g	**protein** 34 g
polyunsaturated fat 1.0 g	**DIETARY EXCHANGES**
monounsaturated fat 2.5 g	1 1/2 starch,
cholesterol 50 mg	2 vegetable, 3 1/2 lean
sodium 348 mg	meat

BEEF PITAS

SERVES 4

This beef patty is even better than your standard hamburger thanks to a simple veggie medley and a special sauce, the latter of which adds a creamy tartness to complement the sweetness from the roasted peppers and tomato.

1 large red bell pepper
1/2 cup fat-free plain Greek yogurt
1 tablespoon plus 1 teaspoon Dijon mustard
    (lowest sodium available)
1/4 teaspoon pepper and 3/4 teaspoon
    pepper, divided use
1 pound extra-lean ground beef
1 tablespoon finely chopped parsley

1 1/2 teaspoons minced garlic
3/4 teaspoon dried oregano, crumbled
1 tablespoon canola or corn oil
3/4 cup chopped onion
1 large tomato, seeded and diced
4 large lettuce leaves
2 6-inch whole-grain pita pockets (lowest
    sodium available), halved

Preheat the broiler.

Put the bell pepper on a baking sheet lined with aluminum foil. Broil 4 to 5 inches from the heat for 7 to 9 minutes, or until the skin is blackened and blistered, turning frequently. Remove the baking sheet from the oven and wrap the foil around the bell pepper. Let stand for 15 to 20 minutes, or until cool enough to handle. Gently peel off the skin under cool running water. Dice the bell pepper.

Meanwhile, in a small bowl, whisk together the yogurt, mustard, and 1/4 teaspoon pepper. Set aside.

In a medium bowl, using your hands or a spoon, combine the beef, parsley, garlic, oregano, and the remaining 3/4 teaspoon pepper. Shape into 4 patties. Put the patties on the broiler pan. Broil 4 to 5 inches from the heat for 3 to 4 minutes on each side, or until they register 160°F on an instant-read thermometer. Set aside.

In a small skillet, heat the oil over medium-high heat, swirling to coat the bottom. Cook the onion for about 3 minutes, or until soft, stirring frequently. Stir in the tomato and roasted bell pepper. Cook for 1 to 2 minutes, or until heated through.

In each pita half, place a lettuce leaf, a beef patty, and 1/4 of the onion mixture. Top with the yogurt mixture.

PER SERVING

calories 312	carbohydrates 27 g
total fat 10.5 g	fiber 5 g
saturated fat 3.0 g	sugars 6 g
trans fat 0.0 g	**protein** 29 g
polyunsaturated fat 1.5 g	**DIETARY EXCHANGES**
monounsaturated fat 4.5 g	1 starch, 2 vegetable,
cholesterol 64 mg	3 1/2 lean meat
sodium 332 mg	

GRILLED MEAT LOAF

SERVES 6

For a twist on burgers on the "barbie," try grilling a meat loaf! Bread soaked in milk is the secret to keeping this meat loaf from drying out as it cooks. Serve with Chile-Lime Grilled Corn *(page 386) or* Caprese Salad with Grilled Zucchini *(page 80).*

1/2 cup fat-free milk
2 slices whole-wheat bread (lowest sodium available), torn into small pieces
Cooking spray
1 pound extra-lean ground beef
2 large egg whites, lightly beaten using a fork
1/2 cup chopped onion
2 teaspoons chopped celery
1 medium tomato, peeled and chopped, or 3/4 cup no-salt-added canned diced tomatoes, drained
2 tablespoons no-salt-added ketchup
1 tablespoon fresh lemon juice
1/8 teaspoon pepper (freshly ground preferred)
1/8 teaspoon dry mustard
1/8 teaspoon dried sage
1/8 teaspoon garlic powder

In a shallow bowl, pour the milk over the bread. Let stand for 5 minutes. Drain well in a colander. Discard any remaining milk.

Lightly spray the grill rack with cooking spray. Preheat the grill on medium high.

In a large bowl, using your hands or a spoon, combine the remaining ingredients. Shape the meat mixture into an oval loaf, about 1 1/2 inches thick.

Grill the meat loaf, covered, for 10 minutes. Using two spatulas, carefully turn over the meat loaf.

Grill, covered, for 10 minutes, or until the meat loaf registers 160°F on an instant-read thermometer.

Remove from the grill. Let stand for 5 to 10 minutes before slicing.

TEX-MEX LASAGNA

SERVES 8

When you're planning a party for a hungry crowd or it's your turn to feed the soccer team, you'll appreciate this easy-to-assemble meal. While the lasagna is baking, serve Edamame Guacamole *(page 15) or* Lots of Layers Dip *(page 15).*

Cooking spray
1 pound extra-lean ground beef
1 14.5-ounce can no-salt-added tomatoes, undrained
1/2 cup salsa (lowest sodium available), such as Salsa Cruda (page 437)
1/4 teaspoon salt
1 cup fat-free ricotta cheese
1 teaspoon chili powder
1 teaspoon ground cumin
16 6-inch corn tortillas, halved
1 cup shredded low-fat Monterey Jack cheese
1 15.5-ounce can no-salt-added pinto beans, rinsed and well drained
1 cup frozen whole-kernel corn, thawed and patted dry
1/4 cup sliced black olives, drained

Preheat the oven to 375°F. Lightly spray a 13 x 9 x 2-inch baking pan with cooking spray.

In a large nonstick skillet, cook the beef over medium-high heat for 8 to 10 minutes, or until browned on the outside and no longer pink in the center, stirring occasionally to turn and break up the beef.

Stir in the tomatoes with liquid, salsa, and salt. Reduce the heat to medium low and cook for 5 minutes, or until heated through, stirring occasionally. Turn off the heat, leaving the skillet on the stove.

In a small bowl, stir together the ricotta, chili powder, and cumin.

Arrange 8 tortilla halves in the baking dish. (The tortillas may overlap slightly, and they won't completely cover the bottom.) Spread half the beef mixture over the tortillas. Sprinkle half the Monterey Jack over the beef mixture. Arrange 8 tortilla halves over the Monterey Jack. Spoon 1-tablespoon mounds of the ricotta mixture over the tortillas. Using a spatula, flatten each mound slightly. Top the ricotta mixture with the beans and corn. Add another layer of 8 tortilla halves. Spread the remaining beef mixture over the tortillas. Sprinkle the remaining Monterey Jack over the beef mixture. Top with a layer of the remaining 8 tortilla halves. Sprinkle the olives over the tortillas.

Bake, covered, for 30 minutes, or until heated through. Transfer the pan to a cooling rack. Let cool for 5 minutes before cutting.

PER SERVING

calories 284	sodium 432 mg
total fat 7.0 g	carbohydrates 31 g
saturated fat 3.0 g	fiber 6 g
trans fat 0.0 g	sugars 4 g
polyunsaturated fat 1.0 g	protein 26 g
monounsaturated fat 2.0 g	DIETARY EXCHANGES
cholesterol 41 mg	2 starch, 3 lean meat

GREEK MEAT LOAF

SERVES 4

This meat loaf has all the makings of a Mediterranean meal—olives, feta, mint, and lemon. While the meat loaf is baking, prepare Yellow Split Pea Dip *(page 12)* or Greek Egg and Lemon Soup (Avgolemono) *(page 35).*

  Cooking spray
  8 ounces extra-lean ground beef
  8 ounces ground lamb or extra-lean ground pork
  1/2 cup plain dry bread crumbs (lowest sodium available)

  1 8-ounce can no-salt-added tomato sauce and 1 8-ounce can no-salt-added tomato sauce, divided use
  1 small onion, chopped
  1 large egg
  1 tablespoon chopped fresh mint
  2 teaspoons dried oregano (Greek preferred), crumbled
  2 teaspoons salt-free lemon pepper
  2 tablespoons crumbled low-fat feta cheese
  1 tablespoon chopped kalamata olives

Preheat the oven to 375°F. Lightly spray a 9 x 5 x 3-inch loaf pan or a baking sheet with cooking spray.

In a large bowl, using your hands or a spoon, combine the beef, lamb, bread crumbs, 8 ounces tomato sauce, onion, egg, mint, oregano, and lemon pepper. Shape into an 8 x 4-inch loaf. Transfer to the pan. Spread the remaining tomato sauce on top. Sprinkle with the feta and olives.

Bake for 45 minutes, or until the meat loaf registers 160°F on an instant-read thermometer. Turn out the loaf onto a cutting board. Let stand for 5 to 10 minutes before slicing.

PER SERVING

calories 226	sodium 266 mg
total fat 7.5 g	carbohydrates 15 g
saturated fat 3.0 g	fiber 3 g
trans fat 0.5 g	sugars 3 g
polyunsaturated fat 1.0 g	protein 25 g
monounsaturated fat 3.0 g	DIETARY EXCHANGES
cholesterol 55 mg	1 starch, 3 lean meat

BEEF AND EGGPLANT CASSEROLE

SERVES 4

If you like eggplant Parmesan, but don't want all the cheese, then try this lighter twist on an Italian favorite. Yogurt—rather than cheese—brings this dish its creaminess. Serve with a spinach salad with Zesty Tomato Dressing *(page 105)* or Chunky Cucumber and Garlic Dressing *(page 106).*

(continued)

Cooking spray
1 pound extra-lean ground beef
1 1/2 medium onions, chopped
1 1/2 tablespoons dried dillweed, crumbled
2 medium garlic cloves, chopped
Pepper to taste (freshly ground preferred)
1 medium eggplant or 3 medium yellow
     summer squash, or a combination, cut
     into vertical slices about 1/8 inch thick
2 cups fat-free plain yogurt

Preheat the oven to 350°F. Lightly spray an 8-inch square casserole dish with cooking spray.

In a medium skillet, cook the beef over medium-high heat for 8 to 10 minutes, or until browned on the outside and no longer pink in the center, stirring occasionally to turn and break up the beef. Stir in the onions, dillweed, garlic, and pepper.

Arrange some of the eggplant slices in a single layer in the casserole dish. Spoon a layer of the beef mixture over the eggplant. Repeat these layers. Top with a layer of eggplant. Spoon the yogurt over all.

Bake for 45 minutes to 1 hour, or until bubbly.

PER SERVING

calories 274	sodium 187 mg
total fat 6.0 g	**carbohydrates** 23 g
saturated fat 2.5 g	fiber 5 g
trans fat 0.0 g	sugars 17 g
polyunsaturated fat 0.5 g	**protein** 33 g
monounsaturated fat 2.5 g	**DIETARY EXCHANGES**
cholesterol 65 mg	2 vegetable, 1 fat-free milk, 3 lean meat

1 small onion, chopped
1/2 medium green bell pepper, chopped
1 pound extra-lean ground beef
2 tablespoons no-salt-added ketchup
1 tablespoon yellow mustard (lowest sodium
     available)
Pepper to taste (freshly ground preferred)
1 28-ounce can no-salt-added diced
     tomatoes, drained
1 tablespoon Worcestershire sauce (lowest
     sodium available)

Prepare the rice using the package directions, omitting the salt and margarine. Set aside.

In a large skillet, heat the oil over medium-high heat, swirling to coat the bottom. Cook the onion and bell pepper for 3 minutes, or until the onion is soft and the bell pepper is tender-crisp, stirring frequently.

Stir in the beef, ketchup, mustard, and pepper. Cook for 3 minutes, or until the beef is browned on the outside, stirring occasionally to turn and break up the beef.

Stir in the tomatoes, Worcestershire sauce, and rice until well blended. Reduce the heat and simmer, covered, for 15 minutes.

PER SERVING

calories 210	**carbohydrates** 26 g
total fat 5.0 g	fiber 3 g
saturated fat 1.5 g	sugars 6 g
trans fat 0.0 g	**protein** 15 g
polyunsaturated fat 1.0 g	**DIETARY EXCHANGES**
monounsaturated fat 2.0 g	1 1/2 starch,
cholesterol 31 mg	1 vegetable, 2 lean
sodium 89 mg	meat

SPANISH RICE

SERVES 8

Also known as Mexican rice, this main-dish version includes ground beef. Serve with Spinach-Chayote Salad with Orange Vinaigrette *(page 68) or* Tex-Mex Cucumber Salad *(page 78).*

1 cup uncooked brown rice
2 teaspoons canola or corn oil

CABBAGE ROLLS WITH SAUERKRAUT

SERVES 6

Sauerkraut adds a bit of a bite to this dish, complementing the mildness of the cabbage and rice. Serve with Rye Bread *(page 445) and* Parmesan Parsnip Puree with Leeks and Carrots *(page 396).*

1 cup uncooked quick-cooking rice

1 large head green cabbage, cored, and
    8 large outer leaves removed

1 pound extra-lean ground beef

1 large egg

2 tablespoons chopped onion

12 ounces sauerkraut (lowest sodium
    available), rinsed and drained

1 8-ounce can no-salt-added tomato sauce

Preheat the oven to 350°F.

Prepare the rice using the package directions, omitting the salt and margarine. Set aside.

In a large saucepan, bring 2 cups water to a boil over high heat.

Meanwhile, cut the heavy stem from the base of each of the 8 cabbage leaves. Put the leaves in the pan. Cover the pan. Turn off the heat and let the leaves steam while preparing the stuffing.

In a large mixing bowl, stir together the beef, egg, onion, and rice.

Carefully remove the cabbage leaves from the pan. Transfer to a flat work surface. Spoon 1 heaping tablespoon of beef mixture in the center of each cabbage leaf. Fold the edges of the leaves toward the center so they slightly overlap. Trying to keep the cabbage rolls fairly tight, roll up from the stem end. Secure with wooden toothpicks.

Place the sauerkraut in a 2-quart casserole dish, arranging it in a single layer. Place each roll with the seam side down on the bed of sauerkraut. Pour the tomato sauce over the rolls. Bake, covered, for 1 hour, or until the rolls are firm.

PER SERVING

calories 200	carbohydrates 20 g
total fat 4.5 g	fiber 3 g
saturated fat 2.0 g	sugars 3 g
trans fat 0.0 g	**protein** 20 g
polyunsaturated fat 0.5 g	**DIETARY EXCHANGES**
monounsaturated fat 2.0 g	1 starch, 1 vegetable,
cholesterol 73 mg	2 1/2 lean meat
sodium 423 mg	

UKRAINIAN STUFFED CABBAGE ROLLS

SERVES 4

These cabbage rolls are a favorite in Ukrainian-heritage households and are served at large gatherings or celebrations. Rice is the most common form of stuffing, but buckwheat is also a favorite. Enjoy with Beet Salad with Red Onions *(page 74).*

Cooking spray

1/2 cup uncooked brown rice

1 large head green cabbage, cored, and
    12 large outer leaves removed

6 ounces extra-lean ground beef

6 ounces extra-lean ground pork

1 cup chopped onion

1 tablespoon chopped fresh dillweed and
    1 tablespoon chopped fresh dillweed,
    divided use

1/4 teaspoon salt

1/4 teaspoon pepper

1 teaspoon canola or corn oil

1 medium garlic clove, minced

1 cup no-salt-added tomato juice

2 teaspoons fresh lemon juice

Preheat the oven to 350°F. Lightly spray a 1 1/2-quart casserole dish with cooking spray.

Prepare the rice using the package directions, omitting the salt and margarine.

In a large saucepan, bring 2 cups water to a boil over high heat.

Cut the heavy stem from the base of each of the 12 cabbage leaves. Put the leaves in the pan. Cover the pan. Turn off the heat and let the leaves steam while preparing the stuffing.

In a large nonstick skillet, cook the beef and pork over medium heat for 3 to 4 minutes, or until partially cooked, stirring frequently to turn and break up the beef and pork. Stir in the onion. Cook for 5 to 6 minutes, or until the beef is no longer pink in the center and the onion is very soft. Stir in the rice, 1 tablespoon dillweed, the salt, and pepper.

(continued)

Spoon 1 to 2 tablespoons of the beef mixture in the center of each cabbage leaf. Fold the edges of the leaves toward the center so they slightly overlap. Trying to keep the cabbage rolls fairly tight, roll up from the stem end. Secure with wooden toothpicks. Transfer the rolls with the seam side down to the casserole dish.

In a small saucepan, heat the oil over medium heat, swirling to coat the bottom. Cook the garlic for 30 seconds to 1 minute, or until fragrant, stirring constantly. Stir in the tomato juice, the remaining 1 tablespoon dillweed, and the lemon juice. Increase the heat to medium high and bring just to a boil. Pour over the cabbage rolls. (The liquid should come halfway up the rolls. If more liquid is needed, add water.) Bake, covered, for 1 hour, or until the rolls are fork-tender.

Cook's Tip: The cabbage rolls and sauce can be made up to 8 hours in advance of serving. Store the rolls and sauce separately. For peak freshness and flavor, though, make the sauce right before the cabbage rolls are baked. Use the remaining cabbage leaves to make Sweet-and-Sour Spring Rolls (page 23), Five-Minute Soup (page 47), or Confetti Coleslaw (page 84).

PER SERVING

calories 250	carbohydrates 20 g
total fat 10.5 g	fiber 3 g
saturated fat 3.5 g	sugars 8 g
trans fat 0.0 g	protein 21 g
polyunsaturated fat 1.5 g	DIETARY EXCHANGES
monounsaturated fat 4.5 g	1/2 starch,
cholesterol 51 mg	2 vegetable, 2 1/2 lean
sodium 233 mg	meat

ONE-SKILLET GREEK BEEF AND SPINACH

SERVES 4

This one-skillet meal couldn't be easier, so it's perfect for rushed midweek evenings. Even the pasta cooks in the same pan, making cleanup a breeze.

1 pound extra-lean ground beef
2 cups fat-free, low-sodium beef broth, such as on page 35

1 14.5-ounce can no-salt-added diced tomatoes, undrained
2 tablespoons chopped kalamata olives
1 teaspoon dried oregano, crumbled
1 teaspoon onion powder
1 teaspoon grated lemon zest
1 teaspoon fresh lemon juice
1/2 teaspoon garlic powder
1/8 teaspoon salt
1/4 teaspoon pepper
4 ounces dried whole-grain rotini
10 ounces frozen chopped spinach, thawed and squeezed dry
1/4 cup crumbled fat-free feta cheese

In a large nonstick skillet, cook the beef over medium-high heat for 8 to 10 minutes, or until no longer pink, stirring occasionally to turn and break up the beef.

Stir in the broth, tomatoes with liquid, olives, oregano, onion powder, lemon zest, lemon juice, garlic powder, salt, and pepper. Bring to a simmer.

Stir in the pasta. Reduce the heat and simmer, covered, for 10 minutes, or until the pasta is tender.

Stir in the spinach. Simmer, covered, for 1 to 2 minutes, or until heated through.

Just before serving, sprinkle with the feta.

PER SERVING

calories 312	carbohydrates 31 g
total fat 7.5 g	fiber 7 g
saturated fat 2.5 g	sugars 5 g
trans fat 0.0 g	protein 32 g
polyunsaturated fat 0.5 g	DIETARY EXCHANGES
monounsaturated fat 3.0 g	1 1/2 starch,
cholesterol 62 mg	2 vegetable, 3 1/2 lean
sodium 443 mg	meat

SHEPHERD'S PIE

SERVES 6

This entrée is for the meat-and-potato lovers in your family. To speed things up, you can cook the sweet potatoes ahead of time and pull them out of the refrigerator when you're ready to start the dish.

1 pound extra-lean ground beef
1 cup fat-free, low-sodium beef broth and
    1/2 cup fat-free, low-sodium beef broth,
    such as on page 35, divided use
1 teaspoon pepper
2 medium dried bay leaves
2 whole cloves
Dash of dried thyme, crumbled
2 medium carrots, thinly sliced
1 large onion, thinly sliced
4 ounces button mushrooms, sliced
2 medium ribs of celery, diced
10 ounces frozen chopped spinach, thawed
    and squeezed dry
Cooking spray
1 tablespoon plus 3/4 teaspoon all-purpose
    flour
1 pound sweet potatoes, peeled, cooked, and
    diced
1/2 cup fat-free milk
1 tablespoon light tub margarine
1 tablespoon very thinly sliced green onion
    (green part only)
3/4 cup shredded low-fat Cheddar cheese

In a large skillet, cook the beef over medium-high heat for 8 to 10 minutes, or until no longer pink, stirring frequently to turn and break up the beef.

Stir in 1 cup broth, the pepper, bay leaves, cloves, and thyme. Reduce the heat and simmer, covered, for 30 minutes.

Stir in the carrots, onion, mushrooms, celery, and spinach. Simmer, covered, for 4 to 5 minutes, or until the vegetables are tender. Discard the bay leaves and cloves.

Meanwhile, preheat the oven to 375°F. Lightly spray a medium casserole dish with cooking spray.

Put the flour in a small bowl. Gradually pour in the remaining 1/2 cup broth, whisking constantly to dissolve the flour and form a smooth paste. Stir into the beef mixture. Simmer for 5 minutes, or until slightly thickened. Pour into the casserole dish.

In a large bowl, mash the sweet potatoes with the milk and margarine.

Stir the green onion into the potatoes. Spread over the beef mixture. Sprinkle the Cheddar on top.

Bake for 10 minutes.

PER SERVING

calories 255	**carbohydrates** 27 g
total fat 6.0 g	fiber 6 g
saturated fat 2.0 g	sugars 8 g
trans fat 0.0 g	**protein** 25 g
polyunsaturated fat 0.5 g	**DIETARY EXCHANGES**
monounsaturated fat 2.0 g	1 starch, 2 vegetable,
cholesterol 45 mg	3 lean meat
sodium 281 mg	

CRUNCHY JÍCAMA TACOS

SERVES 4

Crisp, thin slices of jícama make a nontraditional but refreshing shell for these tacos. The diner picks up the sides of the shell to eat it—similar to a soft taco, but with a crunchy texture. The filling is the more-familiar blend of seasoned beef, fresh tomatoes, and shredded Cheddar cheese. Cilantro-scented sour cream brings it all together.

1 large round jícama (about 12 ounces), cut
    into 8 1/8-inch-thick slices
12 ounces extra-lean ground beef
1/4 cup chopped onion
2 medium garlic cloves, minced
1 teaspoon chili powder and 1/2 teaspoon chili
    powder, divided use
1/2 teaspoon ground cumin
1/4 teaspoon salt
1/8 teaspoon pepper
1/2 cup no-salt-added tomato sauce
1/4 cup fat-free sour cream

(continued)

2 tablespoons chopped fresh cilantro

1/2 teaspoon grated lime zest

1 teaspoon fresh lime juice and 1 tablespoon fresh lime juice, divided use

1 cup shredded romaine

1/4 cup shredded low-fat Cheddar cheese

1 medium Italian plum (Roma) tomato, finely diced

Fill a large bowl with ice-cold water. Soak the jícama slices for 30 minutes, or until pliable. Drain well. Transfer to a work surface. Pat dry with paper towels.

Meanwhile, in a medium nonstick skillet, cook the ground beef and onion over medium-high heat for 6 to 8 minutes, stirring occasionally to turn and break up the beef. Stir in the garlic. Cook for 2 minutes, or until the beef is browned on the outside and no longer pink in the center, stirring occasionally. Stir in 1 teaspoon chili powder, the cumin, salt, and pepper. Cook for 30 seconds, stirring frequently. Stir in the tomato sauce. Reduce the heat to medium. Cook for 5 to 6 minutes, or until the mixture is heated through.

In a small bowl, whisk together the sour cream, cilantro, lime zest, and 1 teaspoon lime juice.

Sprinkle the jícama slices with the remaining 1 tablespoon lime juice and 1/2 teaspoon chili powder. Spoon the meat mixture onto the slices. Sprinkle the romaine, Cheddar, and tomato over the filling. Top with the sour cream mixture and gently fold into a taco shape.

PER SERVING

calories 194	carbohydrates 15 g
total fat 5.0 g	fiber 5 g
saturated fat 2.0 g	sugars 5 g
trans fat 0.0 g	**protein** 23 g
polyunsaturated fat 0.5 g	**DIETARY EXCHANGES**
monounsaturated fat 2.0 g	1/2 starch, 1 vegetable,
cholesterol 51 mg	3 lean meat
sodium 292 mg	

SOUTH-OF-THE-BORDER BEEF TACOS

SERVES 4

Adding coffee granules to this satisfying dish gives it extra-rich color and deep flavor. Serve with Jícama Slaw (page 83).

Cooking spray

12 ounces extra-lean ground beef

1/2 cup fat-free sour cream

1/4 cup chopped fresh cilantro

1 tablespoon fresh lime juice

1 small garlic clove, minced

2 medium green bell peppers, chopped

1 large onion, chopped

1 1/2 cups water

1 14.5-ounce can no-salt-added diced tomatoes, undrained

2 tablespoons chili powder

1 tablespoon instant coffee granules

1 tablespoon sugar

1 1/2 teaspoons ground cumin and 1 teaspoon ground cumin, divided use

1/8 teaspoon salt

8 6-inch corn tortillas

Lightly spray a Dutch oven with cooking spray. Cook the beef over medium-high heat for 8 to 10 minutes, or until no longer pink, stirring frequently to turn and break up the beef. Transfer to a plate.

Meanwhile, whisk together the sour cream, cilantro, lime juice, and garlic.

Lightly spray the pot with cooking spray. Cook the bell peppers and onion, still over medium-high heat, for about 3 minutes, or until the onion is soft, stirring frequently.

Return the beef and any accumulated juices to the pot. Stir in the water, tomatoes with liquid, chili powder, coffee granules, sugar, and 1 1/2 teaspoons cumin. Increase the heat to high and bring to a boil. Reduce the heat and simmer, covered, for 20 minutes. Remove from the heat.

Stir in the salt and the remaining 1 teaspoon cumin. Let stand, covered, for 10 minutes so the flavors blend.

Meanwhile, warm the tortillas using the package directions.

Using a slotted spoon, transfer the beef mixture to the center of each tortilla. Top with the sour cream mixture.

PER SERVING

calories 276	carbohydrates 36 g
total fat 5.5 g	fiber 6 g
saturated fat 2.0 g	sugars 13 g
trans fat 0.0 g	protein 22 g
polyunsaturated fat 1.0 g	DIETARY EXCHANGES
monounsaturated fat 2.0 g	1 1/2 starch,
cholesterol 52 mg	3 vegetable, 2 1/2 lean
sodium 371 mg	meat

BEEF TOSTADAS

SERVES 6

This dish is almost as fast as fast food, but much healthier. The corn tortillas have half the calories and fat of flour tortillas—plus they contain a fraction of the sodium!

6 6-inch corn tortillas
Cooking spray

Filling
1 pound extra-lean ground beef
1 medium onion, finely chopped
1 1/2 to 2 teaspoons chili powder
1/2 teaspoon ground cumin
1/2 teaspoon dried oregano, crumbled
1/2 teaspoon garlic powder
1/4 teaspoon salt
Dash of red hot-pepper sauce

■ ■ ■

2 cups shredded iceberg lettuce
2 medium Italian plum (Roma) tomatoes or
    1 large regular tomato, chopped
3/4 cup salsa (lowest sodium available), such
    as Salsa Cruda (page 437)
3/4 cup shredded fat-free Cheddar cheese

Preheat the oven to 450°F.

Put the tortillas on a baking sheet. Lightly spray the tortillas with cooking spray.

Bake for 8 to 10 minutes, or until crisp.

Meanwhile, in a large nonstick skillet, cook the beef and onion over medium-high heat for 8 to 10 minutes, or until the beef is no longer pink, stirring frequently to turn and break up the beef.

Stir in the remaining filling ingredients. Spread over the tortillas. Top with the remaining ingredients.

PER SERVING

calories 181	carbohydrates 14 g
total fat 4.5 g	fiber 2 g
saturated fat 1.5 g	sugars 4 g
trans fat 0.0 g	protein 22 g
polyunsaturated fat 0.5 g	DIETARY EXCHANGES
monounsaturated fat 1.5 g	1/2 starch, 1 vegetable,
cholesterol 44 mg	3 lean meat
sodium 409 mg	

BEEF AND PASTA SKILLET

SERVES 6

Serve this quick-cooking dish with Marinated Green Beans (page 80), followed by fresh strawberries for dessert.

8 ounces dried tricolor rotini
8 ounces extra-lean ground beef
8 ounces button mushrooms, sliced
1 large onion, chopped
3 medium garlic cloves, minced
1 1/2 teaspoons dried Italian seasoning,
    crumbled
1 1/2 teaspoons dried basil, crumbled
1 cup water
1 6-ounce can no-salt-added tomato paste
2 tablespoons shredded or grated Parmesan
    cheese
2 tablespoons finely chopped fresh parsley
1 teaspoon Worcestershire sauce (lowest
    sodium available)
1/4 teaspoon salt

Prepare the pasta using the package directions, omitting the salt. Drain well in a colander.

(continued)

Meanwhile, in a large skillet, stir together the beef, mushrooms, onion, garlic, Italian seasoning, and basil. Cook, covered, over medium-high heat for 8 to 10 minutes, or until the beef is no longer pink and the mushrooms have released their liquid and are fully cooked, stirring occasionally to turn and break up the beef.

In a small bowl, whisk together the remaining ingredients. Stir the tomato paste mixture and the pasta into the beef mixture. Cook for 5 minutes.

PER SERVING

calories 246	carbohydrates 39 g
total fat 3.0 g	fiber 3 g
saturated fat 1.0 g	sugars 8 g
trans fat 0.0 g	protein 17 g
polyunsaturated fat 0.5 g	**DIETARY EXCHANGES**
monounsaturated fat 1.0 g	2 starch, 2 vegetable,
cholesterol 22 mg	1 lean meat
sodium 182 mg	

MEATBALL WRAP

SERVES 4

If you like meatball Parmesan subs, then you're sure to enjoy this lighter version, too, which cuts out the extra sodium and saturated fat. These homemade meatballs are topped with sauce and cheese, blanketed with fresh spinach, and wrapped all together in a tortilla for a winning combo.

> 1 pound extra-lean ground beef
> 1 medium onion, finely chopped
> 1/4 cup wheat germ
> 1/4 cup fat-free milk
> 1 teaspoon dry mustard
> 1/4 teaspoon garlic powder
> Pepper (freshly ground preferred)

Sauce
> 1 teaspoon canola or corn oil
> 2 tablespoons diced onion
> 1 medium garlic clove, minced
> 1 6-ounce can no-salt-added tomato paste
> 2 8-ounce cans no-salt-added tomato sauce
> 1 teaspoon dried basil, crumbled
> 1 teaspoon dried oregano, crumbled
> 1/4 teaspoon crushed red pepper flakes

. . .

> 1 teaspoon canola or corn oil
> 1/2 cup fat-free, low-sodium beef broth, such as on page 35
> 4 whole-grain tortillas (lowest sodium available)
> 1/4 cup plus 2 tablespoons shredded low-fat mozzarella cheese
> 1/2 cup baby spinach

In a large bowl, using your hands or a spoon, combine the beef, onion, wheat germ, milk, mustard, garlic powder, and pepper. Shape into 12 medium-size meatballs.

In a medium skillet, heat 1 teaspoon oil over medium-high heat, swirling to coat the bottom. Cook the onion for about 3 minutes, or until soft, stirring frequently. Stir in the garlic. Cook for 1 minute, stirring frequently. Stir in the tomato paste. Cook for 1 minute, stirring constantly and scraping the bottom of the skillet. Stir in the tomato sauce, basil, oregano, and red pepper flakes. Bring to a simmer. Reduce the heat and simmer, covered, for 30 minutes.

In a large skillet, heat the remaining 1 teaspoon oil over medium-high heat, swirling to coat the bottom. Cook the meatballs for 5 minutes, turning to brown on all sides. Pour off any drippings from the skillet.

Pour in the broth. Cook, covered, for 20 minutes, or until the meatballs are no longer pink in the center, gently stirring occasionally. Transfer the meatballs to a large plate. Cover to keep warm.

Place the tortillas on a work surface. Place 3 meatballs in a vertical row on the left of each tortilla. Drizzle the sauce over the meatballs. Sprinkle the mozzarella over the sauce. Top with the spinach. Gently roll the tortillas jelly-roll style over the filling, securing with wooden toothpicks.

PER SERVING

calories 385
total fat 11.0 g
  saturated fat 3.0 g
  trans fat 0.0 g
  polyunsaturated fat 2.0 g
  monounsaturated fat 4.5 g
cholesterol 66 mg
sodium 409 mg

carbohydrates 39 g
  fiber 7 g
  sugars 15 g
protein 35 g
DIETARY EXCHANGES
  1 starch, 4 vegetable,
  3 1/2 lean meat

PER SERVING

calories 136
total fat 4.0 g
  saturated fat 1.5 g
  trans fat 0.0 g
  polyunsaturated fat 0.5 g
  monounsaturated fat 1.5 g
cholesterol 42 mg
sodium 97 mg

carbohydrates 8 g
  fiber 2 g
  sugars 4 g
protein 18 g
DIETARY EXCHANGES
  1 vegetable, 3 lean
  meat

CHILI MEATBALLS

SERVES 6

The tomato juice in this recipe is the secret ingredient; it not only keeps the meatballs moist but also infuses them with flavor. Serve with whole-wheat pasta and Fresh Tomato and Roasted Red Bell Pepper Sauce *(page 434) or* Speedy Marinara Sauce *(page 435).*

Cooking spray
1 pound extra-lean ground beef
2 medium onions, minced
1/4 cup wheat germ
2 teaspoons chili powder
1/8 teaspoon garlic powder
1/4 cup low-sodium tomato juice and 3/4 cup
    low-sodium tomato juice or more as
    needed, divided use

Preheat the oven to 350°F. Lightly spray a 1 1/2-quart casserole dish with cooking spray.

In a large bowl, using your hands or a spoon combine the beef, onions, wheat germ, chili powder, garlic powder, and 1/4 cup tomato juice. Shape into 18 meatballs.

Transfer the meatballs to the casserole dish, arranging them in a single layer. Pour the remaining 3/4 cup tomato juice over the meatballs.

Bake, covered, for 1 hour, adding more tomato juice if necessary.

PICADILLO

SERVES 6

Picadillo is a favorite classic in Latin American countries and is probably best described as a stew. The dish is made of ground pork, beef, or veal plus tomatoes, garlic, onions, and other regional ingredients. This is a Cuban version because it's made with raisins, capers, olives, and pimiento.

2 teaspoons light tub margarine
1 medium garlic clove, chopped
1 large onion, chopped
1 medium green bell pepper, chopped
4 sprigs of fresh parsley, chopped
1 1/2 pounds extra-lean ground beef
1/2 cup raisins
1/2 cup no-salt-added tomato paste
1/4 cup sliced almonds
1/4 cup dry red wine (regular or nonalcoholic)
6 pimiento-stuffed green olives, drained,
    chopped
2 teaspoons capers, drained
1 medium dried bay leaf
Pepper (freshly ground preferred)

In a large skillet, melt the margarine over medium heat, swirling to coat the bottom. Cook the garlic for 2 to 3 minutes, or until browned, stirring constantly. Watch carefully so it doesn't burn.

Increase the heat to medium high. Cook the onion, bell pepper, and parsley for 4 minutes, or until the onion is soft and the bell pepper is tender, stirring frequently.

Stir in the beef. Cook for 5 minutes, or until slightly browned on the outside, stirring occasionally to turn and break up the beef.

(continued)

Reduce the heat to medium low. Stir in the remaining ingredients. Simmer, covered, for 10 minutes, stirring occasionally. Discard the bay leaf before serving.

Cook's Tip on Picadillo: In Cuba, this dish is served with rice and black turtle beans. Or, use it as a stuffing as Mexicans frequently do.

HAWAIIAN HAM

SERVES 8

A sweet tangy glaze blankets ham and vegetables as they bake. Serve with baked sweet potatoes and Pan-Roasted Broccoli (page 376). Finish the meal with Coffee-Coconut Custards (page 496) or Spiced Skillet Bananas (page 503).

> 3 cups diced lower-sodium, low-fat cooked ham, all visible fat discarded
> 1 medium onion, cut into thin slices
> 1 small green bell pepper, sliced into rings
> 1 cup canned pineapple chunks, canned in their own juice, drained and juice reserved
> 1/2 cup raisins
> 1/3 cup cider vinegar
> 1/4 cup brown sugar
> 1 tablespoon cornstarch
> 2 teaspoons dry mustard
> 1 teaspoon Worcestershire sauce (lowest sodium available)

Preheat the oven to 350°F.

Put the ham in a 2 1/2-quart casserole dish. Arrange the onion and bell pepper on the ham. Place the pineapple on the onion and bell pepper. Sprinkle the raisins over all.

Add water to the reserved pineapple juice to make 1 cup. Pour into a small saucepan. Whisk in the vinegar, brown sugar, cornstarch, and mustard. Bring to a boil over high heat and boil until the mixture turns clear, whisking constantly. Remove from the heat.

Whisk in the Worcestershire sauce. Pour the glaze over the ham, vegetables, pineapple, and raisins.

Bake for 30 to 40 minutes.

CRUSTLESS HAM AND MUSTARD GREENS TART

SERVES 6

This is a great brunch dish, but it's also perfect for a light lunch or dinner. Serve it with a leafy green salad and Southern Raised Biscuits (page 459).

> Cooking spray
> 2 tablespoons shredded or grated Swiss cheese and 1/4 cup shredded or grated Swiss cheese, divided use
> 1 teaspoon olive oil
> 1 large onion, finely chopped
> 2 medium garlic cloves, minced
> 10 ounces frozen chopped mustard greens, thawed and squeezed dry
> 1 1/2 ounces lower-sodium, low-fat ham, all visible fat discarded, cut into strips
> 1 1/4 cups fat-free milk
> 4 large egg whites
> 1 large egg
> 1 1/2 tablespoons all-purpose flour
> 1 tablespoon finely chopped fresh parsley
> 1/2 teaspoon pepper
> Dash of ground nutmeg

Preheat the oven to 350°F. Lightly spray a 9-inch glass pie pan with cooking spray. Sprinkle with 2 tablespoons Swiss cheese.

In a medium nonstick skillet, heat the oil over medium-high heat, swirling to coat the bottom. Cook the onion for 3 minutes, or until soft, stirring frequently.

Stir in the garlic. Cook for 1 minute, stirring frequently.

Stir in the mustard greens and ham. Spread the mixture in the pie pan.

In a medium bowl, whisk together the milk, egg whites, egg, flour, parsley, pepper, nutmeg, and the remaining 1/4 cup Swiss cheese. Pour over the mustard greens mixture.

Bake for 50 to 55 minutes, or until a knife inserted in the center of the tart comes out clean.

PER SERVING

calories 113	**carbohydrates** 10 g
total fat 4.0 g	fiber 2 g
saturated fat 1.5 g	sugars 5 g
trans fat 0.0 g	**protein** 10 g
polyunsaturated fat 0.5 g	**DIETARY EXCHANGES**
monounsaturated fat 1.5 g	1 vegetable, 1/2 other
cholesterol 41 mg	carbohydrate, 1 lean
sodium 157 mg	meat

BAYOU RED BEANS AND RICE

SERVES 8

This recipe will show you how easy it is to prepare one of Louisiana's most popular comfort foods without the saturated fat and sodium common in most versions.

- 3 15.5-ounce cans no-salt-added red kidney beans, rinsed and drained
- 3 cups fat-free, low-sodium chicken broth, such as on page 36
- 1 14.5-ounce can no-salt-added stewed tomatoes, undrained
- 1 cup chopped lower-sodium, low-fat ham, all visible fat discarded
- 1 large onion, chopped
- 2 medium ribs of celery with leaves, chopped
- 2 teaspoons Louisiana-style hot-pepper sauce
- 1 medium garlic clove, minced
- 1/4 teaspoon pepper
- 1 cup uncooked brown rice

In a Dutch oven, stir together all the ingredients except the rice. Bring to a boil over high heat. Reduce the heat and simmer, covered, for 1 hour, stirring occasionally.

Meanwhile, prepare the rice using the package directions, omitting the salt and margarine.

Using a potato masher, mash about one-fourth of the bean mixture while it's in the pot. Stir the mixture. Cook over low heat for 10 minutes, stirring occasionally. Serve over the rice.

PER SERVING

calories 276	**carbohydrates** 51 g
total fat 1.5 g	fiber 9 g
saturated fat 0.5 g	sugars 7 g
trans fat 0.0 g	**protein** 17 g
polyunsaturated fat 0.5 g	**DIETARY EXCHANGES**
monounsaturated fat 0.5 g	3 starch, 1 vegetable,
cholesterol 8 mg	1 1/2 lean meat
sodium 190 mg	

MARINATED PORK TENDERLOIN

SERVES 4

Steamed snow peas or broccoli go well with this Asian flavored pork. Prep it in the morning and let it marinate while you're at work. Serve it over brown rice.

Marinade
- 1 small onion, grated or minced
- 2 tablespoons soy sauce (lowest sodium available)
- 1 tablespoon toasted sesame oil
- 2 teaspoons grated peeled gingerroot or 3/4 teaspoon ground ginger
- 2 medium garlic cloves, crushed
- 1 teaspoon grated lemon zest

■ ■ ■

(continued)

1 1-pound pork tenderloin, all visible fat discarded
1/4 cup dry white wine (regular or nonalcoholic)
2 tablespoons plus 1 teaspoon honey
1 teaspoon dark brown sugar

In a large glass baking dish, stir together the marinade ingredients. Add the pork, turning to coat. Cover and refrigerate for about 8 hours, turning occasionally.

Preheat the oven to 425°F.

Drain the pork, discarding the marinade. Put the pork in a shallow nonstick baking dish.

In a small bowl, whisk together the remaining ingredients. Pour over the pork, turning to coat.

Roast for 20 to 25 minutes, or until the pork registers 145°F on an instant-read thermometer. Transfer to a cutting board. Let stand for 3 minutes before cutting crosswise into slices.

PER SERVING

calories 169	carbohydrates 12 g
total fat 3.0 g	fiber 0 g
saturated fat 1.0 g	sugars 12 g
trans fat 0.0 g	**protein** 22 g
polyunsaturated fat 0.5 g	**DIETARY EXCHANGES**
monounsaturated fat 1.0 g	1 other carbohydrate,
cholesterol 60 mg	3 lean meat
sodium 243 mg	

HERB-RUBBED PORK TENDERLOIN WITH DIJON-APRICOT MOP SAUCE

SERVES 8

A dry herb rub flavors the pork and creates a crust to keep the pork moist as it bakes. You may want to stop right there, or you can go one step further and add the tangy mop sauce. Serve with Toasted Farro with Caramelized Carrots and Sweet Potatoes (page 420) and steamed green beans.

Rub
1 tablespoon dried rosemary, crushed
1 tablespoon dried thyme, crumbled

1 tablespoon ground cumin
2 teaspoons pepper (coarsely ground preferred)
2 teaspoons paprika
2 teaspoons celery seeds

■ ■ ■

2 1-pound pork tenderloins, all visible fat and silver skin discarded
Cooking spray

Sauce (optional)
1 teaspoon canola or corn oil
1 small onion, finely chopped
1/2 cup cider vinegar
1/4 cup honey
1/4 cup all-fruit apricot spread
2 tablespoons Dijon mustard (lowest sodium available)
1 teaspoon grated lemon zest
1 tablespoon fresh lemon juice

In a small bowl, stir together the rub ingredients. Using your fingertips, gently press the mixture so it adheres to the pork. Set aside.

Preheat the oven to 350°F or lightly spray the grill rack with cooking spray and preheat the grill on medium high.

For the mop sauce, in a small saucepan, heat the oil over medium-high heat, swirling to coat the bottom. Cook the onion for 3 minutes, or until soft, stirring occasionally.

Stir in the remaining sauce ingredients. Bring to a boil. Reduce the heat and simmer for 5 minutes, stirring occasionally. (You may wish to reserve 1/2 cup sauce to use as a dipping sauce for the cooked pork.)

If baking, lightly spray a broiling pan and rack with cooking spray. Put the tenderloins on the rack in the pan. Bake for 30 minutes. Using a pastry brush or basting mop, baste on all sides with the sauce. Bake for 10 minutes. Using a clean pastry brush or basting mop, baste again. Bake for 10 to 15 minutes, or until the pork registers 145°F on an instant-read thermometer.

If grilling, grill the tenderloins for 10 minutes on each side (40 minutes total). Using a pastry brush or basting mop, baste with the sauce. Grill for 2 to 3 minutes on each side, or until the pork registers 145°F on an instant-read thermometer.

Transfer the pork to a cutting board. Let stand for 3 minutes before slicing.

Cook's Tip: Chicken, flank steak, and eye-of-round roast are delicious with both the rub and the mop sauce. Try the mop sauce on its own over vegetable kebabs, beef, poultry, firm fish fillets, or shrimp.

PER SERVING

calories 231	**carbohydrates** 18 g
total fat 6.5 g	fiber 1 g
saturated fat 2.0 g	sugars 14 g
trans fat 0.0 g	**protein** 25 g
polyunsaturated fat 0.5 g	**DIETARY EXCHANGES**
monounsaturated fat 2.5 g	1 other carbohydrate,
cholesterol 75 mg	3 lean meat
sodium 133 mg	

PORK CHOPS WITH DRIED CRANBERRY AND PINE NUT STUFFING

SERVES 4

A slightly sweet, slightly tart filling as well as finishing sauce provides a palate-pleasing dish from the inside out.

4 boneless pork loin chops (about 4 ounces each), all visible fat discarded
1/2 cup dried unsweetened cranberries
2 tablespoons chopped pine nuts, dry-roasted
1 tablespoon brown sugar
1 tablespoon cider vinegar
1 teaspoon dried thyme, crumbled
1/2 cup 100% cranberry juice
1/2 cup fat-free, low-sodium chicken broth, such as on page 36
1 tablespoon honey
1/4 teaspoon pepper

With a sharp knife, make a lengthwise cut into the side of each pork chop to form a pocket for stuffing. Be careful not to cut through to the other side.

In a small bowl, stir together the cranberries, pine nuts, brown sugar, vinegar, and thyme. Spoon about 2 tablespoons of the mixture into the pocket of each pork chop. Secure with wooden toothpicks.

In a large nonstick skillet, cook the pork over medium heat for 1 minute on each side, or until golden brown.

Stir in the remaining ingredients. Increase the heat to medium high and bring to a simmer. Reduce the heat and simmer, covered, for 20 minutes, or until the pork registers 145°F on an instant-read thermometer and the stuffing is heated through. Transfer to a serving plate. Cover to keep warm.

Increase the heat to medium high and bring the cooking liquid to a simmer. Reduce the heat and simmer for 5 minutes, or until reduced to about 1/2 cup. Spoon over the pork.

PER SERVING

calories 232	**carbohydrates** 18 g
total fat 8.0 g	fiber 2 g
saturated fat 2.5 g	sugars 13 g
trans fat 0.0 g	**protein** 24 g
polyunsaturated fat 1.5 g	**DIETARY EXCHANGES**
monounsaturated fat 3.0 g	1/2 fruit, 1/2 other
cholesterol 60 mg	carbohydrate, 3 lean
sodium 61 mg	meat

BRAISED PORK CHOPS WITH TOMATO AND GARLIC SAUCE

SERVES 6

This dish is quick-braised, which allows you to easily get this Italian-style meat and veggie entrée on the table any night of the week. Serve on whole-wheat pasta to help soak up the sauce.

(continued)

2 teaspoons olive oil

6 boneless center-cut pork loin chops (about
4 ounces each, 1 to 1 1/2 inches thick), all
visible fat discarded

2 medium garlic cloves, finely chopped

1/2 teaspoon dried oregano, crumbled

1/2 medium dried bay leaf

1/4 teaspoon dried thyme, crumbled

1/2 cup dry red wine (regular or nonalcoholic)

1 cup canned no-salt-added tomatoes, pureed
until smooth in a food processor or
blender

1 tablespoon no-salt-added tomato paste

2 teaspoons canola or corn oil

1 1/2 large green bell peppers, cut into
2 x 1/4-inch strips

8 ounces button mushrooms, left whole if
small, quartered or sliced if large

In a large, heavy skillet, heat the olive oil over medium-high heat, swirling to coat the bottom. Cook the pork for 3 to 4 minutes on each side, or until it registers 145°F on an instant-read thermometer. Transfer to a plate. Let stand for 3 minutes.

In the same skillet, still over medium-high heat, cook the garlic, oregano, bay leaf, and thyme for 30 seconds, stirring constantly. Pour in the wine. Increase the heat to high and bring to a boil. Boil for 2 minutes, or until the wine is reduced by half (to about 1/4 cup), stirring frequently and scraping to dislodge any browned bits.

Stir in the tomatoes and tomato paste. Reduce the heat to low. Cook the sauce for 5 minutes, or until heated through, stirring occasionally.

Meanwhile, in a separate large skillet, heat the canola oil over medium-high heat, swirling to coat the bottom. Cook the bell peppers for 3 minutes, stirring frequently. Stir in the mushrooms. Cook for 2 minutes, or until beginning to soften. Stir the bell peppers and mushrooms into the sauce. Increase the heat to medium and cook, covered, for 5 minutes, or until the sauce is thick enough to coat a spoon heavily. (If the sauce is too thin, remove the vegetables, in-

crease the heat to high, and boil the sauce down, stirring constantly.)

Arrange the pork on a serving platter. Spoon the sauce over the pork.

PER SERVING

calories 214	carbohydrates 6 g
total fat 9.0 g	fiber 2 g
saturated fat 2.5 g	sugars 4 g
trans fat 0.0 g	protein 24 g
polyunsaturated fat 1.5 g	DIETARY EXCHANGES
monounsaturated fat 4.5 g	1 vegetable, 3 lean
cholesterol 60 mg	meat
sodium 66 mg	

CRUNCHY HERB-CRUSTED PORK CHOPS

SERVES 4

Dunking these pork chops in a mixture of sour cream and herbs keeps them tender and juicy. Crushed cornflakes create a crisp coating while they bake. Serve with Asparagus with Lemon and Capers *(page 373) and a whole grain.*

Cooking spray

1/2 cup fat-free sour cream

1 tablespoon chopped fresh sage or
1 teaspoon dried sage

2 teaspoons chopped fresh thyme or
1 teaspoon dried thyme, crumbled

1/4 teaspoon salt

1/4 teaspoon pepper

1 cup crushed cornflake cereal

4 boneless pork loin chops (about 4 ounces
each), all visible fat discarded

2 teaspoons olive oil

Preheat the oven to 375°F. Lightly spray a baking sheet with cooking spray.

In a shallow bowl, whisk together the sour cream, sage, thyme, salt, and pepper. Put the cornflakes in a separate shallow bowl. Put the bowls and a large plate in a row, assembly-line fashion. Dip the pork in the sour cream mixture, then in the cornflakes, turning to coat at each step and gently shaking off any excess. Using your fingertips, gently press the coating so it adheres to the pork. Put the pork on the plate.

In a large nonstick skillet, heat the oil over medium heat, swirling to coat the bottom. Cook the pork for 2 to 3 minutes on each side, or until golden brown. Transfer the pork to the baking sheet.

Bake the pork for 5 minutes, or until it registers 145°F on an instant-read thermometer. Remove from the oven. Let stand for 3 minutes.

PER SERVING

calories 224	sodium 311 mg
total fat 7.5 g	carbohydrates 17 g
saturated fat 2.0 g	fiber 1 g
trans fat 0.0 g	sugars 3 g
polyunsaturated fat 1.0 g	protein 21 g
monounsaturated fat 3.5 g	**DIETARY EXCHANGES**
cholesterol 62 mg	1 starch, 3 lean meat

LOUISIANA SKILLET PORK

SERVES 4

Deeply browned veggies with a hint of olive oil complement these Cajun-seasoned pork chops. Serve with Baked Fries with Creole Seasoning *(page 401) or* Southern-Style Greens *(page 391).*

> 1 teaspoon salt-free Creole or Cajun
>   seasoning blend, such as on page 401
> 4 boneless center-cut pork chops (about
>   4 ounces each), all visible fat discarded
> Cooking spray
> 1 cup frozen whole-kernel corn, slightly
>   thawed
> 1 medium red bell pepper, chopped
> 1 small zucchini, chopped
> 1/2 cup finely chopped onion
> 1 medium rib of celery, finely chopped
> 1/4 teaspoon pepper
> 1 teaspoon olive oil (extra-virgin preferred)
> 1/4 teaspoon salt

Sprinkle the seasoning blend over both sides of the pork.

Lightly spray a large skillet with cooking spray. Cook the pork over medium-high heat for 6 minutes on each side, or until it registers 145°F on an instant-read thermometer and is no longer pink on the outside. Remove from the heat.

Transfer the pork to a serving plate. Cover to keep warm. Lightly spray any browned bits in the skillet with cooking spray.

Put the corn, bell pepper, zucchini, onion, celery, and pepper in the skillet, stirring to combine. Cook over medium-high heat for 4 minutes, or until the celery is tender-crisp and the vegetables begin to brown on the edges, stirring frequently. Remove from the heat.

Stir in the oil and salt. Spoon the corn mixture over the pork or serve on the side.

Cook's Tip: Be sure to remove the skillet from the heat before adding the olive oil so you get the maximum flavor impact from the oil.

PER SERVING

calories 197	carbohydrates 15 g
total fat 6.5 g	fiber 3 g
saturated fat 1.5 g	sugars 4 g
trans fat 0.0 g	protein 21 g
polyunsaturated fat 1.0 g	**DIETARY EXCHANGES**
monounsaturated fat 2.5 g	1/2 starch, 1 vegetable,
cholesterol 57 mg	3 lean meat
sodium 198 mg	

PORK WITH SPICED SAUERKRAUT

SERVES 8

If you're looking for a holiday roast, look no further. Serve with Winter Fruit Salad with Spinach and Gorgonzola *(page 86).*

> Cooking spray
> 1 teaspoon canola or corn oil
> 1/2 cup chopped onion
> 2 cups cold water
> 12 ounces canned sauerkraut (lowest sodium
>   available), rinsed, drained, and squeezed
>   dry

(continued)

2 teaspoons sugar

2 large potatoes, peeled and grated

6 whole peppercorns

5 whole dried juniper berries

2 medium dried bay leaves

1/4 teaspoon caraway seeds

1 whole allspice

1 1/2 pounds pork tenderloin, all visible fat discarded, cut into 1/2-inch slices

Preheat the oven to 325°F. Lightly spray an 11 x 17-inch casserole dish with cooking spray.

In a large skillet, heat the oil over medium-high heat, swirling to coat the bottom. Cook the onion for 4 to 5 minutes, or until soft and lightly browned, stirring frequently.

Stir in the water, sauerkraut, and sugar. Using a fork, separate the strands of sauerkraut.

Stir in the potatoes. Cook for 5 minutes, stirring occasionally.

Put the peppercorns, juniper berries, bay leaves, caraway seeds, and allspice in a piece of cheesecloth. Tie with kitchen twine.

Transfer the sauerkraut mixture to the casserole dish. Make a well in the center of the sauerkraut. Put the cheesecloth bag in the well.

In the same skillet, still over medium-high heat, cook the pork for 2 minutes on each side, or until browned. Place the pork on the sauerkraut.

Bake, covered, for about 1 hour, or until the pork is no longer pink on the outside.

Bake, uncovered, for 30 minutes, or until the pork registers 145°F on an instant-read thermometer. Transfer the pork to a cutting board. Let stand for 3 minutes.

Time-Saver: Using a covered broilerproof dish, bake the casserole for about 1 hour. Preheat the broiler. Uncover the dish. Broil the casserole about 6 inches from the heat for 3 to 4 minutes, or until the pork registers 145°F on an instant-read thermometer. Transfer the pork to a cutting board. Let stand for 3 minutes.

PER SERVING

calories 175	carbohydrates 19 g
total fat 3.0 g	fiber 3 g
saturated fat 1.0 g	sugars 3 g
trans fat 0.0 g	**protein** 17 g
polyunsaturated fat 0.5 g	**DIETARY EXCHANGES**
monounsaturated fat 1.0 g	1 starch, 1 vegetable,
cholesterol 45 mg	2 1/2 lean meat
sodium 381 mg	

ORANGE PORK MEDALLIONS
SERVES 4

An unusual combination of sweet, spicy, and savory flavors enhances this dish. Try it with Couscous with Vegetables *(page 417).*

Sauce

2/3 to 1 cup fresh orange juice

2 1/2 tablespoons fresh lemon juice

2 tablespoons finely chopped fresh parsley

2 tablespoons all-fruit orange marmalade

1 tablespoon cornstarch

2 teaspoons toasted sesame oil

3/4 teaspoon bottled white horseradish, drained

1/2 teaspoon ground cinnamon

1/2 teaspoon dried rosemary, crushed

1/4 teaspoon pepper

■ ■ ■

1 pound pork tenderloin, all visible fat discarded, cut into slices 1/2 inch thick, flattened to 1/4-inch thickness

4 medium green onions, thinly sliced

1 11-ounce can mandarin orange slices in juice, drained

In a small bowl, whisk together the sauce ingredients.

In a large nonstick skillet, cook the pork over medium-high heat for about 2 minutes on each side, or until browned.

Stir in the green onions. Cook for 1 minute, or until tender.

Stir in the sauce. Cook for 3 to 4 minutes, or until the pork is no longer pink on the outside and the sauce has thickened, stirring constantly.

Spoon the sauce over the pork. Spoon the mandarin oranges over or beside the pork. Sprinkle with the parsley.

PER SERVING

calories 257	sodium 66 mg
total fat 7.5 g	carbohydrates 21 g
saturated fat 2.0 g	fiber 2 g
trans fat 0.0 g	sugars 14 g
polyunsaturated fat 1.5 g	protein 25 g
monounsaturated fat 3.0 g	DIETARY EXCHANGES
cholesterol 75 mg	1 1/2 fruit, 3 lean meat

PORK ROULADES

SERVES 6

Roulade *is a French term for a thin slice of meat rolled around a filling such as bread crumbs and vegetables, browned in a skillet, and then baked. A peppery beef broth mixture is used both as a glaze and finishing sauce.*

Cooking spray
2 teaspoons canola or corn oil and
    1 tablespoon canola or corn oil, divided use
8 ounces button mushrooms
1 tablespoon chopped onion
3 slices whole-grain bread (lowest sodium available), torn into small pieces
2 medium ribs of celery, chopped
1/4 cup chopped walnuts
1 teaspoon chopped fresh parsley
1/2 teaspoon dried thyme, crumbled
1/4 teaspoon salt
Pepper (freshly ground preferred)
2 1-pound pork tenderloins, all visible fat discarded, cut into 6 3 x 4-inch rectangles, then flattened to 1/4-inch thickness

Sauce
2 tablespoons all-purpose flour
1/2 cup fat-free, low-sodium beef broth, such as on page 35

1 tablespoon canola or corn oil
Pepper to taste (freshly ground preferred)

Preheat the oven to 350°F. Lightly spray a Dutch oven with cooking spray. Set aside.

In a medium skillet, heat 2 teaspoons oil over medium-high heat, swirling to coat the bottom. Cook the mushrooms and onion for 4 minutes, or until the onion is soft and beginning to brown, stirring frequently.

In a large bowl, stir together the bread, celery, walnuts, parsley, thyme, salt, and pepper. Stir in the mushroom mixture.

Divide the filling into 6 portions. Place each portion on a piece of pork. Roll the pork around the filling to form a cylinder. Secure with wooden toothpicks.

In the same skillet, still over medium-high heat, heat 1 tablespoon oil, swirling to coat the bottom. Cook the roulades for 5 minutes, turning to brown on all sides. Transfer the roulades to the Dutch oven. Bake, covered, for 1 1/2 hours.

About 30 minutes before the end of the baking time, put the flour in a medium saucepan. Add the broth and the remaining 1 tablespoon oil, whisking to dissolve. Whisk in the pepper. Heat over medium heat, whisking frequently.

About 15 minutes before the end of the baking time, uncover the Dutch oven. Spoon half the sauce over the roulades as a glaze. Return to the oven.

Serve the roulades with the remaining sauce.

PER SERVING

calories 298	sodium 224 mg
total fat 14.0 g	carbohydrates 10 g
saturated fat 2.5 g	fiber 2 g
trans fat 0.0 g	sugars 2 g
polyunsaturated fat 4.0 g	protein 33 g
monounsaturated fat 6.0 g	DIETARY EXCHANGES
cholesterol 80 mg	1/2 starch, 4 lean meat

SWEET-AND-SOUR PORK

SERVES 4

You don't need to have a wok to create this classic Chinese dish at home. You can use a nonstick skillet instead if you prefer. Serve with brown rice to soak up the sauce and Fresh Snow Peas with Water Chestnuts *(page 403).*

1 15-ounce can pineapple chunks in their own juice, drained with juice reserved
1 tablespoon plus 1 teaspoon plain rice vinegar
2 teaspoons dry sherry
2 teaspoons soy sauce (lowest sodium available)
1/8 teaspoon ground ginger
1/8 teaspoon ground allspice
1/8 teaspoon hot chili oil
2 teaspoons cornstarch
1/4 cup water
12 ounces pork tenderloin, all visible fat discarded, cut into 2 x 1/4-inch strips
1/2 cup sliced green bell pepper
1 small onion, sliced
2 tablespoons minced leek or green onions
2 teaspoons chopped fresh parsley
1/8 teaspoon pepper

Add enough water to the reserved pineapple juice to make 1 cup. Set the pineapple aside.

In a small saucepan, whisk together the pineapple juice mixture, vinegar, sherry, soy sauce, ginger, allspice, and hot chili oil. Cook over medium-high heat for 3 to 4 minutes, or until the sauce comes just to a boil, whisking occasionally.

Meanwhile, put the cornstarch in a small bowl. Add the water, whisking until the cornstarch is dissolved.

Whisk the cornstarch mixture into the pineapple juice mixture. Reduce the heat to medium and cook for 1 to 2 minutes, or until the sauce begins to thicken, whisking constantly. Remove from the heat.

In a wok or large nonstick skillet, cook the pork over medium-high heat for 4 to 5 minutes, or until no longer pink on the outside, stirring frequently. Push to the side.

Reduce the heat to medium. Put the bell pepper, onion, and leek in the skillet. Stir together with the pork. Sprinkle the parsley and pepper over all. Cook for 4 to 5 minutes, or until the bell pepper is tender-crisp and the onion is soft, stirring occasionally.

Stir in the sauce and pineapple. Cook for 3 minutes, stirring occasionally.

PER SERVING

calories 199	**carbohydrates** 20 g
total fat 4.0 g	fiber 2 g
saturated fat 1.5 g	sugars 16 g
trans fat 0.0 g	**protein** 19 g
polyunsaturated fat 0.5 g	**DIETARY EXCHANGES**
monounsaturated fat 1.5 g	1 fruit, 1 vegetable,
cholesterol 56 mg	2 1/2 lean meat
sodium 116 mg	

GRILLED PORK MEDALLIONS WITH APPLE CIDER SAUCE

SERVES 8

This succulent entrée requires some planning, because the pork marinates for three days, but the flavor is well worth it. The leftover pork is great in sandwiches or salads.

Marinade
1 cup 100% apple cider
3/4 cup 100% draft cider, 100% apple cider, or cider vinegar
1/2 cup apple-flavored liqueur, draft cider, or apple cider
3 tablespoons sugar
2 tablespoons whole mustard seeds
2 tablespoons olive oil
1 tablespoon chopped fresh rosemary or 1 teaspoon dried rosemary, crushed
2 teaspoons chopped fresh thyme or 1 teaspoon dried thyme, crumbled
3 medium garlic cloves, minced

■ ■ ■

2 pounds pork tenderloin, all visible fat
discarded, cut into 8 medallions
6 cups 100% apple cider

In a medium skillet, stir together the marinade ingredients. Bring to a boil over medium heat. Boil for 4 to 5 minutes. Reduce the heat and simmer for 30 minutes, or until reduced by half (to about 1 cup). Remove from the heat. Let cool for 30 minutes, or until room temperature.

Pour the marinade into a large shallow dish. Add the pork, turning to coat. Cover and refrigerate for three days, turning occasionally.

For the cider sauce, in a medium saucepan, boil 6 cups apple cider over high heat for 40 to 50 minutes, or until reduced to 2/3 cup and thick enough to coat the back of a spoon. Be careful not to let the sauce boil over. If necessary, reduce the heat to medium high.

When the pork has finished marinating, preheat the grill on medium high. Grill the pork for 10 to 12 minutes. Turn over the pork. Grill for 10 to 12 minutes, or until the pork registers 145°F on an instant-read thermometer. Remove from the grill. Let stand for 3 minutes.

Just before serving, drizzle the sauce over the pork.

Cook's Tip: If you prefer, you can replace the pork with eight 4-ounce boneless, skinless chicken breast halves or 2 pounds turkey breast medallions, all visible fat discarded. Reduce the grilling time to 6 to 8 minutes per side, or until the chicken or turkey is no longer pink in the center.

Cook's Tip: You can make the cider sauce up to three days in advance and reheat it in a glass container set in a pan of hot water or in the microwave set on 25 percent power (low) until the sauce is pouring consistency.

PER SERVING

calories 204	sodium 65 mg
total fat 3.0 g	**carbohydrates** 22 g
saturated fat 1.0 g	fiber 0 g
trans fat 0.0 g	sugars 21 g
polyunsaturated fat 0.5 g	**protein** 22 g
monounsaturated fat 1.0 g	**DIETARY EXCHANGES**
cholesterol 60 mg	1 1/2 fruit, 3 lean meat

PORK AND VEGETABLE LO MEIN
SERVES 4

Lo mein, or "tossed noodles," combines noodles with a savory sauce, vegetables, and often meat or tofu. This version is so easy to prepare, you'll be less tempted to order takeout.

4 ounces dried whole grain spaghetti
Cooking spray
12 ounces boneless center-cut pork loin
chops, all visible fat discarded, cut into
thin, bite-size strips
1 8-ounce can sliced water chestnuts, drained
3/4 cup shredded carrot
1 small green bell pepper, diced
1 medium rib of celery, sliced
4 medium green onions, chopped, and
2 medium green onions, chopped,
divided use
2 medium garlic cloves, minced
1 tablespoon cornstarch
1 cup fat-free, low-sodium beef broth, such as
on page 35
1 tablespoon soy sauce (lowest sodium
available)
1 teaspoon grated peeled gingerroot

Prepare the pasta using the package directions, omitting the salt. Drain well in a colander. Set aside.

Meanwhile, lightly spray a large skillet with cooking spray. Cook the pork over medium-high heat for 3 minutes, or until no longer pink on the outside, stirring frequently. Transfer to a medium plate. Set aside.

(continued)

Reduce the heat to medium and cook the water chestnuts, carrot, bell pepper, celery, 4 green onions, and garlic for 4 to 5 minutes, or until the bell pepper and celery are tender, stirring frequently.

Put the cornstarch in a small bowl. Pour in the broth and soy sauce, whisking until the cornstarch is dissolved. Stir the mixture and gingerroot into the water chestnut mixture. Bring to a simmer, still over medium heat, stirring constantly.

Gently stir in the pork and pasta. Cook for 2 to 3 minutes, or until the pork and pasta are heated through. Sprinkle with the remaining 2 green onions.

PER SERVING

calories 245	carbohydrates 32 g
total fat 5.0 g	fiber 6 g
saturated fat 1.0 g	sugars 4 g
trans fat 0.0 g	protein 19 g
polyunsaturated fat 0.5 g	DIETARY EXCHANGES
monounsaturated fat 1.5 g	2 starch, 2 vegetable,
cholesterol 43 mg	2 lean meat
sodium 164 mg	

JAMAICAN JERK PORK AND VEGETABLES WITH MANGO-COCONUT RICE

SERVES 6

Jamaican jerk seasoning infuses this stewed pork dish with its rich, spicy flavor. The sweet mango-coconut rice helps tame the heat.

> 2 teaspoons salt-free Jamaican jerk seasoning
> 1 pound boneless pork loin chops, all visible fat discarded, cut into 3/4-inch cubes
> 1/2 medium onion, cut into 1-inch pieces
> 1 cup fat-free, low-sodium chicken broth, such as on page 36
> 2 teaspoons soy sauce (lowest sodium available)
> 2 15-ounce cans sweet potatoes in light syrup, rinsed and drained
> 3 cups frozen green beans
> 4 medium green onions, cut into 1-inch pieces

> 6 ounces 100% pineapple juice (about 3/4 cup)
> 1/2 cup lite coconut milk
> 1 cup uncooked instant brown rice
> 1 large mango, chopped

Sprinkle the jerk seasoning all over the pork.

Heat a large nonstick saucepan over medium-high heat. Brown the pork for 4 to 6 minutes, stirring occasionally.

Stir in the onion. Cook for about 3 minutes, or until the onion is soft, stirring frequently.

Stir in the broth and soy sauce. Bring to a simmer. Reduce the heat and simmer, covered, for 30 minutes, or until the pork is no longer pink on the outside.

Stir in the sweet potatoes, green beans, and green onions. Simmer, covered, for 8 to 10 minutes, or until the green beans are tender and the mixture is heated through. Set aside.

Meanwhile, in a medium saucepan, bring the pineapple juice and coconut milk to a simmer, covered, over medium-high heat.

Stir in the rice and mango. Reduce the heat and simmer, covered, for 10 minutes. Remove from the heat. Let stand for 5 minutes. Fluff gently with a fork.

Spoon the rice mixture onto plates. Spoon the pork mixture over the rice.

Cook's Tip on Jamaican Jerk Seasoning: Look for Jamaican jerk seasoning in the spice section of the grocery store or mix your own. For about 3 tablespoons total, stir together 1 teaspoon each ground ginger, onion powder, ground allspice, garlic powder, paprika, dried thyme, fennel seeds, black pepper, and ground cloves. This blend will keep in an airtight container for up to six months.

JOLLOF RICE

SERVES 8

Popular in western Africa, jollof rice is a dish that combines rice, tomatoes, and tomato paste with meat, vegetables, and different spices.

Cooking spray

1 pound boneless center-cut pork loin chops (about 4 ounces each), all visible fat discarded, cut into 3/4-inch cubes

1 medium bell pepper, diced (any color)

1 large carrot, thinly sliced

1 medium onion, chopped

2 medium garlic cloves, minced

2 cups fat-free, low-sodium chicken broth, such as on page 36

1 14.5-ounce can no-salt-added diced tomatoes, undrained

1 cup water

1/4 cup no-salt-added tomato paste

1/4 cup diced lower-sodium, low-fat ham (about 2 ounces), all visible fat discarded

1 medium fresh jalapeño, seeds and ribs discarded, diced (see Cook's Tip on Handling Hot Chiles, page 24)

1 teaspoon curry powder

1/4 teaspoon salt

1/4 teaspoon pepper

1 medium dried bay leaf

2 cups uncooked instant brown rice

2 cups frozen green beans

1 cup frozen green peas

Garnishes (optional)

1/4 cup chopped fresh parsley

1 cup chopped cooked cabbage

Whites of 4 large hard-boiled eggs, chopped

Lightly spray a Dutch oven with cooking spray. Cook the pork over medium-high heat for 5 to 6 minutes, or until browned, stirring occasionally.

Stir in the bell pepper, carrot, onion, and garlic. Cook for about 3 minutes, or until the onion is soft, stirring frequently.

Stir in the broth, tomatoes with liquid, water, tomato paste, ham, jalapeño, curry powder, salt, pepper, and bay leaf. Reduce the heat and simmer, covered, for 30 minutes to 1 hour, or until the pork is tender.

Stir in the rice, green beans, and green peas. Increase the heat to medium high and return to a simmer. Simmer, covered, for 10 minutes, or until the rice is tender. Discard the bay leaf. Serve with the garnishes.

BONELESS PORK RIBS WITH BLUEBERRY BARBECUE SAUCE

SERVES 4

If you love tender pork ribs, you'll enjoy this boneless version. Lean pork loin with a zesty rub is braised to perfection and served with a kicked-up fruity barbecue sauce. Serve with Southern-Style Black-Eyed Peas *(page 121) and* Jícama Slaw *(page 83).*

1/2 teaspoon ground cumin

1/2 teaspoon chili powder

1/2 teaspoon onion powder

1/2 teaspoon garlic powder

1/4 teaspoon pepper

1 pound boneless pork loin chops, all visible fat discarded, cut into 16 strips, each about 1 inch wide

(continued)

Cooking spray
8 ounces beer (light or nonalcoholic)
1/4 cup barbecue sauce (lowest sodium available)
1/4 cup all-fruit blueberry spread

In a medium bowl, stir together the cumin, chili powder, onion powder, garlic powder, and pepper. Add the pork, turning to coat.

Lightly spray a large skillet with cooking spray. Cook the pork over medium-high heat for 3 minutes on each side, or until browned.

Pour the beer into the skillet. Bring to a simmer. Reduce the heat and simmer, covered, for 1 hour to 1 hour 30 minutes, or until the pork is tender (no stirring needed). Transfer the pork to a serving plate, leaving the liquid in the skillet. Cover the plate to keep warm.

Stir the barbecue sauce and blueberry spread into the cooking liquid. Increase the heat to medium low and cook for 2 to 3 minutes, or until heated through, stirring occasionally. Spoon the sauce over the pork.

PER SERVING

calories 241	**carbohydrates** 19 g
total fat 6.0 g	fiber 0 g
saturated fat 2.0 g	sugars 14 g
trans fat 0.0 g	**protein** 23 g
polyunsaturated fat 1.0 g	**DIETARY EXCHANGES**
monounsaturated fat 2.5 g	1 other carbohydrate,
cholesterol 60 mg	3 lean meat
sodium 168 mg	

KIBBEE

SERVES 6

This popular Middle Eastern dish combines ground meat, usually lamb, with bulgur and seasonings. Serve with Fattoush Salad (page 70).

1 cup uncooked instant (fine-grain) bulgur
Cooking spray
1 pound ground lamb
1 small onion, minced or grated
1 teaspoon ground cinnamon
Pepper to taste (freshly ground preferred)

1/2 cup water
1/4 cup chopped walnuts or pine nuts, dry-roasted
1 tablespoon light tub margarine
1 1/2 cups fat-free plain yogurt

Put the bulgur in a fine-mesh sieve. Run under cold water. Drain well. Let stand for 10 minutes.

Meanwhile, lightly spray an 8-inch square glass baking dish with cooking spray.

In a medium bowl, stir together the lamb, onion, cinnamon, and pepper. Gradually pour in the water as you stir.

Put half the lamb mixture in the baking dish, smoothing the top and patting it down. Sprinkle the walnuts over the lamb mixture. Pat the remaining lamb mixture over the walnuts. Gently cut the contents of the dish into squares. Dot with the margarine.

Bake for 30 minutes. Serve warm with the yogurt on the side for topping.

PER SERVING

calories 253	**carbohydrates** 25 g
total fat 8.5 g	fiber 5 g
saturated fat 2.0 g	sugars 6 g
trans fat 0.0 g	**protein** 20 g
polyunsaturated fat 3.0 g	**DIETARY EXCHANGES**
monounsaturated fat 3.0 g	1 starch, 1/2 other
cholesterol 42 mg	carbohydrate,
sodium 101 mg	2 1/2 lean meat

PORK STIR-FRY WITH SNOW PEAS

SERVES 4

Stir-fries are an ideal healthy cooking technique on a hurried day because the cooking takes such little time. Just be sure to prep the ingredients in advance if you know your time in the kitchen will be limited! Prepare instant brown rice for a speedy side dish.

2 tablespoons sugar
2 tablespoons soy sauce (lowest sodium available)
2 tablespoons dry sherry or 1 tablespoon

fresh lemon juice and 1 tablespoon
water

1 1/2 tablespoons cider vinegar

1 teaspoon grated peeled gingerroot

1 teaspoon toasted sesame oil

1/8 teaspoon crushed red pepper flakes

1 teaspoon canola or corn oil and 1 teaspoon
canola or corn oil, divided use

12 ounces boneless pork cutlets, all visible fat
discarded, cut into thin slices

1 medium yellow or red bell pepper, cut into
thin strips

1 medium onion, cut into 1/2-inch wedges

1 medium garlic clove, minced

3 ounces snow peas, trimmed

In a small bowl, whisk together the sugar, soy
sauce, sherry, vinegar, gingerroot, sesame oil,
and red pepper flakes until the sugar is dissolved. Set aside.

In a wok or large skillet, heat 1 teaspoon oil, swirling to coat the bottom. Cook the pork for 3 minutes, or until no longer pink on the outside and
beginning to brown, stirring frequently. Transfer
the pork to a separate plate.

Pour the remaining 1 teaspoon oil into the wok
or skillet, swirling to coat the bottom. Cook the
bell pepper, onion, and garlic for 4 minutes, or
until beginning to brown, stirring frequently.

Stir in the snow peas. Cook for 1 minute, stirring
frequently.

Stir in the pork and any accumulated juices.
Cook for 1 minute, stirring frequently.

Transfer the pork mixture to a platter. Whisk the
soy sauce mixture. Spoon over all.

Cook's Tip: Adding the sauce just before serving
allows the concentrated flavors to stay on top
and not get lost in the dish.

PER SERVING

calories 196	carbohydrates 14 g
total fat 6.5 g	fiber 2 g
saturated fat 1.5 g	sugars 11 g
trans fat 0.0 g	**protein** 19 g
polyunsaturated fat 1.5 g	**DIETARY EXCHANGES**
monounsaturated fat 3.0 g	1 vegetable, 1/2 other
cholesterol 49 mg	carbohydrate,
sodium 233 mg	2 1/2 lean meat

ARMENIAN LAMB CASSEROLE

SERVES 4

*Tender chunks of lamb, cubes of vegetables, and po-
tent seasoning make this dish a true winner. Serve
over a bed of freekeh or whole-wheat couscous.*

Cooking spray

1 teaspoon canola or corn oil

1 pound lean lamb from loin or shoulder arm
chop, all visible fat discarded, cut into
bite-size cubes

1 medium onion, sliced

1 medium garlic clove, minced

1 cup canned no-salt-added tomatoes,
undrained

1 medium eggplant, cut into cubes

1 medium green bell pepper, coarsely
chopped

2 medium carrots, sliced

2 small zucchini, cut into cubes

1/2 cup sliced okra (6 to 7 small pods)
(optional)

3 slices lemon

1/2 teaspoon paprika

1/8 teaspoon ground cumin

1/8 teaspoon pepper, or to taste

Lightly spray a stockpot, Dutch oven, or large,
deep skillet with cooking spray. Pour in the oil,
swirling to coat the bottom. Heat over medium-
high heat. Cook the lamb for 10 minutes, or until
browned on all sides, turning occasionally.

Stir in the onion and garlic. Cook for 3 to 4 minutes, or until slightly browned.

Stir in the tomatoes with liquid. Reduce the heat
to low. Cook, covered, for 1 hour, stirring occasionally and adding a small amount of water if
necessary.

Preheat the oven to 350°F.

Stir the remaining ingredients into the lamb
mixture. Increase the heat to high and bring to a
boil. Transfer the mixture to a 3-quart ovenproof
ceramic or glass casserole dish. (Don't use un-
coated cast iron; it will discolor the vegetables.)

(continued)

Bake, covered, for 1 hour, or until the vegetables are tender and the onion is very soft.

MOROCCAN-STYLE LAMB WITH COUSCOUS

SERVES 4

Seasonings such as ginger, cumin, and garlic—along with tart lemon quarters and briny kalamata olives—make this lamb dish so tasty that you'll enjoy preparing it on a regular basis. The savory juices soak into the fluffy couscous, infusing it with flavor.

- 1/4 cup golden raisins
- 3/4 pound lean boneless lamb stew meat (from leg, loin, or shoulder arm chops), all visible fat discarded
- 1 cup baby carrots
- 1 medium onion, quartered
- 1 15.5-ounce can no-salt-added chickpeas, rinsed and drained
- 1 cup fat-free, low-sodium chicken broth, such as on page 36
- 1 medium lemon, cut into 4 wedges and seeded
- 1/4 cup chopped kalamata olives
- 1 cinnamon stick (about 3 inches long)
- 2 medium garlic cloves, minced
- 1 teaspoon paprika
- 1 teaspoon ground cumin
- 1/2 teaspoon ground ginger
- 1/4 teaspoon ground turmeric (optional)
- 1/2 cup coarsely chopped fresh cilantro
- 1 cup uncooked whole-wheat couscous

Soak the raisins in warm water to cover for 1 hour. Drain in a colander, discarding the water. Set aside.

Meanwhile, heat a large nonstick saucepan or Dutch oven over medium-high heat. Cook the lamb for 4 to 5 minutes, or until browned on the outside, stirring occasionally.

Stir in the carrots and onion. Cook for 2 to 3 minutes, or until the carrots are tender-crisp and the onion is soft.

Stir in the chickpeas, broth, lemon wedges, olives, cinnamon stick, garlic, paprika, cumin, ginger, and turmeric. Bring to a simmer.

Reduce the heat and simmer, covered, for 1 hour. Stir in the cilantro and raisins. Simmer for 20 to 30 minutes, or until the lamb is tender.

Meanwhile, prepare the couscous using the package directions, omitting the salt. Fluff with a fork. Spoon the couscous onto plates.

Discard the lemon wedges and cinnamon stick. Ladle the lamb mixture over the couscous.

Vegetarian Entrées

GRILLED VEGETABLE PIZZA

SERVES 6

Fresh basil, goat cheese, and Romano cheese lend a gourmet touch to this pizza you cook on the barbecue. Vary the vegetables to include your favorites or whatever's in season. Good choices include eggplant, asparagus, yellow summer squash, and various colors of bell peppers.

2 1/2 cups white whole-wheat flour, 3 to 4 tablespoons white whole-wheat flour, and 1/4 cup white whole-wheat flour (if needed), divided use
1 tablespoon olive oil
1 teaspoon dried Italian seasoning, crumbled
1 1/4-ounce package fast-rising yeast
1 cup warm water (120°F to 130°F)
Cooking spray
3 medium zucchini, halved lengthwise
2 medium portobello mushrooms, stems discarded
1 medium red onion, halved crosswise
2 medium tomatoes (1 red and 1 yellow preferred), halved
1/4 cup coarsely chopped fresh basil
1 1/2 ounces goat cheese crumbles
2 ounces shredded or grated Romano cheese

Put 2 1/2 cups flour in a large bowl. Whisk in the oil, Italian seasoning, and yeast.

Pour in the water, stirring until the dough starts to pull away from the side of the bowl. (You may need extra flour.)

Using 3 to 4 tablespoons flour, lightly flour a flat surface. Turn out the dough. Knead for 6 to 8 minutes, gradually adding, if needed, enough of the remaining 1/4 cup flour to make the dough smooth and elastic. (The dough shouldn't be dry or stick to the surface. You may not need any of the remaining 1/4 cup flour, or you may need all of it if the dough is sticky.)

Cover the dough with a clean, dry dish towel. Let stand for 20 minutes. (You can cover the bowl with plastic wrap and refrigerate the dough for up to 24 hours. Remove the dough from the refrigerator 1 hour before shaping and grilling.)

While the dough is standing, lightly spray a large grill rack with cooking spray. Preheat the grill on medium high.

Lightly spray all sides of the zucchini, mushrooms, and onion with cooking spray. Lightly spray the cut side of the tomatoes with cooking spray.

Grill the onion for 10 minutes on one side. Turn over the onion. Add the mushrooms with the cap side down. Grill for 5 minutes. Turn over the mushrooms. Add the zucchini with the cut side down. Grill for 3 minutes. Turn over the zucchini. Add the tomatoes with the cut side down. Grill for about 3 minutes, or until the onion and mushrooms are soft and the zucchini and tomatoes are tender.

Transfer the vegetables to a cutting board. Let cool for 5 minutes. Coarsely chop the onion and tomatoes, and thinly slice the mushrooms and zucchini. Transfer to a large bowl.

Gently stir the basil into the vegetables.

Meanwhile, lightly spray a large baking sheet with cooking spray. Using a small amount of flour, lightly flour a flat surface. Roll the dough into a 12-inch circle. Transfer to the baking sheet. Lightly spray the top of the dough with cooking spray. Transfer the dough with the sprayed side down to the grill rack.

Grill, covered, for 3 to 4 minutes (watching carefully so it doesn't burn), or until golden brown. Using two large spatulas (or a spatula and tongs), turn over the crust. Spread the vegetable mixture over the crust. Sprinkle the goat cheese and Romano over the vegetable mixture.

Grill, covered, for 3 to 4 minutes, or until the crust is golden brown on the bottom, the vegetables are heated through, and the goat cheese and Romano are slightly melted.

Using tongs, slide the pizza onto a baking sheet. Transfer the pizza to a cooling rack. Let cool for 5 minutes before slicing.

calories 302	**carbohydrates** 42 g
total fat 8.0 g	fiber 8 g
saturated fat 3.0 g	sugars 7 g
trans fat 0.0 g	**protein** 15 g
polyunsaturated fat 1.0 g	**DIETARY EXCHANGES**
monounsaturated fat 3.0 g	2 starch, 2 vegetable,
cholesterol 10 mg	1 lean meat, 1/2 fat
sodium 200 mg	

ARTICHOKE-TOMATO PIZZA ON A PHYLLO CRUST

SERVES 6

Flaky phyllo dough provides a healthy crust alternative for this pizza. It also bakes more quickly than traditional pizza dough (and no rising time!), so you can have homemade pizza any night of the week.

Olive oil cooking spray
4 medium Italian plum (Roma) tomatoes, seeded and chopped
9 ounces frozen artichoke hearts, thawed, drained, and chopped
1/2 cup thinly sliced red onion
1 teaspoon balsamic vinegar
1 medium garlic clove, minced
6 14 x 9-inch frozen phyllo sheets, thawed
1 cup shredded low-fat mozzarella cheese
2 tablespoons shredded or grated Romano cheese
1/2 teaspoon dried Italian seasoning, crumbled

Preheat the oven to 400°F. Lightly spray a large baking dish with cooking spray.

In a medium bowl, stir together the tomatoes, artichokes, onion, vinegar, and garlic.

Keeping the unused phyllo covered with a damp cloth or damp paper towels to prevent drying, place 1 sheet in the dish. Lightly spray with cooking spray. Working quickly, repeat with the remaining phyllo, layering each sheet on top of the previous one.

Spread the tomato mixture over the phyllo. Sprinkle both cheeses over the tomato mixture. Sprinkle the Italian seasoning on top.

Bake for 10 to 15 minutes, or until both cheeses are bubbly and the crust is golden brown around the edges.

Cook's Tip on Phyllo: These fragile, paper-thin sheets of dough, commonly used in Middle Eastern and Mediterranean cooking, are usually found in the freezer section of the supermarket, near the piecrusts and puff pastry. When baked, the dough becomes flaky and crumbly.

PER SERVING

calories 109	**carbohydrates** 15 g
total fat 2.5 g	fiber 4 g
saturated fat 1.0 g	sugars 2 g
trans fat 0.0 g	**protein** 7 g
polyunsaturated fat 0.0 g	**DIETARY EXCHANGES**
monounsaturated fat 1.0 g	1/2 starch, 1 vegetable,
cholesterol 8 mg	1 lean meat
sodium 217 mg	

PORTOBELLO ALFREDO-BASIL PIZZA

SERVES 4

Meaty portobello mushroom caps step in for the crust, while puréed cannellini beans, pesto, and Parmesan unite to create an Alfredo-style sauce. Topped with cherry tomatoes and creamy mozzarella, this vegetarian meal is sure to be a big hit.

Cooking spray
4 4- to 5-inch portobello mushroom caps, stems discarded and dark gills scraped away
1 cup canned no-salt-added cannellini beans, rinsed and drained
2 tablespoons fat-free, low-sodium vegetable broth, such as on page 36, or fat-free milk
2 tablespoons shredded or grated Parmesan cheese
2 tablespoons finely chopped fresh basil
1/4 teaspoon pepper
1 1/2 teaspoons olive oil
1 small garlic clove, minced
1/2 cup red and yellow cherry tomatoes, thickly sliced crosswise
2 ounces low-fat mozzarella, sliced (about 1/2 cup)

(continued)

Preheat the oven to 450°F. Line a small rimmed baking sheet with aluminum foil. Lightly spray with cooking spray.

Place the mushroom caps with the stem side up on the baking sheet. Bake for 12 to 15 minutes, or until the mushrooms are almost soft. Discard any liquid that forms in the mushroom cap.

Meanwhile, in a food processor or blender, pulse the beans with the broth until smooth. Stir in the Parmesan, basil, and pepper. In a small bowl, whisk together the oil and garlic.

Brush the mushroom caps with the oil mixture. Spread the bean mixture over the caps. Top with the tomatoes and mozzarella.

Bake for 5 to 10 minutes, or until the toppings are hot and the mozzarella is melted.

Cook's Tip: You can substitute 1 tablespoon refrigerated basil pesto for the fresh basil if you prefer. Just reduce the Parmesan to 1 1/2 tablespoons.

PER SERVING

calories 125	carbohydrates 14 g
total fat 4.5 g	fiber 4 g
saturated fat 1.0 g	sugars 2 g
trans fat 0.0 g	protein 9 g
polyunsaturated fat 0.5 g	DIETARY EXCHANGES
monounsaturated fat 2.0 g	1/2 starch, 1 vegetable,
cholesterol 7 mg	1 lean meat
sodium 168 mg	

FLUFFY FONDUE CASSEROLE

SERVES 6

This cheese-flavored egg-white casserole, which puffs up like a soufflé, is a must-have dish for your next brunch. It makes a beautiful presentation when served with fruit salad, such as Berry Explosion Salad *(page 86) or* Ginger-Infused Watermelon and Mixed Berries *(page 87), garnished with sprigs of fresh mint.*

Cooking spray
2 tablespoons light tub margarine

4 slices whole-grain bread (lowest sodium available), toasted
4 large egg whites
1 1/2 cups low-fat cottage cheese
1 1/4 cups fat-free milk
1/4 cup fat-free dry milk
1 heaping tablespoon chopped chives
1 tablespoon dry sherry
1/4 teaspoon dry mustard
1/4 teaspoon paprika
1/4 teaspoon pepper
1/4 teaspoon Worcestershire sauce (lowest sodium available)

Preheat the oven to 350°F.

Lightly spray a 13 x 9 x 2-inch glass baking dish with cooking spray. Spread the margarine over the toast. Cut into cubes. Arrange the cubes in a single layer in the baking dish.

In a large metal or glass mixing bowl, using an electric mixer on high speed, beat the egg whites until stiff peaks form (the peaks don't fall when the beaters are lifted).

In a food processor or blender, process the cottage cheese until smooth and creamy. Add the remaining ingredients. Process until smooth.

Carefully fold the cottage cheese mixture into the egg whites. Pour into the baking dish. Bake for 45 minutes to 1 hour, or until a knife inserted in the center comes out clean.

PER SERVING

calories 151	carbohydrates 14 g
total fat 3.5 g	fiber 1 g
saturated fat 0.5 g	sugars 7 g
trans fat 0.0 g	protein 14 g
polyunsaturated fat 0.5 g	DIETARY EXCHANGES
monounsaturated fat 1.5 g	1/2 starch, 1/2 fat-free
cholesterol 7 mg	milk, 1 lean meat
sodium 367 mg	

SPINACH SOUFFLÉ

SERVES 4

Complement this airy soufflé with a light side soup such as Fresh Mushroom Soup *(page 41).*

> Cooking spray
> 2 tablespoons canola or corn oil
> 2 tablespoons whole-wheat flour
> 1/2 cup fat-free milk
> 10 ounces frozen chopped spinach, cooked, well drained, and squeezed dry
> 2 tablespoons finely chopped onion
> 1/4 heaping teaspoon ground nutmeg
> 1/4 heaping teaspoon pepper, or to taste
> 6 medium egg whites
> 3 tablespoons shredded or grated Parmesan cheese

Preheat the oven to 350°F. Lightly spray a 1 3/4-quart casserole dish with cooking spray. Set aside.

In a small, heavy saucepan, heat the oil over medium-high heat, swirling to coat the bottom. Whisk in the flour. Cook for 1 minute, or until the mixture is smooth and bubbly, whisking constantly. Remove from the heat.

Gradually whisk in the milk. Return to the heat and cook for 1 minute, whisking constantly. Remove from the heat.

In a large bowl, stir together the spinach, onion, nutmeg, and pepper. Stir in the milk mixture.

In a large metal or glass mixing bowl, beat the egg whites until stiff peaks form. Using a rubber scraper, fold gently into the spinach mixture. Gently transfer to the casserole dish. Sprinkle the Parmesan over all.

Bake for 35 minutes, or until the center is set. Serve immediately.

PER SERVING

calories 146	**carbohydrates** 8 g
total fat 9.0 g	fiber 3 g
saturated fat 1.5 g	sugars 3 g
trans fat 0.0 g	**protein** 10 g
polyunsaturated fat 2.0 g	**DIETARY EXCHANGES**
monounsaturated fat 5.0 g	1 vegetable, 1 lean
cholesterol 3 mg	meat, 1 fat
sodium 198 mg	

FARMSTAND FRITTATA

SERVES 4

Frittatas are an Italian creation—basically an omelet that's not folded. Veggies, low-fat cheese, and seasonings are whisked together with the egg substitute. Serve with a cup of Creamy Basil-Tomato Soup *(page 43).*

> 1 1/2 cups egg substitute
> 1/2 cup shredded low-fat mozzarella cheese
> 2 tablespoons fat-free half-and-half
> 2 medium garlic cloves, finely chopped
> 1/2 teaspoon dried Italian seasoning, crumbled
> 1/4 teaspoon crushed red pepper flakes
> 1 medium red bell pepper, chopped
> 1/2 cup chopped onion
> Cooking spray
> 1 6-ounce zucchini, halved lengthwise, then cut crosswise into 1/4-inch slices
> 1 teaspoon olive oil
> 1 tablespoon shredded or grated Parmesan cheese
> Pepper or crushed red pepper flakes to taste (optional)

Preheat the oven to 350°F.

In a medium bowl, whisk together the egg substitute, mozzarella, half-and-half, garlic, Italian seasoning, and red pepper flakes. Set aside.

Heat a 10-inch nonstick skillet with an ovenproof handle (or you can wrap the handle in aluminum foil) over medium-high heat for 2 minutes. Remove the skillet from the burner, leaving the

(continued)

heat on. Spread the bell pepper and onion in the skillet. Lightly spray the mixture with cooking spray. Cook for 3 minutes, or until the onion is just beginning to soften, stirring frequently.

Reduce the heat to medium. Stir in the zucchini. Cook for 4 minutes, or until the zucchini begins to soften and the onion begins to turn golden, stirring frequently.

Reduce the heat to low. Stir in the oil. Spread the mixture in the skillet.

Whisk the egg substitute mixture to recombine. Pour over the bell pepper mixture. Cook for 1 to 2 minutes, or until partially set, lifting the edge of the frittata with a spatula and tilting the skillet so the uncooked portion flows under the edge.

Transfer the skillet to the oven and bake for 5 minutes. Remove from the oven and gently lift the edge of the frittata to allow a little of the uncooked mixture to flow underneath. Bake for 7 to 8 minutes, or until firm, puffy, and golden. Sprinkle with the Parmesan and pepper.

Cook's Tip on Egg Substitute: If you prefer to replace egg substitute with eggs, here's what you should know about the differences in calories, saturated fat, and sodium. One large egg contains 72 calories, 1.6 grams of saturated fat, 71 milligrams of sodium, and 186 milligrams of cholesterol. The egg substitute equivalent (1/4 cup) contains 30 calories, 0 grams of saturated fat, 115 milligrams of sodium, and 0 milligrams of cholesterol.

PER SERVING

calories 120	**sodium** 323 mg
total fat 3.0 g	**carbohydrates** 9 g
saturated fat 1.0 g	fiber 2 g
trans fat 0.0 g	sugars 5 g
polyunsaturated fat 0.0 g	**protein** 15 g
monounsaturated fat 1.5 g	**DIETARY EXCHANGES**
cholesterol 6 mg	1 vegetable, 2 lean meat

ASPARAGUS AND ARTICHOKE QUICHE

SERVES 4

This quiche is a vegetarian pie with a brown rice crust, which is very easy to assemble. Serve the wedges of quiche with chilled slices of honeydew melon.

> 1 1/4 cups fat-free, low-sodium vegetable broth, such as on page 36
> 1 teaspoon salt-free all-purpose seasoning blend
> 1 cup uncooked instant brown rice
> Cooking spray
> 1 large egg white, lightly beaten with a fork
> 8 medium asparagus spears, trimmed and cut into 1/4-inch slices
> 1 cup chopped canned artichoke hearts, drained
> 2 medium Italian plum (Roma) tomatoes, thinly sliced
> 1 cup fat-free half-and-half
> 1/2 cup egg substitute
> 1/4 cup shredded or grated Parmesan cheese
> 1/4 teaspoon pepper

In a medium saucepan, bring the broth and seasoning blend to a simmer over medium-high heat. Stir in the rice. Reduce the heat and simmer, covered, for 10 minutes, or until the rice is tender. Transfer to a medium bowl. Refrigerate for 10 minutes to cool.

Preheat the oven to 400°F. Lightly spray a 9-inch pie pan with cooking spray.

Stir the egg white into the cooled rice. Firmly press the mixture on the bottom and up the sides of the pan, forming a crust.

Bake for 6 to 7 minutes, or until the rice is golden brown. Remove the crust from the oven. Reduce the oven temperature to 325°F.

Arrange the asparagus in the warm crust. Top with the artichokes, then the tomatoes.

In a medium bowl, whisk together the remaining ingredients. Pour over the vegetables.

Bake for 40 to 45 minutes, or until a knife inserted in the center comes out clean. Transfer to a cooling rack. Let cool for 10 minutes before cutting into wedges.

PER SERVING

calories 199	**carbohydrates** 32 g
total fat 2.0 g	fiber 2 g
saturated fat 1.0 g	sugars 6 g
trans fat 0.0 g	**protein** 14 g
polyunsaturated fat 0.5 g	**DIETARY EXCHANGES**
monounsaturated fat 0.5 g	1 1/2 starch,
cholesterol 4 mg	1 vegetable, 1 1/2 lean
sodium 356 mg	meat

SPINACH QUICHE

SERVES 6

This whole-grain crust makes this quiche healthier than those made with ready-made crusts or traditional crusts made with butter. Enjoy it with a fruit salad or soup, such as Ginger-Infused Watermelon and Mixed Berries *(page 87) or* Minted Cantaloupe Soup with Fresh Lime *(page 50).*

Cooking spray
1/4 cup uncooked instant brown rice
1 large egg, lightly beaten using a fork, and 2 large eggs, divided use
1 tablespoon shredded or grated Parmesan cheese and 2 tablespoons shredded or grated Parmesan cheese, divided use
2 teaspoons canola or corn oil
1 medium onion, chopped
10 ounces frozen chopped spinach, thawed and squeezed dry
1 tablespoon fresh lemon juice
1/2 teaspoon ground nutmeg
Pepper to taste (freshly ground preferred)
1 cup fat-free milk

Preheat the oven to 425°F. Lightly spray a 9-inch pie pan with cooking spray.

Prepare the rice using the package directions, omitting the salt and margarine.

In a medium bowl, stir together the beaten egg, 1 tablespoon Parmesan, and the rice. Firmly press the mixture on the bottom and up the sides of the pan, forming a crust.

Bake for 3 minutes. Remove from the oven. Let stand to cool.

In a small skillet, heat the oil over medium-high heat, swirling to coat the bottom. Cook the onion for 5 minutes, or until slightly browned, stirring frequently.

Prepare the spinach using the package directions, omitting the salt and margarine, but adding the lemon juice, nutmeg, and pepper. Stir the onion into the spinach.

Spread the spinach mixture over the crust. Sprinkle the remaining 2 tablespoons Parmesan over the spinach mixture. In a small bowl, whisk together the milk and the remaining 2 eggs. Pour over the spinach mixture.

Bake for 10 minutes. Reduce the oven temperature to 350°F. Bake for 30 minutes, or until a knife inserted in the center comes out clean. Transfer to a cooling rack. Let cool for 10 minutes before cutting into wedges.

PER SERVING

calories 225	**carbohydrates** 36 g
total fat 2.5 g	fiber 7 g
saturated fat 0.5 g	sugars 10 g
trans fat 0.0 g	**protein** 15 g
polyunsaturated fat 0.5 g	**DIETARY EXCHANGES**
monounsaturated fat 1.0 g	2 starch, 1 vegetable,
cholesterol 3 mg	1 1/2 lean meat
sodium 212 mg	

ITALIAN QUICHE

SERVES 6

A classic French quiche is a rich cheese custard tart. This lightened version with its nutty-tasting quinoa crust brims with vegetables and herbs.

(continued)

1/2 cup uncooked quinoa, rinsed and drained

Cooking spray

1 large egg white

1/4 teaspoon salt and 1/4 teaspoon salt, divided use

1 small or 1/2 medium yellow summer squash, chopped

1 large green onion, sliced

2 medium garlic cloves, minced

1 cup fat-free evaporated milk

1/2 cup egg substitute

1/8 teaspoon pepper

2 medium Italian plum (Roma) tomatoes, halved, seeds and liquid discarded, chopped

2 tablespoons chopped fresh basil or dillweed or 1 teaspoon dried basil or dillweed, crumbled

2 tablespoons shredded or grated Parmesan cheese

In a small saucepan, prepare the quinoa using the package directions, omitting the salt. Fluff with a fork.

When the quinoa is almost done, preheat the oven to 375°F.

Lightly spray a 9-inch pie pan with cooking spray. In a medium bowl, stir together the cooked quinoa, the egg white, and 1/4 teaspoon salt. Firmly press the mixture on the bottom and up the sides of the pan, forming a crust.

Bake for 20 minutes. Transfer to a cooling rack. Reduce the oven temperature to 325°F.

Lightly spray a medium skillet with cooking spray. Heat over medium-low heat. Cook the squash, green onion, and garlic for 5 minutes, or until crisp-tender, stirring occasionally. Let cool for 5 minutes.

In a medium bowl, stir together the milk, egg substitute, pepper, and the remaining 1/4 teaspoon salt. Stir in the squash mixture, tomatoes, and basil. Pour into the quinoa crust. Sprinkle the Parmesan over the quiche.

Bake for 35 to 40 minutes, or until a knife inserted in the center comes out clean. Transfer

to a cooling rack. Let cool for 10 minutes before cutting into wedges.

PER SERVING

calories 115	sodium 325 mg
total fat 1.5 g	**carbohydrates** 16 g
saturated fat 0.5 g	fiber 2 g
trans fat 0.0 g	sugars 7 g
polyunsaturated fat 0.5 g	**protein** 9 g
monounsaturated fat 0.5 g	**DIETARY EXCHANGES**
cholesterol 3 mg	1 starch, 1 lean meat

TOMATO QUICHE

SERVES 4

Couscous is usually thought of as a quick side dish, but it also makes a delicious crust for a dill-flavored tomato-and-egg filling. Serve with Yogurt-Fruit Soup (page 48) for a light, summery meal.

Cooking spray

Crust

1/2 cup fat-free, low-sodium vegetable broth, such as on page 36

1/2 cup water

1/2 cup uncooked whole-wheat couscous

1/8 teaspoon ground turmeric

1 medium egg white

Filling

1 teaspoon olive oil

4 ounces button mushrooms, coarsely chopped

6 medium green onions, chopped

2 medium garlic cloves, minced

6 medium Italian plum (Roma) tomatoes, thickly sliced

2 tablespoons shredded or grated Parmesan cheese

3/4 cup egg substitute

1 5-ounce can fat-free evaporated milk

1 tablespoon fresh dillweed or 1 teaspoon dried dillweed, crumbled

1/4 teaspoon pepper

Preheat the oven to 400°F. Lightly spray a 9-inch pie pan with cooking spray.

In a medium saucepan, bring the broth and water to a boil over medium-high heat. Stir in the couscous and turmeric. Remove from the heat. Let stand, covered, for 5 minutes.

Stir the egg white into the couscous. Firmly press the mixture on the bottom and up the sides of the pan, forming a crust.

Bake for 10 minutes. Remove the crust from the oven. Let cool completely, about 30 minutes.

After the crust has been removed, reduce the oven temperature to 350°F.

In a medium nonstick skillet, heat the oil over medium-high heat, swirling to coat the bottom. Cook the mushrooms, green onions, and garlic for 2 to 3 minutes, or until the vegetables are tender.

Arrange the tomato slices on the crust, cover with the mushroom mixture, and sprinkle the Parmesan over all.

In a medium bowl, whisk together the remaining ingredients. Pour over the vegetables.

Bake for 40 to 45 minutes, or until a knife inserted in the center comes out clean. Transfer to a cooling rack. Let cool for 10 minutes before cutting into wedges.

PER SERVING

calories 225	carbohydrates 36 g
total fat 2.5 g	fiber 7 g
saturated fat 0.5 g	sugars 10 g
trans fat 0.0 g	**protein** 15 g
polyunsaturated fat 0.5 g	**DIETARY EXCHANGES**
monounsaturated fat 1.0 g	2 starch, 1 vegetable,
cholesterol 3.0 mg	1 1/2 lean meat
sodium 212 mg	

POACHED EGGS WITH PESTO BULGUR

SERVES 4

This pesto replaces traditional olive oil with vegetable broth and trades the usual pine nuts for walnuts. It combines with a whole grain to create a hearty bed on which delicate poached eggs lie.

> 2/3 cup uncooked instant, or fine-grain, bulgur
> 1 1/3 cups fat-free, low-sodium vegetable broth and 2 tablespoons fat-free, low-sodium vegetable broth, such as on page 36, divided use
> 1 cup tightly packed fresh basil
> 2 tablespoons chopped walnuts, dry-roasted
> 1 small garlic clove, minced
> 1/8 teaspoon salt
> Dash of cayenne
> 1/2 cup finely chopped yellow or red bell pepper
> 1/4 cup thinly sliced green onions
> 4 cups water
> 1 tablespoon white vinegar
> 4 large eggs
> 1 medium lemon, cut into 4 wedges

In a medium saucepan, prepare the bulgur using the package directions, omitting the salt and substituting 1 1/3 cups broth for the water. Fluff with a fork.

Meanwhile, in a food processor or blender, process the basil, walnuts, garlic, salt, cayenne, and the remaining 2 tablespoons broth until smooth. Stir the basil mixture, bell pepper, and green onions into the bulgur.

In a large skillet, bring the water and vinegar to a boil over high heat. Reduce the heat and simmer. Break an egg into a cup and then carefully slip the egg into the simmering water. Repeat with the remaining eggs, placing them in the water so they don't touch. Simmer for 3 to 5 minutes, or until the whites are completely set and the yolks are beginning to set, but aren't hard. Using

(continued)

a slotted spoon, drain the eggs well and place on the bulgur mixture. Serve with the lemon wedges.

Cook's Tip: The vinegar helps the egg whites firm up faster and prevents them from spreading too much.

OPEN-FACE BULGUR AND MUSHROOM BURGERS

SERVES 4

Sunny-side up eggs with runny yolks top these earthy grain-and-veggie burgers that are served open face. For a side salad, try Green Bean and Tomato Toss *(page 79).*

- 1/2 cup fat-free, low-sodium vegetable broth, such as on page 36
- 1/3 cup uncooked instant (fine-grain) bulgur
- 2 teaspoons olive oil
- 1 1/2 cups chopped cremini or baby bella mushrooms
- 1/2 cup sliced green onions
- 1 tablespoon balsamic vinegar
- 1/3 cup chopped walnuts, dry-roasted
- 1/4 cup whole-wheat panko (Japanese-style bread crumbs)
- 3 tablespoons egg substitute
- 1/2 teaspoon dried thyme, crumbled
- 1/4 teaspoon red hot-pepper sauce
- 4 large eggs
- 2 whole-grain round sandwich thins (lowest sodium available), split
- 4 tomato slices

In a small saucepan, bring the broth to a boil over high heat. Stir in the bulgur. Remove from the heat and set aside, covered, for 20 minutes. Drain well.

Meanwhile, in a medium nonstick skillet, heat the oil over medium heat. Cook the mushrooms and green onions for 6 to 8 minutes, or until the mushrooms are tender, stirring occasionally.

Stir in the vinegar. Spread on a plate and let cool to room temperature, about 30 minutes.

Preheat the broiler. Line a baking sheet with aluminum foil.

Put the mushroom mixture and walnuts in a food processor. Pulse until coarsely chopped. Using a rubber scraper, scrape down the side.

Add the bulgur, panko, egg substitute, thyme, and hot-pepper sauce. Process until combined, scraping the side of the bowl as necessary.

Using a heaping 1/3 cup for each, form the bulgur mixture into four 1/2-inch-thick patties (the mixture may seem a little wet). Transfer the patties to the baking sheet.

Broil the patties 4 to 6 inches from the heat for 4 minutes on each side, or until browned.

Meanwhile, in a large nonstick skillet, cook the eggs to the desired doneness.

Toast the sandwich thins. Top each half with a tomato slice. Place the burgers on the tomatoes. Top with the eggs.

Cook's Tip: If you don't cool the mushroom mixture to room temperature, it might start cooking the egg substitute when you blend it in.

CARROT, PARSNIP, AND POTATO PANCAKES

SERVES 6

Inspired by latkes, a Hanukkah staple, these veggie pancakes are an addictive treat any time of year, especially when paired with a creamy, spicy dipping sauce.

Sauce

- 1 cup fat-free sour cream
- 1 tablespoon chopped fresh dillweed
- 1 tablespoon bottled white horseradish, drained
- 1 tablespoon fresh lemon juice
- 1/8 teaspoon salt

■ ■ ■

- 1 pound potatoes (about 3 medium), coarsely grated and squeezed dry
- 1 1/4 cups egg substitute
- 2 medium carrots, coarsely grated and squeezed dry
- 1 medium parsnip, coarsely grated and squeezed dry
- 1 small onion, minced
- 3 tablespoons chopped fresh chives or green onions (green part only)
- 2 tablespoons all-purpose flour
- 2 tablespoons plain dry bread crumbs (lowest sodium available)
- 1/4 teaspoon salt
- Pepper to taste

In a small bowl, whisk together the sauce ingredients. Cover and refrigerate until serving time.

In a large bowl, stir together the remaining ingredients.

Heat a large nonstick griddle or skillet over medium heat. Drop heaping tablespoons of the potato mixture onto the griddle, using the back of a spoon to flatten the pancakes slightly. Cook for 3 to 4 minutes on each side, or until golden brown. Transfer to a serving platter. Stirring to combine between batches as needed, cook the remaining batter. You should get about 24 pancakes.

About 10 minutes before serving time, remove the sauce from the refrigerator. Let stand to bring to room temperature. Serve the pancakes hot or at room temperature with the sauce.

PER SERVING

calories 178	**carbohydrates** 33 g
total fat 0.5 g	fiber 3 g
saturated fat 0.0 g	sugars 8 g
trans fat 0.0 g	**protein** 11 g
polyunsaturated fat 0.0 g	**DIETARY EXCHANGES**
monounsaturated fat 0.0 g	2 starch, 1 vegetable,
cholesterol 7 mg	1 lean meat
sodium 334 mg	

MEATLESS MOUSSAKA

SERVES 8

Traditional moussaka includes layers of sliced eggplant and ground beef or lamb, often with a rich béchamel sauce. This meatless version combines broiled eggplant with a savory tomato sauce and cheesy filling for a rich, satisfying casserole you'll want to make often.

- Cooking spray
- 2 pounds eggplant, peeled and thickly sliced crosswise

Sauce

- 1 teaspoon olive oil
- 1 large onion, finely chopped
- 3 medium garlic cloves, minced
- 1 14.5-ounce can diced no-salt-added tomatoes, undrained
- 1 cup water
- 1 6-ounce can no-salt-added tomato paste
- 2 teaspoons dried rosemary, crushed
- 2 tablespoons chopped fresh parsley
- 2 tablespoons chopped fresh mint

Filling

- 16 ounces fat-free cottage cheese
- 1/2 cup egg substitute
- 2 tablespoons shredded or grated Parmesan cheese
- 1 teaspoon dried rosemary, crushed
- 1/2 teaspoon dried oregano, crumbled
- 1/2 teaspoon pepper, or to taste

(continued)

•••

1/4 cup shredded or grated Parmesan cheese

Preheat the broiler. Lightly spray a 13 x 9 x 2-inch glass baking dish with cooking spray.

Lightly spray both sides of the eggplant slices with cooking spray. Transfer to two large baking sheets.

Broil about 6 inches from the heat for 5 minutes on each side, or until the eggplant is browned and tender.

Preheat the oven to 375°F.

In a large skillet, heat the oil over medium-high heat, swirling to coat the bottom. Cook the onion and garlic for 3 minutes, or until the onion is soft, stirring frequently.

Stir in the tomatoes with liquid, water, tomato paste, and rosemary. Bring to simmer. Reduce the heat and simmer for 10 minutes. Stir in the parsley and mint. Remove from the heat.

In a medium bowl, whisk together the filling ingredients.

In the baking dish, layer as follows: half the sauce, half the eggplant, all the filling, the remaining eggplant, and the remaining sauce. Top with the Parmesan.

Bake, covered, for 45 minutes. Bake, uncovered, for 10 minutes.

PER SERVING

calories 130	carbohydrates 19 g
total fat 2.0 g	fiber 5 g
saturated fat 1.0 g	sugars 11 g
trans fat 0.0 g	protein 12 g
polyunsaturated fat 0.0 g	DIETARY EXCHANGES
monounsaturated fat 1.0 g	3 vegetable 1 1/2 lean
cholesterol 5 mg	meat
sodium 331 mg	

STUFFED PEPPERS
SERVES 4

In this fresh take on a classic, the peppers are roasted first to add a deeper flavor and smoother texture that contrasts well with the crunchy stuffing combination of vegetables, brown rice, and water chestnuts.

Cooking spray
4 large bell peppers, any color or combination, halved lengthwise through the stems, seeds and ribs discarded
1/2 cup uncooked instant brown rice
1 teaspoon olive oil
2 medium tomatoes, chopped
1 medium yellow summer squash, diced
1 medium zucchini, diced
1 medium onion, diced
2 medium garlic cloves, minced
1/2 cup grated low-fat Cheddar cheese
1/4 cup sliced water chestnuts, drained
1 cup no-salt-added tomato juice

Preheat the oven to 400°F.

Lightly spray the bell pepper halves all over with cooking spray. Place in a 13 x 9 x 2-inch baking dish with the cut sides down. Roast for 10 to 15 minutes, or until just tender. Remove from the oven. Let cool slightly. Reduce the oven temperature to 375°F.

Meanwhile, prepare the rice using the package directions, omitting the salt and margarine. Set aside.

In a large skillet, heat the oil over medium heat, swirling to coat the bottom. Cook the tomatoes, yellow squash, zucchini, onion, and garlic for 3 to 4 minutes, or until the zucchini is tender-crisp, stirring occasionally. Don't overcook.

In a medium bowl, stir together the rice, Cheddar, and water chestnuts. Gently stir into the tomato mixture. Turn over the bell pepper halves. Spoon the rice mixture into the bell pepper halves.

Carefully pour the tomato juice around—not over—the bell peppers.

Bake, covered, for 15 to 20 minutes. Uncover and bake for 5 minutes.

PER SERVING

calories 166	**carbohydrates** 29 g
total fat 3.0 g	fiber 7 g
saturated fat 1.0 g	sugars 12 g
trans fat 0.0 g	**protein** 9 g
polyunsaturated fat 0.5 g	**DIETARY EXCHANGES**
monounsaturated fat 1.5 g	1/2 starch, 4 vegetable,
cholesterol 3 mg	1/2 lean meat
sodium 111 mg	

CHILES RELLENOS

SERVES 4

This popular dish is one of the best ways to celebrate the chile. A roasted, peeled, and seeded poblano or Anaheim pepper is stuffed with any of a variety of fillings—cheese, beef, or chicken—and coated with an egg batter. Usually the stuffed pepper is then deep-fried, but this healthier version is baked.

    Cooking spray
    4 medium poblano or Anaheim peppers
        (about 2 ounces each) (see Cook's Tip on
        Handling Hot Chiles, page 24)
    2 ounces shredded queso asadero or low-fat
        Monterey Jack cheese (about 1/2 cup)
    2 ounces requesón or fat-free ricotta cheese
        (about 1/2 cup)
    1/2 teaspoon chili powder
    1/4 to 1/2 teaspoon garlic powder
    1/8 teaspoon ground cumin
    1/8 teaspoon cayenne
    1/8 teaspoon pepper
    3 large egg whites
    1/4 cup all-purpose flour
    1/2 cup yellow cornmeal

Preheat the broiler. Lightly spray the broiler pan with cooking spray.

Using a thin, sharp knife, make a small slit near the stem of each pepper. Broil the peppers on the broiler pan 3 to 4 inches from the heat, turning until the peppers are charred all over. Put the peppers in a bowl and let stand, covered,

for at least 15 minutes. Rinse the peppers with cold water, discarding the skin, ribs, seeds, and stems. Blot the peppers dry with paper towels.

In a small bowl, stir together both cheeses, the chili powder, garlic powder, cumin, cayenne, and pepper. Spoon the mixture into the peppers.

Preheat the oven to 350°F. Lightly spray a baking sheet with cooking spray.

In a medium metal or glass mixing bowl, using an electric mixer on high speed, beat the egg whites until stiff peaks form (the peaks don't fall when the beaters are lifted).

Put the flour and cornmeal in separate shallow dishes. Set the flour, egg whites, and cornmeal in a row, assembly-line fashion. Carefully dip the peppers in the flour, then the egg whites, and finally the cornmeal, turning to coat at each step and gently shaking off any excess. Place the peppers on the baking sheet.

Lightly spray the peppers with cooking spray. Bake for 15 to 20 minutes, or until the top of each pepper is lightly browned.

PER SERVING

calories 178	**carbohydrates** 25 g
total fat 4.5 g	fiber 2 g
saturated fat 2.5 g	sugars 3 g
trans fat 0.0 g	**protein** 10 g
polyunsaturated fat 0.5 g	**DIETARY EXCHANGES**
monounsaturated fat 1.5 g	1 1/2 starch, 1 lean
cholesterol 17 mg	meat
sodium 157 mg	

EGGPLANT PARMESAN

SERVES 4

Cut out lots of saturated fat, cholesterol, and sodium by eating homemade eggplant Parmesan instead of paying more for the far-less-healthy restaurant version.

(continued)

Cooking spray

Eggplant

    2 large egg whites

    2 tablespoons fat-free milk

    1/2 cup plain dry bread crumbs (lowest
        sodium available)

    2 tablespoons shredded or grated Parmesan
        cheese

    1/2 teaspoon dried basil, crumbled

    1/2 teaspoon dried oregano, crumbled

    1 1 1/2-pound eggplant, cut crosswise into
        12 slices

Sauce

    2 teaspoons olive oil

    1 small onion, diced

    1 medium garlic clove, minced

    2 14-ounce cans no-salt-added Italian plum
        (Roma) tomatoes, chopped, undrained

    1/4 teaspoon dried basil, crumbled

    1/4 teaspoon dried oregano, crumbled

■ ■ ■

    1/2 cup shredded low-fat mozzarella cheese

    1 tablespoon shredded or grated Parmesan
        cheese

Preheat the oven to 350°F. Lightly spray a large rimmed baking sheet and a 15 x 10 x 1-inch glass baking dish with cooking spray.

In a shallow dish, whisk together the egg whites and milk. In a separate shallow dish, stir together the bread crumbs, 2 tablespoons Parmesan, 1/2 teaspoon basil, and 1/2 teaspoon oregano. Set the dishes and the baking sheet in a row, assembly-line fashion. Dip the eggplant in the egg white mixture, then in the bread crumb mixture, turning to coat at each step and gently shaking off any excess. Using your fingertips, gently press the coating so it adheres to the eggplant. Place the eggplant slices in a single layer on the baking sheet. Lightly spray the top side of the eggplant with cooking spray.

Bake for 25 to 30 minutes, or until the eggplant is browned on the bottom. Turn over the eggplant. Bake for 10 to 15 minutes, or until

browned. Transfer the baking sheet to a cooling rack. Leave the oven on.

Meanwhile, in a large nonstick skillet, heat the oil over medium-high heat, swirling to coat the bottom. Cook the onion for 3 minutes, or until soft, stirring frequently.

Stir in the garlic. Cook for 1 minute, stirring constantly.

Stir in the tomatoes with liquid, the remaining 1/4 teaspoon basil, and the remaining 1/4 teaspoon oregano. Bring to a boil. Reduce the heat and simmer for 15 minutes, or until the sauce has thickened.

Spread 2 cups sauce in the baking dish. Arrange the eggplant slices in slightly overlapping layers on the sauce. Spoon the remaining sauce over the eggplant. Sprinkle both cheeses over all.

Bake for 15 to 20 minutes, or until the sauce is bubbly and the cheeses have melted.

Cook's Tip: If you don't have a 15 x 10 x 1-inch glass baking dish, use a 13 x 9 x 2-inch glass baking dish and overlap the eggplant slices as needed.

PER SERVING

calories 218	carbohydrates 32 g
total fat 6.0 g	fiber 8 g
saturated fat 1.5 g	sugars 14 g
trans fat 0.0 g	protein 13 g
polyunsaturated fat 1.0 g	DIETARY EXCHANGES
monounsaturated fat 2.5 g	1/2 starch, 4 vegetable,
cholesterol 8 mg	1 lean meat, 1/2 fat
sodium 318 mg	

EGGPLANT ZUCCHINI CASSEROLE
SERVES 8

Put uncooked spaghetti right in the casserole. Everything bakes together—no pasta pot to wash! While the casserole is baking, prepare a salad, such as Spinach Salad with Chickpeas and Cider Vinaigrette *(page 67).*

    Cooking spray

Sauce

    2 8-ounce cans no-salt-added tomato sauce
    2 teaspoons Worcestershire sauce (lowest
        sodium available)
    2 medium garlic cloves, crushed
    1 teaspoon dried oregano, crumbled
    1/2 teaspoon dried basil, crumbled
    1/2 teaspoon dried marjoram, crumbled
    Pepper to taste

■ ■ ■

    1 medium eggplant, peeled and sliced
        crosswise
    2 medium zucchini, sliced crosswise
    4 ounces dried whole-grain spaghetti, broken
        into thirds (about 1 cup)
    3 medium ribs of celery, chopped
    1 medium onion, chopped
    1 medium green bell pepper, chopped
    8 ounces low-fat mozzarella cheese, cut into
        18 small slices

Preheat the oven to 350°F. Lightly spray a 13 x 9 x 2-inch casserole dish with cooking spray.

In a medium bowl, stir together the sauce ingredients.

In the casserole dish, layer as follows: half the eggplant slices arranged in a single layer, and half each of the zucchini, spaghetti, celery, onion, bell pepper, mozzarella, and tomato sauce mixture. Repeat the layers.

Bake, covered, for 1 hour, or until the vegetables are tender.

PER SERVING

calories 159	carbohydrates 23 g
total fat 3.5 g	fiber 6 g
saturated fat 1.0 g	sugars 8 g
trans fat 0.0 g	**protein** 11 g
polyunsaturated fat 0.5 g	**DIETARY EXCHANGES**
monounsaturated fat 1.0 g	1 starch, 2 vegetable,
cholesterol 10 mg	1 lean meat
sodium 230 mg	

KOHLRABI GRATIN

SERVES 4

If you like scalloped potatoes, you'll love this entrée with similar flavors. Although a member of the same family as turnips, kohlrabi is milder and sweeter. To serve the kohlrabi leaves on the side, see the Cook's Tip on Kohlrabi on page 316.

    Cooking spray
    2 medium kohlrabi bulbs (about
        1 1/4 pounds), trimmed, peeled, and cut
        into 1/4-inch slices
    1 cup water
    1 teaspoon olive oil
    2 large shallots, finely chopped
    1 cup fat-free, low-sodium chicken broth, such
        as on page 36
    1/2 cup fat-free evaporated milk
    1 1/2 tablespoons all-purpose flour
    1/4 teaspoon salt
    1/4 teaspoon pepper
    2 tablespoons grated Parmesan cheese
    1 tablespoon chopped fresh dillweed or
        1 teaspoon dried dillweed, crumbled

■ ■ ■

    1/4 cup whole-wheat panko (Japanese-style
        bread crumbs)

Preheat the oven to 350°F. Lightly spray a 1 1/2-quart casserole dish with cooking spray. Set aside.

In a medium saucepan, bring the kohlrabi and water to a boil over high heat. Reduce the heat to medium low and cook, covered, for 5 minutes, or until tender-crisp. Drain well in a colander. Set aside.

Meanwhile, in a separate medium saucepan, heat the oil over medium-low heat, swirling to coat the bottom. Cook the shallots for 1 to 2 minutes, stirring occasionally.

In a medium bowl, whisk together the broth, milk, flour, salt, and pepper. Stir into the shallot mixture. Increase the heat to medium high and

(continued)

bring to a boil, stirring occasionally. Reduce the heat to medium and cook for 1 to 2 minutes, or until the mixture thickens, stirring occasionally.

Stir in the Parmesan and dillweed. Remove from the heat.

Arrange half the kohlrabi in the casserole dish. Spoon half the shallot mixture over the kohlrabi. Repeat the layers.

Bake, covered, for 20 to 25 minutes, or until the kohlrabi is tender. Sprinkle the panko over all. Bake for 10 minutes, or until browned.

Cook's Tip on Kohlrabi: When you buy kohlrabi, look for crisp leaves with no yellow ends. Use the bulbs in recipes such as the one here, then stack the leaves, roll them jelly-roll style, and slice them crosswise into thin strips. Cook about 4 cups sliced leaves with 1/4 cup fat-free, low-sodium chicken broth or water, covered, over medium-low heat for 2 to 3 minutes, or until tender. Season with pepper.

PER SERVING

calories 99	carbohydrates 15 g
total fat 2.0 g	fiber 3 g
saturated fat 0.5 g	sugars 6 g
trans fat 0.0 g	protein 6 g
polyunsaturated fat 0.0 g	DIETARY EXCHANGES
monounsaturated fat 1.0 g	1 vegetable, 1/2 starch,
cholesterol 3 mg	1/2 lean meat
sodium 252 mg	

ITALIAN-STYLE ZUCCHINI

SERVES 6

When summer squash is at its peak, try this layered casserole with an Italian accent. Serve with juicy sliced nectarines and Hot and Spicy Arugula and Romaine Salad *(page 71).*

    Cooking spray
    6 medium zucchini or yellow summer squash, thinly sliced
    1 teaspoon olive oil
    3/4 cup sliced onion
    2 large tomatoes or 4 Italian plum (Roma) tomatoes, thinly sliced

    1 1/4 teaspoons dried basil, crumbled
    1 teaspoon salt-free all-purpose seasoning blend
    3/4 teaspoon dried oregano, crumbled
    4 ounces low-fat mozzarella cheese, shredded (about 1 cup)
    1/3 cup shredded or grated Parmesan cheese
    2 tablespoons finely chopped fresh parsley

Preheat the oven to 375°F. Lightly spray a 2-quart casserole dish with cooking spray. Put the zucchini in a saucepan with water to cover by 1/2 inch. Bring to a boil over high heat. Reduce the heat and simmer for 4 to 5 minutes, or until tender. Drain well in a colander. Transfer to a large bowl.

In a small skillet, heat the oil over medium-high heat, swirling to coat the bottom. Cook the onion for about 3 minutes, or until soft, stirring frequently. Stir into the zucchini.

Stir in the tomatoes, basil, seasoning blend, and oregano.

Spoon half the zucchini mixture into the casserole dish. Sprinkle the mozzarella over the zucchini. Spoon the remaining zucchini mixture on top. Sprinkle the Parmesan over all.

Bake, uncovered, for 25 to 30 minutes. Just before serving, sprinkle with the parsley.

PER SERVING

calories 114	sodium 230 mg
total fat 4.5 g	carbohydrates 11 g
saturated fat 1.5 g	fiber 3 g
trans fat 0.0 g	sugars 7 g
polyunsaturated fat 0.5 g	protein 10 g
monounsaturated fat 1.5 g	DIETARY EXCHANGES
cholesterol 10 mg	2 vegetable, 1 lean meat

STUFFED ZUCCHINI

SERVES 4

Brown rice flecked with color is used to stuff zucchini and transform it from its usual side-dish status to main-dish stardom. The chipotle pepper adds a rich, smoky flavor and a bit of heat to spice up the stuffing.

1/2 cup uncooked instant brown rice

4 small to medium zucchini

2 teaspoons olive oil

1 medium red onion, finely chopped

1 medium tomato, finely chopped

1 chipotle pepper canned in adobo sauce, finely chopped

1 large garlic clove, coarsely chopped

1/8 teaspoon salt

2 cups coarsely chopped spinach (about 2 ounces) or 10 ounces frozen chopped spinach, thawed and squeezed dry

4 large black olives, coarsely chopped

2 tablespoons coarsely chopped fresh cilantro

2 tablespoons white wine vinegar

3/4 teaspoon dried oregano, crumbled

1/4 teaspoon ground cumin

■ ■ ■

1/2 cup shredded low-fat 4-cheese Mexican blend

Prepare the rice using the package directions, omitting the salt and margarine.

Halve the zucchini lengthwise. Scoop out the pulp, leaving a 1/4-inch border of the shell all the way around. Dice the pulp. Set aside.

Place the shells with the cut sides down in a medium glass baking dish. Microwave, covered, on 100 percent power (high) for 4 to 6 minutes, or just until the zucchini is tender. Remove from the microwave. Uncover the dish carefully to avoid steam burns.

Preheat the broiler. Lightly spray a broiler pan with cooking spray.

Meanwhile, in a large, deep skillet, heat the oil over medium-low heat, swirling to coat the bottom. Cook the zucchini pulp, onion, tomato, chipotle, garlic, and salt for 5 to 7 minutes, or until the onion has softened, stirring occasionally.

Stir in the remaining ingredients except the Mexican blend cheese. Cook for 4 minutes, stirring frequently.

Stir the rice into the stuffing mixture. Spoon into the zucchini shells. Sprinkle with the Mexican

blend cheese. Broil about 4 inches from the heat for 1 to 2 minutes, or until the cheese is melted.

Cook's Tip on Chipotle Peppers: Chipotle peppers are dried smoked jalapeños, so expect a little heat. You probably won't use an entire can for any single recipe, but the leftovers freeze nicely. Spread the peppers with sauce in a thin layer on a medium plate covered with cooking parchment or wax paper, then freeze them, uncovered, for about 2 hours, or just until firm. Transfer the peppers to an airtight container or a resealable plastic freezer bag and freeze.

PER SERVING

calories 163	carbohydrates 19 g
total fat 6.5 g	fiber 3 g
saturated fat 2.0 g	sugars 6 g
trans fat 0.0 g	protein 8 g
polyunsaturated fat 0.5 g	DIETARY EXCHANGES
monounsaturated fat 3.0 g	1/2 starch,
cholesterol 9 mg	2 vegetable, 1/2 lean
sodium 292 mg	meat, 1 fat

SPINACH FETA STRUDEL

SERVES 6

The word strudel (a type of layered pastry) evokes thoughts of apples and sugar, but one of the first strudel recipes ever recorded was a savory turnip strudel. In this savory vegetarian entrée, spinach, caraway, and honey blend to make a palate-pleasing vegetarian main course.

8 ounces spinach, leaves torn into bite-size pieces

1 teaspoon light margarine

6 medium green onions, chopped

2 large egg whites

2 tablespoons water

8 14 x 9-inch frozen phyllo sheets, thawed

1 1/2 ounces crumbled low-fat feta cheese

1/2 teaspoon caraway seeds

1/4 teaspoon pepper (freshly ground preferred), or to taste

1 tablespoon honey

(continued)

Preheat the oven to 350°F.

Place the spinach in a medium bowl. Set aside.

In a nonstick skillet, melt the margarine over medium-high heat, swirling to coat the bottom. Stir in the green onions. Cook for 1 to 2 minutes, or until soft, stirring frequently.

Pour the green onions over the spinach. Immediately stir together so the hot green onions will wilt the spinach. Stir to combine.

In a small bowl, using a fork or small whisk, lightly beat the egg whites and water.

Keeping the unused phyllo covered with a damp cloth or damp paper towels to prevent drying, lightly brush 4 sheets of phyllo with the egg white mixture. Stack all the phyllo sheets, alternating the brushed and unbrushed sheets. Reserve the remaining egg white mixture.

Spread the spinach mixture over the phyllo, leaving a 1-inch border on all sides. Crumble the feta over the spinach. Sprinkle the caraway seeds and pepper over all. Drizzle with the honey.

Starting with a long side, roll up the phyllo, jelly-roll style. Place with the seam side down on a nonstick baking sheet, making sure that the ends of the roll are tucked under.

Brush the top lightly with the remaining egg white mixture. At 1 1/2-inch intervals, cut through the pastry to the spinach to create vents for steam to escape. Bake for 20 to 30 minutes, or until a light golden brown and a knife inserted in the center of the strudel comes out clean.

Cook's Tip: This recipe freezes well. Prepare as directed, but omit the final brushing and the baking. Freeze overnight on a baking sheet, then wrap well in freezer paper or foil. To prevent the pastry from getting soggy, don't defrost before baking. Place on a baking sheet, brush with egg white wash, and bake at 350°F for 35 to 45 minutes, or until light golden brown.

Cook's Tip on Phyllo: Phyllo is a paper-thin dough, available frozen in most large supermarkets and specialty groceries. Thaw the phyllo in the refrigerator. Unopened, the thawed dough will keep for a month if refrigerated. Refreezing can make the dough crumbly.

PER SERVING

calories 99	carbohydrates 17 g
total fat 1.5 g	fiber 2 g
saturated fat 0.5 g	sugars 4 g
trans fat 0.0 g	protein 5 g
polyunsaturated fat 0.5 g	DIETARY EXCHANGES
monounsaturated fat 0.5 g	1/2 starch, 1/2 other
cholesterol 3 mg	carbohydrate, 1/2 lean
sodium 213 mg	meat

GREEN PEPPER TOSTADAS

SERVES 4

A traditional tostada is usually made with a corn tortilla that's fried; this version uses broiling—a healthier cooking method—to create the crunch.

> Cooking spray
> 2 teaspoons canola or corn oil
> 2 medium green bell peppers, diced
> 3 medium tomatoes, diced
> 1 medium onion, diced
> 1/4 cup low-fat whipped cream cheese
> 4 6-inch corn tortillas
> 1/2 cup shredded or grated low-fat
>   mozzarella cheese
> 1/2 cup shredded romaine

Preheat the broiler. Lightly spray a broiler pan with cooking spray.

In a medium skillet, heat the oil over medium-high heat, swirling to coat the bottom. Cook the bell peppers, tomatoes, and onion for 3 minutes, or until the bell peppers are tender-crisp and the onion is soft, stirring frequently.

Stir in the cream cheese. Cook for 5 minutes, stirring frequently.

Broil the tortillas 4 to 6 inches from the heat for 2 minutes, or until slightly crisp. (The tortillas will curl up and form a pocket.) Transfer to a work surface.

Spoon the bell pepper mixture into each tortilla. Sprinkle the mozzarella over the bell pepper mixture. Return to the broiler for 1 minute to melt the mozzarella.

Serve the tostadas topped with the romaine.

PER SERVING

calories 140	carbohydrates 17 g
total fat 6.0 g	fiber 4 g
saturated fat 1.5 g	sugars 7 g
trans fat 0.0 g	protein 7 g
polyunsaturated fat 1.0 g	DIETARY EXCHANGES
monounsaturated fat 2.5 g	1/2 starch,
cholesterol 10 mg	2 vegetable, 1/2 lean
sodium 178 mg	meat, 1 fat

SPANAKOPITA

SERVES 6

This updated version of Greek spinach pie adds popular greens—kale and chard—for extra nutrition and flavor. While the entrée is baking, prepare Greek Yogurt with Honey and Walnuts (page 498) for dessert.

Cooking spray
1 teaspoon olive oil
1 cup chopped onion
2 large garlic cloves, minced
1/2 cup fat-free cottage cheese
1/4 cup crumbled low-fat feta cheese
1 large egg
1 large egg white
2 tablespoons chopped fresh dillweed or
    2 teaspoons dried dillweed, crumbled
1 tablespoon all-purpose flour
1/4 teaspoon pepper
10 ounces frozen chopped spinach, thawed
    and squeezed dry
2 cups chopped kale, tough stems discarded
2 cups chopped chard, tough stems discarded
1/2 cup water
11 14 x 9-inch frozen phyllo sheets, thawed

Preheat the oven to 375°F. Lightly spray a 9-inch pie pan with cooking spray.

In a large nonstick skillet, heat the oil over medium heat, swirling to coat the bottom. Cook the onion for 3 minutes, or until almost soft, stirring frequently. Stir in the garlic. Cook for 1 minute, or until fragrant, stirring constantly. Transfer the mixture to a large bowl. Stir the cottage cheese, feta, egg, egg white, dillweed, flour, and pepper into the onion mixture until combined. Stir in the spinach.

Put the kale, chard, and water in the skillet. Bring to a boil over medium heat. Cook, covered, for 3 minutes, or until the greens are wilted. Increase the heat to high. Cook, uncovered, for 1 to 2 minutes, or until the water has evaporated. Stir the greens into the spinach mixture.

Keeping the unused phyllo covered with a damp cloth or damp paper towels to prevent drying, and working quickly, place one sheet across the pie pan, letting it hang over the edges. Lightly spray the sheet with cooking spray. Place a second sheet crosswise over the first sheet. Lightly spray with cooking spray. Continue layering 4 more sheets of phyllo on top, lightly spraying each layer and alternating the position of the sheets to cover the pie pan. Spoon the spinach mixture into the pan, gently smoothing it with the back of a spoon to spread it out. Top with the remaining 5 sheets of phyllo, lightly spraying each one and alternating the direction of the sheets. Loosely crumple the overhanging pieces of the phyllo to create a free-form edge for the crust.

Bake for 35 minutes, or until the phyllo is golden brown and a knife inserted in the center of the pie comes out clean.

PER SERVING

calories 156	carbohydrates 23 g
total fat 3.5 g	fiber 3 g
saturated fat 1.0 g	sugars 3 g
trans fat 0.0 g	protein 10 g
polyunsaturated fat 0.5 g	DIETARY EXCHANGES
monounsaturated fat 1.5 g	1 starch, 1 vegetable,
cholesterol 34 mg	1 lean meat
sodium 330 mg	

COLLARD GREENS AND ARTICHOKE GRATIN

SERVES 6

Greens, artichokes, and cheese—a tasty trio. As the gratin bakes to bubbly richness, prepare steamed carrots and a tossed salad with a healthy dressing (pages 105–106) to complete your meal.

Cooking spray
16 ounces fat-free ricotta cheese
1/2 cup egg substitute
3 tablespoons shredded or grated Parmesan cheese
1 tablespoon fresh lemon juice
1/8 teaspoon pepper (white preferred)
1/8 teaspoon ground nutmeg
1/8 teaspoon red hot-pepper sauce
20 ounces frozen chopped collard greens, thawed and squeezed dry
3 medium green onions, thinly sliced (green part only)
9 ounces frozen artichoke hearts, thawed, drained, halved, and patted dry
1/2 cup shredded low-fat Cheddar cheese

Preheat the oven to 375°F. Lightly spray a 1 1/2-quart glass baking dish with cooking spray.

In a food processor or blender, process the ricotta, egg substitute, Parmesan, lemon juice, pepper, nutmeg, and hot-pepper sauce until smooth. Transfer to a large bowl.

Stir the collard greens and green onions into the ricotta mixture. Spread half in the baking dish.

Arrange the artichoke hearts in a single layer on the ricotta mixture. Sprinkle the Cheddar over all. Cover with the remaining ricotta mixture.

Bake, covered, for 25 minutes, or until the Cheddar is melted and the gratin is heated through.

PER SERVING

calories 153
total fat 2.0 g
  saturated fat 1.0 g
  trans fat 0.0 g
  polyunsaturated fat 0.0 g
  monounsaturated fat 0.5 g
cholesterol 10 mg
sodium 352 mg

carbohydrates 12 g
  fiber 6 g
  sugars 4 g
protein 18 g
DIETARY EXCHANGES
  2 vegetable, 2 lean meat

PORTOBELLOS WITH POLENTA AND TOMATOES

SERVES 4

Layered meaty mushrooms, velvety polenta, and juicy red tomato slices give this vegetarian entrée an intriguing texture. Two mushrooms make a satisfying main dish for one person, or you can serve one mushroom each as a side dish for eight.

1 teaspoon olive oil, 1 teaspoon olive oil, and 1 teaspoon olive oil, divided use
8 large portobello mushrooms (each about 4 1/2 inches in diameter), stems and gills discarded
1/8 teaspoon salt
1/3 cup finely diced onion
1 medium garlic clove, minced
2 cups fat-free, low-sodium vegetable broth, such as on page 36
1/4 teaspoon dried basil, crumbled
1/2 cup yellow cornmeal
1/3 cup shredded or grated Parmesan cheese and 2 tablespoons shredded or grated Parmesan cheese, divided use
1/8 teaspoon pepper
1 large tomato, cut into 8 slices

In a large nonstick skillet, heat 1 teaspoon oil over medium-high heat, swirling to coat the bottom. Cook 4 of the mushrooms, covered, for 6 to 8 minutes, or until tender, turning once halfway through. Arrange the mushrooms with the cap side down in a single layer in a broiler-safe baking pan (a rimmed metal baking sheet works well). Repeat with 1 teaspoon oil and the remaining 4 mushrooms. Sprinkle the salt over all the mushrooms.

Meanwhile, preheat the broiler.

In a medium saucepan, heat the remaining 1 teaspoon oil over medium heat, swirling to coat the bottom. Cook the onion for 4 minutes, or until soft, stirring frequently. Stir in the garlic. Cook for 1 minute, stirring occasionally.

Stir in the broth and basil. Increase the heat to high and bring to a boil. Using a long-handled whisk, carefully stir the broth mixture to create a swirl. Slowly pour the cornmeal in a steady stream into the swirl, whisking constantly. Holding the pan steady, continue whisking for 1 to 2 minutes, or until the polenta is very thick. Remove from the heat. Stir in 1/3 cup Parmesan and the pepper.

Spoon 1/4 cup polenta into each mushroom cap. Top each with a tomato slice. Sprinkle with the remaining 2 tablespoons Parmesan.

Broil about 5 inches from the heat for 1 to 2 minutes, or until the Parmesan melts. Serve immediately for the best texture.

Cook's Tip: You can give this dish a smoky flavor by grilling the mushrooms. To save time when you are preparing dinner, you can grill them a day ahead and refrigerate them in an airtight container. Microwave the mushrooms to reheat them before filling them with the polenta.

PER SERVING

calories 175	carbohydrates 24 g
total fat 7.0 g	fiber 3 g
saturated fat 2.0 g	sugars 4 g
trans fat 0.0 g	protein 8 g
polyunsaturated fat 1.0 g	**DIETARY EXCHANGES**
monounsaturated fat 3.5 g	1 starch, 2 vegetable,
cholesterol 7 mg	1/2 lean meat, 1 fat
sodium 241 mg	

BARLEY RISOTTO WITH MUSHROOMS AND ASPARAGUS

SERVES 4

The fiber-rich barley in this creamy combination has a satisfying nutlike taste and offers more nutritional value than the Arborio rice usually used for risottos. If asparagus isn't in season, try sliced zucchini, yellow summer squash, or bell peppers instead.

> 4 cups fat-free, low-sodium vegetable broth, such as on page 36
> 1 1/2 cups water
> 2 teaspoons olive oil
> 2 cups diced onion
> 1 pound button mushrooms, sliced
> 1 1/4 cups uncooked pearl barley
> 1 pound asparagus spears, trimmed and cut into 2-inch pieces
> 3/4 cup shredded or grated Parmesan cheese
> 1/2 teaspoon pepper

In a large saucepan, heat the broth and water over medium-high heat for about 5 minutes, or until hot. Reduce the heat to low to keep the broth hot.

Meanwhile, in a separate large saucepan, heat the oil over medium-high heat, swirling to coat the bottom. Cook the onion for 3 minutes, or until soft, stirring frequently.

Stir the mushrooms together with the onion. Cook for 8 minutes, or until they exude their liquid, stirring occasionally. Stir in the barley.

Ladle 1/2 cup broth into the pan. Cook for 1 to 2 minutes, or until the broth is absorbed, stirring occasionally. Repeat, adding 1/2 cup broth at a time and cooking until the broth is absorbed after each addition, stirring in the asparagus after 15 minutes of cooking time. (The total cooking time will be about 30 minutes.) Remove from the heat.

Stir in the Parmesan and pepper. Serve immediately for the best texture.

(continued)

Cook's Tip: To remove the tough ends from asparagus spears, bend one spear at a time until you find the point where it naturally snaps in two, usually about 1 inch from the bottom.

PER SERVING

calories 389	carbohydrates 66 g
total fat 7.5 g	fiber 15 g
saturated fat 3.0 g	sugars 9 g
trans fat 0.0 g	protein 19 g
polyunsaturated fat 1.0 g	DIETARY EXCHANGES
monounsaturated fat 3.0 g	3 1/2 starch,
cholesterol 11 mg	3 vegetable, 1 lean
sodium 282 mg	meat

BARLEY WITH BRAISED SQUASH AND SWISS CHARD

SERVES 4

Although it is so nutritious—high in fiber, vitamins, and minerals—chard may not have made it into your cooking repertory yet. This dish would be a great introduction to this member of the beet family.

4 cups water

3/4 cup uncooked pearl barley

1 tablespoon olive oil

1/4 cup sliced shallots

3 medium garlic cloves, minced

1/8 teaspoon crushed red pepper flakes

1 pound butternut squash, peeled and cut into 1/2-inch cubes

1 cup fat-free, low-sodium vegetable broth, such as on page 36

1 small bunch Swiss chard (about 12 ounces), stems discarded and leaves coarsely chopped

1/4 cup shredded or grated Parmesan cheese

In a medium saucepan, bring the water to a boil over high heat. Stir in the barley. Reduce the heat and simmer, covered, for 45 to 50 minutes, or until the barley is tender. Drain well. Transfer to plates.

Meanwhile, about 30 minutes after the barley starts cooking, in a large skillet, heat the oil over medium heat, swirling to coat the bottom. Cook the shallots for 2 minutes, stirring occasionally.

Stir in the garlic and red pepper flakes. Cook for 30 seconds.

Stir in the squash and broth. Increase the heat to medium high and bring to a boil. Reduce the heat and simmer, covered, for 8 to 10 minutes, or until the squash is just tender.

Stir in the chard. Cook, covered, for 4 to 6 minutes, or until wilted. Using a slotted spoon, spoon over the barley. Sprinkle with the Parmesan.

Cook's Tip on Swiss Chard: Known for its crinkly green leaves and celery-like stalks, chard is available all year long but best during the summer months. The greens can be prepared like spinach. Store it wrapped in a plastic bag in the refrigerator for up to three days.

PER SERVING

calories 262	carbohydrates 48 g
total fat 5.5 g	fiber 10 g
saturated fat 1.5 g	sugars 5 g
trans fat 0.0 g	protein 9 g
polyunsaturated fat 0.5 g	DIETARY EXCHANGES
monounsaturated fat 3.0 g	3 starch, 1 vegetable,
cholesterol 4 mg	1/2 fat
sodium 284 mg	

PORTOBELLO MUSHROOM WRAP WITH YOGURT CURRY SAUCE

SERVES 8

Enhanced by a creamy, curry-flavored sauce, this wrap features rice and a garden of fresh veggies as its main attractions. Feta cheese adds briny richness.

Sauce

8 ounces fat-free plain yogurt

2 teaspoons fresh lemon juice

1 teaspoon sugar

1 teaspoon curry powder

■ ■ ■

2 tablespoons balsamic vinegar

1 tablespoon olive oil

2 medium garlic cloves, minced

2 medium portobello mushrooms, each cut into 8 slices

3/4 cup uncooked instant (fine-grain) bulgur

2 medium green onions, thinly sliced

1/4 cup crumbled fat-free feta cheese

1 medium Italian plum (Roma) tomato, diced

1 teaspoon light brown sugar

1 teaspoon plain rice vinegar

8 6-inch whole-wheat tortillas (lowest sodium available)

16 medium asparagus spears, trimmed and cooked until tender-crisp

In a small bowl, whisk together the sauce ingredients. Cover and refrigerate for 30 minutes to two days.

In a shallow glass dish, stir together the balsamic vinegar, oil, and garlic. Add the mushrooms, turning to coat. Cover and refrigerate for 10 to 15 minutes.

Meanwhile, prepare the bulgur using the package directions, omitting the salt.

Preheat the grill on medium high.

In a medium bowl, gently stir together the bulgur, green onions, feta, tomato, brown sugar, and rice vinegar.

Drain the mushrooms, discarding the marinade, but leaving what clings to the mushrooms.

Grill the mushrooms for 1 to 2 minutes on each side, or until tender.

Put a tortilla on a microwaveable plate. Put 2 mushroom slices in the center of the tortilla. Top with 2 asparagus spears and 1/4 cup bulgur mixture. Microwave on 100 percent power (high) for 30 seconds. Roll up the tortilla jelly-roll style. Repeat with the remaining ingredients. Serve with the sauce.

PER SERVING

calories 181
total fat 3.0 g
　saturated fat 0.5 g
　trans fat 0.0 g
　polyunsaturated fat 1.0 g
　monounsaturated fat 2.0 g
cholesterol 1 mg

sodium 299 mg
carbohydrates 32 g
　fiber 6 g
　sugars 8 g
protein 8 g
DIETARY EXCHANGES
　2 starch, 1 vegetable

CHEESY VEGGIE QUINOA

SERVES 4

You'll enjoy more than two servings of vegetables and a serving of whole grains in this entrée bathed in a rich fresh herb, two-cheese sauce. You can also halve the serving size to make this a side dish.

1 cup uncooked quinoa, rinsed and drained

1 large carrot, sliced into half-rounds

4 ounces broccoli florets (about 1 cup)

4 ounces cauliflower florets (about 1 cup)

1 medium zucchini, sliced into half-rounds

1 medium yellow summer squash, sliced into half-rounds

Sauce

2 tablespoons fat-free, low-sodium vegetable broth, such as on page 36

2 medium shallots, finely chopped

1 cup fat-free milk

2 tablespoons all-purpose flour

1/8 teaspoon pepper (white preferred)

2 ounces low-fat mozzarella cheese, shredded (about 1/2 cup)

2 tablespoons shredded or grated Parmesan cheese

1 tablespoon finely chopped fresh basil

1/2 teaspoon finely chopped fresh parsley

Prepare the quinoa using the package directions, omitting the salt. Fluff with a fork. Transfer to a large serving platter.

In a medium saucepan, add water to a depth of 1 inch. Put the carrot in a collapsible steamer basket. Place the steamer in the pan. Make sure the

(continued)

water doesn't touch the bottom of the steamer. Steam the carrot, covered, for 5 minutes, or until tender-crisp.

Add the broccoli, cauliflower, zucchini, and yellow squash. Steam, covered, for 10 minutes. Remove from the heat. Carefully uncover the pan away from you (to prevent steam burns). Drain the vegetables well in a colander, discarding any cooking water. Pat dry with paper towels. Arrange the vegetables on the quinoa. Cover to keep warm.

Meanwhile, in a medium saucepan, heat the broth over medium heat. Cook the shallots for 2 to 3 minutes, stirring occasionally.

Whisk in the milk, flour, and pepper. Increase the heat to medium high and bring to a boil. Boil for 3 to 4 minutes, or until the mixture thickens, stirring frequently.

Reduce the heat to low. Stir in the remaining ingredients. Cook for 1 to 2 minutes, or until the mozzarella melts, stirring constantly. Pour the sauce over the vegetables.

PER SERVING

calories 274	carbohydrates 43 g
total fat 5.0 g	fiber 6 g
saturated fat 1.5 g	sugars 9 g
trans fat 0.0 g	**protein** 16 g
polyunsaturated fat 1.5 g	**DIETARY EXCHANGES**
monounsaturated fat 1.5 g	2 starch, 2 vegetable,
cholesterol 8 mg	1 lean meat
sodium 205 mg	

MEDITERRANEAN TOASTED QUINOA AND SPINACH

SERVES 4

Feta cheese and lemon give a Mediterranean twist to this dish, made colorful with shreds of deep green spinach and slivers of red onion.

1 1/2 cups uncooked quinoa, rinsed and drained
3 cups fat-free, low-sodium vegetable broth, such as on page 36
4 cups shredded spinach, stems discarded

1 ounce low-fat feta cheese, crumbled
1/2 teaspoon grated lemon zest
1 tablespoon fresh lemon juice
1 tablespoon olive oil
1/4 teaspoon pepper
1/4 cup slivered red onion

In a large nonstick skillet, dry-roast the quinoa over medium-high heat for about 3 to 4 minutes, or until lightly toasted and any excess water has evaporated, stirring frequently (the quinoa won't turn golden brown).

In a medium saucepan, bring the broth to a boil over high heat. Stir in the quinoa. Return to a boil. Reduce the heat and simmer for 15 to 20 minutes, or until the broth is absorbed and the quinoa is tender.

Stir in the remaining ingredients except the onion. Just before serving, sprinkle with the onion.

Cook's Tip on Quinoa: Dry-roasting the quinoa really enhances its flavor. Although most packaged quinoa has already been rinsed, it's a good idea to rinse it yourself to be sure the bitter coating is removed. One way is to swirl it around in a bowl of water and drain it in a fine-mesh strainer. Replacing the water each time, repeat several times until the water runs clear.

PER SERVING

calories 292	sodium 129 mg
total fat 8.0 g	**carbohydrates** 44 g
saturated fat 1.5 g	fiber 5 g
trans fat 0.0 g	sugars 4 g
polyunsaturated fat 2.5 g	**protein** 12 g
monounsaturated fat 3.5 g	**DIETARY EXCHANGES**
cholesterol 3 mg	3 starch, 1 fat

QUINOA WITH BLACK BEANS AND SEARED BELL PEPPER

SERVES 4

Pine nuts add a bit of crunch and pizzazz to this filling and fiber-rich dish. Its flavors match well with Spinach-Chayote Salad with Orange Vinaigrette (page 68).

1 1/3 cups water

2/3 cup uncooked quinoa, rinsed and drained

1 15.5-ounce can no-salt-added black beans, rinsed and drained

3/4 cup frozen whole-kernel corn, thawed

Cooking spray

2 medium onions, cut into thin strips

1 large red bell pepper, cut into thin strips

1 medium garlic clove, minced

2 tablespoons pine nuts, dry-roasted

1 tablespoon olive oil (extra-virgin preferred)

1 teaspoon ground cumin

1/2 teaspoon salt

1/4 teaspoon crushed red pepper flakes

In a medium saucepan, bring the water to a boil over high heat. Stir in the quinoa. Return to a boil. Reduce the heat and simmer, covered, for about 12 minutes, or until the water is absorbed and the quinoa is just tender.

Stir in the beans and corn. Remove from the heat. Cover to keep warm.

Meanwhile, lightly spray a large skillet with cooking spray. Cook the onions, bell pepper, and garlic over medium-high heat for 8 minutes, or until deeply browned, stirring frequently.

Stir the onion mixture and the remaining ingredients into the quinoa mixture.

Cook's Tip on Dry-Roasting Pine Nuts: To dry roast pine nuts, heat a small skillet over medium-high heat. Dry-roast the pine nuts for 1 to 2 minutes, or until they begin to brown lightly, stirring constantly. Watch carefully so the nuts don't burn.

PER SERVING

calories 316	carbohydrates 52 g
total fat 7.5 g	fiber 10 g
saturated fat 1.0 g	sugars 13 g
trans fat 0.0 g	**protein** 13 g
polyunsaturated fat 2.0 g	**DIETARY EXCHANGES**
monounsaturated fat 3.5 g	3 starch, 2 vegetable,
cholesterol 0 mg	1 fat
sodium 302 mg	

QUINOA PILAF WITH TOFU AND VEGETABLES

SERVES 4

Quinoa, with its delicate flavor, is a welcome whole grain in this Asian-inspired pilaf. Have Chai-Spiced Flans with Blueberries *(page 496) for dessert.*

1/2 cup uncooked quinoa, rinsed and drained

16 ounces frozen mixed stir-fry vegetables

12 ounces light firm tofu, drained, patted dry, and cubed

1 cup fat-free, low-sodium vegetable broth, such as on page 36

2 teaspoons soy sauce (lowest sodium available)

1 teaspoon chili paste

1 teaspoon toasted sesame oil

2 tablespoons slivered almonds, dry-roasted

In a large nonstick skillet, dry-roast the quinoa over medium-high heat for 3 to 4 minutes, or until lightly toasted and any excess water has evaporated, stirring occasionally (the quinoa won't turn golden brown).

Stir in the remaining ingredients except the almonds. Bring to a simmer. Reduce the heat and simmer, covered, for 15 minutes, or until the quinoa is tender.

Stir in the almonds. Fluff the mixture with a fork.

PER SERVING

calories 204	carbohydrates 24 g
total fat 6.0 g	fiber 5 g
saturated fat 0.5 g	sugars 5 g
trans fat 0.0 g	**protein** 13 g
polyunsaturated fat 2.5 g	**DIETARY EXCHANGES**
monounsaturated fat 2.0 g	1 starch, 2 vegetable,
cholesterol 0 mg	1 lean meat, 1/2 fat
sodium 174 mg	

QUINOA, BEAN, AND VEGGIE LOAF

SERVES 6

When you're craving comfort food, nothing beats a slice of this hearty loaf paired with Mashed Potatoes with Parmesan and Green Onions *(page 399)* or Basil-Ricotta Mashed Cauliflower *(page 383). The combination of lentils, quinoa, and beans provides plenty of protein to keep you satisfied.*

Cooking spray
3 cups fat-free, low-sodium vegetable broth, such as on page 36
1/2 cup dried lentils, sorted for stones and shriveled lentils, rinsed, and drained
1/2 cup uncooked quinoa, rinsed and drained
1 15.5-ounce can no-salt-added kidney beans, rinsed, drained, and mashed with a fork
1 medium zucchini, shredded and squeezed dry
1/2 cup diced red bell pepper
1/2 cup shredded carrot
1/2 cup diced red onion
1/2 cup shredded or grated Parmesan cheese
1 large egg
2 large egg whites
2 medium garlic cloves, minced, and 1 medium garlic clove, minced, divided use
1 teaspoon dried sage
1 teaspoon dried oregano, crumbled
1/2 teaspoon salt
1/4 teaspoon pepper
1 8-ounce can no-salt-added tomato sauce
1 tablespoon light brown sugar
1 teaspoon dried basil, crumbled

Preheat the oven to 350°F. Fold an 18-inch-long piece of aluminum foil lengthwise into thirds. Place the foil in an 8 x 4 x 2-inch loaf pan so it runs the length of the pan and hangs over the two short sides. (The foil will help you remove the cooked meat loaf from the pan later.) Lightly spray the foil and the inside of the pan with cooking spray. Set aside.

In a medium saucepan, bring the broth and lentils to a boil over high heat. Reduce the heat and simmer, covered, for 15 minutes. Stir in the quinoa. Simmer, covered, for 15 minutes, or until the lentils and quinoa are tender. Drain in a colander.

Transfer the lentil mixture to a medium bowl. Set aside for 10 minutes, or until cooled.

Add the beans, zucchini, bell pepper, carrot, red onion, Parmesan, egg, egg whites, 2 garlic cloves, the sage, oregano, salt, and pepper to the lentil mixture. Using your hands or a spoon, combine the mixture. Press the mixture into the pan. Bake for 30 minutes, or until the loaf is set in the center (it bounces back when lightly pressed).

Meanwhile, in a small bowl, whisk together the tomato sauce, brown sugar, basil, and the remaining garlic clove. Remove the loaf from the oven.

Increase the oven temperature to 375°F. Pour the tomato sauce over the loaf. Bake for 5 minutes, or until the sauce mixture has thickened into a glaze. Grasping the ends of the foil, carefully lift the loaf from the pan. Transfer to a cutting board. Cover loosely. Let stand for 5 minutes before slicing.

PER SERVING

calories 263	carbohydrates 42 g
total fat 4.0 g	fiber 8 g
saturated fat 1.5 g	sugars 9 g
trans fat 0.0 g	protein 18 g
polyunsaturated fat 1.0 g	DIETARY EXCHANGES
monounsaturated fat 1.0 g	2 1/2 starch,
cholesterol 36 mg	1 vegetable, 2 lean
sodium 361 mg	meat

THREE-CHEESE VEGETABLE AND WHITE BEAN STRUDEL

SERVES 4

Dinner is all wrapped up when vegetables are cooked quickly in a skillet, seasoned and combined with beans, rolled in wafer-thin layers of phyllo dough, and baked to a golden brown.

1 teaspoon olive oil
16 ounces frozen mixed vegetables (any combination)

1/4 cup coarsely chopped fresh basil

2 tablespoons chopped fresh dillweed

1/4 teaspoon salt-free lemon pepper

1 15.5-ounce can no-salt-added navy beans, rinsed and drained

1 cup fat-free ricotta cheese

1 cup shredded low-fat mozzarella cheese

1/4 cup shredded or grated Romano cheese

6 14 x 18-inch sheets frozen phyllo dough, thawed

Cooking spray

In a large nonstick skillet, heat the oil over medium-high heat, swirling to coat the bottom. Cook the vegetables for 8 to 10 minutes, or until tender and heated through, stirring occasionally. (If there is excess liquid in the pan, increase the heat to high. Leaving the vegetables in the pan, cook for 2 to 3 minutes, or until the liquid has almost evaporated, stirring occasionally.) Remove from the heat.

Stir in the basil, dillweed, and lemon pepper. Let cool for 5 minutes.

In a medium bowl, stir together the beans, ricotta, mozzarella, and Romano. Stir in the vegetable mixture. Set aside.

Preheat the oven to 350°F.

Place one sheet of phyllo dough on a cutting board. Lightly spray the top with cooking spray. Place another sheet of phyllo on top. Lightly spray with cooking spray. Repeat with a third sheet of phyllo. Leaving a 2-inch border along one wide end of the phyllo, spoon half the filling along that end. Fold the edge closest to the filling over the filling. Fold the short ends slightly toward the center and roll up from the wide end to enclose the filling. Transfer the strudel with the seam side down to a large nonstick baking sheet. Repeat with the remaining phyllo and filling, placing the second strudel about 2 inches from the first.

Lightly spray the top and sides of the strudels with cooking spray. Cut diagonal slits in the top of each strudel about 2 inches apart and about 1/2 inch deep.

Bake for 30 to 35 minutes, or until the crust is golden brown and a knife inserted in the center of the strudels comes out clean.

PER SERVING

calories 391	**carbohydrates** 58 g
total fat 6.0 g	fiber 9 g
saturated fat 1.5 g	sugars 11 g
trans fat 0.0 g	**protein** 28 g
polyunsaturated fat 0.5 g	**DIETARY EXCHANGES**
monounsaturated fat 2.5 g	3 starch, 3 vegetable,
cholesterol 18 mg	2 1/2 lean meat
sodium 524 mg	

VEGETABLE CREOLE

SERVES 4

Louisiana is the birthplace of Creole cuisine, and this stew, with its swirl of colorful veggies, gets its kick from Louisiana-style hot sauce. Southern Raised Biscuits (page 459) are the perfect accompaniment.

1 1/2 cups uncooked brown rice

1 tablespoon canola or corn oil

1/2 cup diced celery

1/3 cup diced green bell pepper

1/3 cup sliced onion

2 1/2 cups canned no-salt-added diced tomatoes, drained

1 teaspoon chopped fresh basil

1 teaspoon celery seeds

1/2 teaspoon chopped fresh rosemary

Pepper to taste (freshly ground preferred)

2 cups cooked green peas

1/2 cup canned no-salt-added kidney beans, rinsed and drained

1/4 teaspoon Louisiana-style hot-pepper sauce

Prepare the rice using the package directions, omitting the salt and margarine. Set aside.

In a large skillet, heat the oil over medium heat, swirling to coat the bottom. Cook the celery, bell pepper, and onion over medium heat for 3 to 5 minutes, or until the celery and bell pepper are tender and the onion is soft.

(continued)

Stir in the tomatoes, basil, celery seeds, rosemary, and pepper. Cook for about 20 minutes, stirring occasionally.

Stir in the green peas and beans. Cook, covered, for 5 minutes, or until heated through. Stir in the hot sauce. Serve the vegetable mixture over the rice.

PER SERVING

calories 416	carbohydrates 77 g
total fat 6.0 g	fiber 10 g
saturated fat 1.0 g	sugars 11 g
trans fat 0.0 g	protein 13 g
polyunsaturated fat 2.0 g	DIETARY EXCHANGES
monounsaturated fat 3.0 g	4 1/2 starch,
cholesterol 0 mg	2 vegetable, 1/2 fat
sodium 118 mg	

VEGETABLE AND PINTO BEAN ENCHILADAS

SERVES 8

These filling enchiladas offer not only vitamin-rich spinach and protein-packed pinto beans but also julienned vegetables. Chilled slices of fresh jicama with a squeeze of lime and a sprinkle of chili powder make a crisp accompaniment.

16 6-inch corn tortillas

1 teaspoon olive oil

1 medium carrot, cut into matchstick-size strips

2 medium leeks (white part only), thinly sliced, or 1/2 cup sliced onion

1 medium zucchini, cut into matchstick-size strips

1 15.5-ounce can no-salt-added pinto beans, rinsed and drained

10 ounces frozen chopped spinach, cooked, well drained, and squeezed dry

4 ounces light tub cream cheese

1/2 cup salsa (lowest sodium available), such as Salsa Cruda (page 437)

1 teaspoon fresh lime juice

1/4 teaspoon salt

1/2 cup fat-free half-and-half

1 teaspoon ground cumin

1 cup shredded or grated low-fat Cheddar cheese

Preheat the oven to 350°F.

Wrap the tortillas in aluminum foil.

Bake for 5 minutes, or until heated through. Set aside, still in the foil, to keep warm.

Meanwhile, in a large nonstick skillet, heat the oil over medium-high heat, swirling to coat the bottom. Cook the carrot and leeks for 2 to 3 minutes, or until the carrot is tender-crisp, stirring occasionally.

Stir in the zucchini. Cook for 2 to 3 minutes, or until the zucchini is tender-crisp.

Stir in the beans, spinach, cream cheese, salsa, lime juice, and salt. Reduce the heat to medium low. Cook for 2 to 3 minutes, or until heated through, stirring occasionally.

Spoon about 1/4 cup filling down the center of a tortilla. Roll up jelly-roll style and place with the seam side down in a nonstick 13 x 9 x 2-inch baking pan. Repeat with the remaining filling and tortillas.

In a small bowl, whisk together the half-and-half and cumin. Pour over the enchiladas. Sprinkle the Cheddar over all.

Bake for 15 to 20 minutes, or until heated through.

PER SERVING

calories 218	carbohydrates 32 g
total fat 5.0 g	fiber 6 g
saturated fat 2.0 g	sugars 7 g
trans fat 0.0 g	protein 12 g
polyunsaturated fat 0.5 g	DIETARY EXCHANGES
monounsaturated fat 1.5 g	1 1/2 starch,
cholesterol 12 mg	1 vegetable, 1 lean
sodium 380 mg	meat

ENCHILADA BAKE

SERVES 6

Plenty of vegetables, creamy sauce, beans, and tortillas are all the right components to make a tasty Mexican casserole that's even better the day after you prepare it. Serve with Zesty Corn Relish (page 78).

Sauce

1 teaspoon light tub margarine
1 medium onion, chopped
1/2 medium green bell pepper, chopped
8 ounces button mushrooms, quartered
1 to 2 medium garlic cloves, minced
2 cups canned no-salt-added black or pinto
        beans, rinsed and drained
1 14.5-ounce can no-salt-added stewed
        tomatoes, undrained
1/2 cup dry red wine (regular or nonalcoholic)
2 to 3 teaspoons chili powder
1 to 2 teaspoons ground cumin
1/4 teaspoon salt

■ ■ ■

Cooking spray
3/4 cup fat-free ricotta cheese
1/2 cup fat-free plain yogurt
6 6-inch corn tortillas, quartered
1/2 cup grated low-fat Monterey Jack cheese
6 medium black olives, sliced

In a large saucepan, melt the margarine over medium-high heat, swirling to coat the bottom. Cook the onion, bell pepper, mushrooms, and garlic for about 3 minutes, or until the onion is soft, stirring frequently.

Stir in the remaining sauce ingredients. Reduce the heat and simmer for 30 minutes.

Preheat the oven to 350°F. Lightly spray a 1 1/2-quart casserole dish with cooking spray.

In a small bowl, whisk together the ricotta and yogurt.

In the casserole dish, layer as follows: 3 tortillas (12 quarters), half the sauce, half the Monterey Jack, and half the ricotta mixture. Repeat the layers. Sprinkle the olives on top.

Bake, covered, for 15 to 20 minutes, or until heated through.

PER SERVING

calories 224	**carbohydrates** 32 g
total fat 2.5 g	fiber 7 g
saturated fat 0.5 g	sugars 11 g
trans fat 0.0 g	**protein** 15 g
polyunsaturated fat 0.5 g	**DIETARY EXCHANGES**
monounsaturated fat 1.0 g	1 1/2 starch,
cholesterol 6 mg	2 vegetable, 1 lean
sodium 327 mg	meat

CHEESE-TOPPED ANAHEIM PEPPERS WITH PINTO RICE

SERVES 4

Instead of stuffing peppers as is done in the classic version, you simply place the halved peppers on top of the filling in this dish. A splash of fresh lime juice adds just the right amount of tartness.

1 cup uncooked instant brown rice
Cooking spray
1 15.5-ounce can no-salt-added pinto beans,
        rinsed and drained
3/4 cup finely chopped green onions
1 tablespoon chili powder
2 teaspoons ground cumin
1/8 teaspoon salt and 1/8 teaspoon salt,
        divided use
4 medium fresh Anaheim or poblano
        peppers, halved lengthwise, stems,
        seeds, and ribs discarded (see Cook's Tip
        on Handling Hot Chiles, page 24)
1 cup shredded low-fat Cheddar cheese
1 medium lime, cut into 4 wedges

Prepare the rice using the package directions, omitting the salt and margarine.

Meanwhile, preheat the oven to 350°F. Lightly spray an 11 x 7 x 2-inch baking pan with cooking spray.

In the pan, stir together the rice, beans, green onions, chili powder, cumin, and 1/8 teaspoon salt. Alternating the wide and narrow ends, arrange the peppers with the cut side down on the rice mixture. Sprinkle the Cheddar over all.

(continued)

Bake, covered, for 45 minutes, or until the peppers are tender when pierced with a fork.

Sprinkle with the remaining 1/8 teaspoon salt. Squeeze the lime juice over all.

Cook's Tip: If the peppers are too long for the pan, cut off any excess and use the pieces for another dish or freeze them.

PER SERVING

calories 264	carbohydrates 42 g
total fat 3.5 g	fiber 8 g
saturated fat 1.5 g	sugars 7 g
trans fat 0.0 g	protein 16 g
polyunsaturated fat 0.5 g	DIETARY EXCHANGES
monounsaturated fat 1.0 g	2 1/2 starch,
cholesterol 6 mg	1 vegetable, 1 1/2 lean
sodium 368 mg	meat

BEAN AND BULGUR CHILI

SERVES 12

This Mexican-style chili is perfect for a potluck supper or a Super Bowl party. Serve with Corn Bread Muffins *(page 464) and* Spinach-Chayote Salad with Orange Vinaigrette *(page 68).*

1 cup instant (fine-grain) bulgur

2 teaspoons canola or corn oil

2 teaspoons chili powder

1 teaspoon dried oregano, crumbled (Mexican preferred)

1/2 teaspoon ground cumin

1/8 teaspoon cayenne

3 medium ribs of celery, chopped

1 1/2 large green bell peppers, chopped

2 medium onions, chopped

1 medium garlic clove, finely chopped

4 medium tomatoes, chopped

1 medium fresh jalapeño, seeds and ribs discarded, chopped (see Cook's Tip on Handling Hot Chiles, page 24)

3 cups canned no-salt-added red kidney beans, rinsed and drained

1/2 teaspoon salt

4 medium green onions, chopped

1/4 cup shredded low-fat 4-cheese Mexican blend

Prepare the bulgur using the package directions, omitting the salt. Transfer to a medium bowl. Fluff with a fork. Set aside.

In a large skillet, heat the oil over medium heat, swirling to coat the bottom. Stir in the chili powder, oregano, cumin, and cayenne. Cook for 2 minutes, stirring constantly.

Increase the heat to medium high. Stir in the celery, bell peppers, onions, and garlic. Cook for 5 minutes, or until the onions are very soft and the celery and bell peppers are tender, stirring frequently.

Stir in the tomatoes and jalapeño. Increase the heat to high and bring to a boil. Reduce the heat to medium high. Stir in the beans. Cook for 3 minutes, or until heated through, stirring occasionally. Stir in the bulgur and salt.

Just before serving, sprinkle the chili with the green onions and Mexican-blend cheese.

PER SERVING

calories 135	carbohydrates 26 g
total fat 1.5 g	fiber 7 g
saturated fat 0.5 g	sugars 5 g
trans fat 0.0 g	protein 7 g
polyunsaturated fat 0.5 g	DIETARY EXCHANGES
monounsaturated fat 0.5 g	1 1/2 starch,
cholesterol 1 mg	1 vegetable, 1/2 lean
sodium 140 mg	meat

TOSTADAS

SERVES 6

Enjoy saucy, spicy beans and tomatoes over warm, crisp corn tortillas. Serve with Mexican Fried Rice *(page 421) and* Jícama Slaw *(page 83).*

Sauce

6 medium tomatoes, seeded and chopped

1 cup finely chopped onion

1/2 cup red wine vinegar

1 teaspoon dried oregano, crumbled (Mexican preferred)

1 teaspoon honey

1 medium garlic clove, minced

■ ■ ■

2 teaspoons olive oil
1 medium onion, chopped
2 medium garlic cloves, minced
1 teaspoon ancho powder
Pinch of cayenne
1 15.5-ounce can no-salt-added pinto beans,
    rinsed and drained
2 medium tomatoes, chopped

■ ■ ■

12 6-inch corn tortillas
3 cups shredded romaine
1/4 cup plus 2 tablespoons queso fresco or
    farmer cheese

In a large bowl, stir together the sauce ingredients. Set aside.

Preheat the oven to 350°F.

In a large skillet, heat the oil over medium-high heat, swirling to coat the bottom. Cook the onion for about 3 minutes, or until soft, stirring frequently. Stir in the garlic, ancho powder, and cayenne. Cook for 1 minute, stirring frequently.

Stir in the beans and tomatoes. Cook for 3 minutes, using the back of a fork to mash the beans and stirring and turning over the beans gently.

Place the tortillas directly on the oven rack. Bake for 8 to 10 minutes, or until crisp. Transfer to a work surface.

Spread the bean mixture on the tortillas. Spoon the sauce over the bean mixture. Sprinkle with the romaine and queso fresco.

PER SERVING

calories 219	carbohydrates 39 g
total fat 4.0 g	fiber 8 g
saturated fat 1.0 g	sugars 11 g
trans fat 0.0 g	protein 10 g
polyunsaturated fat 0.5 g	DIETARY EXCHANGES
monounsaturated fat 1.5 g	2 starch, 2 vegetable,
cholesterol 5 mg	1/2 lean meat
sodium 85 mg	

ROOT VEGETABLE AND KIDNEY BEAN STEW

SERVES 6

Get to the root of good taste with this chunky stew, featuring three root vegetables. A hint of barley adds a toothsome texture. Serve with crusty whole-grain bread to soak up the juices.

4 cups fat-free, low-sodium vegetable broth,
    such as on page 36
1 15.5-ounce can no-salt-added kidney beans,
    rinsed and drained
1 14.5-ounce can no-salt-added stewed
    tomatoes, undrained
1 large rutabaga (about 12 ounces), peeled
    and cut into 2-inch cubes
2 medium turnips (about 8 ounces), peeled
    and cut into 2-inch cubes
2 large parsnips (about 6 ounces), peeled and
    cut into 2-inch pieces
2 tablespoons uncooked pearl barley
1 teaspoon celery seeds
1 teaspoon dried thyme, crumbled
1 teaspoon bottled white horseradish,
    drained (optional)
1/2 teaspoon dried sage
1/4 teaspoon salt
1/4 teaspoon pepper

In a large stockpot or Dutch oven, stir together all the ingredients. Bring to a simmer over medium-high heat, stirring occasionally. Reduce the heat and simmer, covered, for 40 to 45 minutes, or until the vegetables and barley are tender.

PER SERVING

calories 156	carbohydrates 33 g
total fat 0.5 g	fiber 8 g
saturated fat 0.0 g	sugars 9 g
trans fat 0.0 g	protein 7 g
polyunsaturated fat 0.0 g	DIETARY EXCHANGES
monounsaturated fat 0.0 g	1 starch, 3 vegetable,
cholesterol 0 mg	1/2 lean meat
sodium 153 mg	

BLACK BEAN POLENTA WITH AVOCADO SALSA

SERVES 6

The Mexican-seasoned polenta combines with the beans and bakes to perfection. While the polenta is chilling, prepare Watermelon-Cilantro Sorbet *(page 504) for dessert.*

Polenta

4 cups water

1 teaspoon olive oil

1/2 teaspoon ground cumin

1/2 teaspoon ancho powder

1/4 teaspoon salt

1 1/2 cups yellow cornmeal

1 15.5-ounce can no-salt-added black beans, rinsed and drained

Salsa

2 medium avocados, finely chopped

1/4 cup finely chopped red onion

2 tablespoons chopped fresh cilantro

2 tablespoons fresh lime juice

1/4 teaspoon salt

In a medium saucepan, stir together the water, oil, cumin, ancho powder, and salt. Bring to a boil over high heat.

Using a wooden spoon, carefully stir the water to create a swirl. Slowly pour the cornmeal in a steady stream into the swirl, stirring constantly. When all the cornmeal is incorporated, reduce the heat and simmer for 5 minutes, stirring occasionally. Remove the pan from the heat.

Stir in the beans. Spread the mixture in an 8-inch square baking pan. Let cool to room temperature, about 30 minutes, then cover and refrigerate for at least 2 hours.

Preheat the broiler. Line a baking sheet with aluminum foil. Cut the polenta into 8 pieces. Transfer to the baking sheet.

Broil the polenta 4 to 6 inches from the heat for 4 to 5 minutes on each side, or until the pieces are lightly browned and heated through.

Meanwhile, in a medium bowl, stir together the salsa ingredients. Spoon over the polenta.

PER SERVING

calories 303
total fat 11.5 g
  saturated fat 1.5 g
  trans fat 0.0 g
  polyunsaturated fat 1.5 g
  monounsaturated fat 7.5 g
cholesterol 0 mg

sodium 209 mg
carbohydrates 47 g
  fiber 10 g
  sugars 4 g
protein 8 g
DIETARY EXCHANGES
  3 starch, 2 fat

CUBAN BLACK BEANS

SERVES 8

The cumin and vinegar give this dish its Cuban flavor. If you have leftover beans and sometimes eat meat, save a cup of them and give Southwestern Pork Salad *(page 99) a try.*

2 cups dried black beans (about 1 pound), sorted for stones and shriveled beans, rinsed, and drained

Cooking spray

1 teaspoon light tub margarine

2 medium onions, chopped

1/2 medium rib of celery, diced

1/2 medium lemon, quartered

1 tablespoon chopped fresh savory or 1 teaspoon dried savory, crumbled

2 medium garlic cloves, minced

1 medium dried bay leaf

1 teaspoon ground cumin

1/2 teaspoon salt

1 1/2 cups uncooked brown rice

4 medium green onions, chopped (optional)

3 tablespoons red wine vinegar (optional)

2 medium oranges, sliced (optional)

Soak the beans using the package directions. Drain well in a colander.

Lightly spray a stockpot with cooking spray. Heat the margarine over medium-high heat, swirling to coat the bottom. Cook the onions and celery for about 3 minutes, or until the onions are soft, stirring frequently.

Add the beans, lemon, savory, garlic, bay leaf, cumin, and salt. Add water to cover by 2 inches. Stir well. Increase the heat to high and bring to a boil. Reduce the heat and simmer, covered, for

1 hour to 1 hour 30 minutes, or until the beans are tender. Discard the lemon and bay leaf.

Meanwhile, prepare the rice using the package directions, omitting the salt and margarine.

Spoon the rice into bowls. Spoon the beans over the rice. Sprinkle with the green onions and vinegar, or garnish with the orange slices.

PER SERVING

calories 305	sodium 158 mg
total fat 1.5 g	carbohydrates 60 g
saturated fat 0.0 g	fiber 7 g
trans fat 0.0 g	sugars 7 g
polyunsaturated fat 0.5 g	protein 13 g
monounsaturated fat 0.5 g	DIETARY EXCHANGES
cholesterol 0 mg	4 starch, 1 lean meat

BLACK BEAN STUFFED SWEET POTATOES

SERVES 4

Serve this Mexican adaptation of a loaded baked potato as part of your Cinco de Mayo *feast. Start the evening off with* Tortilla Pinwheels *(page 17) and* Jalapeño Poppers *(page 24).*

Cooking spray
4 medium sweet potatoes
1 cup fat-free sour cream
3/4 cup no-salt-added canned black beans, rinsed and drained
4 or 5 medium green onions, thinly sliced
1/2 cup queso fresco, crumbled
1/4 cup chopped avocado (about 1/2 medium avocado)
1/4 cup chopped fresh cilantro (optional)

Preheat the oven to 400°F. Lightly spray a large baking sheet with cooking spray.

Pierce the sweet potatoes with a fork. Bake for 1 hour. Remove from the oven. Transfer to a cooling rack. Let stand for 15 to 20 minutes, or until cool enough to handle.

Halve the sweet potatoes lengthwise. Using a spoon, scoop out the pulp, leaving about an 1/8-inch shell. Transfer the pulp to a medium bowl. Using a potato masher or fork, mash the pulp. Stir in the sour cream, black beans, and green onions until well combined. Spoon the sweet potato mixture into the shells.

Bake for 15 minutes, or until the sweet potato mixture is heated through.

Just before serving, sprinkle with the queso fresco, avocado, and cilantro.

PER SERVING

calories 368	carbohydrates 67 g
total fat 5.0 g	fiber 10 g
saturated fat 2.0 g	sugars 17 g
trans fat 0.0 g	protein 13 g
polyunsaturated fat 0.5 g	DIETARY EXCHANGES
monounsaturated fat 2.0 g	4 1/2 starch, 1 lean
cholesterol 21 mg	meat
sodium 296 mg	

RED BEANS AND COUSCOUS

SERVES 4

Try a modern twist on the classic red beans and rice with this quick and easy recipe. Serve with Creole Squash *(page 406).*

1 teaspoon olive oil
1/2 medium green bell pepper, chopped
1 medium rib of celery, chopped
1/2 medium onion, chopped
2 medium garlic cloves, chopped
2 cups fat-free, low-sodium vegetable broth, such as on page 36
1 15-ounce can no salt added small red beans, rinsed and drained
2 ounces meatless Canadian bacon, chopped
1 1/2 to 2 teaspoons salt-free Creole or Cajun seasoning blend, such as on page 401
1 1/2 cups uncooked whole-wheat couscous

In a medium nonstick saucepan, heat the oil over medium-high heat, swirling to coat the bottom. Cook the bell pepper, celery, onion, and garlic for 3 to 4 minutes, or until the bell pepper and celery are tender and the onion is soft, stirring frequently.

(continued)

Stir in the broth, beans, Canadian bacon, and seasoning blend. Bring to a simmer. Reduce the heat and simmer for 1 to 2 minutes, or until the Canadian bacon is tender.

Stir in the couscous. Remove from the heat. Let stand, covered, for 5 minutes, or until the couscous has absorbed the liquid. Fluff with a fork.

PER SERVING

calories 442	carbohydrates 85 g
total fat 3.0 g	fiber 15 g
saturated fat 0.5 g	sugars 3 g
trans fat 0.0 g	**protein** 22 g
polyunsaturated fat 0.5 g	**DIETARY EXCHANGES**
monounsaturated fat 1.0 g	5 1/2 starch, 1 lean
cholesterol 0 mg	meat
sodium 167 mg	

BLACK BEAN CAKES WITH GREENS

SERVES 4

Sautéing the greens with onion and garlic gives the bean cakes a rich flavor and texture. A topping of bright Fresh Herb Chimichurri Sauce (page 437) adds color and freshness.

1 teaspoon olive oil and 1 tablespoon olive oil, divided use
1/2 cup chopped onion
2 medium garlic cloves, minced
2 cups chopped spinach, stems discarded
2 cups chopped kale, tough stems and ribs discarded
2 teaspoons chopped fresh thyme or 1/2 teaspoon dried thyme, crumbled
1/4 teaspoon salt
1/4 teaspoon pepper (freshly ground preferred)
1 15.5-ounce can no-salt-added black beans, rinsed and drained
1 large egg, lightly beaten using a fork
1/2 cup Fresh Herb Chimichurri Sauce (page 437)

In a large, nonstick skillet, heat 1 teaspoon oil over medium-high heat, swirling to coat the bottom. Cook the onion for about 3 minutes or until soft, stirring frequently. Stir in the gar-

lic. Cook for 1 minute or until fragrant, stirring frequently. Stir in the spinach, kale, thyme, salt, and pepper. Cook for 1 to 2 minutes or until the greens are wilted. Transfer the mixture to a food processor. Let cool slightly for 5 minutes. Wipe the skillet with paper towels.

Add the beans to the greens mixture in the food processor. Process until slightly chunky. Transfer the mixture to a large bowl. Add the egg, stirring to combine. Using your hands or a spoon, combine the ingredients. Shape into 4 patties. Transfer to a medium plate.

In the same skillet, heat the remaining 1 tablespoon oil over medium heat, swirling to coat the bottom. Cook the patties for 3 to 4 minutes on each side, or until golden brown. Transfer to serving plates. Spoon the sauce over the patties.

PER SERVING

calories 212	carbohydrates 26 g
total fat 8.0 g	fiber 6 g
saturated fat 1.5 g	sugars 6 g
trans fat 0.0 g	**protein** 10 g
polyunsaturated fat 1.0 g	**DIETARY EXCHANGES**
monounsaturated fat 5.0 g	1 1/2 starch,
cholesterol 47 mg	1 vegetable, 1 lean
sodium 273 mg	meat, 1/2 fat

BULGUR, BROWN RICE, AND BEANS

SERVES 4

Two kinds of whole grains envelop these sautéed veggies and white beans seasoned with Italian flavor. Try Creamy Basil-Tomato Soup (page 43) on the side.

2 cups water
1/2 cup uncooked instant brown rice
1/2 cup uncooked instant (fine-grain) bulgur
1 teaspoon olive oil and 1 tablespoon olive oil (extra-virgin preferred), divided use
1 large red bell pepper, chopped
4 cups baby spinach, chopped
1 15.5-ounce can no-salt-added cannellini beans, rinsed and drained
1/3 cup pine nuts, dry-roasted

1 tablespoon finely chopped fresh oregano or
     1 teaspoon dried oregano, crumbled
2 medium garlic cloves, minced
3/4 teaspoon finely chopped fresh rosemary
     or 1/4 teaspoon dried rosemary, crushed
1/2 teaspoon salt
4 sprigs of fresh rosemary (optional)

In a medium saucepan, bring the water to a boil over high heat. Stir in the rice and bulgur. Reduce the heat and simmer, covered, for 10 minutes, or until most of the water has evaporated. Remove from the heat.

Meanwhile, in a separate medium saucepan, heat 1 teaspoon oil over medium-high heat. Cook the bell pepper for 4 minutes, or until beginning to brown on the edges, stirring frequently. Stir in the spinach, stirring until wilted. Stir the bell pepper mixture into the rice mixture.

Stir in the remaining ingredients except the sprigs of rosemary. Garnish with the rosemary.

PER SERVING

calories 302	**carbohydrates** 42 g
total fat 11.5 g	fiber 10 g
saturated fat 1.5 g	sugars 4 g
trans fat 0.0 g	**protein** 12 g
polyunsaturated fat 3.5 g	**DIETARY EXCHANGES**
monounsaturated fat 6.0 g	2 1/2 starch,
cholesterol 0 mg	1 vegetable, 1/2 lean
sodium 360 mg	meat, 1 1/2 fat

RATATOUILLE WITH CANNELLINI BEANS AND BROWN RICE

SERVES 6

This chunky, hearty French stew is a simple yet delicious combination of vegetables and legumes. Serve with Whole-Wheat French Bread (page 443).

Ratatouille
1 teaspoon olive oil
8 ounces button mushrooms, sliced
1/2 medium onion (sweet onion, such as
     Vidalia, Maui, or Oso Sweet preferred),
     sliced into rings and halved
2 medium zucchini, cut into 1/4-inch slices
3 medium garlic cloves, minced

2 14.5-ounce cans no-salt-added stewed
     tomatoes, undrained
1 15.5-ounce can no-salt-added cannellini
     beans, rinsed and drained
1 small eggplant (about 1/2 pound), peeled
     and diced
1/2 large red bell pepper, diced
1/4 cup shredded or grated Parmesan cheese
2 teaspoons dried oregano, crumbled
1 teaspoon dried basil, crumbled
1/2 teaspoon dried thyme, crumbled
1/8 teaspoon pepper

■ ■ ■

2 cups uncooked instant brown rice
1 3/4 cups fat-free, low-sodium vegetable
     broth, such as on page 36
2 tablespoons shredded or grated Parmesan
     cheese
Crushed red pepper flakes (optional)

In a large, heavy nonstick skillet, heat the oil over medium-high heat, swirling to coat the bottom. Cook the mushrooms and onion for 5 to 7 minutes, or until the onion begins to brown, stirring occasionally. Stir in the zucchini and garlic. Cook for 8 to 10 minutes, or until the zucchini is soft, stirring frequently.

Stir in the remaining ratatouille ingredients, breaking up the tomatoes into smaller pieces. Simmer for 15 to 20 minutes, or until the bell pepper and eggplant are tender, stirring occasionally to prevent sticking.

Meanwhile, prepare the rice using the package directions, omitting the salt and margarine and substituting the broth for the water. Spoon into bowls and top with the ratatouille, the remaining 2 tablespoons Parmesan, and the red pepper flakes.

PER SERVING

calories 279	**carbohydrates** 49 g
total fat 4.0 g	fiber 9 g
saturated fat 1.0 g	sugars 11 g
trans fat 0.0 g	**protein** 12 g
polyunsaturated fat 0.5 g	**DIETARY EXCHANGES**
monounsaturated fat 1.5 g	2 1/2 starch,
cholesterol 4 mg	2 vegetable, 1/2 lean
sodium 143 mg	meat

HOPPIN' JOHN

SERVES 4

Hoppin' John always combines black-eyed peas with rice, onion, and herbs. Less certain is the history of the name and whether eating Hoppin' John on New Year's Day really brings good luck throughout the year. Regardless, your family will definitely feel lucky when you serve this southern dish.

1 cup uncooked instant brown rice

1 teaspoon canola or corn oil

1 medium rib of celery, diced

1 small onion, sliced

2 1/2 cups canned no-salt-added tomatoes, undrained

1 teaspoon chopped fresh basil or
    1/4 teaspoon dried basil, crumbled

1/2 teaspoon dried rosemary, crushed

Pepper to taste

1 15.5-ounce can no-salt-added black-eyed peas, rinsed and drained

Prepare the rice using the package directions, omitting the salt and margarine.

Meanwhile, in a large skillet, heat the oil over medium heat, swirling to coat the bottom. Cook the celery and onion for about 3 minutes, or until the onion is almost soft, stirring frequently.

Stir in the remaining ingredients except the peas. Reduce the heat and simmer for 20 minutes, stirring occasionally.

Stir in the peas. Cook, covered, over low heat for 5 minutes, or until heated through. Serve the peas over the rice.

Cook's Tip on Mortar and Pestle: The mortar is a heavy bowl, and the pestle is a grinding tool—a handle with a large knob on one end. Put spices such as caraway seeds or herbs such as rosemary in the mortar and mash them against the bottom and side with the pestle until they are as fine as you want.

PER SERVING

calories 233	carbohydrates 44 g
total fat 2.0 g	fiber 9 g
saturated fat 0.0 g	sugars 10 g
trans fat 0.0 g	protein 10 g
polyunsaturated fat 0.5 g	DIETARY EXCHANGES
monounsaturated fat 1.0 g	2 1/2 starch,
cholesterol 0 mg	2 vegetable, 1/2 lean
sodium 77 mg	meat

CHICKPEA PILAF

SERVES 6

Quinoa replaces the usual rice in this protein-rich pilaf. Serve with Creamy Cauliflower Soup (page 39) or Spiralized Cucumbers with Yogurt-Dill Dressing (page 79).

1/2 to 3/4 cup dry-packed sun-dried tomatoes

1 cup boiling water

1 cup uncooked quinoa, rinsed and drained

1 1/2 teaspoons olive oil

10 ounces frozen green peas, thawed

1 large garlic clove, minced

1 to 1 1/2 teaspoons dried oregano, crumbled

1/2 teaspoon crushed red pepper flakes

1 15.5-ounce can no-salt-added chickpeas, rinsed and drained

3 ounces fat-free feta cheese

Put the tomatoes in a small bowl. Pour in the boiling water. Set aside for about 10 minutes to soften. Drain the tomatoes, saving the liquid in a 2-cup measuring cup. Chop the tomatoes and set aside. Add enough water to the tomato liquid to equal 2 cups. Pour into a medium saucepan.

In a large skillet, dry-roast the quinoa over medium-high heat for about 3 to 4 minutes, or until it is lightly toasted and any excess water has evaporated, stirring frequently (the quinoa won't turn golden brown).

Stir the quinoa into the tomato liquid. Bring to a boil over high heat. Reduce the heat and simmer, covered, for 15 minutes, or until all the liquid is absorbed.

Meanwhile, in a large nonstick skillet, heat the oil over medium heat, swirling to coat the bottom. Cook the peas, garlic, oregano, and red pepper flakes for 2 minutes, stirring occasionally.

Stir in the chickpeas. Cook for 5 minutes, or until heated through.

In a large bowl, stir together the tomatoes, quinoa, and chickpea mixture. Crumble the feta on top.

PER SERVING

calories 259	**carbohydrates** 42 g
total fat 4.0 g	fiber 8 g
saturated fat 0.5 g	sugars 6 g
trans fat 0.0 g	**protein** 14 g
polyunsaturated fat 1.0 g	**DIETARY EXCHANGES**
monounsaturated fat 1.5 g	2 1/2 starch,
cholesterol 0 mg	1 vegetable, 1 lean
sodium 293 mg	meat

FALAFEL WITH QUICK-PICKLED GARLIC CUCUMBERS

SERVES 4

This version of a Middle Eastern classic eliminates the deep-frying but still provides a crispy crust and moist center by first browning the falafels in a skillet and then baking them. For dessert, try Cashew and Cardamom Cookies *(page 486) or* Chai-Spiced Flans with Blueberries *(page 496).*

1 15.5 ounce can no-salt-added chickpeas, rinsed and drained

1 large egg

1 tablespoon fresh lemon juice

2 teaspoons ground cumin

2 large garlic cloves, minced, and 1 large garlic clove, sliced, divided use

1 teaspoon baking powder

1/4 teaspoon pepper

1/4 cup chopped fresh cilantro

3 tablespoons minced red onion

2 tablespoons chopped fresh Italian (flat-leaf) parsley

3 unpeeled seedless baby cucumbers, thinly sliced (about 1 cup)

1/4 teaspoon crushed red pepper flakes

1/4 cup plain rice vinegar

2 tablespoons water

Cooking spray

2 teaspoons olive oil and 2 teaspoons olive oil, divided use

In a food processor or blender, process the chickpeas until finely chopped. Add the egg, lemon juice, cumin, minced garlic, baking powder, and pepper. Pulse until well combined and almost smooth. Add the cilantro, onion, and parsley. Pulse until smooth.

Transfer the falafel mixture to a medium bowl. Cover and refrigerate for 30 minutes.

Meanwhile, in a small bowl, stir together the cucumbers, red pepper flakes, and the remaining sliced garlic.

In a small microwaveable bowl, microwave the vinegar and water on 100 percent power (high) for 30 to 50 seconds, or until hot. Pour over the cucumber mixture. Let stand for 30 minutes, or until room temperature. Drain well in a colander.

Meanwhile, preheat the oven to 350°F. Line a large baking sheet with aluminum foil. Lightly spray the foil with cooking spray.

In a large nonstick skillet, heat 2 teaspoons of oil over medium-high heat, swirling to coat the bottom. Place four 1/4-cup mounds of the falafel mixture in the skillet. Using the back of a spoon, gently press down on the mounds, spreading them to make patties 3 inches in diameter. Cook the patties for 3 to 4 minutes, or until well browned on the bottom. (Be sure they're well browned before they're turned or they may fall apart.) Gently turn over the patties. Cook for 1 minute. Transfer the patties to the baking sheet. Repeat the process with the remaining 2 teaspoons oil and falafel mixture.

Bake for 5 to 8 minutes, or until the patties are hot in the center. Serve with the cucumbers.

(continued)

Cook's Tip: If the chickpea mixture sticks to the spoon when shaping the patties, wet the spoon with a little water.

stantly. Stir in the remaining ingredients except the yogurt. Increase the heat to medium-high and bring just to a boil. Reduce the heat to low and simmer for 20 to 30 minutes, or until the potatoes are tender and the liquid is slightly thickened. Garnish the stew with the yogurt.

CHANA MASALA

SERVES 4

This aromatic, easy-to-make version of the traditional Indian stew, combines chickpeas with spices, tomatoes, and potatoes for a quick dinner. If desired, serve over brown rice and garnish with lime wedges.

> 1 teaspoon canola or corn oil
> 1 cup chopped onion
> 2 teaspoons minced peeled gingerroot
> 2 medium garlic cloves, minced
> 2 15.5-ounce cans no-salt-added chickpeas, rinsed and drained
> 2 cups chopped tomatoes
> 12 ounces unpeeled baby red potatoes, cut into 3/4-inch pieces
> 1 1/2 cups water
> 1/2 to 1 small fresh serrano pepper, finely chopped, seeds and ribs discarded (see Cook's Tip on Handling Hot Chiles, page 24)
> 1 1/2 teaspoons ground cumin
> 1 1/2 teaspoons ground coriander
> 1 teaspoon garam masala
> 1/4 teaspoon salt
> 1/4 cup fat-free plain Greek yogurt

In a large pot, heat the oil over medium heat, swirling to coat the bottom. Cook the onion for 4 to 5 minutes, or until beginning to brown, stirring frequently. Stir in the gingerroot and garlic. Cook for 1 minute, or until fragrant, stirring con-

BROCCOLI RABE AND CHICKPEAS OVER PARMESAN TOASTS

SERVES 6

You can serve this interesting one-dish meal of broccoli rabe and chickpeas over whole-grain penne instead of toast, for a change. If you can't find broccoli rabe, use broccolini instead.

> 2 medium bunches broccoli rabe, trimmed and coarsely chopped
> 1 tablespoon plus 2 teaspoons olive oil (extra-virgin preferred)
> 3 large garlic cloves, coarsely chopped
> 1 teaspoon fennel seeds
> 1/4 teaspoon crushed red pepper flakes
> 1/4 teaspoon salt
> Pepper to taste
> 4 15.5-ounce cans no-salt-added chickpeas, rinsed and drained
> 6 slices whole-grain Italian or French bread, 1/2 inch thick (regular size, not baguette)
> 1 1/2 tablespoons shredded or grated Parmesan cheese

In a large saucepan, add water to a depth of 1 inch. Put the broccoli rabe in a collapsible steamer basket (you might have to do this in batches). Place the steamer in the pan. Steam the broccoli rabe, covered, for 5 minutes, or until tender-crisp. Remove from the heat. Carefully uncover the pan away from you (to prevent steam burns). Drain well in a colander.

In a stockpot, heat the oil over medium-low heat, swirling to coat the bottom. Cook the broccoli rabe, garlic, fennel seeds, red pepper flakes, salt, and pepper, covered, for 10 minutes, stirring occasionally.

Stir the chickpeas into the broccoli rabe mixture. Cook, covered, for 10 to 15 minutes, or until the broccoli rabe is tender, stirring occasionally. Remove from the heat. Leave covered to keep warm.

Meanwhile, preheat the broiler.

Put the bread on a broilerproof baking sheet. Sprinkle the Parmesan over the bread. Broil about 4 inches from the heat for about 1 minute, or until the bread is golden brown and the Parmesan has melted.

Transfer the toasts to a large, deep serving platter. Spoon the broccoli rabe mixture and cooking liquid over the toasts.

Cook's Tip on Chickpeas: If you prefer to use dried chickpeas, prepare 1 pound chickpeas using the package directions, omitting the salt. Drain well and proceed as directed.

Cook's Tip on Broccoli Rabe: Known by several other names—broccoli raab, American gai lan, and rapini—broccoli rabe (*rahb*) is a bitter vegetable with a lemon-pepper taste. Look for deep, dark green leaves and buds (which look like tiny broccoli buds) with no trace of yellow (a sign of age).

PER SERVING

calories 434	carbohydrates 70 g
total fat 7.5 g	fiber 12 g
saturated fat 1.0 g	sugars 3 g
trans fat 0.0 g	protein 22 g
polyunsaturated fat 2.0 g	DIETARY EXCHANGES
monounsaturated fat 4.0 g	4 1/2 starch,
cholesterol 1 mg	1 vegetable, 1 1/2 lean
sodium 383 mg	meat

LENTIL LOAF

SERVES 6

This vegetarian version of meatloaf is so good you won't even notice it's meatless! If you prefer a saucier loaf, prepare a sauce, such as Bourbon Barbecue Sauce *(page 431) or* Fresh Tomato and Roasted Red Bell Pepper Sauce *(page 434), while the loaf is baking.*

> Cooking spray
> 1 large onion, chopped
> 1 cup dried lentils, sorted for stones and
>   shriveled lentils, rinsed, and drained
> 1/2 cup chopped walnuts
> 1/2 cup crushed cornflakes or whole-wheat
>   bread crumbs (lowest sodium available)
> 1/2 cup fat-free evaporated milk
> 1 large egg or 2 large egg whites
> 1 teaspoon ground cumin
> 1/4 teaspoon dried thyme, crumbled
> 3 medium lemons, cut into 4 wedges each

Preheat the oven to 350°F. Lightly spray a 9 x 5 x 3-inch loaf pan with cooking spray.

In a large bowl, stir together all the remaining ingredients except the lemon wedges until well blended.

Transfer to the pan. Bake for 30 minutes. Serve with the lemon wedges.

PER SERVING

calories 257	carbohydrates 35 g
total fat 7.5 g	fiber 6 g
saturated fat 1.0 g	sugars 8 g
trans fat 0.0 g	protein 16 g
polyunsaturated fat 5.0 g	DIETARY EXCHANGES
monounsaturated fat 1.0 g	2 1/2 starch, 1 1/2 lean
cholesterol 32 mg	meat
sodium 103 mg	

MEDITERRANEAN LENTILS AND RICE

SERVES 4

Middle Eastern cuisine often combines sweet ingredients, such as cinnamon and currants, with more savory ingredients, such as cumin and onion. That sweet and savory pairing makes this dish especially enticing. Although the currants are so small that they aren't readily apparent, they add an important depth and richness.

1 medium onion, minced

2 teaspoons ground cumin

2 teaspoons ground cinnamon

1/2 teaspoon cayenne

2 cups fat-free, low-sodium vegetable broth and 2 cups fat-free, low-sodium vegetable broth, such as on page 36, or 2 cups water and 2 cups water, divided use

3/4 cup dried lentils, sorted for stones and shriveled lentils, rinsed, and drained

1 14.5-ounce can no-salt-added crushed tomatoes, undrained

1 cup uncooked brown rice

1/2 cup water

1/3 cup dried currants

1/4 cup crumbled fat-free feta cheese

In a large nonstick skillet, cook the onion, cumin, cinnamon, and cayenne over medium heat for 10 minutes, stirring occasionally.

Stir in 2 cups broth and the lentils. Increase the heat to medium high and bring to a boil. Reduce the heat and simmer, covered, for 20 minutes.

Stir in the tomatoes with liquid, rice, 1/2 cup water, the currants, and the remaining 2 cups broth. Increase the heat to medium high and bring to a boil. Reduce the heat and simmer, covered, for 20 minutes, or until the rice and lentils are tender. Just before serving, sprinkle with the feta.

PER SERVING

calories 406
total fat 1.5 g
  saturated fat 0.5 g
  trans fat 0.0 g
  polyunsaturated fat 0.5 g
  monounsaturated fat 0.5 g
cholesterol 0 mg
sodium 190 mg

carbohydrates 81 g
  fiber 12 g
  sugars 17 g
protein 20 g
DIETARY EXCHANGES
  4 starch, 2 vegetable, 1/2 fruit, 1 1/2 lean meat

CUMIN AND GINGER LENTILS ON QUINOA

SERVES 4

Ground cumin is the key ingredient in this dish, tying all the other flavors together. Serve as a meatless entrée for four or as a side dish for eight with grilled lamb chops or pork.

1 teaspoon olive oil

1 1/2 cups diced onions

1 cup thinly sliced carrots

1/2 cup thinly sliced celery

2 medium garlic cloves, minced

2 cups water and 1 1/4 cups water, divided use

1/2 cup dried lentils, sorted for stones and shriveled lentils, rinsed and drained

1/2 cup uncooked quinoa, rinsed and drained

1/4 cup finely chopped green onions

1/3 cup pine nuts, dry-roasted

2 teaspoons grated peeled gingerroot

3/4 to 1 teaspoon ground cumin

1/2 teaspoon salt

1/8 teaspoon cayenne (optional)

In a large nonstick skillet, heat the oil over medium-high heat, swirling to coat the bottom. Cook the onions, carrots, and celery for 6 minutes, or until beginning to brown on the edges, stirring frequently.

Stir in the garlic. Cook for 15 seconds.

Stir in 2 cups water and the lentils. Bring to a boil, still over medium-high heat. Reduce the heat and simmer, covered, for 25 minutes, or until the lentils are tender. Remove from the heat.

Meanwhile, in a medium saucepan, bring the remaining 1 1/4 cups water to a boil over high heat.

Stir in the quinoa. Return to a boil. Reduce the heat and simmer, covered, for 10 to 12 minutes, or until the water is absorbed and the quinoa is just tender. Remove from the heat.

Stir the green onions into the quinoa. Set aside, uncovered.

When the lentil mixture is cooked, gently stir in the remaining ingredients.

Spoon the quinoa mixture onto a serving plate. Spoon the lentil mixture over the quinoa. Serve immediately for peak flavor.

PER SERVING

calories 267	carbohydrates 39 g
total fat 8.0 g	fiber 10 g
saturated fat 1.0 g	sugars 8 g
trans fat 0.0 g	**protein** 13 g
polyunsaturated fat 3.0 g	**DIETARY EXCHANGES**
monounsaturated fat 3.0 g	2 starch, 2 vegetable,
cholesterol 0 mg	1/2 lean meat, 1 fat
sodium 337 mg	

LENTIL, SQUASH, AND CARAMELIZED ONION CROQUETTES

SERVES 4

Two kinds of squash add not only extra vegetables but also moisture to these patties. Serve on a bed of steamed spinach or Basil Spinach *(page 404).*

3/4 cup dried brown lentils, sorted for stones and shriveled lentils, rinsed, and drained

1 teaspoon olive oil, 2 teaspoons olive oil, and 2 teaspoons olive oil, divided use

1 medium onion, thinly sliced

1/2 cup uncooked oatmeal

1 large egg

1/2 teaspoon curry powder

1/8 teaspoon ground allspice

1/2 cup shredded butternut squash

1/3 cup shredded zucchini

1/4 cup sliced green onions (green part only)

3/4 cup whole-wheat panko (Japanese-style bread crumbs)

In a medium saucepan, bring 2 1/4 cups water to a boil over high heat. Stir in the lentils. Reduce the heat and simmer, covered, for 30 minutes, or until tender. Drain well in a fine-mesh sieve.

Meanwhile, in a small nonstick skillet, heat 1 teaspoon oil over medium heat, swirling to coat the bottom. Reduce the heat to low. Cook the onion, covered, for 5 minutes. Cook, uncovered, for 3 to 5 minutes, or until golden brown, stirring frequently.

In a food processor or blender, pulse the lentils until coarsely chopped. Add the oatmeal. Pulse until coarsely ground. Add the onion, egg, curry powder, and allspice. Pulse until almost smooth. Add the squash, zucchini, and green onions. Process until well blended.

Transfer the lentil mixture to a medium bowl. Cover and refrigerate for 1 to 2 hours, or until chilled.

Put the panko in a shallow dish. Put 1/4 cup of the lentil mixture in the panko, turning to coat completely. Shape into a 4 x 2-inch oval. Transfer the croquette to a large plate. Repeat with the remaining lentil mixture and panko.

In a large nonstick skillet, heat 2 teaspoons of oil, swirling to coat the bottom. Cook 4 croquettes over medium heat for 7 to 10 minutes, or until browned, turning once halfway through.

Transfer the croquettes to a large serving platter. Cover to keep warm.

Repeat with the remaining 2 teaspoons of oil and 4 croquettes.

PER SERVING

calories 315	carbohydrates 47 g
total fat 8.0 g	fiber 9 g
saturated fat 1.5 g	sugars 6 g
trans fat 0.0 g	**protein** 17 g
polyunsaturated fat 1.0 g	**DIETARY EXCHANGES**
monounsaturated fat 5.0 g	3 starch, 1 lean meat,
cholesterol 47 mg	1/2 fat
sodium 41 mg	

PALAK PANEER

SERVES 4

This velvety dish of spinach and aromatic spices paired with chunks of fresh Indian cheese (paneer) is served over basmati rice and topped with yogurt.

1 cup uncooked brown basmati rice
2 teaspoons canola or corn oil
1 cup chopped onion
3 large garlic cloves, minced
2 teaspoons minced peeled gingerroot
1 1/2 teaspoons ground coriander
1 teaspoon ground cumin
1/4 teaspoon crushed red pepper flakes
1 medium tomato, chopped
20 ounces frozen chopped spinach, thawed
    and squeezed dry
2 1/2 ounces paneer, cut into 1/2-inch cubes
1 teaspoon garam masala
1/2 to 3/4 cup water
1/3 cup fat-free plain yogurt and
    2 tablespoons fat-free plain yogurt,
    divided use

Prepare the rice using the package directions, omitting the salt and margarine. Set aside.

Meanwhile, in a large saucepan, heat the oil over medium heat, swirling to coat the bottom. Add the onion. Cook for 2 minutes, or until beginning to soften, stirring frequently. Stir in the garlic and gingerroot. Cook for 2 to 3 minutes, or until the mixture begins to brown, stirring frequently. Reduce the heat to low if necessary. Stir in the coriander, cumin, and red pepper flakes. Cook for 30 seconds to 1 minute, or until fragrant, stirring constantly.

Stir in the tomato. Cook for 1 to 2 minutes, or until softened. Stir in the spinach. Cook for 2 to 3 minutes, or until hot. Stir in the paneer and garam masala. Pour in 1/2 cup water. Bring to a boil. Cook for 1 to 2 minutes, or until the mixture is hot and creamy, adding additional water if necessary. Remove from the heat.

Stir in 1/3 cup yogurt. Spoon the rice onto plates. Serve the palak paneer over the rice. Garnish with the remaining 2 tablespoons yogurt.

Cook's Tip on Paneer: Paneer is a fresh unripened cheese with a firm texture. It can be found in well-stocked grocery stores, cheese markets, or Indian grocers. If it's not available, you can substitute farmer cheese or firm tofu, well drained and patted dry.

PER SERVING

calories 324	carbohydrates 50 g
total fat 9.5 g	fiber 8 g
saturated fat 3.5 g	sugars 7 g
trans fat 0.0 g	protein 15 g
polyunsaturated fat 2.0 g	DIETARY EXCHANGES
monounsaturated fat 3.0 g	2 1/2 starch,
cholesterol 18 mg	2 vegetable, 1 lean
sodium 140 mg	meat, 1 fat

GREEN CHILE AND RICE PIE

SERVES 4

This quiche-like pie has south-of-the-border flair. Start your meal with a cup of Gazpacho *(page 49).*

Cooking spray

Pie

1 teaspoon olive oil
2 cups sliced button mushrooms
1/2 cup chopped onion
2 medium garlic cloves, minced
1 1/2 cups fat-free milk
1 14.5-ounce can no-salt-added diced
    tomatoes, well drained, patted dry with
    paper towels
1 cup uncooked instant brown rice
1/2 cup shredded low-fat 4-cheese Mexican
    blend
1/2 cup egg substitute
1 4-ounce can diced green chiles, drained
1/4 cup shredded or grated Parmesan cheese
3/4 teaspoon ground cumin

Topping

1/4 cup fat-free sour cream
1 tablespoon plus 1 teaspoon salsa (lowest
    sodium available), such as Salsa Cruda
    (page 437)
1 tablespoon plus 1 teaspoon chopped fresh
    cilantro

Preheat the oven to 350°F. Lightly spray a 9-inch deep pie pan with cooking spray.

In a large nonstick skillet, heat the oil over medium-high heat, swirling to coat the bottom. Cook the mushrooms and onion for 3 minutes, or until the mushrooms and onion are soft, stirring frequently.

Stir in the garlic. Cook for 30 seconds, stirring frequently.

Pour in the milk. Cook for 1 1/2 to 2 minutes, or until hot but not boiling, stirring occasionally. Remove from the heat.

Stir in the remaining pie ingredients. Carefully pour into the pie pan.

Bake for 30 to 35 minutes, or until a knife inserted in the center comes out clean, the top is golden, and the edges are browned. Spoon the sour cream and salsa on top. Sprinkle with the cilantro.

PER SERVING

calories 266	carbohydrates 35 g
total fat 6.5 g	fiber 3 g
saturated fat 2.5 g	sugars 11 g
trans fat 0.0 g	protein 17 g
polyunsaturated fat 0.5 g	DIETARY EXCHANGES
monounsaturated fat 2.5 g	1 1/2 starch,
cholesterol 17 mg	2 vegetable, 1 1/2 lean
sodium 452 mg	meat

EDAMAME, CABBAGE, AND BROWN RICE STIR-FRY

SERVES 4

Edamame provides snap and protein in this classic stir-fry. If you can't find napa cabbage, substitute regular green cabbage.

1 cup uncooked instant brown rice
3 tablespoons soy sauce (lowest sodium available)
2 1/2 teaspoons sugar
1 teaspoon Worcestershire sauce (lowest sodium available)

4 cups shredded napa cabbage (about 8 ounces)
2 cups frozen shelled edamame, thawed
1 large onion, chopped
1 9-ounce can sliced water chestnuts, rinsed and drained
1 8-ounce can bamboo shoots, rinsed and drained
1 medium carrot, shredded
2 medium garlic cloves, minced
1 teaspoon grated peeled gingerroot
1 tablespoon canola or corn oil

Prepare the rice using the package directions, omitting the salt and margarine. Set aside.

In a small bowl, whisk together the soy sauce, sugar, and Worcestershire sauce until the sugar is dissolved. Set aside.

In a large bowl, stir together the remaining ingredients except the oil.

In a wok or large skillet, heat the oil over high heat, swirling to coat the wok. Cook the cabbage mixture for 2 minutes, stirring constantly.

Stir in the cooked rice. Cook for 2 minutes, stirring constantly. Remove from the heat.

Stir in the soy sauce mixture.

PER SERVING

calories 301	carbohydrates 42 g
total fat 8.0 g	fiber 10 g
saturated fat 0.5 g	sugars 13 g
trans fat 0.0 g	protein 15 g
polyunsaturated fat 3.0 g	DIETARY EXCHANGES
monounsaturated fat 4.0 g	2 starch 3 vegetable,
cholesterol 0 mg	1 lean meat, 1 fat
sodium 337 mg	

BUTTERNUT, BROCCOLI, AND BROWN RICE STIR-FRY

SERVES 4

This unusual combo packs in flavor and nutrients from colorful veggies, whole grain, and omega-rich sunflower seeds. The warm lemon-honey mixture that tops the dish is infused with just a hint of vanilla and nutmeg.

> 1/2 cup uncooked instant brown rice
> 1 cup fat-free, low-sodium vegetable broth, such as on page 36
> 1 cup frozen shelled edamame
> 2 teaspoons olive oil
> 6 ounces broccoli florets
> 10 ounces frozen cubed butternut squash, thawed
> 1 teaspoon grated lemon zest
> 2 tablespoons fresh lemon juice
> 2 tablespoons honey
> 1/2 teaspoon vanilla extract
> 1/4 teaspoon pepper
> 1/8 teaspoon ground nutmeg
> 2 tablespoons shelled unsalted sunflower seeds

Prepare the rice using the package directions, omitting the salt and margarine and substituting the broth for the water.

In a medium saucepan, bring about 2 cups of water to a boil over high heat. Stir in the edamame. Reduce the heat to medium high and cook for 5 minutes, or until tender. Drain well in a colander.

Meanwhile, in a large nonstick skillet, heat the oil over medium-high heat, swirling to coat the bottom. Cook the broccoli for 3 to 4 minutes, or until tender-crisp, stirring constantly.

Gently stir in the butternut squash and edamame, being careful not to mash the squash. Cook for 3 to 5 minutes, or until heated through, stirring occasionally. Reduce the heat to low to keep warm, stirring occasionally.

In a small microwaveable bowl, whisk together the remaining ingredients except the sunflower

seeds. Microwave on 100 percent power (high) for 20 to 30 seconds, or until heated through.

Spoon the rice into shallow dishes or onto plates. Top with the butternut squash mixture. Drizzle the lemon juice mixture over all. Sprinkle with the sunflower seeds.

Cook's Tip on Butternut Squash: If your supermarket doesn't carry frozen diced butternut squash, feel free to substitute a 10-ounce package of frozen cooked winter squash. Cook as directed above. Although the texture will be different and not as attractive, the flavor of the dish will be just as delicious.

PER SERVING

calories 238	carbohydrates 36 g
total fat 7.5 g	fiber 6 g
saturated fat 1.0 g	sugars 12 g
trans fat 0.0 g	protein 9 g
polyunsaturated fat 3.0 g	DIETARY EXCHANGES
monounsaturated fat 2.5 g	2 starch, 1 vegetable,
cholesterol 0 mg	1 fat
sodium 26 mg	

PENNE AND RICOTTA CASSEROLE

SERVES 5

This is a healthier version of the baked ziti that you'd find at your favorite neighborhood Italian restaurant. It has the gooey cheese and classic Italian herbs, but not an excess of sodium and saturated fat. Enjoy with a dark green, leafy salad with Zesty Tomato Dressing (page 105) and a crusty whole-grain roll.

> Olive oil cooking spray
> 1 15-ounce can tomato puree
> 1 cup fat-free, low-sodium vegetable broth, such as on page 36, or water
> 1 1/2 teaspoons dried Italian seasoning, crumbled
> 1/2 teaspoon garlic powder and 1/2 teaspoon garlic powder, divided use
> 1/4 teaspoon crushed red pepper flakes
> 15 ounces low-fat ricotta cheese
> 1/2 teaspoon onion powder
> 8 ounces dried whole-grain penne

2 ounces low-fat mozzarella cheese,
shredded or sliced

Preheat the oven to 350°F. Lightly spray an 8-inch square glass casserole dish with cooking spray.

In a small bowl, stir together the tomato purée, broth, Italian seasoning, 1/2 teaspoon garlic powder, and the red pepper flakes.

In a separate small bowl, stir together the ricotta cheese, onion powder, and the remaining 1/2 teaspoon garlic powder.

Layer in the casserole dish as follows: 1 cup tomato purée mixture, spread over the bottom; half the pasta; all the ricotta mixture, dolloped, then spread as well as possible; 1 cup tomato purée mixture; the remaining pasta; and the remaining tomato purée mixture.

Bake, covered, for 1 hour for al dente pasta (longer if you prefer softer pasta). Remove from the oven. Top with the mozzarella. Bake, uncovered, for 5 minutes.

PER SERVING

calories 300	carbohydrates 46 g
total fat 5.0 g	fiber 5 g
saturated fat 2.5 g	sugars 7 g
trans fat 0.0 g	protein 18 g
polyunsaturated fat 0.5 g	DIETARY EXCHANGES
monounsaturated fat 1.5 g	2 1/2 starch,
cholesterol 25 mg	2 vegetable, 1 1/2 lean
sodium 182 mg	meat

PASTA PRIMAVERA

SERVES 4

Pasta primavera *simply means "spring pasta," and this simple, verdant recipe uses the best of the season's bounty.*

12 ounces dried whole-grain linguine
6 ounces thin asparagus, trimmed and cut
    into 1 1/2-inch pieces
3 cups kale, stems removed and leaves
    roughly chopped, or 5 ounces baby
    spinach

1 cup frozen shelled edamame
1 tablespoon olive oil (extra-virgin preferred)
1 medium spring onion, thinly sliced, or 1 large
    green onion, thinly sliced
3 medium garlic cloves
1 cup fat-free plain yogurt (not Greek)
1/2 cup fat-free ricotta
1 tablespoon grated lemon zest
2 tablespoons fresh lemon juice, or to taste
Pepper to taste
1 tablespoon plus 1 teaspoon shredded or
    grated Parmesan cheese

Prepare the pasta using the package directions, omitting the salt. Three minutes before the pasta is done, add the asparagus, kale, and edamame. Drain well in a colander.

Meanwhile, in a large skillet, heat the oil over medium heat, swirling to coat the bottom. Cook the spring onion and garlic for 2 minutes, or until the garlic is golden, stirring constantly. Don't let it brown. Remove from the heat. Stir in the pasta mixture, ricotta, lemon zest, lemon juice, and pepper, tossing gently until combined.

Just before serving, sprinkle with the Parmesan.

Cook's Tip: Leftovers make an amazing cold pasta salad, so you might want to make extra.

PER SERVING

calories 489	carbohydrates 80 g
total fat 8.5 g	fiber 14 g
saturated fat 1.0 g	sugars 12 g
trans fat 0.0 g	protein 27 g
polyunsaturated fat 2.0 g	DIETARY EXCHANGES
monounsaturated fat 4.0 g	4 1/2 starch,
cholesterol 5 mg	1 vegetable, 1/2 fat-
sodium 159 mg	free milk, 1 lean meat

ZUCCHINI LINGUINE WITH WALNUTS

SERVES 4

The generous amount of toasted walnuts gives this one-dish meal a warm and rustic character—just right for a cold or rainy night.

8 ounces dried whole-grain linguine
Olive oil cooking spray
2 medium zucchini, sliced
1 medium onion, thinly sliced
8 ounces button mushrooms, sliced
1 tablespoon dried oregano, crumbled
4 medium garlic cloves, minced
1/4 teaspoon crushed red pepper flakes
1/2 cup chopped walnuts, dry-roasted
2 teaspoons olive oil (extra-virgin preferred)
1/4 teaspoon salt

Prepare the pasta using the package directions, omitting the salt. Drain well in a colander, reserving 1/2 cup pasta water.

Meanwhile, lightly spray a large skillet or Dutch oven with cooking spray. Cook the zucchini and onion over medium-high heat for 8 minutes, or until beginning to lightly brown on the edges, stirring frequently. Remove the skillet from the heat. Transfer the zucchini mixture to a plate.

Lightly spray the same skillet with cooking spray. Cook the mushrooms, oregano, garlic, and red pepper flakes, still over medium-high heat, for 4 minutes, or until the mushrooms begin to lightly brown, stirring occasionally.

Stir the zucchini mixture into the mushroom mixture. Stir in the pasta and reserved pasta water. Cook for 30 seconds, or until most of the liquid has evaporated. Remove from the heat.

Stir in the walnuts, oil, and salt.

PER SERVING

calories 367	carbohydrates 53 g
total fat 14.0 g	fiber 10 g
saturated fat 1.5 g	sugars 8 g
trans fat 0.0 g	protein 13 g
polyunsaturated fat 8.0 g	DIETARY EXCHANGES
monounsaturated fat 3.5 g	3 starch, 2 vegetable,
cholesterol 0 mg	2 fat
sodium 159 mg	

PECAN-TOPPED PASTA WITH VEGETABLES

SERVES 4

This dish gets a double dose of nutty flavor from cumin and pecans. Spiral-shaped pasta is piled high with several types of sizzling veggies and has a crunch from a sprinkling of toasted nuts on top.

8 ounces dried whole-grain rotini
1 1/2 cups finely chopped onions
1 medium red bell pepper, thinly sliced
1 cup matchstick-size carrot strips
6 ounces button mushrooms, thinly sliced
1/2 teaspoon ground cumin
1/4 teaspoon salt
1 1/2 ounces finely chopped pecans, dry-roasted

Prepare the pasta using the package directions, omitting the salt. Drain well in a colander.

Put the onions, bell pepper, carrots, and mushrooms in a large nonstick skillet. Cook over medium-high heat for 10 to 12 minutes, or until the onions are deeply browned, stirring frequently.

Stir in the cumin and salt. Cook for 30 seconds. Serve the vegetable mixture over the pasta. Sprinkle with the pecans.

PER SERVING

calories 331	carbohydrates 55 g
total fat 9.5 g	fiber 10 g
saturated fat 0.5 g	sugars 9 g
trans fat 0.0 g	protein 11 g
polyunsaturated fat 3.0 g	DIETARY EXCHANGES
monounsaturated fat 4.5 g	3 starch, 2 vegetable,
cholesterol 0 mg	1 fat
sodium 174 mg	

SPAGHETTI WITH SPINACH AND TOASTED HAZELNUTS

SERVES 4

This Italian-flavored pasta dish is full of cheesiness and crunch. Serve with Marinated Tomato Salad (page 81).

8 ounces dried whole-grain spaghetti, broken into small pieces

1 cup fat-free ricotta cheese

10 ounces frozen chopped spinach, thawed and squeezed dry

2 medium green onions (green part only), sliced

2 tablespoons shredded or grated Parmesan cheese

2 tablespoons fat-free milk

1/2 teaspoon dried Italian seasoning, crumbled

1 tablespoon light tub margarine

Pepper to taste

1/4 cup chopped hazelnuts, dry-roasted

Prepare the pasta using the package directions, omitting the salt. Drain well in a colander.

Meanwhile, in a medium bowl, stir together the ricotta, spinach, green onions, Parmesan, milk, and Italian seasoning.

In the same pot used for the pasta, melt the margarine over medium-low heat, swirling to coat the bottom. Return the pasta to the pot. Stir. When the pasta is warm, stir in the ricotta mixture. Cook for 3 to 4 minutes, or until heated through, stirring occasionally. Stir in the pepper. Sprinkle with the hazelnuts.

PER SERVING

calories 341	carbohydrates 49 g
total fat 8.0 g	fiber 9 g
saturated fat 1.0 g	sugars 6 g
trans fat 0.0 g	**protein** 20 g
polyunsaturated fat 1 5 g	**DIETARY EXCHANGES**
monounsaturated fat 4.5 g	3 starch, 1 vegetable,
cholesterol 7 mg	1 1/2 lean meat
sodium 243 mg	

SPAGHETTI WITH ZESTY MARINARA SAUCE

SERVES 8

This aromatic sauce that cooks low and slow turns any meal into an Italian feast. While the sauce is simmering, bake Focaccia (page 443).

Sauce

1 teaspoon olive oil

1 large onion, finely chopped

2 large garlic cloves, crushed

1 6-ounce can no-salt-added tomato paste

2 tablespoons minced fresh parsley

2 teaspoons sugar

1 1/4 teaspoons dried Italian seasoning, crumbled

1/2 teaspoon dried basil, crumbled

1/4 teaspoon pepper, or to taste

1/8 teaspoon crushed red pepper flakes, or to taste

1/8 teaspoon salt

1 14.5-ounce can no-salt-added crushed tomatoes, undrained

1 cup water

1 8-ounce can no-salt-added tomato sauce

1/4 cup dry red wine (regular or nonalcoholic)

1 medium dried bay leaf

■ ■ ■

16 ounces dried whole-grain spaghetti

1/2 cup shredded or grated Parmesan cheese

In a medium saucepan, heat the oil over medium-high heat, swirling to coat the bottom. Cook the onion and garlic for 3 minutes, or until the onion is soft, stirring frequently.

Whisk in the tomato paste, parsley, sugar, Italian seasoning, basil, pepper, red pepper flakes, and salt. Reduce the heat to medium low. Cook for 4 minutes, stirring frequently.

Stir in the remaining sauce ingredients. Increase the heat to high and bring to a boil. Reduce the heat and simmer, partially covered, for 1 hour to 1 hour 30 minutes, stirring occasionally. Discard the bay leaf.

Meanwhile, prepare the pasta using the package directions, omitting the salt. Drain well in a colander. Transfer to a large serving bowl.

Stir in the Parmesan. Top with the sauce.

Cook's Tip: Because the sauce freezes well, you might want to cook half the amount of spaghetti

(continued)

to serve four and then freeze the remaining half of the sauce for a later use; it'll keep for up to six months.

PER SERVING

calories 293	sodium 148 mg
total fat 3.5 g	carbohydrates 55 g
saturated fat 1.0 g	fiber 9 g
trans fat 0.0 g	sugars 10 g
polyunsaturated fat 0.5 g	protein 12 g
monounsaturated fat 1.5 g	**DIETARY EXCHANGES**
cholesterol 4 mg	3 starch, 2 vegetable

SESAME-PEANUT PASTA

SERVES 4

While the pasta is cooking, you can prepare the simple seven-ingredient sauce and have this dish put together in minutes! Enjoy with a cup of Thai-Style Lemon and Spinach Soup *(page 44).*

8 ounces dried whole-grain spaghetti
1/2 cup fat-free, low-sodium vegetable broth, such as on page 36
2 medium green onions, thinly sliced
3 tablespoons low-sodium peanut butter
1 tablespoon plus 1 teaspoon cider vinegar or plain rice vinegar
1 teaspoon toasted sesame oil
1/8 to 1/4 teaspoon cayenne
1/8 teaspoon salt

Prepare the pasta using the package directions, omitting the salt. Drain well in a colander. Transfer to a serving bowl.

Meanwhile, in a medium bowl, whisk together the remaining ingredients. Stir into the pasta. Serve for a hot entrée or cover and refrigerate for a cold entrée.

PER SERVING

calories 290	sodium 101 mg
total fat 8.5 g	carbohydrates 45 g
saturated fat 1.0 g	fiber 7 g
trans fat 0.0 g	sugars 4 g
polyunsaturated fat 2.5 g	protein 10 g
monounsaturated fat 4.0 g	**DIETARY EXCHANGES**
cholesterol 0 mg	3 starch, 1 fat

SPAGHETTI WITH PERFECT PESTO

SERVES 6

This sauce includes the traditional pesto ingredients plus adds spinach—a nutrition bonus—to boost the vitamins and minerals in this dish. Prepare Green Bean and Tomato Toss *(page 79) as a side salad.*

12 ounces dried whole-grain thin spaghetti
Pesto
2 cups tightly packed spinach (3 to 4 ounces)
1/2 cup tightly packed fresh basil
1/2 cup tightly packed fresh parsley
1/4 cup fat-free, low-sodium vegetable broth, such as on page 36
1/4 cup shredded or grated Parmesan cheese, or 2 tablespoons shredded or grated Parmesan cheese and 2 tablespoons shredded or grated Romano cheese
2 tablespoons pine nuts, dry-roasted
1 tablespoon olive oil (extra-virgin preferred)
2 medium garlic cloves
Pepper to taste
1 to 2 tablespoons water (if needed)

Prepare the pasta using the package directions, omitting the salt. Drain well in a colander. Transfer to a large serving bowl.

Meanwhile, in a food processor or blender, process the pesto ingredients except the water until almost smooth. If the mixture is too thick, add the water. Serve over the pasta.

Cook's Tip on Pine Nuts: Native to many parts of the world, pine nuts are the seeds found in particular varieties of pine trees. The difficulty in harvesting makes them rather expensive, but you use them in small quantities. Pine nuts—also called *pignoli* or *piñons*—are traditionally used in pesto sauce and are also very popular in southwestern cuisine. Store them in the refrigerator or freezer to keep them from turning rancid.

calories 257
total fat 6.0 g
   saturated fat 1.0 g
   trans fat 0.0 g
   polyunsaturated fat 1.5 g
   monounsaturated fat 3.0 g
cholesterol 2 mg

sodium 73 mg
carbohydrates 43 g
   fiber 7 g
   sugars 2 g
protein 10 g
DIETARY EXCHANGES
   3 starch, 1 fat

MEDITERRANEAN LINGUINE

SERVES 4

If you're a fan of Italian ingredients, you'll rave about this all-in-one dinner. Roasted vegetables add a deeper flavor to this pasta dish.

   Cooking spray
   6 ounces dried whole-grain linguine
   1 medium green bell pepper, thinly sliced
   1 medium red bell pepper, thinly sliced
   1 medium onion, cut into 1/4-inch wedges
   1 medium zucchini, cut lengthwise into
      eighths, then crosswise into 2-inch
      pieces
   8 dry-packed sun-dried tomato halves,
      chopped
   1/4 cup finely chopped fresh parsley
   12 kalamata olives, chopped
   3 tablespoons capers, drained
   1 1/2 tablespoons dried basil, crumbled
   1 medium garlic clove, minced
   3/4 cup shredded low-fat mozzarella cheese
   2 tablespoons shredded or grated Parmesan
      cheese

Preheat the broiler. Lightly spray a broiler pan with cooking spray.

Prepare the pasta using the package directions, omitting the salt. Drain well in a colander, reserving 1/2 cup pasta water.

Meanwhile, arrange the bell peppers, onion, and zucchini in a single layer in the broiler pan. Lightly spray the vegetables with cooking spray.

Broil for 10 minutes. Stir. Broil for 4 minutes, or until the edges are beginning to look deeply browned.

Meanwhile, in a small bowl, stir together the tomatoes, parsley, olives, capers, basil, and garlic.

In a large shallow dish, gently stir together the pasta, reserved pasta water, bell pepper mixture, and tomato mixture. Gently stir in the mozzarella and Parmesan.

calories 297
total fat 7.5 g
   saturated fat 1.5 g
   trans fat 0.0 g
   polyunsaturated fat 1.0 g
   monounsaturated fat 3.5 g
cholesterol 9 mg
sodium 579 mg

carbohydrates 46 g
   fiber 9 g
   sugars 9 g
protein 15 g
DIETARY EXCHANGES
   2 1/2 starch,
   2 vegetable, 1 lean
   meat, 1/2 fat

DOUBLE CHEESY NOODLES

SERVES 4

Creamy, cheesy noodles combined with kale provide a super nutritious and delicious meal. Serve with thick, juicy tomato slices drizzled with Zesty Tomato Dressing (page 105)

   Cooking spray
   8 ounces dried whole-grain noodles
   1 1/2 cups fat-free sour cream
   1 medium onion, finely diced
   1 cup fat-free cottage cheese, drained
   10 ounces frozen chopped kale, thawed and
      squeezed dry
   1/4 cup fat-free milk
   2 medium garlic cloves, minced
   1 teaspoon Worcestershire sauce (lowest
      sodium available)
   1/8 teaspoon pepper (white preferred)
   1/4 cup shredded or grated Parmesan cheese
   1 tablespoon poppy seeds

Preheat the oven to 350°F. Lightly spray a 2-quart casserole dish with cooking spray.

Prepare the noodles using the package directions, omitting the salt. Drain well in a colander.

(continued)

Meanwhile, in a large bowl, stir together the sour cream, onion, cottage cheese, kale, milk, garlic, Worcestershire sauce, and pepper.

Stir in the noodles. Spoon into the casserole dish.

Bake for 25 minutes. Sprinkle the Parmesan and poppy seeds over the casserole. Bake for 5 minutes.

PER SERVING

calories 404	carbohydrates 69 g
total fat 4.0 g	fiber 9 g
saturated fat 1.0 g	sugars 14 g
trans fat 0.0 g	protein 25 g
polyunsaturated fat 1.5 g	DIETARY EXCHANGES
monounsaturated fat 1.0 g	4 starch, 2 vegetable,
cholesterol 21 mg	2 lean meat
sodium 400 mg	

THREE-CHEESE BAKED PASTA

SERVES 6

This jazzed-up version of an old favorite is easy to put together. You don't even have to cook the pasta before adding it to the casserole.

> Cooking spray
> 1 1/2 10.75-ounce cans tomato puree
> 1 cup water
> 2 teaspoons dried Italian seasoning, crumbled
> 2 medium garlic cloves, minced, and
>   1 medium garlic clove, minced, divided use
> 24 ounces low-fat cottage cheese
> 1 large shallot, finely chopped
> 8 ounces dried whole-grain pasta (about 2 cups)
> 1 tablespoon shredded or grated Parmesan cheese
> 1 ounce low-fat mozzarella cheese, shredded (about 1/4 cup)

Preheat the oven to 350°F. Lightly spray a 9-inch square casserole dish with cooking spray.

In a medium bowl, stir together the tomato puree, water, Italian seasoning, and 2 garlic cloves.

In another medium bowl, stir together the cottage cheese, shallot, and the remaining 1 garlic clove.

Spread one-third of the tomato mixture in the casserole dish. In order, layer half the pasta, all the cottage cheese mixture, one-third of the tomato mixture, all the Parmesan, the remaining pasta, and the remaining tomato mixture.

Bake, covered, for 1 hour. Uncover and sprinkle the mozzarella on top. Bake, uncovered, for 5 minutes, or until the mozzarella has melted. Let stand for 10 minutes before serving.

PER SERVING

calories 248	carbohydrates 36 g
total fat 2.0 g	fiber 4 g
saturated fat 1.0 g	sugars 5 g
trans fat 0.0 g	protein 22 g
polyunsaturated fat 0.0 g	DIETARY EXCHANGES
monounsaturated fat 0.5 g	2 starch, 1 vegetable,
cholesterol 7 mg	2 lean meat
sodium 375 mg	

TORTELLINI AND VEGETABLE KEBABS WITH ITALIAN PESTO SALSA

SERVES 4

These make-ahead kebabs of pasta and vegetables are just right for dinner on a busy weeknight. Once assembled, the kebabs are ready to go without any last-minute cooking.

Kebabs
> 24 fresh cheese tortellini (about 4 1/2 ounces)
> 24 small broccoli florets
> 24 cherry tomatoes

Salsa
> 1 14.5-ounce can no-salt-added diced tomatoes, undrained
> 1/2 cup loosely packed fresh basil
> 4 tablespoons pine nuts or chopped walnuts, dry-roasted
> 2 tablespoons shredded or grated Parmesan cheese
> 1 tablespoon balsamic vinegar
> 1 medium garlic clove, minced

Prepare the tortellini using the package directions, omitting the salt. One minute before the end of their cooking time, stir in the broccoli. Cook for 1 minute, or until the broccoli is tender-crisp. Drain well in a colander.

Using twelve 8-inch wooden skewers, thread each skewer with 2 tortellini, 2 broccoli florets, and 2 cherry tomatoes. (Cover and refrigerate the kebabs at this point for up to two days if desired.)

In a food processor or blender, process the salsa ingredients for 30 to 40 seconds, or until slightly chunky. Serve the salsa with the kebabs.

PER SERVING

calories 209	carbohydrates 30 g
total fat 7.0 g	fiber 5 g
saturated fat 2.0 g	sugars 9 g
trans fat 0.0 g	**protein** 11 g
polyunsaturated fat 2.5 g	**DIETARY EXCHANGES**
monounsaturated fat 2.0 g	1 starch, 3 vegetable,
cholesterol 14 mg	1/2 lean meat, 1 fat
sodium 256 mg	

KALE RICOTTA ROLLS

SERVES 4

In this recipe, you'll create individual servings of lasagna. Lasagna noodles are rolled up to encase a cheesy kale filling then smothered in a zesty tomato sauce. Serve with Green Beans Oregano *(page 390).*

> 8 dried whole-grain lasagna noodles
> Olive oil cooking spray

Sauce
> 1 teaspoon olive oil
> 1 small or medium onion, finely chopped
> 2 large garlic cloves, minced
> 2 cups fat-free, low-sodium vegetable broth, such as on page 36
> 1 6-ounce can no-salt-added tomato paste
> 1 tablespoon dried basil, crumbled
> 1/4 to 1/2 teaspoon crushed red pepper flakes
> 1/8 teaspoon salt

Filling
> 20 ounces frozen chopped kale, thawed and squeezed dry
> 1 cup fat-free ricotta cheese
> 1/2 cup shredded low-fat mozzarella cheese
> 2 tablespoons shredded or grated Parmesan cheese
> 1/4 teaspoon pepper (white preferred)
> 1/8 teaspoon ground nutmeg

Prepare the noodles using the package directions, omitting the salt. Drain well in a colander. Pat dry. Arrange in a single layer on wax paper. Set aside.

Preheat the oven to 350°F. Lightly spray an 8-inch square glass baking dish with cooking spray.

In a small nonstick saucepan, heat the oil over medium-high heat, swirling to coat the bottom. Cook the onion and garlic for about 3 minutes, or until the onion is soft, stirring frequently.

Stir in the remaining sauce ingredients. Reduce the heat and simmer for 5 minutes, or until slightly thickened, stirring occasionally. Remove from the heat. Set aside.

In a large bowl, stir together the filling ingredients.

Spread the filling lengthwise down each noodle, leaving a border on all sides. Roll up each noodle from a short end and place it on its side in the baking dish. (The rolled noodles shouldn't touch each other.) Pour the sauce over the noodles.

Bake, covered, for 25 to 30 minutes, or until heated through.

PER SERVING

calories 390	carbohydrates 63 g
total fat 5.5 g	fiber 12 g
saturated fat 1.0 g	sugars 11 g
trans fat 0.0 g	**protein** 26 g
polyunsaturated fat 1.0 g	**DIETARY EXCHANGES**
monounsaturated fat 2.0 g	3 starch, 4 vegetable,
cholesterol 12 mg	2 lean meat
sodium 389 mg	

MEATLESS LASAGNA WITH ZUCCHINI AND RED WINE

SERVES 9

After enjoying a meal of this hearty lasagna, freeze single portions of any that is left over. You'll be ready for dinner on those busy days or for lunch anytime.

Cooking spray
8 ounces dried whole-grain lasagna noodles
1 teaspoon olive oil and 1 tablespoon plus
    2 teaspoons olive oil (extra-virgin
    preferred), divided use
2 medium zucchini, thinly sliced
1 medium onion, chopped
4 medium garlic cloves, minced
3 8-ounce cans no-salt-added tomato sauce
1/3 cup dry red wine (regular or nonalcoholic)
1 tablespoon cider vinegar
2 teaspoons dried Italian seasoning, crumbled
1/4 teaspoon crushed red pepper flakes
    (optional)
1 cup fat-free ricotta cheese
1 large egg white
2 tablespoons dried basil, crumbled
8 ounces vegetarian sausage patties or links
    (soy- or bean-based, about 6), finely
    chopped
1/8 teaspoon salt and 1/4 teaspoon salt,
    divided use
1 cup shredded low-fat mozzarella cheese
1/3 cup shredded or grated Parmesan cheese

Preheat the oven to 350°F. Lightly spray a 13 x 9 x 2-inch baking pan with cooking spray.

Prepare the noodles using the package directions, omitting the salt. Drain well in a colander. Pat dry. Arrange in a single layer on wax paper. Set aside.

Meanwhile, in a large nonstick skillet, heat 1 teaspoon oil over medium heat, swirling to coat the bottom. Cook the zucchini for 4 minutes, or until just beginning to brown, stirring frequently.

Stir in the onion. Cook for 3 minutes, stirring frequently.

Stir in the garlic. Cook for 15 seconds.

Stir in the tomato sauce, wine, vinegar, Italian seasoning, and red pepper flakes. Increase the heat to medium high and bring to a boil. Reduce the heat and simmer for 5 minutes. Remove from the heat.

Stir in the remaining 1 tablespoon plus 2 teaspoons oil.

In a small bowl, whisk together the ricotta, egg white, and basil.

In the pan, layer as follows: one-third of the noodles, one-third of the tomato sauce mixture, half the ricotta mixture (use a teaspoon for more even distribution), and half the vegetarian sausage. Repeat the layers. Top with the remaining noodles, remaining sauce, 1/8 teaspoon salt, and the mozzarella.

Bake, covered, for 40 minutes, or until the mozzarella melts. Let stand, uncovered, on a cooling rack for 10 minutes. Sprinkle with the remaining 1/4 teaspoon salt, then the Parmesan.

PER SERVING

calories 260	**carbohydrates** 33 g
total fat 7.5 g	fiber 7 g
saturated fat 1.5 g	sugars 8 g
trans fat 0.0 g	**protein** 18 g
polyunsaturated fat 1.5 g	**DIETARY EXCHANGES**
monounsaturated fat 3.5 g	1 1/2 starch,
cholesterol 9 mg	2 vegetable, 2 lean
sodium 499 mg	meat

EDAMAME FRIED RICE

SERVES 4

Our modern meatless version of classic fried rice substitutes edamame for peas, which doubles the protein, and adds a hint of cilantro for a bright flavor boost. Try this as a bed for Cantonese Vegetables (page 412).

1/2 cup uncooked brown rice
1 teaspoon toasted sesame oil
1 medium garlic clove, minced
2/3 cup egg substitute
1 1/2 cups frozen shelled edamame, thawed

1/2 cup slivered red bell pepper

1/2 cup shredded carrot

1/2 cup water

1 tablespoon soy sauce (lowest sodium available)

1/4 cup sliced green onions

1 tablespoon chopped fresh cilantro

Prepare the rice using the package directions, omitting the salt and margarine. Set aside.

In a large nonstick skillet, heat the oil over medium heat, swirling to coat the bottom. Cook the garlic for 1 minute, stirring frequently.

Pour in the egg substitute. Cook for 2 to 3 minutes, or until the egg mixture is no longer wet, stirring constantly. Transfer the mixture to a cutting board and coarsely chop. Set aside.

Wipe the skillet with paper towels. Put the edamame, bell pepper, carrot, and water in the skillet. Stir together. Cook over medium-high heat for 5 to 6 minutes, or until the vegetables are tender and the water has almost evaporated, stirring occasionally.

Stir in the rice and soy sauce. Cook for 2 to 3 minutes, or until heated through, stirring frequently. Stir in the chopped egg substitute mixture, green onions, and cilantro.

PER SERVING

calories 163	carbohydrates 18 g
total fat 4.0 g	fiber 4 g
saturated fat 0.0 g	sugars 5 g
trans fat 0.0 g	**protein** 13 g
polyunsaturated fat 1.5 g	**DIETARY EXCHANGES**
monounsaturated fat 1.5 g	1 starch, 1 1/2 lean
cholesterol 0 mg	meat
sodium 201 mg	

MUSHROOM STROGANOFF

SERVES 4

The meaty texture of mushrooms plays well with the traditional flavor profile of a classic beef stroganoff dish. The creamy sauce packs a protein punch with a surprise ingredient: tofu.

4 ounces dried whole-grain egg noodles

1 tablespoon olive oil

4 cups sliced mushrooms, such as button, chanterelle, brown (cremini), oyster, morel, or shiitake (stems discarded), or any combination

1 medium onion, sliced

1/4 cup fat-free, low-sodium vegetable broth and 1 cup fat-free, low sodium vegetable broth, such as on page 36, divided use

2 medium garlic cloves, minced

2 tablespoons all-purpose flour

1/2 cup dry white wine (regular or nonalcoholic)

1 tablespoon Worcestershire sauce (lowest sodium available)

1 tablespoon soy sauce (lowest sodium available)

1 1/2 teaspoons fresh thyme or 1/2 teaspoon dried thyme, crumbled

1 teaspoon dried marjoram, crumbled

12 ounces light soft tofu, drained and patted dry, pureed until smooth

2 medium Italian plum (Roma) tomatoes, peeled and chopped

1/2 cup fat-free sour cream

Prepare the noodles using the package directions, omitting the salt. Drain well in a colander. Set aside.

In a large nonstick skillet, heat the oil over medium-high heat, swirling to coat the bottom. Cook the mushrooms, onion, and 1/4 cup broth for 8 to 10 minutes, or until the vegetables are soft, stirring frequently.

Stir in the garlic. Cook for 1 minute, stirring occasionally. Stir in the flour. Cook for 1 minute, or until the flour is absorbed, stirring constantly.

Stir in the wine, Worcestershire sauce, soy sauce, thyme, marjoram, and the remaining 1 cup broth. Gently stir in the tofu and tomatoes. Cook, covered, for 3 to 4 minutes, or until the sauce has thickened, stirring occasionally.

(continued)

Stir in the noodles. Reduce the heat to medium. Cook for 1 to 2 minutes, or until the stroganoff is heated through.

EDAMAME, SQUASH, AND CHERRY TOMATO STIR-FRY

SERVES 4

Jade-green edamame and vibrant cherry tomatoes really make this a showstopper—and a nutritious one to boot. Serve on a bed of Asian Linguine *(page 418).*

> 1/2 cup fat-free, low-sodium vegetable broth, such as on page 36
> 1 tablespoon hoisin sauce (lowest sodium available)
> 2 teaspoons soy sauce (lowest sodium available)
> 1 1/2 teaspoons cornstarch
> 1 teaspoon wasabi powder
> 1 teaspoon toasted sesame oil
> 1 teaspoon canola or corn oil
> 1 cup diced baby pattypan squash
> 1/2 cup matchstick-size carrot strips, halved lengthwise
> 16 ounces frozen shelled edamame, thawed
> 1 cup cherry tomatoes
> 2 medium green onions, thinly sliced

In a small bowl, whisk together the broth, hoisin sauce, soy sauce, cornstarch, wasabi powder, and sesame oil until the cornstarch is dissolved. Set aside.

Meanwhile, in a wok or large nonstick skillet, heat the canola oil over medium-high heat, swirling to coat the bottom. Cook the squash

and carrot for 2 to 3 minutes, or until tender-crisp, stirring constantly.

Stir in the broth mixture and edamame. Cook for 4 minutes, or until the mixture has thickened, stirring occasionally. Remove from the heat.

Stir in the tomatoes and green onions.

CURRIED CAULIFLOWER AND TOFU WITH BASMATI RICE

SERVES 6

The light and delicate curry flavor along with the unusual combination of ingredients such as mango chutney, apple, cauliflower, green beans, and tofu make this dish a must-try. Serve with Baked Ginger Pears *(page 502) for dessert.*

> 1 cup uncooked basmati rice
> 1 tablespoon plus 2 teaspoons olive oil
> 1 small head cauliflower, coarsely chopped
> 12 medium asparagus spears, trimmed and cut into 1-inch pieces
> 12 green beans, trimmed and cut into 1-inch pieces
> 2 large tomatoes, cut into 1-inch wedges
> 1 large sweet onion, such as Vidalia, Maui, or Oso Sweet, coarsely chopped
> 1/4 cup coarsely chopped fresh Italian (flat-leaf) parsley
> 1 tablespoon curry powder, or to taste
> 1/8 teaspoon cayenne, or to taste
> 1 cup fat-free evaporated milk
> 1 medium apple (Fuji preferred), finely diced
> 2 tablespoons mango chutney or honey
> 1/4 teaspoon salt
> Pepper to taste

1 pound light firm tofu, drained, patted dry,
and cut into 1/2-inch cubes
1 cup frozen green peas
1/4 cup coarsely chopped fresh cilantro
2 tablespoons cashews, dry-roasted

Prepare the rice using the package directions, omitting the salt and margarine.

In a stockpot, heat the oil over medium-low heat, swirling to coat the bottom. Put the cauliflower, asparagus, green beans, tomatoes, onion, parsley, curry, and cayenne in the pot, stirring to combine. Cook, covered, for 15 minutes, or until the vegetables exude their liquids, stirring occasionally.

Stir the evaporated milk, apple, chutney, salt, and pepper into the cauliflower mixture. Cook, covered, for 10 to 12 minutes, or until the green beans are tender-crisp, stirring occasionally.

Gently stir in the tofu, green peas, and cilantro. Cook, uncovered, for 5 minutes. Spoon over the rice. Just before serving, sprinkle with the cashews.

PER SERVING

calories 330	carbohydrates 53 g
total fat 7.0 g	fiber 7 g
saturated fat 1.0 g	sugars 17 g
trans fat 0.0 g	protein 16 g
polyunsaturated fat 1.5 g	DIETARY EXCHANGES
monounsaturated fat 4.0 g	2 starch, 2 vegetable,
cholesterol 2 mg	1 other carbohydrate,
sodium 218 mg	1 lean meat, 1 fat

KOREAN TOFU AND GREENS STIR-FRY

SERVES 4

This protein-packed stir-fry comes together fast on a busy night. The two types of greens are blanched first, so they can quickly be added at the end of the quick-cooking meal.

Sauce

2 tablespoons soy sauce (lowest sodium
available)
1 tablespoon fresh lemon juice

1 1/2 teaspoons toasted sesame oil
1/2 teaspoon crushed red pepper flakes

■ ■ ■

8 ounces collard greens, any large stems
discarded, chopped
4 ounces kale, any large stems discarded,
chopped
1 teaspoon canola or corn oil
14 ounces firm or extra-firm tofu, drained
and patted dry, cut into 1-inch cubes
1 teaspoon toasted sesame oil
1 medium red bell pepper, cut into 1-inch
squares
2 small carrots, thinly sliced diagonally (about
1/2 cup)
1/3 cup sliced green onions
1 tablespoon minced garlic
1 teaspoon sesame seeds, dry-roasted

In a small bowl, whisk together the sauce ingredients. Set aside.

In a large saucepan or Dutch oven, bring 10 to 12 cups water to a boil over high heat. Add the collard greens. Return to a boil for 3 minutes. Add the kale. Return to a boil for 2 minutes, or until the greens are tender. Run under ice cold water to stop the cooking process. Drain well in a colander. Squeeze out any excess moisture. Pat the greens dry with paper towels. Set aside.

In a wok or large nonstick skillet, heat the canola oil over medium-high heat, swirling to coat the bottom. Cook the tofu for 8 to 10 minutes, turning occasionally to brown on all sides. Transfer to a plate.

In the same wok or skillet, still over medium-high heat, heat the sesame oil, swirling to coat the bottom. Cook the bell pepper, carrots, green onions, and garlic for 2 to 3 minutes, or until the vegetables are tender-crisp, stirring constantly. Stir in the greens. Cook for 1 minute, or until the greens are warm. Add the tofu. Pour in the sauce. Reduce the heat to medium. Bring to a boil, stirring gently to combine. Just before serving, sprinkle with the sesame seeds.

(continued)

Cook's Tip: Crushed red pepper flakes stand in for traditional Korean chili flakes because this ingredient can be difficult to find. If you do use Korean chili flakes, be sure to start with a small amount and add more to taste; they're hotter than crushed red pepper flakes.

PER SERVING

calories 181	**carbohydrates** 14 g
total fat 9.5 g	fiber 5 g
saturated fat 1.0 g	sugars 4 g
trans fat 0.0 g	**protein** 12 g
polyunsaturated fat 4.5 g	**DIETARY EXCHANGES**
monounsaturated fat 3.5 g	3 vegetable, 1 lean
cholesterol 0 mg	meat, 1 fat
sodium 282 mg	

THAI SWEET CHILI–GLAZED TOFU WITH ASPARAGUS AND RICE

SERVES 4

Pressing the tofu gives it a meatier texture. Teaming it with fragrant jasmine rice and fresh asparagus tossed with a spicy sauce makes this dish a feast for the senses.

- 12 ounces light extra-firm tofu, drained and patted dry
- 3/4 cup brown jasmine rice
- 2 tablespoons soy sauce (lowest sodium available)
- 2 tablespoons dry sherry
- 1 tablespoon plain rice vinegar
- 2 medium garlic cloves, minced
- 1 teaspoon grated peeled gingerroot
- 1 teaspoon toasted sesame oil
- 1/2 teaspoon crushed red pepper flakes
- 1/4 teaspoon pepper (white preferred)
- 1 teaspoon canola or corn oil and 1 tablespoon canola or corn oil, divided use
- 1 pound asparagus, trimmed and cut into 2-inch pieces
- 1 tablespoon Thai sweet red chili sauce (lowest sodium available)
- 4 medium green onions, cut into 1-inch pieces

Put the tofu on a cutting board lined with four layers of paper towels. Cover with four layers of paper towels. Place a large, heavy baking dish on top. Let stand for 30 minutes so the tofu releases its excess moisture, replacing the paper towels if necessary. Cut the tofu into 1/2-inch slices.

Meanwhile, prepare the rice using the package directions, omitting the salt and margarine. Set aside.

In a medium bowl, whisk together the soy sauce, sherry, vinegar, garlic, gingerroot, sesame oil, red pepper flakes, and pepper. Add the tofu, stirring gently to coat.

Heat a wok or large skillet over medium-high heat. Pour in 1 teaspoon oil, swirling to coat the wok. Cook the asparagus for 1 minute, or until tender-crisp, stirring constantly. Transfer to a medium bowl. Add the chili sauce, stirring to coat.

In the same wok, pour in the remaining 1 tablespoon oil, swirling to coat the wok. Cook the tofu mixture for 3 to 4 minutes, or until light golden brown, stirring frequently.

Return the asparagus mixture to the wok. Stir in the green onions. Cook for 30 seconds, stirring constantly. Serve the tofu mixture over the rice.

PER SERVING

calories 286	**carbohydrates** 39 g
total fat 8.0 g	fiber 5 g
saturated fat 0.5 g	sugars 5 g
trans fat 0.0 g	**protein** 13 g
polyunsaturated fat 3.0 g	**DIETARY EXCHANGES**
monounsaturated fat 4.5 g	2 starch, 2 vegetable,
cholesterol 0 mg	1 lean meat, 1 fat
sodium 311 mg	

TOFU RANCHEROS TOSTADAS

SERVES 4

Turmeric transforms the color of tofu, giving it the appearance of scrambled eggs so this dish resembles huevos rancheros. The tostadas are topped with classic Mexican ingredients. Enjoy with Gazpacho (page 49).

Cooking spray

12 ounces light firm silken tofu, drained and patted dry

4 6-inch corn tortillas

1 teaspoon canola or corn oil and 1/2 teaspoon canola or corn oil, divided use

1/2 teaspoon ground turmeric

1/4 teaspoon smoked paprika

1/4 cup sliced green onions (green part only)

2/3 cup canned no-salt-added black beans, rinsed and drained

1/2 teaspoon ground cumin

1/2 cup quartered grape tomatoes

1/2 cup low-fat 4-cheese Mexican blend

1/4 cup chopped fresh cilantro

1/2 medium avocado, sliced

Preheat the oven to 375°F. Line a large rimmed baking sheet with aluminum foil. Lightly spray the foil with cooking spray.

Put the tofu in a medium bowl. Using a fork, break up the tofu to resemble scrambled eggs.

Place 1 tortilla in a medium nonstick skillet. Heat over medium-high heat for 30 seconds to 1 minute, or until hot, turning once halfway through. Transfer to the baking sheet. Repeat with the remaining tortillas.

Reduce the heat to medium. In the same skillet, heat 1 teaspoon oil, swirling to coat the bottom. Cook the tofu, turmeric, and paprika for 2 to 3 minutes, until the tofu is hot, stirring gently. Stir in the green onions until combined. Spoon the tofu mixture over the tortillas.

Heat the remaining 1/2 teaspoon oil, swirling to coat the bottom. Cook the beans and cumin for 2 to 3 minutes, or until the beans are hot. Spoon over the tofu mixture. Cook the tomatoes for 1 to 2 minutes, or until just beginning to soften, stirring occasionally. Spoon over the bean mixture. Sprinkle the Mexican-blend cheese over the tomatoes.

Bake the tostadas for 3 to 5 minutes, or until the cheese has melted. Just before serving, sprinkle with the cilantro. Garnish with the avocado.

PER SERVING

calories 206	carbohydrates 19 g
total fat 9.5 g	fiber 5 g
saturated fat 2.5 g	sugars 3 g
trans fat 0.0 g	protein 13 g
polyunsaturated fat 1.5 g	DIETARY EXCHANGES
monounsaturated fat 4.5 g	1 1/2 starch, 1 1/2 lean
cholesterol 9 mg	meat, 1 fat
sodium 211 mg	

THAI TOFU AND WINTER SQUASH STEW

SERVES 4

Some days call for a comforting bowl of stew, and this dish is sure to fit the bill. Butternut squash provides an autumnal feel and a creamy texture that's brightened by the unique flavor notes of gingerroot, garlic, lemongrass, and Thai red chili paste.

1 stalk lemongrass, 1 teaspoon lemongrass paste, 1 teaspoon ground dried lemongrass, or 2 teaspoons grated lemon zest

1 tablespoon olive oil

2 teaspoons minced peeled gingerroot

4 medium garlic cloves, minced

1 medium red bell pepper, diced

2 cups cubed butternut squash

2 cups fat-free, low-sodium vegetable broth, such as on page 36

12 ounces light extra-firm tofu, drained and patted dry, diced

1/2 cup lite coconut milk

1 tablespoon Thai red chili paste

3/4 cup uncooked brown jasmine rice

8 ounces green beans, trimmed and cut into 1-inch pieces

1/2 cup loosely packed fresh basil (Thai basil preferred), coarsely chopped

Trim about 6 inches off the slender green end of the lemongrass stalk and discard. Remove the outer layer of leaves from the root of the stalk. Halve the stalk lengthwise. (Lemongrass stalks are slightly tough, so be careful as you slice.)

(continued)

In a large saucepan or Dutch oven, heat the oil over medium heat, swirling to coat the bottom. Cook the gingerroot and garlic for 10 seconds, or until fragrant, stirring constantly. Stir in the bell pepper. Cook for 2 to 3 minutes, or until tender-crisp, stirring occasionally. Stir in the squash, broth, tofu, coconut milk, chili paste, and lemongrass. Increase the heat to medium high and bring to a simmer. Reduce the heat and simmer, covered, for 10 minutes (no stirring needed).

Meanwhile, prepare the rice using the package directions, omitting the salt and margarine. Remove from the heat. Cover to keep warm.

Stir the green beans into the stew. Return to a simmer. Simmer, covered, for 5 minutes, or until the green beans and squash are tender. Discard the lemongrass stalk. Stir in the basil.

Transfer the rice to bowls. Spoon the stew over the rice.

PER SERVING

calories 300	carbohydrates 47 g
total fat 7.5 g	fiber 6 g
saturated fat 1.5 g	sugars 5 g
trans fat 0.0 g	protein 12 g
polyunsaturated fat 1.5 g	DIETARY EXCHANGES
monounsaturated fat 3.5 g	2 1/2 starch,
cholesterol 0 mg	2 vegetable, 1 lean
sodium 139 mg	meat, 1/2 fat

SPICY TOFU WITH EGGPLANT AND BELL PEPPERS

SERVES 4

This vegetable stew features tofu marinated in a spicy paprika-lemon marinade. Serve over a whole grain.

> 14 ounces light firm tofu, drained and patted dry, cut into 1-inch cubes
> 2 tablespoons fresh lemon juice
> 1 teaspoon paprika
> 1/2 teaspoon crushed red pepper flakes
> 1 1-pound eggplant, peeled and cut into 1-inch squares (about 3 cups)

> 1 1/2 teaspoons olive oil and 1/2 teaspoon olive oil, divided use
> 1 1/2 cups chopped onions
> 3 large garlic cloves, minced
> 2 cups medium red or yellow bell peppers (or a combination), cut into 1-inch squares
> 3 cups chopped tomatoes
> 1 teaspoon dried fennel seeds, crushed using a mortar and pestle
> 1/4 teaspoon pepper
> 1/2 cup chopped fresh basil
> 1/2 cup chopped fresh parsley

Arrange the tofu on a large shallow plate. Drizzle the lemon juice over the tofu. Sprinkle the paprika and red pepper flakes over the tofu. Cover and refrigerate for 30 minutes, turning occasionally.

Meanwhile, put the eggplant in a large microwaveable bowl. Pour 1/4 cup water over the eggplant. Microwave, covered, on 100 percent power (high) for 1 to 2 minutes, or until tender. Drain well in a colander. Set aside.

In a Dutch oven, heat 1 1/2 teaspoons oil over medium-high heat, swirling to coat the bottom. Drain the tofu, reserving the marinade. Cook the tofu for 5 minutes or until golden, turning to brown on all sides. Transfer to a large plate. Cover to keep warm.

Reduce the heat to medium. In the same pot, heat the remaining 1/2 teaspoon oil, swirling to coat the bottom. Cook the onions for 3 minutes, or until beginning to soften, stirring frequently. Stir in the garlic. Cook for 30 seconds, or until fragrant, stirring constantly. Stir in the bell peppers. Cook for 1 minute.

Stir in the eggplant, tomatoes, fennel seeds, pepper, and the reserved marinade. Increase the heat to high and bring to a boil. Reduce the heat to low. Cook, covered, for 10 minutes, stirring occasionally. Stir in the tofu, basil, and parsley. Cook for 1 minute, or until the tofu is hot.

Cook's Tip: To marinate the tofu for a longer time to deepen its flavor, cover and refrigerate it for up to 24 hours.

calories 173	carbohydrates 23 g
total fat 5.0 g	fiber 7 g
saturated fat 0.5 g	sugars 12 g
trans fat 0.0 g	protein 12 g
polyunsaturated fat 1.5 g	DIETARY EXCHANGES
monounsaturated fat 2.0 g	4 vegetable, 1 lean
cholesterol 0 mg	meat, 1/2 fat
sodium 53 mg	

VEGETABLE SUKIYAKI

SERVES 6

Sukiyaki, a popular Japanese stir-fry, is often prepared at the table. The traditional way to eat this dish in Japan is for diners to dip each bite into a beaten raw egg. Here, the cooking is done at the stove for convenience, the meat has been left out for a vegetarian version, and no eggs are used since consuming raw eggs can be harmful. But it's just as delicious as the original.

> 1 cup dried shirataki noodles
>
> 1 1/2 teaspoons canola or corn oil
>
> 1 head Chinese cabbage, chopped crosswise into 1-inch pieces
>
> 12 medium green onions, sliced into 2-inch pieces
>
> 2 medium carrots, sliced
>
> 8 ounces button mushrooms, sliced
>
> 1 medium green bell pepper, sliced
>
> 1 medium onion, thinly sliced
>
> 6 ounces light firm tofu, drained, patted dry, and cut into bite-size pieces
>
> 1/4 cup soy sauce (lowest sodium available)
>
> 1 tablespoon sugar

Prepare the noodles using the package directions, omitting the salt. Drain well in a colander.

In a wok or large skillet, heat the oil over medium-high heat, swirling to coat the bottom. Stir in the cabbage, green onions, carrots, mushrooms, bell pepper, and onion. Cook for 3 minutes, stirring frequently.

Stir in the tofu. Cook for 3 minutes, gently stirring frequently, or until the tofu is heated through; the cabbage, carrots, and bell pepper are tender-crisp; and the green onions, mushrooms, and onion are soft.

Stir in the noodles, soy sauce, and sugar. Cook for 2 minutes, stirring occasionally.

Cook's Tip on Shirataki Noodles: Shirataki noodles are thin, translucent traditional Japanese noodles made from the Konjac yam. They're low in calories and carbohydrates and have no real flavor, making them perfect in a stir-fry. As these noodles have increased in popularity, some grocery stores now carry them. Look for them in the refrigerator case. You can also find them in Asian markets and online.

calories 190	carbohydrates 37 g
total fat 2.0 g	fiber 6 g
saturated fat 0.0 g	sugars 11 g
trans fat 0.0 g	protein 7 g
polyunsaturated fat 1.0 g	DIETARY EXCHANGES
monounsaturated fat 1.0 g	1 1/2 starch,
cholesterol 0 mg	3 vegetable, 1/2 lean
sodium 393 mg	meat

PAD THAI WITH TOFU AND GREENS

SERVES 4

A healthier spin on pad Thai, the popular noodle dish from Thailand, this entrée features supermarket-friendly ingredients to re-create similar flavors. Powerhouse vegetables—leafy green spinach and Swiss chard—add extra nutrients to the meal, and a sprinkling of unsalted peanuts provides texture.

> 6 ounces dried fettuccine noodles or dried flat rice sticks (see Cook's Tip on Rice Sticks, page 360)
>
> 4 cups baby spinach
>
> 4 cups Swiss chard leaves, coarsely chopped, or baby spinach

(continued)

Sauce

2 tablespoons fresh lime juice

2 tablespoons soy sauce (lowest sodium available)

1 tablespoon sugar

1 tablespoon dry sherry (optional)

■ ■ ■

Cooking spray

2 large eggs, beaten, or 1/2 cup egg substitute

1 teaspoon canola or corn oil

1 large red bell pepper, thinly sliced

2 medium garlic cloves, minced

1/2 teaspoon crushed red pepper flakes

14 ounces light tofu (firm or extra-firm), diced

2 medium green onions, cut into 1-inch pieces

2 tablespoons chopped unsalted peanuts, crushed

1 medium lime, cut into 4 wedges

Prepare the pasta using package directions, omitting the salt. Two minutes before the pasta is done, stir in the spinach and Swiss chard. Drain well in a colander. Set aside.

Meanwhile, in a small bowl, whisk together the sauce ingredients until the sugar is dissolved. Set aside.

Lightly spray a medium skillet with cooking spray. Heat over medium heat. Pour the eggs into the skillet, tilting to cover the bottom. Cook for 20 to 30 seconds, or until the egg is set (doesn't jiggle when the skillet is gently shaken).

Using a spatula, scramble the eggs, still over medium heat, for 10 to 15 seconds, or until cooked through. Transfer to a plate. Set aside.

Increase the heat to medium high. In the same skillet, heat the oil, swirling to coat the bottom. Cook the bell pepper, garlic, and red pepper flakes for 1 minute, or until the bell pepper is tender, stirring occasionally.

Stir in the tofu and green onions. Cook for 2 to 3 minutes, or until the tofu is lightly browned and heated through, stirring occasionally.

Stir in the reserved sauce. Cook for 15 seconds.

Stir in the pasta mixture and the scrambled eggs. Cook for 1 to 2 minutes, or until heated through, stirring occasionally.

Just before serving, sprinkle with the peanuts. Garnish with the lime wedges.

Cook's Tip on Rice Sticks: Made of rice flour and water, rice sticks (or rice-flour noodles) are available in Asian grocery stores, health food stores, and sometimes even in the Asian section of supermarkets. To use flat rice sticks in this recipe, soak 6 ounces of dried noodles in hot water for 15 to 20 minutes. (You'll need to cook the spinach and Swiss chard separately in boiling water for 2 minutes.) Drain the noodles and add them to the dish with the scrambled eggs, spinach, and chard. Be careful not to overcook rice noodles, or they will become mushy.

PER SERVING

calories 337	carbohydrates 46 g
total fat 8.5 g	fiber 5 g
saturated fat 1.5 g	sugars 9 g
trans fat 0.0 g	protein 21 g
polyunsaturated fat 3.0 g	DIETARY EXCHANGES
monounsaturated fat 3.0 g	2 1/2 starch,
cholesterol 93 mg	2 vegetable, 2 lean
sodium 373 mg	meat

ONE-SKILLET BOK CHOY AND SNOW PEAS WITH TOFU

SERVES 4

Popular ingredients of Thai cuisine—such as lemongrass and Thai basil—flavor whole-grain pasta in this one-skillet dish.

1 teaspoon canola or corn oil

1/2 medium red bell pepper, cut into 1-inch squares

1 cup sliced mushrooms, such as shiitake (stems discarded if using shiitake)

2 medium shallots, coarsely chopped

1 1/2 cups fat-free, low-sodium vegetable broth, such as on page 36

2 teaspoons soy sauce (lowest sodium available)

2 teaspoons fresh lime juice

1 teaspoon light brown sugar

1 teaspoon ground dried lemongrass, or
   1 tablespoon finely chopped fresh
   lemongrass (cut from bottom end of
   stalk) (optional)

1/4 to 1/2 teaspoon crushed red pepper flakes

3 ounces dried whole-grain angel hair

12 ounces light firm tofu, drained and patted
   dry, cut into 1/2-inch cubes

2 medium stalks of bok choy, stems and
   leaves coarsely chopped

1 cup fresh or frozen snow peas, trimmed
   if fresh

2 tablespoons chopped fresh Thai basil

In a large skillet, heat the oil over medium-high heat, swirling to coat the bottom. Cook the bell pepper, mushrooms, and shallots for 2 to 3 minutes, or until the bell pepper is tender-crisp, stirring occasionally.

Stir in the broth, soy sauce, lime juice, brown sugar, lemongrass, and red pepper flakes. Bring to a simmer. Reduce the heat and simmer, covered, for 3 minutes.

Stir in the pasta. Simmer, covered, for 4 to 5 minutes, or until the pasta is tender.

Gently stir in the tofu, bok choy, snow peas, and Thai basil. Simmer, covered, for 1 to 2 minutes, or until the tofu is heated through and the bok choy and snow peas are tender-crisp.

Cook's Tip on Thai Basil: Thai basil has a thin green leaf with a purplish cast, and its flavor is spicy and licorice-like. Look for it in Asian markets or specialty grocery stores, as well as at your local farmers' market. If it's not available, you can substitute sweet Italian basil, but the flavor will be different.

PER SERVING

calories 167	carbohydrates 24 g
total fat 3.5 g	fiber 4 g
saturated fat 0.5 g	sugars 5 g
trans fat 0.0 g	**protein** 12 g
polyunsaturated fat 1.5 g	**DIETARY EXCHANGES**
monounsaturated fat 1.0 g	1 starch, 1 vegetable,
cholesterol 0 mg	1 lean meat
sodium 106 mg	

MOO SHU MUSHROOMS

SERVES 4

The popular moo shu style of cooking originated in northern China. In America, this dish is often served with thin pancakes brushed with a small amount of hoisin sauce. The pancakes are easy to make, but if you prefer, you can substitute packaged crêpes, frozen Mandarin pancakes, or even 6-inch whole-wheat flour tortillas (lowest sodium available).

1 1/4 cups white whole-wheat flour and 1 to
   2 tablespoons white whole-wheat flour,
   divided use

1/2 cup boiling water and (if needed)
   1 tablespoon boiling water, divided use

1 teaspoon toasted sesame oil

1 1/2 teaspoons cornstarch

1/2 cup fat-free, low-sodium vegetable broth,
   such as on page 36

2 tablespoons soy sauce (lowest sodium
   available)

1 tablespoon canola or corn oil

2 medium garlic cloves, minced

1 teaspoon grated peeled gingerroot

2 cups sliced mushrooms, such as shiitake
   (stems discarded), brown (cremini),
   button, oyster, or enoki

1 cup shredded red cabbage

1 medium carrot, shredded

1/2 medium red bell pepper, cut into
   matchstick-size strips

8 ounces soy crumbles, thawed if frozen

4 medium green onions, cut into 1-inch pieces

■ ■ ■

2 tablespoons plus 2 teaspoons hoisin sauce
   (lowest sodium available)

Put 1 1/4 cups flour in a medium bowl. Make a well in the center. Pour 1/2 cup boiling water into the well. Using a fork, gradually stir the water together with the flour to combine. Stir in the remaining 1 tablespoon water if the dough seems too dry. Lightly flour a flat work surface with the remaining 1 to 2 tablespoons flour. Turn out the dough onto the floured surface. Knead

(continued)

for 5 to 7 minutes, or until smooth and elastic (the dough springs back when you push against it with your fingers). Return the dough to the bowl. Cover with plastic wrap. Let stand for 20 minutes.

Roll the dough into an 8-inch-long cylinder. Cut the cylinder crosswise into 1-inch pieces. Using your hands, roll each piece into a ball. Using your palm or the bottom of a glass, flatten slightly to a 3-inch diameter. Using a pastry brush, lightly brush 1 teaspoon sesame oil over the tops of the circles. With the oiled sides facing each other, press 2 circles together. Using a rolling pin, lightly roll out these joined circles to form a large pancake, 5 to 6 inches in diameter. Repeat with the remaining dough circles, keeping the unused ones covered with a slightly damp paper towel to prevent drying.

Heat a small nonstick or cast-iron skillet over medium heat. Cook one pancake for 2 minutes on each side, or until lightly browned. Transfer to a plate. Let cool slightly. Gently and carefully peel the two sides apart to create two pancakes (they should separate relatively easily). Repeat this process with the remaining pancakes. Cover to keep warm. Set aside.

Put the cornstarch in a small bowl. Pour in the broth and soy sauce, whisking until the cornstarch is dissolved. Set aside.

In a wok or large skillet, heat the canola oil over medium-high heat, swirling to coat the bottom. Cook the garlic and gingerroot for 10 seconds, stirring constantly. Stir in the mushrooms. Cook for 2 to 3 minutes, or until soft, stirring constantly. Stir in the cabbage, carrot, and bell pepper. Cook for 2 minutes, or until tender-crisp, stirring constantly. Stir in the soy crumbles and green onions. Cook for 1 minute, stirring constantly.

Make a well in the center of the wok. Pour the broth mixture into the well (don't stir). Cook for 1 to 2 minutes, or until the sauce is thickened, stirring just the sauce occasionally. Stir together the sauce and mushroom mixture. Cook for

1 to 2 minutes, or until heated through, stirring frequently.

Just before serving, spread the hoisin sauce on each pancake. Top each with the mushroom mixture.

Cook's Tip: Look for Mandarin pancakes in the freezer section of Asian groceries or specialty markets.

PER SERVING

calories 302	**carbohydrates** 41 g
total fat 7.0 g	fiber 10 g
saturated fat 0.5 g	sugars 9 g
trans fat 0.0 g	**protein** 19 g
polyunsaturated fat 2.5 g	**DIETARY EXCHANGES**
monounsaturated fat 3.5 g	2 1/2 starch,
cholesterol 0 mg	1 vegetable, 1 1/2 lean
sodium 512 mg	meat

JAPANESE EGGPLANT BOATS

SERVES 4

Slender Japanese eggplants provide perfect portion control when stuffed with a mixture of Asian-spiced vegetables and soy crumbles. A topping of crunchy chopped peanuts echoes the nutty flavor of the miso paste in the stuffing.

Cooking spray
2 medium Japanese eggplants
1 tablespoon olive oil
2 medium leeks, chopped (white part only)
1 medium carrot, shredded
1/2 cup shredded red cabbage
1 medium garlic clove, minced
8 ounces frozen soy crumbles, thawed
1 tablespoon soy sauce (lowest sodium available)
1 tablespoon miso paste (lowest sodium available)
1/4 teaspoon pepper (white preferred)
2 tablespoons chopped peanuts or sliced almonds, dry-roasted

Preheat the oven to 375°F. Lightly spray a shallow baking dish with cooking spray.

Halve the eggplants lengthwise. Scoop out the pulp, leaving a 1/2-inch border of the shell all the way around. Transfer the shells with the cut side up to the baking dish. Transfer the pulp to a cutting board. Coarsely chop the pulp.

In a large nonstick skillet, heat the oil over medium-high heat, swirling to coat the bottom. Cook the leeks, carrot, cabbage, and garlic for 2 to 3 minutes, or until the vegetables are tender-crisp, stirring occasionally. Stir in the eggplant pulp. Cook for 4 to 6 minutes, or until the pulp is tender, stirring occasionally. Stir in the soy crumbles, soy sauce, miso paste, and pepper.

Spoon the stuffing into the shells. Bake for 20 to 30 minutes, or until the eggplant is tender when pierced with a fork and the stuffing is cooked through (registers 155°F on an instant-read thermometer). Just before serving, sprinkle with the peanuts.

Cook's Tip on Leeks: To prepare leeks, cut off and discard the roots on the white bulb. Cut off the tougher dark green leaves. Chop the leeks. Transfer them to a small colander. Rinse them well under cold water. Drain them well. If necessary, repeat the process to clean off all the sandy grit.

PER SERVING

calories 217	**carbohydrates** 27 g
total fat 6.0 g	fiber 10 g
saturated fat 0.5 g	sugars 12 g
trans fat 0.0 g	**protein** 16 g
polyunsaturated fat 1.5 g	**DIETARY EXCHANGES**
monounsaturated fat 3.5 g	1/2 starch,
cholesterol 0 mg	4 vegetable, 1 1/2 lean
sodium 544 mg	meat

TEMPEH KEBABS

SERVES 4

The kebabs can marinate in just an hour, or for up to 12 hours if you want to prepare them in the morning for dinner that night. Serve the kebabs over brown rice or other whole grain. Before shutting off the grill, toss some fruit on it, such as watermelon or Grilled Pineapple (page 502), for your dessert.

8 ounces tempeh, cut into 12 cubes

Marinade
2/3 cup coarsely chopped fresh cilantro
1/2 cup sliced green onions
1/4 cup fresh orange juice
3 tablespoons fresh lime juice (about 2 medium limes)
2 teaspoons chopped peeled gingerroot
2 teaspoons olive oil
3 medium garlic cloves, coarsely chopped
1 small fresh serrano pepper, seeds and ribs discarded, coarsely chopped (see Cook's Tip on Handling Hot Chiles, page 24)

■ ■ ■

1 medium zucchini, cut crosswise into 12 slices
1 medium red bell pepper, cut into 12 squares
6 medium button mushrooms, halved
1 medium onion, cut into 12 wedges
Cooking spray

In a large saucepan, bring about 1 cup of water to a boil over high heat. Put the tempeh cubes in a collapsible steamer basket. Place the steamer basket in the pan. Make sure the water doesn't touch the bottom of the steamer. Simmer for 15 minutes, or until the tempeh is hot and tender. Remove from the heat. Cool to room temperature.

Meanwhile, soak four 14- to 16-inch bamboo skewers for at least 10 minutes in cold water to keep them from charring, or use metal skewers.

In a food processor or blender, process the marinade ingredients until smooth.

For each kebab, thread each skewer with 3 tempeh cubes, 3 zucchini slices, 3 bell pepper squares, 3 mushroom halves, and 3 onion wedges. Place the kebabs on a large rimmed baking sheet. Pour the marinade over the kebabs, brushing to coat all sides. Cover and refrigerate for 1 to 12 hours.

Lightly spray the grill rack with cooking spray. Preheat the grill on medium.

(continued)

Lightly spray the kebabs with cooking spray. Grill for 6 to 8 minutes, or until the tempeh is browned and the vegetables are tender-crisp, turning once halfway through and brushing with any remaining marinade.

PER SERVING

calories 164	carbohydrates 15 g
total fat 7.5 g	fiber 2 g
saturated fat 1.5 g	sugars 6 g
trans fat 0.0 g	protein 13 g
polyunsaturated fat 2.5 g	DIETARY EXCHANGES
monounsaturated fat 2.5 g	1/2 starch,
cholesterol 0 mg	2 vegetable, 1 1/2 lean
sodium 17 mg	meat, 1/2 fat

GRILLED TEMPEH BURGERS

SERVES 4

Steaming the tempeh before grilling improves its flavor by reducing bitterness and also makes it easier for the tempeh to absorb the flavors in the garlic-infused soy sauce marinade. Enjoy this meatless burger complete with all the fixings. Serve with Caprese Salad with Grilled Zucchini (page 80) or Chile-Lime Grilled Corn (page 386).

8 ounces tempeh, halved lengthwise, then each piece halved crosswise to form 4 square patties

2 tablespoons soy sauce (lowest sodium available)

2 tablespoons fat-free, low-sodium vegetable broth, such as on page 36

1/2 teaspoon dried thyme, crumbled

1/2 teaspoon garlic powder

2 tablespoons light mayonnaise

2 tablespoons fat-free plain yogurt

2 tablespoons chopped fresh herbs, such as basil, tarragon, chives, rosemary, and/ or sage

1 medium garlic clove, minced

1/8 teaspoon cayenne

4 ultra-thin Colby-Jack cheese slices

1 small to medium sweet onion, such as Vidalia, Maui, or Oso Sweet, cut crosswise into 8 slices, leaving the skin on

4 whole-grain round sandwich thins (lowest sodium available)

1 medium tomato, cut into 8 slices

8 large Boston lettuce leaves

In a large saucepan, bring about 1 cup of water to a boil over high heat. Put the tempeh patties in a collapsible steamer basket. Place the steamer basket in the pan. Make sure the water doesn't touch the bottom of the steamer. Simmer for 15 minutes, or until the tempeh is hot and tender.

Meanwhile, in a shallow glass dish, whisk together the soy sauce, broth, thyme, and garlic powder. Add the tempeh, turning to coat. Cover and refrigerate for 30 minutes, turning occasionally. (The tempeh can also be covered and refrigerated overnight.)

In a small bowl, stir together the mayonnaise, yogurt, herbs, garlic, and cayenne. Set aside.

Preheat the grill on medium heat.

Drain the tempeh, reserving the marinade. Brush the tempeh with the remaining marinade. Grill for 5 minutes, or until lightly browned. Turn over the tempeh. Grill for 2 to 3 minutes, or until lightly browned. Top each patty with a slice of the cheese during the last 30 seconds of grilling.

While the tempeh is grilling, place the onion on the grill. Grill for 5 to 8 minutes, or until browned and lightly charred, turning once halfway through.

Grill the sandwich thins for 30 seconds to 1 minute, or until toasted.

To assemble each burger, spread the mayonnaise mixture on the inside of both the top and bottom halves of the sandwich thins. Place 1 patty, 2 onion slices, 2 tomato slices, and 2 lettuce leaves on the bottom half. Place the top half of the sandwich thin on the lettuce.

Cook's Tip on Grilling Onion Slices: When grilling onion slices, leave the skin on to help the slices hold together and to protect the outer rings from burning. Remove the skin before serving.

ROASTED SEITAN AND VEGETABLES WITH CRANBERRY– RED WINE SAUCE

SERVES 6

Seitan, *a meat substitute made from wheat gluten, is an ideal vegetarian dupe for chicken because of its similar texture. An herb rub covers the seitan before it roasts to enhance its taste. A sweet-tart sauce blankets the dish for an added flavor boost.*

Cooking spray

1 large onion, cut into 1-inch wedges

2 large carrots, halved crosswise, each half quartered lengthwise

6 2-ounce red potatoes, quartered

4 ounces brown (cremini) mushrooms, halved

1 teaspoon olive oil and 2 teaspoons olive oil, divided use

2 sprigs of fresh rosemary or thyme

2 teaspoons dried thyme, crumbled

2 teaspoons paprika

1 teaspoon garlic powder

1/4 teaspoon pepper

24 ounces seitan (2 12-ounce blocks or loaves), patted dry

1/4 cup dry red wine and 1/4 cup dry red wine (regular or nonalcoholic), divided use

1/2 cup fat-free, low-sodium vegetable broth and 1 cup fat-free, low-sodium vegetable broth, such as on page 36, divided use

1/3 cup sweetened dried cranberries

1/8 teaspoon ground allspice

2 teaspoons cornstarch

2 teaspoons water

Preheat the oven to 425°F. Lightly spray a shallow roasting pan with cooking spray.

Put the onion, carrots, potatoes, and mushrooms in the pan. Drizzle 1 teaspoon oil over the vegetables. Add the sprigs of rosemary. Bake for 30 minutes, or until the vegetables are browned and tender-crisp.

Meanwhile, in a medium bowl, stir together the thyme, paprika, garlic powder, and pepper. Add the seitan, turning to coat. Using your fingertips, gently press the mixture so it adheres to the seitan.

In a medium nonstick skillet, heat the remaining 2 teaspoons oil over medium-high heat, swirling to coat the bottom. Cook the seitan for 3 to 5 minutes, turning to brown on all sides, and adjusting the heat if necessary. Transfer the seitan to a plate. Set aside the skillet, reserving any browned bits.

When the vegetables are roasted, reduce the oven temperature to 350°F. Move the vegetables to the sides of the pan. Place the seitan in the center. Pour 1/2 cup broth over the seitan and vegetables. Bake, covered, for 30 minutes, or until the seitan is hot and the vegetables are tender.

Transfer the seitan and vegetables to a serving platter. Discard the sprigs of rosemary. Loosely cover the platter with aluminum foil. Let stand for 5 minutes.

In the same medium nonstick skillet, over medium-high heat, bring 1/4 cup wine to a boil for 30 seconds to 1 minute, or until reduced by half, scraping the bottom to dislodge any browned bits. Pour in the remaining 1 cup broth. Stir in the cranberries. Bring the mixture to a boil and boil for 1 to 2 minutes, or until slightly thickened. Stir in the allspice.

Pour the remaining 1/4 cup wine into the roasting pan, scraping the bottom to dislodge any browned bits. Stir the wine mixture from the pan into the wine mixture in the skillet. Bring just to a boil over medium-high heat.

Meanwhile, put the cornstarch in a small bowl. Add the water, whisking until the cornstarch is

(continued)

dissolved. When the wine mixture in the skillet has come just to a boil, gradually add the cornstarch mixture. Cook for 1 to 2 minutes, or until the sauce is thickened to the desired consistency, whisking frequently.

Cut the seitan into slices. Spoon the sauce over the seitan and vegetables.

PER SERVING

calories 288	**carbohydrates** 28 g
total fat 5.0 g	fiber 4 g
saturated fat 0.5 g	sugars 12 g
trans fat 0.0 g	**protein** 31 g
polyunsaturated fat 1.5 g	**DIETARY EXCHANGES**
monounsaturated fat 2.5 g	1 starch, 1 vegetable,
cholesterol 0 mg	1/2 fruit, 4 lean meat
sodium 460 mg	

VEGGIE TACOS WITH SEITAN

SERVES 4

A creamy, spicy cilantro sauce envelops tender squash and meaty seitan in these tacos. Round out your meal with Jicama Slaw (page 83) or Mexican Fried Rice (page 421).

> 1 tablespoon canola or corn oil
> 1 medium yellow summer squash, cut into 1/2-inch pieces
> 1 medium zucchini, cut into 1/2-inch pieces
> 1 medium onion, thinly sliced
> 1/2 cup diced red bell pepper
> 2 medium garlic cloves, minced
> 8 ounces seitan cubes or strips
> 1 teaspoon chili powder
> 1 teaspoon ground cumin
> 1/4 teaspoon salt
> 1/8 teaspoon pepper
> 1/4 cup fat-free half-and-half
> 2 tablespoons chopped fresh cilantro
> 1 tablespoon fresh lime juice
> 8 6-inch corn tortillas
> 2 medium Italian plum (Roma) tomatoes, diced
> 1/2 cup shredded fat-free Cheddar cheese

In a large nonstick skillet, heat the oil over medium-high heat, swirling to coat the bottom. Cook the summer squash, zucchini, onion, and bell pepper for 4 to 5 minutes, or until the squashes are tender-crisp and the onion is soft, stirring occasionally. Stir in the garlic. Cook for 1 minute, stirring occasionally.

Stir in the seitan, chili powder, cumin, salt, and pepper. Cook for 3 to 4 minutes, or until the mixture is heated through, stirring occasionally.

Stir in the half-and-half, cilantro, and lime juice. Cook for 1 minute, stirring once or twice.

Warm the tortillas using the package directions.

For each taco, spoon 1/2 cup squash mixture down the center of a tortilla. Top with the tomato. Sprinkle with the Cheddar.

PER SERVING

calories 252	**carbohydrates** 28 g
total fat 6.0 g	fiber 5 g
saturated fat 0.5 g	sugars 9 g
trans fat 0.0 g	**protein** 23 g
polyunsaturated fat 2.0 g	**DIETARY EXCHANGES**
monounsaturated fat 3.0 g	1 1/2 starch,
cholesterol 3 mg	2 vegetable, 2 1/2 lean
sodium 580 mg	meat

LOUISIANA GUMBO WITH SEITAN

SERVES 4

Browning the flour and combining it with broth helps thicken the stew and avoids adding the extra saturated fat and calories that are typically part of a classic roux. Serve with Corn Bread Muffins (page 464).

> 3/4 cup uncooked brown rice
> 1/2 cup flour
> 1 cup fat-free, low-sodium vegetable broth and 3 cups fat-free, low-sodium vegetable broth, such as on page 36, divided use
> 1 tablespoon olive oil
> 1 cup chopped onion
> 1 medium green bell pepper, chopped
> 2 medium ribs of celery, chopped

2 medium garlic cloves, minced

1 14.5-ounce can no-salt-added diced tomatoes, undrained

1 small eggplant, peeled and diced

1 medium yellow summer squash, chopped

1 medium zucchini, chopped

1 cup fresh or frozen okra, thawed if frozen, cut into 1/2-inch slices

8 ounces seitan cubes

1 tablespoon salt-free Creole or Cajun seasoning blend

4 cups chopped mustard greens, stems and ribs discarded

1 teaspoon gumbo filé powder or several dashes of red hot-pepper sauce

Preheat the oven to 400°F.

Prepare the rice using the package directions, omitting the salt and margarine. Set aside.

In a large skillet, cook the flour over medium heat for 6 to 8 minutes, or until golden brown, stirring frequently. Let cool for 5 minutes. Pour the flour into a medium bowl. Pour in 1 cup broth, whisking to combine. Set aside.

In a large saucepan or Dutch oven, heat the oil over medium-high heat, swirling to coat the bottom. Cook the onion, bell pepper, and celery for 6 to 8 minutes, or until the onion is soft and the bell pepper and celery are tender, stirring occasionally.

Stir in the garlic. Cook for 1 minute, or until fragrant, stirring frequently. Stir in the flour mixture, tomatoes with liquid, eggplant, summer squash, zucchini, okra, seitan, seasoning blend, and the remaining 3 cups broth. Bring to a simmer. Reduce the heat and simmer, covered, for 15 minutes, or until the eggplant, summer squash, zucchini, and okra are tender, stirring occasionally.

Stir in the mustard greens. Cook over medium heat for 10 minutes, or until the greens are tender and the mixture has thickened.

Ladle the gumbo over the rice. Sprinkle with the filé powder.

Vegetables and Side Dishes

ACORN SQUASH STUFFED WITH CRANBERRIES AND WALNUTS

SERVES 6

A bounty of ingredients, including wine-red dried cranberries, fills mellow squash for a delectable dish. Pair with Crispy Baked Chicken *(page 185) for a meal that will warm your heart on a cold night.*

Stuffing

> 1/4 cup uncooked instant brown rice
> 1 cup unseasoned croutons (lowest sodium available), coarsely crushed
> 1 medium onion, finely chopped
> 1/2 cup fat-free, low-sodium chicken broth, such as on page 36
> 1/4 cup sweetened dried cranberries
> 2 tablespoons chopped walnuts, dry-roasted
> 1 tablespoon light tub margarine
> 1 teaspoon dried sage
> 1/2 teaspoon dried thyme, crumbled
> 1/4 teaspoon dried oregano, crumbled
> 1/4 teaspoon salt
> 1/4 teaspoon pepper

■ ■ ■

> 3 small acorn squash (about 4 inches in diameter), halved lengthwise, seeds and strings discarded

Prepare the rice using the package directions, omitting the salt and margarine.

Preheat the oven to 400°F.

In a large bowl, stir together the rice and the remaining stuffing ingredients. Fill the squash halves loosely with the stuffing mixture.

Pour about 1/4 cup water into a 13 x 9 x 2-inch casserole dish. Place the squash halves with the filled side up in the dish.

Bake for 1 hour, or until the squash is tender when pierced with the tip of a sharp knife.

MICROWAVE METHOD
Put the acorn squash halves (unstuffed) with the cut side down in a microwaveable dish. Pour about 1/4 cup water around the squash halves.

Microwave, covered, on 100 percent power (high) for 5 minutes. Carefully remove the covering away from you to avoid steam burns. Remove the squash from the dish, leaving the water. Fill the squash halves loosely with the stuffing mixture. Return to the dish. Microwave, covered, on 100 percent power (high) for 10 to 12 minutes, or until the squash is tender when pierced with the tip of a sharp knife.

PER SERVING

calories 171	**sodium** 171 mg
total fat 3.0 g	**carbohydrates** 37 g
saturated fat 0.0 g	fiber 4 g
trans fat 0.0.g	sugars 10 g
polyunsaturated fat 1.5 g	**protein** 4 g
monounsaturated fat 0.5 g	**DIETARY EXCHANGES**
cholesterol 0 mg	2 starch, 1/2 fruit

GINGERED ACORN SQUASH

SERVES 4

This sweet and savory side dish is ideal for fall and winter evenings when there's a chill in the air. The pineapple will warm you up with thoughts of the tropics.

> Cooking spray
> 2 medium acorn squash (about 3/4 pound each), halved lengthwise, seeds and strings discarded
> 1 8-ounce can pineapple tidbits in their own juice, drained
> 3 tablespoons raisins (optional)
> 2 tablespoons light brown sugar
> 1 tablespoon light tub margarine, melted
> 1 teaspoon grated peeled gingerroot

Preheat the oven to 400°F. Lightly spray a 13 x 9 x 2-inch baking dish with cooking spray.

Put the squash halves with the cut side up in the baking dish.

In a small bowl, stir together the remaining ingredients. Spoon the mixture into the cavity of each squash. Carefully pour a small amount of water around, but not over, the squash.

Bake, covered, for 45 minutes to 1 hour, or until the squash is tender when pierced with the tip of a sharp knife.

Cook's Tip on Winter Squash: To make a hard winter squash easier to cut, pierce it in several places with the tip of a sharp knife. Put the squash on a paper towel and microwave it on 100 percent power (high) for about 2 minutes, or until the skin softens. Carefully transfer it to a cutting board. Let it stand for 3 to 5 minutes, or until it's cool enough to handle.

PER SERVING

calories 107	**sodium** 32 mg
total fat 1.5 g	**carbohydrates** 26 g
saturated fat 0.0 g	fiber 2 g
trans fat 0.0 g	sugars 15 g
polyunsaturated fat 0.5 g	**protein** 1 g
monounsaturated fat 0.5 g	**DIETARY EXCHANGES**
cholesterol 0 mg	1 starch, 1 fruit

ARTICHOKE HEARTS RIVIERA

SERVES 6

This French-style side dish is ready in minutes, and it pairs well with nearly any roasted entrée, including Roast Chicken with Grapes *(page 181) or* Filet of Beef with Herbes de Provence *(page 245). You can prepare the garlicky wine sauce while the artichoke hearts cook.*

18 ounces frozen artichoke hearts

Sauce

  1/2 cup dry white wine (regular or nonalcoholic)

  2 tablespoons light tub margarine

  1 tablespoon chopped fresh parsley

  1 tablespoon fresh lemon juice

  1 medium garlic clove, crushed

  1/2 teaspoon dry mustard

  1/2 teaspoon dried tarragon, crumbled

  Pepper to taste (white preferred)

■ ■ ■

Chopped fresh parsley (optional)

Prepare the artichoke hearts using the package directions, omitting the salt and margarine. Drain well in a colander. Transfer to a serving bowl.

Meanwhile, in a small saucepan, whisk together the sauce ingredients. Bring to a boil over medium-high heat. Reduce the heat and simmer, covered, for 5 minutes.

Pour the sauce over the artichoke hearts. Sprinkle with the remaining chopped parsley.

PER SERVING

calories 71	**sodium** 77 mg
total fat 1.5 g	**carbohydrates** 9 g
saturated fat 0.0 g	fiber 6 g
trans fat 0.0 g	sugars 1 g
polyunsaturated fat 0.5 g	**protein** 2 g
monounsaturated fat 1.0 g	**DIETARY EXCHANGES**
cholesterol 0 mg	2 vegetable, 1/2 fat

ASPARAGUS WITH LEMON AND CAPERS

SERVES 4

Tender asparagus is enhanced by the classic pairing of lemon and capers in this Mediterranean culinary delight.

  1 pound medium asparagus spears, trimmed

  1 tablespoon olive oil (extra-virgin preferred)

  1 tablespoon capers, drained

  1/2 teaspoon grated lemon zest

  2 teaspoons fresh lemon juice

  1/4 teaspoon pepper

In a large skillet, bring about 1/2 cup of water to a boil over medium-high heat. Add the asparagus. Reduce the heat and simmer, covered, for 3 to 5 minutes, or just until tender-crisp. Drain, discarding the water and leaving the asparagus in the skillet. Gently stir the remaining ingredients together with the asparagus.

Cook's Tip on Asparagus: Try to use crisp asparagus spears that are about as big around as your little finger. If the spears are thicker and tougher

(continued)

than you'd like, use a vegetable peeler to remove the outer layer.

PER SERVING

calories 54
total fat 3.5 g
  saturated fat 0.5 g
  trans fat 0.0 g
  polyunsaturated fat 0.5 g
  monounsaturated fat 2.5 g
cholesterol 0 mg

sodium 66 mg
carbohydrates 5 g
  fiber 3 g
  sugars 2 g
protein 3 g
DIETARY EXCHANGES
  1 vegetable, 1 fat

ASPARAGUS WITH GARLIC AND PARMESAN BREAD CRUMBS

SERVES 6

Cheesy herbed bread crumbs blanket steamed asparagus spears in this easy side dish. Try it with Lemon Baked Chicken (page 183).

Crumbs
  2 slices whole-grain bread (lowest sodium available), torn into 1-inch pieces
  1 tablespoon light tub margarine
  2 medium garlic cloves, minced
  1 1/2 teaspoons dried oregano, crumbled
  2 tablespoons shredded or grated Parmesan cheese

■ ■ ■

  1 1/4 pounds medium asparagus spears, trimmed
  1/8 teaspoon salt
  Butter-flavor cooking spray

Put the bread in a food processor or blender and pulse until fine crumbs are formed.

In a large nonstick skillet, melt the margarine over medium-high heat, swirling to coat the bottom. Cook the garlic for 10 seconds, stirring constantly.

Stir in the bread crumbs and oregano. Cook for 5 minutes, or until the crumbs are golden brown, stirring frequently. Remove from the heat.

Stir in the Parmesan.

Meanwhile, in a medium saucepan, steam the asparagus for 3 minutes, or until just tender-crisp.

Arrange the asparagus on a platter. Sprinkle with the salt. Lightly spray with the cooking spray. Top with the bread crumb mixture.

PER SERVING

calories 58
total fat 1.5 g
  saturated fat 0.5 g
  trans fat 0.0 g
  polyunsaturated fat 0.5 g
  monounsaturated fat 0.5 g
cholesterol 1 mg

sodium 127 mg
carbohydrates 8 g
  fiber 3 g
  sugars 2 g
protein 4 g
DIETARY EXCHANGES
  1/2 starch, 1 vegetable, 1/2 fat

MIXED SQUASH WITH GARLIC AND LEMON BREAD CRUMBS

Substitute 2 medium yellow summer squash, thinly sliced, and 2 medium zucchini, thinly sliced, for the asparagus, and 1 tablespoon grated lemon zest for the Parmesan cheese.

PER SERVING

calories 54
total fat 1.5 g
  saturated fat 0.0 g
  trans fat 0.0 g
  polyunsaturated fat 0.5 g
  monounsaturated fat 0.5 g
cholesterol 0 mg

sodium 103 mg
carbohydrates 9 g
  fiber 2 g
  sugars 4 g
protein 3 g
DIETARY EXCHANGES
  1/2 starch, 1 vegetable, 1/2 fat

REFRIED BEANS

SERVES 5

Canned fat-free refried beans tend to be high in sodium. Make this simple version instead—it's low in saturated fat and sodium, but the seasonings make it high in taste.

  1 teaspoon canola or corn oil
  2 tablespoons finely chopped onion
  2 medium garlic cloves, minced, or 1 teaspoon bottled minced garlic
  2 15.5-ounce cans no-salt-added pinto beans, well drained, 1/2 cup liquid reserved
  1 tablespoon no-salt-added ketchup
  2 tablespoons canned diced green chiles, drained

In a large nonstick skillet, heat the oil over medium heat, swirling to coat the bottom. Cook the onion for 5 minutes, or until soft, stirring frequently.

Stir in the garlic. Cook for 2 to 3 minutes, stirring frequently. Set aside.

In a shallow bowl, mash the beans using a potato masher or fork. Add the reserved bean liquid and ketchup, mashing to combine.

Add the bean mixture and chiles to the onion mixture, stirring well to combine. Cook over medium heat, or until heated through, stirring constantly.

PER SERVING

calories 153	**sodium** 43 mg
total fat 1.0 g	**carbohydrates** 27 g
saturated fat 0.0 g	fiber 8 g
trans fat 0.0 g	sugars 1 g
polyunsaturated fat 0.5 g	**protein** 8 g
monounsaturated fat 0.5 g	**DIETARY EXCHANGES**
cholesterol 0 mg	2 starch, 1/2 lean meat

ROASTED BEETS

SERVES 4

Roasting beets really intensifies their natural sweetness, which is complemented in this dish by a few simple seasonings. Save any leftovers (or roast extra beets) to use in Beet Salad with Red Onions *(page 74) or* Roasted Beet Salad *(page 74).*

    2 pounds beets, greens trimmed to about
        1 inch, beets peeled and cut into 1/2-inch
        cubes
    2 medium shallots, coarsely chopped
    1 tablespoon olive oil
    1/2 teaspoon dried thyme or dried Italian
        seasoning, crumbled
    1/4 teaspoon pepper
    1/8 teaspoon salt

Preheat the oven to 400°F.

Arrange the beets and shallots in a single layer on a large rimmed baking sheet. Drizzle with the oil. Stir to coat.

Sprinkle the thyme, pepper, and salt over the vegetables.

Roast for 35 to 45 minutes, or until the beets are tender and the edges are just beginning to brown and caramelize, stirring once halfway through.

PER SERVING

calories 101	**sodium** 192 mg
total fat 3.5 g	**carbohydrates** 16 g
saturated fat 0.5 g	fiber 4 g
trans fat 0.0 g	sugars 11 g
polyunsaturated fat 0.5 g	**protein** 3 g
monounsaturated fat 2.5 g	**DIETARY EXCHANGES**
cholesterol 0.0 mg	3 vegetable, 1 fat

STIR-FRIED BOK CHOY WITH GREEN ONION SAUCE

SERVES 8

Vitamin-rich bok choy is cooked quickly, then stirred together with an Asian-influenced pesto-like sauce. This side dish is great with dishes such as Teriyaki Halibut *(page 145) or* Grilled Lemongrass Flank Steak *(page 249).*

Sauce
    4 medium green onions, thinly sliced
    1/4 cup fat-free, low-sodium chicken broth,
        such as on page 36
    2 tablespoons chopped fresh cilantro or
        parsley
    1 tablespoon slivered almonds, dry-roasted
    1 teaspoon toasted sesame oil
    1 teaspoon soy sauce (lowest sodium
        available)
    1/2 teaspoon cornstarch
    1/2 teaspoon red chili paste (optional)

■ ■ ■

    1 teaspoon canola or corn oil
    8 medium stalks of bok choy (green and
        white parts), cut into 1-inch pieces

In a food processor or blender, process the sauce ingredients for 10 to 15 seconds, or until almost smooth.

(continued)

In a large nonstick skillet, heat the oil over medium-high heat, swirling to coat the bottom. Cook the bok choy for 2 to 3 minutes, or until tender-crisp, stirring constantly.

Stir in the sauce. Cook for 1 to 2 minutes, or until the sauce is slightly thickened, stirring constantly.

PER SERVING

calories 23
total fat 1.5 g
  saturated fat 0.0 g
  trans fat 0.0 g
  polyunsaturated fat 0.5 g
  monounsaturated fat 1.0 g
cholesterol 0 mg

sodium 29 mg
carbohydrates 2 g
  fiber 1 g
  sugars 1 g
protein 1 g
DIETARY EXCHANGES
  1/2 fat

PAN-ROASTED BROCCOLI

SERVES 4

Fresh broccoli doesn't need much to make it tender and delicious—just a few pantry staples and a few minutes of time. Serve with Mock Hollandaise Sauce *(page 433).*

> 2 broccoli crowns (about 1 pound), separated into florets, stems cut off and into 2-inch pieces
> 2 teaspoons canola or corn oil
> 1 tablespoon minced onion
> 1 medium garlic clove, minced
> 1 tablespoon fresh lemon juice
> Pepper to taste (freshly ground preferred)

Blanch the broccoli. (Boil the stems for 2 to 3 minutes. Add the florets. Boil for 2 minutes.) Plunge the broccoli into cold water to stop the cooking process.

In a medium skillet, heat the oil over medium-high heat, swirling to coat the bottom. Cook the onion and garlic for 3 minutes, or until soft, stirring frequently.

Stir in the broccoli. Cook for 2 minutes, or until tender-crisp, stirring gently. Transfer to a serving bowl. Sprinkle with the lemon juice and pepper. Serve immediately for peak texture and flavor.

PER SERVING

calories 62
total fat 3.0 g
  saturated fat 0.0 g
  trans fat 0.0 g
  polyunsaturated fat 0.5 g
  monounsaturated fat 1.5 g
cholesterol 0 mg

sodium 38 mg
carbohydrates 8 g
  fiber 3 g
  sugars 2 g
protein 3 g
DIETARY EXCHANGES
  2 vegetable, 1/2 fat

PECAN BROCCOLI

SERVES 6

It only takes a few dry-roasted nuts to add a crunchy punch to vegetables, such as this citrusy broccoli.

> 1 pound fresh or frozen broccoli florets
> 1/2 teaspoon grated orange zest
> 2 tablespoons fresh orange juice
> 1/8 teaspoon salt
> 1/4 cup chopped pecans, dry-roasted

In a medium saucepan, steam the broccoli for 6 to 8 minutes, or until tender-crisp.

Meanwhile, in a medium bowl, stir together the orange zest, orange juice, and salt. Gently stir in the broccoli. Sprinkle with the pecans.

PER SERVING

calories 60
total fat 3.5 g
  saturated fat 0.5 g
  trans fat 0.0 g
  polyunsaturated fat 1.0 g
  monounsaturated fat 2.0 g
cholesterol 0 mg

sodium 74 mg
carbohydrates 6 g
  fiber 2 g
  sugars 2 g
protein 3 g
DIETARY EXCHANGES
  1 vegetable, 1 fat

CRUNCHY BROCCOLI CASSEROLE

SERVES 8

Tired of steamed broccoli but short on time? This creamy casserole can be prepared ahead of time and then baked while you're cooking the entrée.

> Cooking spray
> 1 3/4 pounds broccoli crowns, any tough stems peeled, stems and florets cut into 4-inch pieces

Sauce

- 2 tablespoons fat-free, low-sodium chicken broth and 2 cups fat-free, low-sodium chicken broth, such as on page 36, divided use
- 1 large onion, finely chopped
- 1/2 medium red bell pepper, diced
- 1/4 cup all-purpose flour
- 1 cup fat-free milk
- 1/4 cup shredded or grated Romano or Parmesan cheese
- 1 tablespoon finely chopped fresh basil or 1 teaspoon dried basil, crumbled
- 1/8 teaspoon salt
- 1/8 teaspoon ground nutmeg
- 1/8 teaspoon pepper (white preferred)

■ ■ ■

- 1 cup unseasoned croutons (lowest sodium available), coarsely crushed
- 2 tablespoons finely chopped walnuts, dry-roasted

Preheat the oven to 400°F. Lightly spray a 13 x 9 x 2-inch glass baking dish with cooking spray.

In a large saucepan, steam the broccoli for 4 minutes. Arrange in vertical rows in the baking dish. Set aside.

In a medium saucepan, heat 2 tablespoons broth over medium-high heat. Cook the onion and bell pepper for about 3 minutes, or until the onion is soft.

Put the flour in a small bowl. Pour in the milk, whisking until the flour is dissolved. Whisk the flour mixture and the remaining 2 cups broth into the onion mixture. Reduce the heat to medium and cook until thickened, whisking constantly.

Whisk in the remaining sauce ingredients. Pour over the broccoli.

Sprinkle the croutons and walnuts over the broccoli and sauce.

Bake for 20 to 25 minutes, or until the sauce is bubbly.

PER SERVING

calories 108	carbohydrates 18 g
total fat 2.0 g	fiber 4 g
saturated fat 0.5 g	sugars 5 g
trans fat 0.0 g	protein 7 g
polyunsaturated fat 1.0 g	DIETARY EXCHANGES
monounsaturated fat 0.0 g	1/2 starch, 2 vegetable,
cholesterol 2 mg	1/2 fat
sodium 144 mg	

MAPLE-GLAZED BUTTERNUT SQUASH

SERVES 4

The light touch of maple syrup and cinnamon makes nutritious squash a real winner. Enjoy as a side dish to Roast Chicken with Grapes *(page 181)* or Yemeni Lemon Chicken *(page 181)*

- 1 1- to 1 1/2-pound butternut squash, halved lengthwise, seeds and strings discarded
- 2 teaspoons light tub margarine
- 1 tablespoon plus 1 teaspoon pure maple syrup
- 1/4 teaspoon ground cinnamon

Preheat the oven to 425°F.

Put the squash with the cut side up in a shallow baking pan. Put 1 teaspoon margarine in the cavity of each half.

In a small bowl, stir together the maple syrup and cinnamon. Pour into the cavities.

Bake the squash for 40 to 50 minutes, or until tender when tested with the tip of a sharp knife. When cool enough to handle, cut each piece in half lengthwise. Brush with the maple syrup mixture from the pan.

PER SERVING

calories 63	sodium 20 mg
total fat 1.0 g	carbohydrates 15 g
saturated fat 0.0 g	fiber 3 g
trans fat 0.0 g	sugars 6 g
polyunsaturated fat 0.0 g	protein 1 g
monounsaturated fat 0.5 g	DIETARY EXCHANGES
cholesterol 0 mg	1 starch

GARLICKY BROCCOLINI WITH CHARRED CHERRY TOMATOES

SERVES 4

Broccolini, *sometimes known as baby broccoli, is actually a cross between broccoli and Chinese kale. Its bright green color is a welcome addition to any meal, along with its fresh, light, and slightly peppery taste. This simple preparation is table-ready in about 10 minutes.*

> 6 ounces broccolini, thick stalks halved lengthwise
> 1 teaspoon olive oil
> 1/2 cup halved cherry tomatoes
> 2 large garlic cloves, minced
> 1/4 teaspoon pepper

Bring a large stockpot of water to a boil over high heat. Boil the broccolini for 2 to 3 minutes, or until the stems are tender-crisp. Drain well in a colander. Pat dry with paper towels.

In a large nonstick skillet, heat the oil over medium-high heat, swirling to coat the bottom. Cook the broccolini and tomatoes for 2 to 3 minutes, or until hot and slightly charred, adjusting the heat as necessary and stirring frequently. Reduce the heat to medium. Stir in the garlic and pepper. Cook for 30 seconds, or until fragrant, stirring constantly. Serve immediately for peak flavor and texture.

Cook's Tip on Broccolini: The broccolini can be blanched ahead of time. Just drain it and transfer it to a bowl of ice water to stop the cooking process and set the color. Then pat it dry and cover and refrigerate it until you're ready to cook it.

PER SERVING

calories 33	sodium 17 mg
total fat 1.5 g	carbohydrates 5 g
saturated fat 0.0 g	fiber 2 g
trans fat 0.0 g	sugars 2 g
polyunsaturated fat 0.0 g	protein 2 g
monounsaturated fat 1.0 g	**DIETARY EXCHANGES**
cholesterol 0 mg	1 vegetable

ROASTED BRUSSELS SPROUTS

SERVES 4

Roasting brussels sprouts really enhances their flavor. Give these a try with Fish Fillets in Foil *(page 137).*

> Cooking spray
> 1 tablespoon olive oil
> 2 teaspoons balsamic vinegar
> 3 medium garlic cloves, minced
> 1/4 teaspoon dried thyme, crumbled
> 1/8 teaspoon salt
> 1/8 teaspoon pepper
> 1 pound brussels sprouts (about 16), trimmed, halved lengthwise, and loose outer leaves discarded

Preheat the oven to 400°F. Lightly spray a medium baking sheet with cooking spray.

In a medium bowl, stir together all the ingredients except the brussels sprouts. Add the brussels sprouts, stirring to coat. Arrange on the baking sheet in a single layer with the cut side up.

Roast for 15 to 20 minutes, or until browned on the outside and tender on the inside, turning over halfway through.

Cook's Tip: Portions of the brussels sprouts may become very dark, appearing almost burned; actually, those spots are caramelized and add flavor. After making this dish a time or two, you may decide to cook the sprouts longer, until they are even darker and have crisper outer leaves.

PER SERVING

calories 85	sodium 102 mg
total fat 3.5 g	carbohydrates 12 g
saturated fat 0.5 g	fiber 4 g
trans fat 0.0 g	sugars 3 g
polyunsaturated fat 0.5 g	protein 4 g
monounsaturated fat 2.5 g	**DIETARY EXCHANGES**
cholesterol 0 mg	2 vegetable, 1 fat

BRUSSELS SPROUTS AND PISTACHIOS

SERVES 8

A crunchy topping covers tender brussels sprouts enveloped in a creamy, nutty sauce. Serve these with Stuffed Chicken with Blue Cheese *(page 193).*

  Cooking spray
  1 1/2 pounds fresh brussels sprouts, trimmed, and loose outer leaves discarded, or 20 ounces frozen brussels sprouts

Sauce
  1 cup fat-free, low-sodium chicken broth, such as on page 36
  2/3 cup fat-free evaporated milk
  1/4 cup all-purpose flour
  1/4 teaspoon salt
  1/8 teaspoon pepper
  2 tablespoons chopped pistachios, dry-roasted

■ ■ ■

  2 teaspoons chopped fresh rosemary, or 1/2 teaspoon dried rosemary, crushed
  1/2 cup whole-wheat panko (Japanese-style bread crumbs)

Preheat the oven to 400°F. Lightly spray a 1 1/2-quart casserole dish with cooking spray.

In a medium saucepan, steam the fresh brussels sprouts for 6 to 8 minutes, or until tender, uncovering briefly after 2 to 3 minutes to release the odor, or prepare the frozen sprouts using the package directions, omitting the salt and margarine. Transfer to the casserole dish.

In the same saucepan, whisk together the sauce ingredients except the pecans. Cook over medium-high heat for 3 to 4 minutes, or until the sauce comes to a boil and thickens, whisking occasionally. Remove from the heat.

Whisk the pistachios into the sauce. Pour over the brussels sprouts, stirring to coat. Sprinkle the rosemary and panko over all. Lightly spray with cooking spray.

Bake for 10 minutes, or until the topping is lightly browned.

PER SERVING

calories 107	**carbohydrates** 19 g
total fat 1.5 g	fiber 4 g
saturated fat 0.5 g	sugars 5 g
trans fat 0.0 g	**protein** 7 g
polyunsaturated fat 0.5 g	**DIETARY EXCHANGES**
monounsaturated fat 0.5 g	1/2 starch,
cholesterol 1 mg	2 vegetable, 1/2 fat
sodium 171 mg	

BUTTERNUT MASH

SERVES 8

Savory spices and a spark of lime boost the flavor of yellow-orange butternut squash. Serve this side dish with a pork roast.

  1 medium butternut squash (about 2 1/2 pounds), halved lengthwise, seeds and strings discarded
  1/4 cup fat-free half-and-half
  2 teaspoons fresh lime juice
  1 teaspoon ground cumin
  2 medium garlic cloves, minced
  1 teaspoon olive oil
  1/4 teaspoon salt
  1/4 teaspoon pepper

Place the squash with the cut side up in a large microwaveable container. Pour about 1 cup water around the squash. Microwave, covered, on 100 percent power (high) for 14 to 15 minutes, or until the squash is tender. Let cool for 3 to 4 minutes.

Meanwhile, in a small saucepan, cook the remaining ingredients over low heat for 2 to 3 minutes, stirring occasionally. Cover the pan.

Scoop the flesh from the squash into a medium bowl. Pour in the half-and-half mixture. Mash with a potato masher until smooth.

Cook's Tip: To roast the squash instead, cut it in half lengthwise, discarding the seeds and

(continued)

strings. Preheat the oven to 350°F. Place the squash with the cut side up on a nonstick baking sheet. Bake for 1 hour, or until tender.

PER SERVING

calories 51	**sodium** 85 mg
total fat 0.5 g	**carbohydrates** 12 g
saturated fat 0.0 g	fiber 3 g
trans fat 0.0 g	sugars 3 g
polyunsaturated fat 0.0 g	**protein** 2 g
monounsaturated fat 0.5 g	**DIETARY EXCHANGES**
cholesterol 0 mg	1 starch

CABBAGE WITH MUSTARD-CARAWAY SAUCE

SERVES 8

The distinctive flavor of caraway combines with spicy mustard and tangy yogurt in a sauce that complements both cabbage and brussels sprouts. Poached fish or chicken is a good culinary contrast to this robust dish. Try with Fish in Crazy Water *(page 134) or* Poached Chicken Three Ways *(page 192).*

8 cups coarsely shredded cabbage (about 1 2-pound head or 1 1-pound package shredded cabbage) or 1 1/2 pounds fresh brussels sprouts, trimmed and loose outer leaves discarded

Sauce

2 cups fat-free, low-sodium chicken broth, such as on page 36

1 tablespoon plus 1 teaspoon spicy brown mustard (lowest sodium available)

1 tablespoon cornstarch (2 tablespoons for brussels sprouts)

1/2 teaspoon caraway seeds, crushed

1/3 cup fat-free plain yogurt

1/2 teaspoon grated lemon zest

1/4 teaspoon salt

1/4 teaspoon pepper

In a medium saucepan, steam the cabbage for 5 minutes (6 to 8 minutes for brussels sprouts), or until tender-crisp. Remove the steamer from the saucepan. Set aside.

Meanwhile, in a large saucepan, whisk together the broth, mustard, cornstarch, and caraway seeds until the cornstarch is dissolved. Bring to a boil over medium-high heat, stirring occasionally. Cook for 1 to 2 minutes, or until thickened.

Stir in the remaining sauce ingredients. Reduce the heat to low. Cook for 2 to 3 minutes.

Stir in the cabbage until well coated. Cook for 2 to 3 minutes, or until heated through. Don't overcook.

Cook's Tip on Caraway Seeds: The fruit of an herb in the carrot family, caraway seeds are very popular in German, Austrian, and Hungarian foods. To release their flavor, crush them in a mortar and pestle. In many recipes, you can substitute other seeds, such as fennel, cumin, or dill.

PER SERVING

calories 33	**sodium** 125 mg
total fat 0.0 g	**carbohydrates** 6 g
saturated fat 0.0 g	fiber 2 g
trans fat 0.0 g	sugars 3 g
polyunsaturated fat 0.0 g	**protein** 2 g
monounsaturated fat 0.0 g	**DIETARY EXCHANGES**
cholesterol 0 mg	1 vegetable

SPICED RED CABBAGE

SERVES 4

Celebrate Oktoberfest or any other fall or winter occasion with this festive dish of red cabbage, apples, and spices. Try it with a pork entrée, such as Grilled Pork Medallions with Apple Cider Sauce *(page 292) or* Herb-Rubbed Pork Tenderloin with Dijon-Apricot Mop Sauce *(page 286).*

3 cups shredded red cabbage (about 12 ounces)

1/2 cup water (plus more as needed)

1/4 cup cider vinegar

1/4 teaspoon ground allspice

1/4 teaspoon ground cinnamon

1/8 teaspoon ground nutmeg

2 medium tart apples, peeled and diced

1 tablespoon sugar

In a large saucepan, stir together the cabbage, water, vinegar, allspice, cinnamon, and nutmeg. Cook, covered, over low heat for 15 minutes, stirring occasionally and adding 2 to 3 tablespoons water if needed during cooking.

Stir in the apples. Cook, covered, for 5 minutes. If necessary, uncover and cook until all the moisture has cooked away.

Stir in the sugar.

Cook's Tip on Apples: Tart apples include Granny Smith and Gravenstein. Among the varieties that are tart but have a hint of sweetness are Braeburn, Jonathan, McIntosh, pippin (or Newton pippin), and Winesap.

PER SERVING

calories 71	sodium 16 mg
total fat 0.0 g	carbohydrates 18 g
saturated fat 0.0 g	fiber 2 g
trans fat 0.0 g	sugars 13 g
polyunsaturated fat 0.0 g	protein 1 g
monounsaturated fat 0.0 g	DIETARY EXCHANGES
cholesterol 0 mg	1 fruit, 1 vegetable

MAPLE-GLAZED CARROTS

SERVES 4

A sweet and tart glaze enhances the natural sweetness of carrots in this dish.

10 to 12 small carrots (about 12 ounces total)
2 tablespoons light tub margarine
1 tablespoon fresh orange juice
1 tablespoon pure maple syrup
1/8 teaspoon ground cinnamon
1/16 teaspoon ground allspice

In a large saucepan, bring about 2 cups of water to a boil over high heat. Reduce the heat to medium high. Cook the carrots for 15 minutes, or until tender. Drain well in a colander.

Dry the pan. Reduce the heat to medium. Melt the margarine, swirling to coat the bottom. Stir in the remaining ingredients and carrots. Reduce the heat to low. Cook for 2 to 3 minutes, stirring frequently to coat the carrots with the glaze.

PER SERVING

calories 70	sodium 104 mg
total fat 2.5 g	carbohydrates 12 g
saturated fat 0.0 g	fiber 2 g
trans fat 0.0 g	sugars 8 g
polyunsaturated fat 0.5 g	protein 1 g
monounsaturated fat 1.5 g	DIETARY EXCHANGES
cholesterol 0 mg	2 vegetable, 1/2 fat

GINGERED CARROTS

SERVES 5

Try these sweet and peppery carrots with Crunchy Herb-Crusted Pork Chops *(page 288).*

1 pound carrots, peeled and cut into 1/4-inch slices
2 teaspoons light tub margarine
2 teaspoons sugar
1 teaspoon grated peeled gingerroot
2 tablespoons finely chopped fresh parsley

In a large saucepan, steam the carrots, covered, for 15 minutes, or until barely tender. Drain well.

In a large skillet, melt the margarine over medium heat until it bubbles, swirling to coat the bottom. Add the carrots, sugar, and gingerroot, stirring to coat. Cook for 1 to 2 minutes. Just before serving, sprinkle with the parsley.

PER SERVING

calories 50	sodium 76 mg
total fat 1.0 g	carbohydrates 11 g
saturated fat 0.0 g	fiber 3 g
trans fat 0.0 g	sugars 6 g
polyunsaturated fat 0.0 g	protein 1 g
monounsaturated fat 0.5 g	DIETARY EXCHANGES
cholesterol 0 mg	2 vegetable

CARROTS BRAISED IN CARROT JUICE

SERVES 4

Braising carrots in carrot juice provides a more "carroty" taste and a deeper color. The fresh citrus and herbs brighten the dish.

1 tablespoon canola or corn oil

1 medium shallot, minced

3 cups carrots, peeled and sliced diagonally into 3/4-inch-thick slices (about 6 medium)

1 cup 100% carrot juice (fresh or bottled)

1/2 teaspoon grated lemon zest

1 tablespoon fresh lemon juice

1/8 teaspoon nutmeg (freshly ground preferred)

1/8 teaspoon pepper (freshly ground preferred)

1 tablespoon chopped fresh mint

1 tablespoon finely sliced fresh chives (optional)

In a medium saucepan, heat the oil over medium-high heat, swirling to coat the bottom. Cook the shallot for 3 minutes, or until soft, stirring frequently. Stir in the carrots. Cook for 3 to 5 minutes, or until lightly browned, stirring frequently. Stir in the carrot juice, lemon zest, and lemon juice. Reduce the heat to medium low. Simmer, covered, for 6 to 8 minutes, or until the carrots are just tender, stirring occasionally.

Cook, uncovered, for 5 to 6 minutes, or until the sauce is reduced by half (to about 1/2 cup). Stir in the nutmeg and pepper. Serve warm or at room temperature. Sprinkle with the mint and chives.

Cook's Tip: You can change the flavors in this versatile side dish. Substitute orange zest and orange juice for the lemon zest and lemon juice. Add fresh rosemary, thyme, or parsley for the herbs, if desired.

PER SERVING

calories 93	**sodium** 109 mg
total fat 4.0 g	**carbohydrates** 14 g
saturated fat 0.5 g	fiber 3 g
trans fat 0.0 g	sugars 8 g
polyunsaturated fat 1.0 g	**protein** 2 g
monounsaturated fat 2.0 g	**DIETARY EXCHANGES**
cholesterol 0 mg	3 vegetable, 1 fat

BAKED CAULIFLOWER AND CARROTS WITH NUTMEG

SERVES 4

Nutmeg gives a mellow, slightly nutty taste to this dish without overpowering the other flavors. Once you pop this vegetable combo in the oven, you can forget it for 45 minutes.

8 ounces cauliflower florets, broken into bite-size pieces

2 medium carrots, thinly sliced

2 tablespoons water

2 tablespoons light tub margarine

1/8 teaspoon ground nutmeg

Dash of cayenne (optional)

1/8 teaspoon salt

Preheat the oven to 375°F.

In a 9-inch or 2-quart glass baking dish, stir together the cauliflower and carrots. Spoon the water on top. Dot with small pieces of the margarine. Sprinkle the nutmeg and cayenne over all.

Bake, covered, for 45 minutes, or until the vegetables are tender. Just before serving, sprinkle with the salt.

PER SERVING

calories 49	**sodium** 160 mg
total fat 2.5 g	**carbohydrates** 6 g
saturated fat 0.0 g	fiber 2 g
trans fat 0.0 g	sugars 3 g
polyunsaturated fat 0.5 g	**protein** 1 g
monounsaturated fat 1.5 g	**DIETARY EXCHANGES**
cholesterol 0 mg	1 vegetable, 1/2 fat

CAULIFLOWER AND ROASTED CORN WITH CHILI POWDER AND LIME

SERVES 8

The roasted corn combined with the spiciness of the chili powder and the tanginess of the lime juice provides your palate with an intense flavor sensation. Try this side dish with Fish Tacos with Watermelon-Mango Pico de Gallo *(page 135).*

2 medium ears of corn, husks and silk discarded
4 cups cauliflower florets (about 1/2 medium head)
1/4 cup fat-free, low-sodium chicken broth, such as on page 36
1 2-ounce jar diced pimiento, drained
1 tablespoon fresh lime juice
1 tablespoon light tub margarine
1/4 teaspoon chili powder
1/4 teaspoon salt
1/8 teaspoon pepper

Preheat the oven to 400°F.

Put the corn on a baking sheet. Roast for 15 minutes. Let cool on a cooling rack for 5 to 10 minutes. Slice the corn off the cobs. Discard the cobs. Set the kernels aside.

Meanwhile, in a large saucepan, bring the cauliflower and broth to a boil over medium-high heat. Reduce the heat to medium low. Cook, covered, for 10 to 15 minutes, or until the cauliflower is tender. Discard any remaining liquid.

In a small bowl, stir together the remaining ingredients.

Stir the pimiento mixture and roasted corn into the cauliflower. Cook, uncovered, over medium-low heat for 1 to 2 minutes, or until heated through, stirring occasionally.

Cook's Tip on Corn: To remove the kernels from the cob without making a mess, invert a small bowl inside a large bowl. Stand the cob on the small bowl, and using a sharp knife, slowly slice down the cob, letting the kernels fall into the large bowl.

PER SERVING

calories 43	sodium 107 mg
total fat 1.0 g	carbohydrates 8 g
saturated fat 0.0 g	fiber 2 g
trans fat 0.0 g	sugars 3 g
polyunsaturated fat 0.5 g	protein 2 g
monounsaturated fat 0.5 g	DIETARY EXCHANGES
cholesterol 0 mg	1/2 starch

BASIL-RICOTTA MASHED CAULIFLOWER

SERVES 4

Cauliflower blended with Italian cheeses, mild sweet onions, citrus, and fresh basil pairs well with Baked Parmesan Chicken *(page 186).*

2 teaspoons canola or corn oil
2 medium shallots, thinly sliced
1 medium head cauliflower, leaves and stems discarded, cut into 1-inch florets
3 tablespoons fresh orange juice
1/4 teaspoon freshly grated nutmeg
1/3 cup fat-free ricotta cheese
2 tablespoons shredded or grated Parmesan cheese
Chiffonade of 6 fresh basil leaves

In a small nonstick skillet, heat the oil over medium-high heat, swirling to coat the bottom. Add the shallots. Reduce the heat to medium. Cook the shallots for 4 to 5 minutes, or until soft and just beginning to brown, stirring frequently. Remove from the heat. Set aside.

Put the cauliflower in a medium saucepan. Pour in water to cover. Increase the heat to medium high and bring to a boil. Reduce the heat to low. Cook for about 4 to 5 minutes, or until the cauliflower is very tender. Drain well in a colander.

Transfer the cauliflower to a food processor or blender. Add the orange juice and nutmeg. Process for 4 to 5 minutes, or until smooth. Return the cauliflower mixture to the pan. Cook over low heat for 3 to 4 minutes. Add the ricotta and Parmesan, stirring until well blended. Remove

(continued)

from the heat. Just before serving, fold in the basil.

PER SERVING

calories 95
total fat 3.5 g
  saturated fat 0.5 g
  trans fat 0.0 g
  polyunsaturated fat 0.5 g
  monounsaturated fat 1.5 g
cholesterol 4 mg
sodium 128 mg

carbohydrates 11 g
  fiber 3 g
  sugars 5 g
protein 7 g
DIETARY EXCHANGES
  2 vegetable, 1/2 lean
  meat, 1/2 fat

CREOLE CELERY AND PEAS

SERVES 10

Although both Creole and Cajun cuisines are popular in New Orleans and share the "holy trinity" of onion, bell pepper, and celery, Creole dishes are less spicy and use more tomatoes. Serve this with Bronzed Catfish with Remoulade Sauce (page 140) or Salmon Cakes with Creole Aïoli (page 151).

1 teaspoon light tub margarine
1 medium onion, chopped
1/2 medium green bell pepper, chopped
1 14.5-ounce can no-salt-added tomatoes, drained, liquid reserved
1/2 teaspoon red hot-pepper sauce
1/4 teaspoon dried thyme, crumbled
8 medium ribs of celery, cut diagonally into bite-size pieces
10 ounces frozen green peas

In a large skillet, melt the margarine over medium-high heat, swirling to coat the bottom. Cook the onion and bell pepper for about 3 minutes, or until the onion is soft, stirring frequently.

Stir the liquid from the tomatoes (set the tomatoes aside), hot-pepper sauce, and thyme into the onion. Bring to a boil.

Stir in the celery and peas. Reduce the heat and simmer, covered, for 10 minutes, or until the celery is barely tender.

Stir in the tomatoes, crushing slightly with a spoon. Cook until heated through.

PER SERVING

calories 41
total fat 0.5 g
  saturated fat 0.0 g
  trans fat 0.0 g
  polyunsaturated fat 0.0 g
  monounsaturated fat 0.0 g
cholesterol 0 mg

sodium 66 mg
carbohydrates 8 g
  fiber 3 g
  sugars 4 g
protein 2 g
DIETARY EXCHANGES
  1/2 starch

SAUTÉED RED SWISS CHARD

SERVES 4

With its pretty green leaves and ruby-hued stems, Swiss chard is an especially attractive vegetable. This simple preparation brings out its mild flavor, which makes it an excellent accompaniment to nearly any entrée.

1 tablespoon olive oil
1 bunch Swiss chard (about 12 ounces), stems cut crosswise into 1/2-inch slices and leaves coarsely chopped
1 medium garlic clove, minced
1/4 teaspoon salt-free lemon pepper

In a large skillet, heat the oil over medium heat, swirling to coat the bottom. Cook the chard stems and garlic for 4 to 5 minutes, or until the stems are tender-crisp, stirring frequently.

Add the leaves. Using tongs, combine with the stems. Cook for 4 to 5 minutes, or until the leaves are wilted, turning several times with the tongs.

Sprinkle with the lemon pepper, using the tongs to combine.

PER SERVING

calories 47
total fat 3.5 g
  saturated fat 0.5 g
  trans fat 0.0 g
  polyunsaturated fat 0.5 g
  monounsaturated fat 2.5 g
cholesterol 0 mg

sodium 181 mg
carbohydrates 3 g
  fiber 1 g
  sugars 1 g
protein 2 g
DIETARY EXCHANGES
  1 fat

ROASTED CHAYOTE SQUASH

SERVES 4

Assertive seasonings, such as the lemon and the red pepper flakes in this dish, are great complements to the very mild, slightly sweet chayote squash.

2 8-ounce chayote squash, halved lengthwise, seeds discarded, and skin pierced in several places with a fork
Cooking spray
1 tablespoon plus 1 teaspoon olive oil (extra-virgin preferred)
1/2 teaspoon grated lemon zest
2 teaspoons fresh lemon juice
1/2 teaspoon dried oregano, crumbled
1/8 teaspoon crushed red pepper flakes
1/8 teaspoon salt

Preheat the oven to 400°F. Cover a baking sheet with aluminum foil.

Lightly spray both sides of the squash with cooking spray. Place with the cut side down on the baking sheet.

Bake for 40 to 45 minutes, or until tender when the skin is pierced with a fork. Transfer the squash with the cut side up to plates.

In a small bowl, stir together the remaining ingredients except the salt. Spoon into the cavity of each squash half. Sprinkle with the salt.

PER SERVING

calories 63	sodium 75 mg
total fat 4.5 g	carbohydrates 5 g
saturated fat 0.5 g	fiber 2 g
trans fat 0.0 g	sugars 2 g
polyunsaturated fat 0.5 g	**protein** 1 g
monounsaturated fat 3.5 g	**DIETARY EXCHANGES**
cholesterol 0 mg	1 fat

CAJUN CORN

SERVES 4

Richly browned onions are simmered with sweet yellow corn and served with Cajun-spiced margarine in this dish guaranteed to spice up any simple entrée.

1 1/2 tablespoons light tub margarine
1/2 teaspoon paprika
1/4 teaspoon dried thyme, crumbled
1/8 teaspoon pepper
1/8 teaspoon cayenne
Cooking spray
1 1/2 large onions, chopped
1/4 teaspoon sugar
3 cups frozen whole-kernel corn, thawed and drained

In a small bowl, stir together the margarine, paprika, thyme, pepper, and cayenne. Set aside.

Lightly spray a large skillet, preferably cast iron, with cooking spray. Heat over high heat for 1 minute. Cook the onions for 2 minutes, stirring constantly. Reduce the heat to medium.

Stir in the sugar. Cook for 3 minutes, or until the onions are golden-brown, stirring frequently.

Stir in the corn. Cook for 3 minutes, stirring occasionally. Remove from the heat.

Stir in the margarine mixture.

PER SERVING

calories 167	carbohydrates 36 g
total fat 2.5 g	fiber 5 g
saturated fat 0.0 g	sugars 10 g
trans fat 0.0 g	**protein** 5 g
polyunsaturated fat 1.0 g	**DIETARY EXCHANGES**
monounsaturated fat 1.0 g	2 starch, 1 vegetable,
cholesterol 0 mg	1/2 fat
sodium 43 mg	

SOUTHWESTERN CORN

Substitute dried oregano, crumbled, for the thyme, and add 1/4 teaspoon ground cumin to the margarine mixture. Add 2 seeded and finely chopped medium fresh jalapeño peppers (see Cook's Tip on Handling Hot Chiles, page 24) when stirring in the corn.

PER SERVING

calories 170	**sodium** 43 mg
total fat 2.5 g	**carbohydrates** 37 g
saturated fat 0.0 g	fiber 5 g
trans fat 0.0 g	sugars 10 g
polyunsaturated fat 1.0 g	**protein** 5 g
monounsaturated fat 1.0 g	**DIETARY EXCHANGES**
cholesterol 0 mg	2 starch, 1 vegetable, 1/2 fat

CHILE-LIME GRILLED CORN

SERVES 4

Nothing says summer like grilled corn on the cob. In this recipe, spicy chili powder and tart lime juice enhance the sweetness of the fresh corn. It's the perfect side dish to serve with grilled entrées such as Grilled Salmon with Cilantro Sauce *(page 150).*

4 small ears of corn, husks and silk discarded
Cooking spray
2 tablespoons light tub margarine, melted
1 tablespoon chili powder, or to taste
1 teaspoon grated lime zest
1 tablespoon fresh lime juice
1/8 teaspoon pepper
1/8 teaspoon salt
1 tablespoon chopped fresh cilantro

Put the corn in a large bowl. Fill with cold water to cover the corn. Soak for 30 minutes. Drain well.

Meanwhile, lightly spray the grill rack with cooking spray. Preheat the grill on medium high.

Stir together the remaining ingredients except the cilantro. Brush the corn generously with the mixture, reserving any that remains.

Grill the corn for 10 to 12 minutes, or until tender, turning to grill evenly and brushing frequently

with the margarine mixture. Just before serving, sprinkle with the cilantro.

PER SERVING

calories 90	**sodium** 162 mg
total fat 3.5 g	**carbohydrates** 15 g
saturated fat 0.5 g	fiber 2 g
trans fat 0.0 g	sugars 5 g
polyunsaturated fat 1.0 g	**protein** 3 g
monounsaturated fat 1.5 g	**DIETARY EXCHANGES**
cholesterol 0 mg	1 starch, 1/2 fat

SOUTHWESTERN CREAMY CORN

SERVES 6

Try this creamy dish, flecked with color from red bell peppers, green chiles, and cilantro, as a side for Beef Tostadas *(page 281) or* Southwestern Chicken *(page 195).*

1 teaspoon light tub margarine
1/2 large onion, finely chopped
1/2 medium red bell pepper, diced
4 ounces fat-free brick cream cheese
1/4 cup canned diced green chiles, drained
1/4 cup fat-free milk
1/2 teaspoon pepper
1/2 teaspoon chili powder
2 cups frozen whole-kernel corn
2 teaspoons finely chopped fresh cilantro

In a large nonstick skillet, melt the margarine over medium-high heat, swirling to coat the bottom. Cook the onion and bell pepper for about 3 minutes, or until the onion is soft, stirring frequently.

Reduce the heat to low. Stir in the cream cheese, green chiles, milk, pepper, and chili powder. Cook for 2 to 3 minutes, or until the mixture is smooth, stirring constantly.

Stir in the corn. Cook for 2 to 3 minutes, or just until the corn is heated through. Stir in the cilantro.

calories 93
total fat 1.0 g
  saturated fat 0.0 g
  trans fat 0.0 g
  polyunsaturated fat 0.5 g
  monounsaturated fat 0.5 g
cholesterol 4 mg

sodium 188 mg
carbohydrates 18 g
  fiber 2 g
  sugars 5 g
protein 5 g
DIETARY EXCHANGES
  1 starch, 1/2 lean meat

calories 101
total fat 2.5 g
  saturated fat 0.5 g
  trans fat 0.0 g
  polyunsaturated fat 1.0 g
  monounsaturated fat 1.0 g
cholesterol 0 mg
sodium 112 mg

carbohydrates 20 g
  fiber 4 g
  sugars 7 g
protein 4 g
DIETARY EXCHANGES
  1 starch, 1 vegetable,
  1/2 fat

"ZOODLES" WITH CORN AND TOMATOES

SERVES 6

This traditional Mexican side dish, seasoned not only with fresh cilantro (also known as coriander or Chinese parsley) but also with crushed coriander seeds, is updated with zucchini noodles. If you don't own a spiralizer, use a vegetable peeler to cut the zucchini into ribbons.

  2 teaspoons canola or corn oil
  1 medium onion, sliced
  2 medium garlic cloves, minced
  1 pound zucchini, spiralized or cut into
    ribbons
  2 cups fresh or frozen whole-kernel corn,
    thawed if frozen
  2 large tomatoes, peeled if desired, seeded,
    and diced
  1/4 cup fat-free, low-sodium chicken broth,
    such as on page 36
  1/4 teaspoon salt
  1/4 teaspoon ground coriander seeds
  1/8 teaspoon pepper
  1 tablespoon chopped fresh cilantro

In a large skillet, heat the oil over medium-high heat, swirling to coat the bottom. Cook the onion and garlic for 3 minutes, or until the onion is soft, stirring frequently.

Stir in the remaining ingredients except the cilantro. Bring to a simmer, still over medium-high heat. Reduce the heat and simmer, partially covered, for 4 to 5 minutes, or until the zucchini and corn are tender-crisp. Remove from the heat.

Stir in the cilantro.

EDAMAME WITH WALNUTS

SERVES 6

This delicious and nutritious side dish will become one of your go-to recipes. It's quick, it complements almost any entrée, and the ingredients are easy to keep on hand.

  1 tablespoon olive oil
  16 ounces frozen shelled edamame
  3 medium garlic cloves, minced
  1/4 cup whole-wheat panko (Japanese-style
    bread crumbs)
  1/4 cup chopped walnuts
  1/4 teaspoon pepper
  1/8 teaspoon salt

In a large skillet, heat the oil over medium heat, swirling to coat the bottom. Cook the edamame and garlic for 8 to 10 minutes, or just until tender, stirring occasionally.

Stir in the panko and walnuts. Cook for 3 to 4 minutes, or until the crumbs are golden, stirring occasionally.

Stir in the pepper and salt.

calories 155
total fat 8.5 g
  saturated fat 0.5 g
  trans fat 0.0 g
  polyunsaturated fat 4.0 g
  monounsaturated fat 3.5 g
cholesterol 0 mg
sodium 57 mg

carbohydrates 10 g
  fiber 4 g
  sugars 3 g
protein 10 g
DIETARY EXCHANGES
  1/2 starch, 1 lean meat,
  1 fat

EGGPLANT HUNAN STYLE

SERVES 4

Eggplant, an ancient vegetable, is popular throughout Asia. This spicy dish brings out its best.

1 tablespoon canola or peanut oil and
　　1/2 teaspoon canola or peanut oil,
　　divided use
1 1-pound Japanese eggplant, unpeeled, cut
　　into 1-inch pieces
4 medium garlic cloves, minced
1 tablespoon chili garlic sauce or chili paste
1 1/2 teaspoons minced peeled gingerroot
1/2 cup fat-free, low-sodium chicken broth,
　　such as on page 36
1 tablespoon soy sauce (lowest sodium
　　available)
2 teaspoons sugar
2 teaspoons sake, mirin, or dry sherry
　　(optional)
1 tablespoon plain rice vinegar
2 tablespoons chopped green onion
1 teaspoon toasted sesame oil

Heat a nonstick wok or large, heavy skillet over medium heat. Pour in 1 tablespoon canola oil, swirling to coat the wok. Cook the eggplant for 3 minutes, or until soft, stirring constantly. Using a slotted spoon, transfer the eggplant to a bowl. Set aside.

Heat the remaining 1/2 teaspoon canola oil, still over medium heat, swirling to coat the wok. Cook the garlic, chili garlic sauce, and gingerroot for about 15 seconds, stirring constantly. Stir in the broth, soy sauce, sugar, and sake. Bring to a boil. Stir in the eggplant and vinegar. Cook for 1 minute, or until the eggplant has absorbed most of the sauce. Stir in the green onion and sesame oil.

Cook's Tip: If you'd like to add meat to make this an entrée dish, cook 3 ounces ground pork in a medium skillet over medium heat for about 5 minutes, or until no longer pink, stirring occasionally to turn and break up the pork. Add to the wok with the garlic, chili garlic sauce, and gingerroot, then proceed as directed.

PER SERVING

calories 94	sodium 191 mg
total fat 5.5 g	carbohydrates 11 g
saturated fat 0.5 g	fiber 3 g
trans fat 0.0 g	sugars 7 g
polyunsaturated fat 1.5 g	protein 2 g
monounsaturated fat 3.0 g	DIETARY EXCHANGES
cholesterol 0 mg	2 vegetable, 1 fat

DILLED GREEN BEANS

SERVES 6

The secret's in the broth. The green beans absorb the vegetable broth, infused with bell pepper, onion, and dill seeds, which have a more intense flavor than dillweed.

1 cup fat-free, low-sodium vegetable broth,
　　such as on page 36
1/4 medium green bell pepper, chopped
2 tablespoons chopped onion
1/2 teaspoon dill seeds
18 ounces frozen cut green beans

In a large saucepan, cook all the ingredients except the green beans over medium heat for 3 to 4 minutes, or until heated through, stirring occasionally.

Stir in the green beans. Cook, covered, for 5 to 8 minutes, or until the green beans are tender-crisp. Serve hot or cover and refrigerate to serve chilled.

Cook's Tip: This recipe is not only quick and easy but versatile as well. Experiment with different herbs and seeds to find out just how adaptable it is. Substitute any of the following for the dill seeds: caraway, fennel, or coriander seeds; crumbled dried marjoram or oregano; or crushed dried rosemary.

PER SERVING

calories 29	sodium 99 mg
total fat 0.0 g	carbohydrates 6 g
saturated fat 0.0 g	fiber 2 g
trans fat 0.0 g	sugars 2 g
polyunsaturated fat 0.0 g	protein 1 g
monounsaturated fat 0.0 g	DIETARY EXCHANGES
cholesterol 0 mg	1 vegetable

GREEN BEANS WITH MUSHROOMS

SERVES 4

Green beans get a flavor boost when combined with lemony sautéed mushrooms. Try this delectable duo with Orange Pecan Chicken *(page 212).*

9 ounces frozen cut green beans
2 teaspoons canola or corn oil
1 medium green onion, finely chopped, or
1 tablespoon finely chopped shallots
4 ounces button mushrooms, sliced
1 teaspoon fresh lemon juice
1 teaspoon paprika
1 teaspoon all-purpose flour

Prepare the green beans using the package directions, omitting the salt and margarine. Drain well in a colander. Transfer to a serving dish.

In a medium skillet, heat the oil over medium heat, swirling to coat the bottom. Cook the green onion for 2 minutes, or until soft. Stir in the mushrooms and lemon juice. Cook for 3 minutes, or until the mushrooms are soft, stirring constantly.

In a small bowl, stir together the paprika and flour. Sprinkle over the mushroom mixture. Cook for 1 minute, stirring constantly.

Stir the mushroom mixture into the green beans. Serve immediately for peak texture and flavor.

PER SERVING

calories 53	**sodium** 76 mg
total fat 2.5 g	**carbohydrates** 6 g
saturated fat 0.0 g	fiber 2 g
trans fat 0.0 g	sugars 2 g
polyunsaturated fat 0.5 g	**protein** 2 g
monounsaturated fat 1.5 g	**DIETARY EXCHANGES**
cholesterol 0 mg	1 vegetable, 1/2 fat

GREEN BEANS WITH LEMON AND GARLIC

SERVES 4

These beans offer a flavor fusion thanks to the Cajun trinity of celery, bell pepper, and onion, as well as the Italian staples of garlic, tomato, and oregano. The combination with a burst of citrus takes ordinary green beans to the extraordinary.

1 pound green beans, trimmed
1 teaspoon olive oil
2 teaspoons light tub margarine
1 large garlic clove, minced
1/2 to 1 teaspoon crushed red pepper flakes
(optional)
1 tablespoon grated lemon zest
1 tablespoon fresh lemon juice
1/8 teaspoon salt
1/8 teaspoon pepper
1 medium lemon, cut into 4 wedges

In a large saucepan over high heat, bring to a boil enough water to cover the green beans. Add the green beans and boil for 4 minutes. Drain the green beans and plunge them into a large bowl of ice water to stop the cooking process. Drain well.

In a large skillet, heat the oil and margarine over medium heat, swirling to coat the bottom. Cook the garlic and red pepper flakes for 30 seconds, or until fragrant, stirring constantly. Stir in the remaining ingredients except the lemon wedges. Cook for 3 to 5 minutes, or until the green beans are tender-crisp, stirring occasionally. Serve with the lemon wedges.

PER SERVING

calories 55	**sodium** 95 mg
total fat 2.0 g	**carbohydrates** 9 g
saturated fat 0.0 g	fiber 3 g
trans fat 0.0 g	sugars 4 g
polyunsaturated fat 0.5 g	**protein** 2 g
monounsaturated fat 1.0 g	**DIETARY EXCHANGES**
cholesterol 0 mg	2 vegetable, 1/2 fat

GREEN BEANS AND RICE WITH HAZELNUTS

SERVES 8

Combining a vegetable and whole grain in one dish makes it easy to get dinner on the table. The mild flavors pair well with seafood dishes such as Broiled Marinated Fish Steaks *(page 133) or* Mushroom-Stuffed Fish Rolls *(page 136).*

> 1/2 cup uncooked instant brown rice
> 9 ounces frozen French-style green beans
> 1 1/2 tablespoons light tub margarine
> 3 tablespoons sliced green onions
> 1/2 to 1 teaspoon fresh lemon juice
> 1/4 teaspoon salt
> Pepper to taste
> 1/4 cup chopped or sliced hazelnuts, dry-roasted
> 1/4 cup chopped roasted red bell peppers, drained if bottled

Prepare the rice using the package directions, omitting the salt and margarine.

Prepare the green beans using the package directions, omitting the salt and margarine. Drain well in a colander.

In a large saucepan, melt the margarine over medium heat, swirling to coat the bottom. Stir in the green beans, rice, green onions, lemon juice, salt, and pepper. Cook until heated through, stirring occasionally. Just before serving, sprinkle with the hazelnuts and roasted peppers.

Cook's Tip on Hazelnuts: Traditional in many European dishes, hazelnuts (also called filberts) have a bitter brown skin that you'll want to remove. Put the nuts in a single layer on a baking pan and dry-roast in a preheated 350°F oven for about 10 minutes. Let them cool for 1 to 2 minutes. While the hazelnuts are still warm, put a handful in a dish towel and rub them to remove their skins.

PER SERVING

calories 64	sodium 96 mg
total fat 3.0 g	carbohydrates 7 g
saturated fat 0.0 g	fiber 2 g
trans fat 0.0 g	sugars 1 g
polyunsaturated fat 0.5 g	protein 1 g
monounsaturated fat 2.0 g	DIETARY EXCHANGES
cholesterol 0 mg	1/2 starch, 1/2 fat

GREEN BEANS OREGANO

SERVES 4

These Italian-style green beans have a bit of New Orleans flair thanks to the green pepper, onions, tomatoes, and celery—staples of Creole cooking. Try with entrées such as Bronzed Catfish with Remoulade Sauce *(page 140) or* Roast Chicken with Grapes *(page 181).*

> 1 1/2 medium tomatoes, diced
> 1 medium rib of celery, diced
> 1/3 cup water
> 1/4 medium green bell pepper, diced
> 2 tablespoons chopped onion
> 1/2 teaspoon garlic powder
> 1/2 teaspoon onion powder
> 1/2 teaspoon dried oregano, crumbled
> 1/8 teaspoon pepper (white preferred)
> 1/8 teaspoon salt
> 9 ounces frozen green beans (Italian preferred)

In a medium saucepan, stir together all the ingredients except the green beans. Bring to a boil over high heat. Reduce the heat and simmer, covered, for 10 minutes.

Increase the heat to medium. Add the green beans, separating them with a fork. Cook for 5 to 8 minutes, or until the green beans are tender-crisp, stirring occasionally.

PER SERVING

calories 55	sodium 95 mg
total fat 2.0 g	carbohydrates 9 g
saturated fat 0.0 g	fiber 3 g
trans fat 0.0 g	sugars 4 g
polyunsaturated fat 1.0 g	protein 2 g
monounsaturated fat 0.0 g	DIETARY EXCHANGES
cholesterol 0 mg	2 vegetable, 1/2 fat

SOUTHERN-STYLE GREENS

SERVES 4

This updated version of Southern greens decreases the cooking time, keeping the greens bright and flavorful. Blanching is the key; cooked briefly in boiling water, quick-cooled, and then sautéed, these greens are a snap to make but still tender, colorful, and tasty.

- 6 ounces collard greens, tough stems discarded, leaves coarsely chopped
- 6 ounces kale, tough stems discarded, leaves coarsely chopped
- 4 ounces Swiss chard, tough stems discarded, leaves coarsely chopped
- 1 teaspoon canola or corn oil
- 2 slices turkey bacon, chopped
- 1/3 cup chopped onion
- 2 tablespoons balsamic vinegar
- 1 teaspoon pure maple syrup
- 2 tablespoons chopped pecans, dry-roasted

Pour 3 to 3 1/2 quarts of water into a large stockpot. Bring to a boil over high heat. Boil the collard greens for 5 minutes. Add the chard. Boil for 2 to 3 minutes, or until the greens are tender. Transfer to a colander. Run under very cold water. Drain well. Gently squeeze out the excess water. Pat the greens dry with paper towels.

In a large nonstick skillet, heat the oil over medium heat, swirling to coat the bottom. Cook the bacon and onion for 3 to 4 minutes, or until the bacon is lightly browned, stirring frequently. Stir in the greens. Cook for 1 to 2 minutes, or until hot. Add the vinegar and maple syrup, stirring until the greens are coated. Just before serving, sprinkle with the pecans.

Cook's Tip: You can substitute mustard greens for the Swiss chard.

PER SERVING

calories 109	sodium 247 mg
total fat 5.5 g	carbohydrates 12 g
saturated fat 1.0 g	fiber 3 g
trans fat 0.0 g	sugars 4 g
polyunsaturated fat 1.5 g	protein 5 g
monounsaturated fat 3.0 g	DIETARY EXCHANGES
cholesterol 5 mg	2 vegetable, 1 fat

ROSEMARY KALE WITH ALMONDS

SERVES 6

This earthy nutrient-rich vegetable absorbs flavors from broth, onion, and rosemary as it cooks; it peaks when mixed with two oils and nuts before serving.

- 2 pounds fresh kale, ribs and any tough stems discarded, coarsely chopped, or 20 ounces frozen leaf kale, thawed and drained
- 1/2 cup fat-free, low-sodium vegetable broth, such as on page 36
- 2 tablespoons chopped red onion
- 1/2 teaspoon sugar
- 1 teaspoon dried rosemary, crushed
- 1/4 teaspoon salt
- Pepper to taste (freshly ground preferred)
- 1 teaspoon olive oil
- 1 teaspoon toasted sesame oil
- 1/4 cup sliced almonds, dry-roasted

In a large saucepan, stir together the kale, broth, onion, sugar, and rosemary. Cook, covered, over medium-high heat for 10 minutes, or until the kale is tender, stirring occasionally. Remove from the heat.

Stir in the salt and pepper.

Just before serving, stir in the oils. Sprinkle with the almonds.

PER SERVING

calories 113	sodium 156 mg
total fat 5.0 g	carbohydrates 15 g
saturated fat 0.5 g	fiber 4 g
trans fat 0.0 g	sugars 1 g
polyunsaturated fat 1.5 g	protein 7 g
monounsaturated fat 2.0 g	DIETARY EXCHANGES
cholesterol 0 mg	3 vegetable, 1 fat

CREAMY KALE WITH RED BELL PEPPER

SERVES 4

The creamy sauce in this dish complements the mild cabbage-like flavor of kale. Like other greens, kale goes well with pork dishes, such as Orange Pork Medallions *(page 290), or try it with a braised eye-of-round roast.*

1 1/2 pounds kale, ribs and any tough stems
    discarded, leaves torn into small pieces
1 medium red bell pepper, diced
2 tablespoons water
1 tablespoon plus 1 teaspoon light tub
    margarine
1 tablespoon plus 1 teaspoon all-purpose flour
3/4 cup fat-free milk
1/8 teaspoon salt
1/8 teaspoon pepper
1/4 cup fat-free half-and-half
1/2 teaspoon sugar

Put the kale and bell pepper in a large saucepan over medium-high heat. Add the water. Reduce the heat to low. Cook, covered, for 5 to 6 minutes, or until the kale is wilted.

Meanwhile, in a separate large saucepan, melt the margarine over medium-high heat, swirling to coat the bottom. Whisk in the flour. Cook for 1 minute, whisking constantly.

Whisk in the milk, salt, and pepper. Bring to a boil, whisking constantly. Remove from the heat.

Stir in the kale mixture, half-and-half, and sugar.

Cook's Tip on Kale: Kale has deep green frilly leaves, usually tinged with blue or purple. The best kale is available in the wintertime. Massaging the leaves before using them in a salad can tone down their bitterness and make them more tender.

PER SERVING

calories 143
total fat 3.0 g
  saturated fat 0.0 g
  trans fat 0.0 g
  polyunsaturated fat 1.0 g
  monounsaturated fat 1.0 g
cholesterol 1 mg
sodium 203 mg

carbohydrates 24 g
  fiber 4 g
  sugars 5 g
protein 10 g
DIETARY EXCHANGES
  3 vegetable, 1/2 starch,
  1/2 fat

COCOA-CAYENNE KALE CRISPS

SERVES 4

Small pieces of kale baked until crisp make a nice accompaniment to a sandwich or other entrée— and even do double duty as a healthy snack. Try them as an alternative to french fries with Creole Tuna Steak Sandwich with Caper Tartar Sauce *(page 165) or tortilla chips with* South-of-the-Border Beef Tacos *(page 280).*

Cooking spray
8 ounces kale, any large stems and ribs
    discarded, greens chopped (about
    5 cups)
1 tablespoon olive oil
2 teaspoons unsweetened cocoa powder
1 teaspoon sugar
1/8 to 1/4 teaspoon cayenne
1/8 teaspoon salt

Place a rack on the lowest shelf of the oven. Preheat the oven to 350°F. Lightly spray a large rimmed baking sheet with cooking spray.

Thoroughly dry the kale in a salad spinner or by blotting with paper towels or dish towels. (Moisture will prevent the kale from becoming crisp.) Transfer the kale to a large bowl.

Add the oil to the kale, stirring to coat. Spread the kale in a single layer on the baking sheet. Lightly spray the top side of the kale with cooking spray.

Bake for 10 minutes. Transfer the baking sheet to a cooling rack.

Meanwhile, in a small bowl, stir together the cocoa powder, sugar, cayenne, and salt. Sprinkle over the kale, stirring gently to combine thoroughly.

Bake for 15 to 20 minutes, or until the desired crispness, turning with tongs every 5 minutes. As the pieces become crisp, remove them from the baking sheet and continue baking the remaining kale. Serve immediately for maximum crispness.

PER SERVING

calories 66	sodium 94 mg
total fat 4.0 g	carbohydrates 7 g
saturated fat 0.5 g	fiber 1 g
trans fat 0.0 g	sugars 1 g
polyunsaturated fat 0.5 g	protein 3 g
monounsaturated fat 2.5 g	**DIETARY EXCHANGES**
cholesterol 0 mg	1 vegetable, 1 fat

LEMON KALE CRISPS

Omit the cocoa powder mixture. In a small bowl, stir together 1 tablespoon lemon juice, the oil, and salt. Use the mixture in place of the oil, and bake the kale for 25 to 30 minutes as directed.

PER SERVING

calories 59	sodium 94 mg
total fat 4.0 g	carbohydrates 5 g
saturated fat 0.5 g	fiber 1 g
trans fat 0.0 g	sugars 0 g
polyunsaturated fat 0.5 g	protein 2 g
monounsaturated fat 2.5 g	**DIETARY EXCHANGES**
cholesterol 0 mg	1 vegetable, 1 fat

TACO-SPICED KALE CRISPS

Instead of the cocoa powder mixture, stir together 2 teaspoons salt-free taco seasoning mix, 1/2 teaspoon grated lime zest, and the salt. Bake as directed.

PER SERVING

calories 58	sodium 94 mg
total fat 4.0 g	carbohydrates 5 g
saturated fat 0.5 g	fiber 1 g
trans fat 0.0 g	sugars 0 g
polyunsaturated fat 0.5 g	protein 2 g
monounsaturated fat 2.5 g	**DIETARY EXCHANGES**
cholesterol 0 mg	1 vegetable, 1 fat

MEDITERRANEAN LIMA BEANS
SERVES 4

The delicate taste of lima beans, also called butter beans because of their texture, works perfectly in this Mediterranean side. Garlic, tomatoes, onion, and mint flavor the beans.

> 10 ounces frozen lima beans
> 1 teaspoon light tub margarine
> 1/4 cup chopped onion
> 1 medium garlic clove, crushed or minced
> 1 cup canned no-salt-added tomatoes, undrained
> 1/2 teaspoon dried mint, crumbled

Prepare the lima beans using the package directions, omitting the salt and margarine. Drain well in a colander.

In a medium skillet, melt the margarine over medium-high heat, swirling to coat the bottom. Cook the onion and garlic for 3 minutes, or until the onion is soft, stirring frequently.

Stir in the beans, tomatoes with liquid, and mint. Cook until heated through, stirring occasionally.

PER SERVING

calories 98	sodium 137 mg
total fat 0.5 g	carbohydrates 18 g
saturated fat 0.0 g	fiber 4 g
trans fat 0.0 g	sugars 3 g
polyunsaturated fat 0.0 g	protein 4 g
monounsaturated fat 0.0 g	**DIETARY EXCHANGES**
cholesterol 0 mg	1 starch, 1 vegetable

MUSHROOMS WITH RED WINE
SERVES 4

Dress up mushrooms in a snap by cooking them quickly, then letting them absorb a delicate red wine sauce. If you prefer, you can use brown (cremini) or roughly chopped portobello mushrooms instead.

(continued)

1 pound medium button mushrooms,
   quartered
2 tablespoons dry red wine (regular or
   nonalcoholic)
2 teaspoons (2 packets) salt-free instant beef
   bouillon
1 medium garlic clove, minced
1/2 teaspoon sugar
1/2 teaspoon dried thyme, crumbled
1/4 cup chopped fresh parsley
2 teaspoons olive oil (extra-virgin preferred)
1/8 teaspoon salt

In a large nonstick skillet, cook the mushrooms over medium-high heat for 4 minutes, or until soft.

Meanwhile, in a small bowl, whisk together the wine, bouillon, garlic, sugar, and thyme until the sugar is dissolved.

Stir the wine mixture into the mushrooms. Increase the heat to high and bring to a boil. Remove from the heat.

Stir in the parsley, oil, and salt. Let stand, covered, for 3 minutes before serving.

PER SERVING

calories 61	sodium 84 mg
total fat 2.5 g	carbohydrates 6 g
saturated fat 0.5 g	fiber 1 g
trans fat 0.0 g	sugars 3 g
polyunsaturated fat 0.5 g	protein 4 g
monounsaturated fat 1.5 g	DIETARY EXCHANGES
cholesterol 0 mg	1 vegetable, 1/2 fat

MUSHROOMS WITH WHITE WINE AND SHALLOTS

SERVES 4

Cook succulent mushrooms with shallots and white wine, then reduce the juices to intensify the flavor. Serve as a side dish or spoon the mushrooms over lean broiled or grilled steak.

2 tablespoons light tub margarine
1/2 cup finely chopped shallots (about 8 large)
1 pound medium button mushrooms,
   quartered
1/2 cup dry white wine (regular or
   nonalcoholic)
1 tablespoon finely chopped fresh parsley
Pepper to taste

In a large nonstick skillet, melt the margarine over medium-high heat, swirling to coat the bottom. Cook the shallots for about 3 minutes, stirring constantly.

Stir in the mushrooms and wine. Reduce the heat to medium. Cook, covered, for 7 to 9 minutes. Increase the heat to high. Cook, uncovered, for 5 to 6 minutes, or until the juices have evaporated.

Stir in the parsley and pepper.

PER SERVING

calories 80	sodium 55 mg
total fat 2.5 g	carbohydrates 7 g
saturated fat 0.0 g	fiber 2 g
trans fat 0.0 g	sugars 4 g
polyunsaturated fat 0.5 g	protein 4 g
monounsaturated fat 1.5 g	DIETARY EXCHANGES
cholesterol 0 mg	1 vegetable, 1/2 fat

BAKED OKRA BITES

SERVES 4

Once you've enjoyed these crisp okra bites as a side dish with grilled fish or as part of a southern-style menu, try them also as "croutons" for a spinach and romaine salad or sprinkle them on top of baked casseroles.

Cooking spray
1/4 cup egg substitute
1/2 cup yellow cornmeal
1/4 cup all-purpose flour
1/2 teaspoon onion powder
1/2 teaspoon garlic powder

1/2 teaspoon salt-free Creole or Cajun
seasoning blend, such as on page 401,
or 1/2 teaspoon salt-free spicy seasoning
blend
8 ounces fresh okra, stems discarded, cut into
1/2-inch slices, or 2 cups frozen sliced
okra, thawed

Preheat the oven to 400°F. Lightly spray a large
baking sheet with cooking spray.

Put the egg substitute in a medium bowl. In a
shallow dish, stir together the cornmeal, flour,
onion powder, garlic powder, and seasoning
blend. Put the bowl, dish, and baking sheet in a
row, assembly-line fashion. Add the okra to the
egg substitute, stirring to coat. Using a slotted
spoon, transfer the okra in batches to the cornmeal mixture, stirring to coat and gently shaking
off any excess. Arrange the okra in a single layer
on the baking sheet (leave space between the
pieces so they brown evenly). Lightly spray the
okra with cooking spray.

Bake for 20 to 25 minutes, or until crisp on the
outside and tender on the inside. Transfer the
baking sheet to a cooling rack. Let the okra cool
for 2 to 3 minutes before serving.

PER SERVING

calories 118	sodium 36 mg
total fat 0.5 g	carbohydrates 25 g
saturated fat 0.0 g	fiber 3 g
trans fat 0.0 g	sugars 1 g
polyunsaturated fat 0.0 g	protein 5 g
monounsaturated fat 0.0 g	DIETARY EXCHANGES
cholesterol 0 mg	1 1/2 starch,
	1 vegetable

OVEN-FRIED ONION RINGS

SERVES 4

*Crumbled melba toasts make these onion rings so
crisp your family will think they're fried.*

Cooking spray
2 tablespoons white whole-wheat flour
1/2 teaspoon paprika

1/8 teaspoon cayenne
3 large egg whites
3/4 teaspoon red hot-pepper sauce
16 unsalted whole-grain melba toasts,
processed to fine crumbs
2 large sweet onions, cut into 1/2-inch slices
and separated into 24 large rings
(reserve small inner rings for another
use)

Preheat the oven to 400°F. Line two large
rimmed baking pans with aluminum foil. Place a
cooling rack in each pan. Lightly spray the racks
with cooking spray.

In a large shallow dish, stir together the flour,
paprika, and cayenne. In a separate shallow
dish, whisk together the egg whites and hot-
pepper sauce. Put the melba toast crumbs in
a third shallow dish. Put the dishes and baking
pans in a row, assembly-line fashion. Dip the
onion rings, a few at a time, in the flour mixture,
then in the egg white mixture, and finally in the
crumbs, turning to coat at each step and gently
shaking off any excess. Using your fingertips,
gently press the coating so it adheres to the
rings. Transfer the rings to the racks in the baking pans, arranging them in a single layer. Lightly
spray the rings with cooking spray.

Bake for 12 to 15 minutes, or until browned (don't
turn over the onion rings).

PER SERVING

calories 133	sodium 204 mg
total fat 0.5 g	carbohydrates 27 g
saturated fat 0.0 g	fiber 4 g
trans fat 0.0 g	sugars 6 g
polyunsaturated fat 0.5 g	protein 6 g
monounsaturated fat 0.0 g	DIETARY EXCHANGES
cholesterol 0 mg	1 starch, 1 vegetable

PARMESAN PARSNIP PUREE WITH LEEKS AND CARROTS

SERVES 6

Sweet, slightly peppery parsnips blended with carrots, leeks, and Parmesan cheese create a pale gold side dish similar in texture to mashed potatoes.

1 pound parsnips, peeled and cut crosswise into 1/2-inch pieces

2 large leeks (white part only), thinly sliced

2 small carrots, cut crosswise into 1/2-inch pieces

1/2 cup fat-free, low-sodium chicken broth and 1/2 cup fat-free, low-sodium chicken broth, such as on page 36, divided use

2 tablespoons shredded or grated Parmesan cheese

1 tablespoon light tub margarine

1/4 teaspoon salt

2 tablespoons thinly sliced almonds, dry-roasted

In a large saucepan, bring the parsnips, leeks, carrots, and 1/2 cup broth to a boil over high heat. Reduce the heat to medium low. Cook, covered, for 10 minutes, or until tender. Remove from the heat. Let cool for 5 minutes.

In a food processor or blender, process the parsnip mixture, Parmesan, margarine, salt, and the remaining 1/2 cup broth until smooth. Sprinkle with the almonds.

Cook's Tip on Parsnips: Parsnips look like pale carrots and are in the same family. Whether you bake, sauté, roast, steam, or boil them, parsnips are sweet and aromatic. Be careful not to overcook them, though, as they tend to turn mushy quickly. Look for firm parsnips without pitting. Don't worry if they're large—bigger size doesn't mean parsnips won't be tender. Wrapped in plastic wrap and refrigerated, parsnips will keep for several weeks to several months.

PER SERVING

calories 108	**carbohydrates** 20 g
total fat 2.5 g	fiber 5 g
saturated fat 0.5 g	sugars 6 g
trans fat 0.0 g	**protein** 3 g
polyunsaturated fat 0.5 g	**DIETARY EXCHANGES**
monounsaturated fat 1.0 g	1 starch, 1 vegetable,
cholesterol 1 mg	1/2 fat
sodium 169 mg	

FRENCH PEAS

SERVES 6

Tender peas, wilted lettuce, and crunchy water chestnuts provide a variety of textures in this side dish. For Paris in a meal, serve with Burgundy Chicken with Mushrooms *(page 212) or* Chicken in White Wine and Tarragon *(page 211).*

10 ounces frozen green peas

1 tablespoon canola or corn oil

1 cup finely shredded lettuce

2 medium green onions, diced

1 teaspoon all-purpose flour

3 tablespoons fat-free, low-sodium chicken broth, such as on page 36

1 8-ounce can sliced water chestnuts, drained

Pepper to taste

Prepare the green peas using the package directions, omitting the salt and margarine. Drain well in a colander. Set aside.

Meanwhile, in a large saucepan, heat the oil over low heat, swirling to coat the bottom. Cook the lettuce and green onions for 1 to 2 minutes, stirring occasionally.

Put the flour in a small bowl. Add the broth, whisking until the flour is dissolved. Stir into the lettuce mixture. Increase the heat to medium. Cook for 2 to 3 minutes, or until thickened, stirring occasionally.

Stir in the green peas, water chestnuts, and pepper. Cook until heated through, stirring occasionally.

calories 76
total fat 2.5 g
    saturated fat 0.0 g
    trans fat 0.0 g
    polyunsaturated fat 0.5 g
    monounsaturated fat 1.5 g
cholesterol 0 mg
sodium 57 mg

carbohydrates 11 g
    fiber 4 g
    sugars 3 g
protein 3 g
DIETARY EXCHANGES
1/2 starch, 1 vegetable, 1/2 fat

MINTED PEAS

SERVES 4

Fresh citrus and mint bring a pop of brightness to tender peas. A mild onion provides a bit of bite. This super simple side dish goes well with poultry and beef entrées.

    10 ounces frozen green peas
    2 tablespoons water
    1 to 2 tablespoons chopped fresh mint
    1 to 2 green onions (green part only), thinly sliced
    1 teaspoon light tub margarine
    1 teaspoon grated lemon zest
    1/4 teaspoon salt
    1/4 teaspoon pepper

Put the peas and water in a medium saucepan. Bring to a boil over high heat. Reduce the heat and simmer, covered, for 3 to 5 minutes, or until tender-crisp. Remove from the heat.

Gently stir in the mint, green onions, margarine, lemon zest, salt, and pepper.

PER SERVING

calories 63
total fat 0.5 g
    saturated fat 0.0 g
    trans fat 0.0 g
    polyunsaturated fat 0.0 g
    monounsaturated fat 0.0 g
cholesterol 0 mg

sodium 233 mg
carbohydrates 11 g
    fiber 4 g
    sugars 4 g
protein 4 g
DIETARY EXCHANGES
1/2 starch

BASIL ROASTED PEPPERS

SERVES 8

Serve these on top of grilled chicken breasts or burgers, diced and mixed with brown rice or steamed spinach, or in salads.

    Cooking spray
    6 firm medium red bell peppers
    1/4 cup plus 1 tablespoon olive oil
    1/4 cup red wine vinegar
    2 tablespoons finely chopped fresh basil
    3 or 4 medium garlic cloves, minced
    1/2 teaspoon pepper, or to taste
    1/4 teaspoon salt

Preheat the broiler. Lightly spray a broiler pan and rack with cooking spray.

Broil the bell peppers on the rack about 4 inches from the heat for 1 to 2 minutes on each side, or until lightly charred. Transfer to a large bowl. Cover with plastic wrap. Let cool for 5 to 10 minutes. (It won't hurt the peppers to stand for as long as 20 minutes.) Rinse the peppers with cold water, removing and discarding the skin, stem, ribs, and seeds. Blot the peppers dry with paper towels. Cut into strips 1/2 inch wide.

In a medium bowl, stir together the remaining ingredients. Stir in the peppers. Cover and refrigerate for 30 minutes to 8 hours. Drain well in a colander, discarding the marinade. Refrigerate the drained peppers in an airtight container for up to five days or freeze for up to four months.

PER SERVING

calories 28
total fat 0.5 g
    saturated fat 0.0 g
    trans fat 0.0 g
    polyunsaturated fat 0.0 g
    monounsaturated fat 0.0 g
cholesterol 0 mg

sodium 76 mg
carbohydrates 5 g
    fiber 2 g
    sugars 4 g
protein 1 g
DIETARY EXCHANGES
1 vegetable

POTATOES WITH LEEKS AND FRESH HERBS

SERVES 8

While this one-skillet side dish simmers, it will fill your kitchen with a tantalizing aroma. And the dish tastes even better than it smells.

Olive oil cooking spray
2 medium leeks (white part only), sliced
2 medium garlic cloves, crushed
1 cup fat-free, low-sodium chicken broth, such as on page 36
1/2 cup chopped fresh parsley
1 2-ounce jar diced pimiento, rinsed and drained (about 1/4 cup)
1/4 cup dry white wine (regular or nonalcoholic) (optional)
2 tablespoons chopped fresh dillweed
1 tablespoon chopped fresh sage or thyme
2 teaspoons grated lemon zest
Pepper to taste
6 medium potatoes (about 2 pounds), peeled and thinly sliced

Lightly spray a large skillet with cooking spray. Heat over medium heat. Cook the leeks and garlic for 2 to 3 minutes, or until soft, stirring occasionally.

Stir in the remaining ingredients except the potatoes. Remove from the heat.

Arrange the potatoes on the leek mixture.

Increase the heat to medium high. Bring the potato mixture to a boil. Reduce the heat and simmer, covered, for 20 minutes, or until the potatoes are tender.

Cook's Tip: If you have any of these potatoes left over, combine them with lightly cooked sliced mushrooms and egg substitute or egg whites to make a delicious frittata.

TWICE-BAKED POTATOES

SERVES 8

This creamy, cheesy side dish pairs perfectly with Rosemary Chicken (page 192) or Swiss Steak (page 252)—both entrées cook at the same temperature as the potatoes.

Cooking spray
4 medium potatoes (russet preferred), baked, halved lengthwise
1 cup fat-free cottage cheese
1/2 cup fat-free milk
1 tablespoon minced onion
Pepper to taste (freshly ground preferred)
1/8 teaspoon paprika
1/4 cup chopped fresh parsley

Preheat the oven to 350°F. Lightly spray a rimmed baking sheet with cooking spray.

Using a spoon or melon baller, scoop out the potato pulp, leaving the skins intact. Transfer the pulp to a large bowl. Lightly chop the pulp. Place the skins with the cut sides up on the baking sheet.

In a food processor or blender, pulse the pulp, cottage cheese, milk, and onion until somewhat smoother, but with some texture remaining. Spoon the mixture back into the skins.

Sprinkle the paprika and parsley, in order, over the potatoes. Bake for 10 minutes, or until just golden.

calories 111	**carbohydrates** 22 g
total fat 0.0 g	fiber 2 g
saturated fat 0.0 g	sugars 3 g
trans fat 0.0 g	**protein** 6 g
polyunsaturated fat 0.0 g	**DIETARY EXCHANGES**
monounsaturated fat 0.0 g	1 1/2 starch, 1/2 lean
cholesterol 2 mg	meat
sodium 120 mg	

SCALLOPED POTATOES

SERVES 6

Just out of the oven, these potatoes are a beautiful golden brown with a slight crunch on top. Serve with lean grilled pork chops and Asparagus with Lemon and Capers (page 373) or take to a potluck for plenty of rave reviews.

Cooking spray
2 tablespoons light tub margarine
1 large onion, finely chopped
1/4 cup all-purpose flour
2 cups fat-free milk
1/4 cup fat-free half-and-half
3 tablespoons finely chopped fresh parsley
1/8 teaspoon salt and 1/8 teaspoon salt, divided use
1/8 to 1/4 teaspoon pepper and 1/8 teaspoon pepper (white preferred), divided use
2 pounds baking potatoes, peeled and thinly sliced
2 tablespoons shredded or grated Romano or Parmesan cheese

Preheat the oven to 325°F. Lightly spray an 8-inch square glass baking dish with cooking spray. Set aside.

In a medium saucepan, melt the margarine over medium-high heat, swirling to coat the bottom. Cook the onion for about 3 minutes, or until soft, stirring frequently.

Whisk in the flour. Cook for 1 minute.

Whisk in the milk. Cook for 3 to 4 minutes, or until the sauce has thickened, whisking constantly.

Whisk in the half-and-half, parsley, 1/8 teaspoon salt, and 1/8 to 1/4 teaspoon pepper. Remove from the heat.

Arrange the potatoes in the baking dish. Sprinkle the remaining 1/8 teaspoon salt and 1/8 teaspoon pepper over the potatoes. Pour the sauce over the potatoes. Sprinkle the Romano over the sauce.

Bake for 1 hour 30 minutes.

calories 198	**carbohydrates** 39 g
total fat 2.0 g	fiber 3 g
saturated fat 0.0 g	sugars 8 g
trans fat 0.0 g	**protein** 7 g
polyunsaturated fat 0.5 g	**DIETARY EXCHANGES**
monounsaturated fat 1.0 g	2 1/2 starch, 1/2 lean
cholesterol 3 mg	meat
sodium 194 mg	

MASHED POTATOES WITH PARMESAN AND GREEN ONIONS

SERVES 4

The secret to the super creaminess of these spuds is fat-free evaporated milk rather than fat-free milk. Keeping the skin on the potatoes adds pops of red, perfectly complementing the bits of green onions.

8 ounces red potatoes, unpeeled, cut into 1/2-inch cubes
2 medium green onions, finely chopped
1/4 cup plus 2 tablespoons fat-free evaporated milk
1/8 teaspoon pepper
1 tablespoon plus 1 teaspoon light tub margarine, melted
1/8 teaspoon salt
2 teaspoons shredded or grated Parmesan cheese

In a medium saucepan, steam the potatoes for 8 to 10 minutes, or until tender. Drain well in a colander. If you have a hand mixer or immersion (or handheld) blender, return the potatoes to the pan (off the heat) and beat or blend until no

(continued)

lumps remain (the skins will keep the mixture from being smooth). Otherwise, transfer them to a large mixing bowl. Using an electric mixer on medium speed, beat the potatoes until almost smooth.

Set 2 tablespoons of the green onions aside. Add the milk, pepper, and the remaining green onions to the potatoes. Beat until well blended. Transfer to a serving bowl. Drizzle the potatoes with the margarine. Sprinkle with, in order, the salt, Parmesan, and the reserved 2 tablespoons green onions.

PER SERVING

calories 80	**sodium** 157 mg
total fat 2.0 g	**carbohydrates** 13 g
saturated fat 0.0 g	fiber 2 g
trans fat 0.0 g	sugars 4 g
polyunsaturated fat 0.5 g	**protein** 3 g
monounsaturated fat 1.0 g	**DIETARY EXCHANGES**
cholesterol 2 mg	1 starch

RUSTIC POTATO PATTIES

SERVES 5

Black pepper and cayenne spice up these potato patties, which get their texture from the skins. The spiciness will cut the richness of beef, making these a perfect accompaniment to dishes such as Filet of Beef with Herbes de Provence *(page 245).*

> 1 pound red potatoes, unpeeled, diced
> 1/2 cup minced onion
> 1/4 cup plus 2 tablespoons fat-free
>   evaporated milk
> 1 large egg white
> 1/4 teaspoon salt
> 1/8 teaspoon pepper
> 1/8 teaspoon cayenne
> 1/4 cup all-purpose flour
> 1 1/2 teaspoons canola or corn oil and
>   1 1/2 teaspoons canola or corn oil,
>   divided use

Preheat the oven to warm or 140°F.

In a medium saucepan, steam the potatoes for 8 to 10 minutes, or until tender. Drain well in a colander. If you have a hand mixer or immersion (handheld) blender, return the potatoes to the pan (off the heat) and beat or blend until no lumps remain (the skins will keep the mixture from being smooth). Otherwise, transfer the potatoes to a large mixing bowl. Using an electric mixer on medium speed, beat the potatoes until almost smooth.

Beat in the onion, milk, egg white, salt, pepper, and cayenne until well blended.

Beat in the flour.

In a large nonstick skillet, heat 1 1/2 teaspoons oil over medium-high heat for about 2 minutes, or until hot, swirling to coat the bottom. Spoon five 1/3-cup mounds of the potato mixture (about half) into the skillet. Using the back of a fork, flatten slightly until about 1/2 inch thick. Cook for about 9 minutes, turning once halfway through. Transfer the patties to an ovenproof platter. Put in the oven.

Heat the remaining 1 1/2 teaspoons oil, still over medium-high heat, for 30 seconds, swirling to coat the bottom. Repeat the process, making 5 more patties.

Time-Saver: Since you'll beat the cooked potatoes, you may wonder why you dice them first. It doesn't take long to dice them in the food processor, and using small pieces saves cooking time.

PER SERVING

calories 136	**sodium** 166 mg
total fat 3.0 g	**carbohydrates** 23 g
saturated fat 0.5 g	fiber 2 g
trans fat 0.0 g	sugars 4 g
polyunsaturated fat 1.0 g	**protein** 5 g
monounsaturated fat 2.0 g	**DIETARY EXCHANGES**
cholesterol 1 mg	1 1/2 starch, 1/2 fat

BAKED FRIES WITH CREOLE SEASONING

SERVES 4

These spice-flecked, crisp fries will perk up your taste buds. Serve them with Grilled Hamburgers with Vegetables and Feta *(page 272).*

4 medium unpeeled russet potatoes (1 1/4 to 1 1/2 pounds total)

Creole or Cajun Seasoning Blend
    1/2 teaspoon chili powder
    1/2 teaspoon ground cumin
    1/2 teaspoon onion powder
    1/2 teaspoon garlic powder
    1/2 teaspoon paprika
    1/2 teaspoon pepper
    1/8 teaspoon cayenne (optional)

■ ■ ■

Cooking spray

Cut the potatoes into long strips about 1/2 inch wide. Put them in a large bowl. Pour in enough cold water to cover by 1 inch. Soak for 15 minutes.

Meanwhile, in a small bowl, stir together the seasoning blend ingredients.

Preheat the oven to 450°F. Lightly spray a large baking sheet with cooking spray.

Drain the potatoes. Pat dry. Spread the potatoes in a single layer on the baking sheet. Lightly spray with cooking spray. Sprinkle the seasoning blend over the potatoes.

Bake for 30 to 35 minutes, or until crisp.

Cook's Tip on Creole or Cajun Seasoning: To save time in the future, double or triple the seasonings in this recipe and keep the blend in a container with a shaker top. This seasoning blend is excellent sprinkled on seafood, poultry, meat, and vegetables. Or use it in recipes such as Baked Okra Bites (page 394), Catfish with Zesty Slaw Topping (page 141), or Bronzed Catfish with Remoulade Sauce (page 140).

PER SERVING

calories 129	**sodium** 15 mg
total fat 0.5 g	**carbohydrates** 29 g
saturated fat 0.0 g	fiber 2 g
trans fat 0.0 g	sugars 1 g
polyunsaturated fat 0.0 g	**protein** 4 g
monounsaturated fat 0.0 g	**DIETARY EXCHANGES**
cholesterol 0 mg	2 starch

GARLIC POTATOES

SERVES 4

This country-style recipe is made for garlic lovers. If you use boiling (more waxy) potatoes, your results will be creamier. If you use baking potatoes, the dish will be fluffier. Don't be tempted to make this recipe in the food processor—it's meant to have lots of texture.

1 pound boiling or baking potatoes, with or without skin
3 large garlic cloves, peeled but left whole
1 1/2 teaspoons olive oil
1 teaspoon fresh lemon juice
1/2 teaspoon white balsamic vinegar (optional)
1/4 teaspoon chopped fresh rosemary
1/4 teaspoon chopped fresh oregano
1/8 teaspoon salt
1/8 teaspoon pepper (white preferred)

In a large saucepan, bring enough water to cover the potatoes to a boil over high heat.

Meanwhile, cut the boiling potatoes in half or the baking potatoes in quarters. Add the potatoes and garlic to the boiling water and return to a boil. Boil for about 30 minutes, or until the potatoes are soft all the way through when tested with a knife. Using a slotted spoon, transfer the potatoes to a medium bowl and the garlic to a small plate, reserving the cooking water.

Mash the garlic cloves. Add to the potatoes, combining lightly with a potato masher or large

(continued)

fork until coarse-textured (don't use a food processor). Stir in the remaining ingredients, adding a little hot cooking water if needed for the desired consistency. The texture should remain coarse.

Cook's Tip: For a taste change, substitute other fresh herbs for the rosemary and/or oregano. Parsley and sage are just two possibilities. This recipe doubles well.

STIR-FRIED SUGAR SNAP PEAS

SERVES 4

Crisp peas simmered with an Asian-style sauce and garnished with toasted nuts are a snap to make. Serve with grilled pork or poached fish, as well as with Asian entrées.

3 tablespoons fat-free, low-sodium chicken broth, such as on page 36
1 teaspoon soy sauce (lowest sodium available)
1/2 teaspoon cornstarch
1/2 teaspoon light brown sugar
1/4 teaspoon toasted sesame oil
1/8 teaspoon crushed red pepper flakes (optional)
8 ounces sugar snap peas, trimmed
1 medium garlic clove, minced
1 tablespoon sliced almonds, dry-roasted

In a small bowl, whisk together the broth, soy sauce, cornstarch, brown sugar, oil, and red pepper flakes until the cornstarch is dissolved.

In a medium nonstick skillet, cook the peas and garlic over medium-high heat for 1 to 2 minutes, or until tender-crisp, stirring constantly.

Pour the broth mixture into the skillet. Reduce the heat and simmer until thickened, stirring occasionally. Sprinkle with the almonds.

SWEET LEMON SNOW PEAS

SERVES 4

Chinese snow pea pods are quickly steamed (just two minutes), then splashed with a spicy-sweet, lemony soy sauce mixture.

2 tablespoons sugar
2 tablespoons soy sauce (lowest sodium available)
1 teaspoon grated lemon zest
2 tablespoons fresh lemon juice
1/4 teaspoon crushed red pepper flakes
9 ounces fresh or frozen snow peas, trimmed if fresh

In a small bowl, stir together all the ingredients except the snow peas until the sugar is dissolved.

In a medium saucepan, steam the snow peas for 2 minutes, or until just tender-crisp. Transfer to a rimmed plate or shallow dish.

Pour the sauce over the snow peas. Don't stir.

Cook's Tip on Lemon Zest: You can grate the zest of several lemons at one time—especially when they're on sale—and freeze what you don't use. Having zest on hand whenever you need it will save you time and money.

FRESH SNOW PEAS WITH WATER CHESTNUTS

SERVES 6

Wondering what to serve with an Asian entrée besides steamed rice? Here's your answer. Try it with Teriyaki Halibut *(page 145) or* Five-Spice Turkey Medallions *(page 236).*

> 1 1/2 teaspoons canola or corn oil
> 1 teaspoon hot chili oil
> 1 1/2 pounds snow peas, trimmed and cut diagonally into 1 1/2-inch pieces
> 1 8-ounce can sliced water chestnuts, drained
> 1 tablespoon sesame seeds, dry-roasted
> 1/4 teaspoon salt

In a large skillet, heat the oils over medium-high heat, swirling to coat the bottom. Cook the peas for 2 to 3 minutes, or until almost tender-crisp, stirring frequently.

Stir in the water chestnuts. Cook for 1 minute, stirring constantly.

Stir in the sesame seeds and salt. Cook until heated through, stirring constantly.

Cook's Tip on Water Chestnuts: Grown in water and frequently used in Chinese cooking, water chestnuts are the underground stems of a marsh plant. Fresh and unpeeled, they do resemble chestnuts. You can find the fresh ones in Chinese markets. Peel them and use them either raw or cooked to add crunch to salads and stir-fry dishes. Canned whole or sliced water chestnuts are also available.

ASIAN SPINACH AND MUSHROOMS

SERVES 4

Just a little sesame oil adds rich flavor to this speedy vegetable combo. Use it as a bed for Five-Spice Turkey Medallions *(page 236) or serve it with* Crisp Pan Seared Trout with Green Onions *(page 162).*

> 2 teaspoons toasted sesame oil
> 1 cup sliced button mushrooms
> 1/4 cup chopped shallots
> 1 tablespoon grated peeled gingerroot
> 1 tablespoon plain rice vinegar
> 8 cups loosely packed spinach, stems discarded
> 1/4 teaspoon pepper
> 1/8 teaspoon salt

In a large skillet, heat the oil over medium heat, swirling to coat the bottom. Cook the mushrooms, shallots, gingerroot, and vinegar for 4 to 5 minutes, or until the mushrooms are soft, stirring occasionally.

Using tongs, combine the spinach with the mushroom mixture. Cook for 2 to 3 minutes, or just until the spinach is wilted, turning frequently with the tongs. Don't overcook.

Add the pepper and salt, turning the vegetables to combine.

BASIL SPINACH

SERVES 4

The addition of basil and garlic gives this ultra-quick side dish the taste of Italy in a matter of seconds. The spinach makes a delicious bed for grilled or broiled chicken breasts or salmon fillets.

2 tablespoons light tub margarine
1 teaspoon dried basil, crumbled
1 medium garlic clove, minced
9 ounces baby spinach

In a large nonstick skillet, heat the margarine, basil, and garlic over medium-high heat, stirring until the margarine is melted.

Stir in the spinach. Cook for 45 seconds, or until just wilted, stirring constantly. Don't overcook. Remove from the heat.

PER SERVING

calories 37	sodium 96 mg
total fat 2.5 g	carbohydrates 3 g
saturated fat 0.0 g	fiber 2 g
trans fat 0.0 g	sugars 0 g
polyunsaturated fat 0.5 g	protein 2 g
monounsaturated fat 1.5 g	DIETARY EXCHANGES
cholesterol 0 mg	1/2 fat

BROWN RICE PILAF WITH SUMMER SQUASH

SERVES 10

This whole-grain and veggie cold side dish is a tasty complement to any grilled entrée. Pair it with Grilled Lemon-Sage Chicken (page 202) or Grilled Meat Loaf (page 274).

1 cup uncooked long-grain brown rice
3 medium yellow summer squash, thinly sliced
1/2 cup unsalted shelled sunflower seeds, dry-roasted
3 medium green onions, thinly sliced
3 tablespoons olive oil (extra-virgin preferred)
2 tablespoons garlic wine vinegar

2 teaspoons dried dillweed, crumbled
Pepper to taste (freshly ground preferred)

Prepare the rice using the package directions, omitting the salt and margarine.

In a medium saucepan, steam the squash over medium-high heat for 3 to 5 minutes, or until tender. Drain well. Let stand for 2 minutes to cool.

In a large bowl, gently stir together the sunflower seeds, green onions, rice, and squash, being careful not to break up the squash.

In a small bowl, whisk together the oil, vinegar, dillweed, and pepper. Pour over the rice mixture, tossing gently until well blended. Cover and refrigerate until serving time.

PER SERVING

calories 156	sodium 7 mg
total fat 8.0 g	carbohydrates 19 g
saturated fat 1.0 g	fiber 3 g
trans fat 0.0 g	sugars 2 g
polyunsaturated fat 3.0 g	protein 4 g
monounsaturated fat 4.0 g	DIETARY EXCHANGES
cholesterol 0 mg	1 1/2 starch, 1 fat

PATTYPAN SQUASH WITH APPLE-NUT STUFFING

SERVES 4

Here's a summertime version of stuffed squash. Like its wintertime counterpart, acorn squash, pattypan squash goes especially well with poultry and pork.

4 medium pattypan squash, unpeeled, halved crosswise, seeds discarded
2 medium baking apples, such as Rome Beauty, chopped
1/4 cup sweetened dried cranberries
2 1/2 tablespoons light brown sugar
2 tablespoons chopped walnuts or pecans
Butter-flavor cooking spray

Preheat the oven to 350°F.

Put the squash with the cut side down in a 13 × 9 × 2-inch glass baking dish.

Bake for 30 minutes.

Meanwhile, in a small bowl, stir together the remaining ingredients except the spray margarine. Spoon into the squash halves. Lightly spray with the cooking spray.

Bake with the stuffed side up for 30 minutes, or until tender when tested with the tip of a sharp knife or a fork.

Cook's Tip on Pattypan Squash: A white, yellow, or pale green summer squash, pattypan looks something like a scalloped flying saucer with a stem. Its unique shape makes it perfect for stuffing. (You may need to cut a slice from the bottom so the squash won't rock.) Use it as you would yellow summer squash or zucchini.

PER SERVING

calories 149	carbohydrates 32 g
total fat 3.0 g	fiber 4 g
saturated fat 0.5 g	sugars 26 g
trans fat 0.0 g	**protein** 3 g
polyunsaturated fat 2.0 g	**DIETARY EXCHANGES**
monounsaturated fat 0.5 g	2 fruit, 1 vegetable,
cholesterol 0 mg	1/2 fat
sodium 4 mg	

YELLOW SUMMER SQUASH CASSEROLE

SERVES 6

Tender cooked and mashed yellow summer squash enhanced with fresh sage and combined with soft bread crumbs pairs perfectly with Crunchy Herb-Crusted Pork Chops (page 288), which bake at the same temperature.

Olive oil cooking spray
1/2 teaspoon olive oil and 1 teaspoon olive oil, divided use
1/2 large onion, thinly sliced
1 pound yellow summer squash, diced
2 tablespoons fat-free, low-sodium chicken broth, such as on page 36
3/4 teaspoon chopped fresh sage, or
 1/4 teaspoon dried sage
1 medium garlic clove, minced
1/8 teaspoon salt
1/8 teaspoon pepper
1 1/4 cups soft whole-grain bread crumbs (lowest sodium available)
2 tablespoons shredded or grated Parmesan cheese

Lightly spray a medium saucepan with cooking spray. Heat 1/2 teaspoon oil over medium-high heat, swirling to coat the bottom. Cook the onion for 8 to 10 minutes, or until golden, stirring occasionally.

Stir in the squash, broth, sage, garlic, salt, and pepper. Bring to a simmer. Reduce the heat and simmer, covered, for 10 to 12 minutes, or until the squash is tender.

Meanwhile, preheat the oven to 375°F.

In a medium bowl, stir together the bread crumbs, Parmesan, and the remaining 1 teaspoon oil.

Using a potato masher, mash the squash mixture until slightly chunky. Pour into an 8-inch square baking dish. Spread the bread crumb mixture over the squash. Lightly spray with cooking spray.

Bake for 25 to 30 minutes, or until the topping is golden brown and the squash mixture is heated through.

PER SERVING

calories 66	carbohydrates 9 g
total fat 2.0 g	fiber 2 g
saturated fat 0.5 g	sugars 3 g
trans fat 0.0 g	**protein** 3 g
polyunsaturated fat 0.5 g	**DIETARY EXCHANGES**
monounsaturated fat 1.0 g	1/2 starch, 1 vegetable,
cholesterol 1 mg	1/2 fat
sodium 126 mg	

CREOLE SQUASH

SERVES 4

Unlike its Cajun cousin, Creole cuisine usually isn't spicy. This layered vegetable casserole is a super side with Creole Tuna Steak Sandwich with Caper Tartar Sauce *(page 165).*

1 teaspoon canola or corn oil and 1 teaspoon
    canola or corn oil, divided use
1 medium button mushroom, sliced
1 tablespoon chopped onion
1 tablespoon chopped green bell pepper
1 cup canned no-salt-added stewed
    tomatoes, drained, or 1 large tomato,
    chopped
Pepper to taste

■ ■ ■

3 medium yellow summer squash, cubed
Cooking spray
1/4 cup whole-wheat panko (Japanese-style
    bread crumbs)
1 1/2 teaspoons light tub margarine

In a small saucepan, heat 1 teaspoon oil over low heat, swirling to coat the bottom. Cook the mushroom, onion, and bell pepper for 5 minutes, stirring occasionally. Stir in the tomatoes and pepper. Simmer for 30 minutes, or until the sauce has thickened, stirring occasionally.

Meanwhile, in a medium skillet, heat the remaining 1 teaspoon oil, swirling to coat the bottom. Cook the squash for 4 to 5 minutes, or just until tender, stirring occasionally.

Preheat the oven to 350°F. Lightly spray an 8-inch square baking dish with cooking spray.

To assemble, alternate the layers of squash and sauce in the casserole dish, starting with the squash and ending with the sauce. Sprinkle the panko over all. Dot the margarine on top.

Bake for 30 minutes, or until bubbling.

Cook's Tip: This recipe is also delicious with eggplant. Substitute about 3/4 pound eggplant, sliced or cubed, for the squash and proceed as directed on page 405.

PER SERVING

calories 87	sodium 28 mg
total fat 3.5 g	carbohydrates 12 g
saturated fat 0.0 g	fiber 3 g
trans fat 0.0 g	sugars 6 g
polyunsaturated fat 1.0 g	protein 3 g
monounsaturated fat 2.0 g	**DIETARY EXCHANGES**
cholesterol 0 mg	2 vegetable, 1/2 fat

SCALLOPED SQUASH

SERVES 6

This summery side cooks quickly and complements grilled entrées, which also cook fast. Serve this herb-flecked dish with Turkey Cutlets with Fresh Herbs *(page 236) or* Grilled Tuna with Smoky-Sweet Fruit Salsa *(page 164).*

1 teaspoon light tub margarine
1 large onion, finely chopped
1 1/2 pounds yellow summer squash, sliced
2/3 cup fat-free, low-sodium chicken broth,
    such as on page 36
1 teaspoon dried basil, crumbled
1 teaspoon dried thyme, crumbled
1 teaspoon dried marjoram, crumbled
1/4 teaspoon salt
1 3/4 cups unseasoned croutons (lowest
    sodium available), crushed
1/4 cup chopped fresh chives

In a large saucepan, melt the margarine over medium-high heat, swirling to coat the bottom. Cook the onion for about 3 minutes, or until soft, stirring frequently.

Stir in the squash, broth, basil, thyme, marjoram, and salt. Reduce the heat to medium. Cook, covered, for 10 minutes, or until the squash is tender.

Stir in the croutons. If the mixture is too dry, stir in a small amount of hot water. Stir in the chives.

PER SERVING

calories 76	sodium 194 mg
total fat 0.5 g	carbohydrates 16 g
saturated fat 0.0 g	fiber 2 g
trans fat 0.0 g	sugars 5 g
polyunsaturated fat 0.0 g	protein 3 g
monounsaturated fat 0.0 g	**DIETARY EXCHANGES**
cholesterol 0 mg	1/2 starch, 1 vegetable

BAKED SWEET POTATO CHIPS

SERVES 4

Elevate baked sweet potatoes to a new level with spices and herbs and bake them at a high temperature so they become crisp; they bake at the same temperature as Crispy Baked Fillet of Sole *(page 153).*

Cooking spray
1 teaspoon dried rosemary, crushed
1 teaspoon dried parsley, crumbled
1/2 teaspoon dry mustard
1/4 teaspoon paprika
1/4 teaspoon salt
1/4 teaspoon pepper
2 medium sweet potatoes, unpeeled, cut crosswise into 1/8-inch-thick slices

Preheat the oven to 450°F. Lightly spray a baking sheet with cooking spray.

In a small bowl, stir together the remaining ingredients except the sweet potatoes.

Arrange the sweet potatoes in a single layer on the baking sheet. Lightly spray with cooking spray. Sprinkle the rosemary mixture over the sweet potatoes.

Bake for 25 minutes, or until tender-crisp.

PER SERVING

calories 77	sodium 193 mg
total fat 0.5 g	carbohydrates 18 g
saturated fat 0.0 g	fiber 3 g
trans fat 0.0 g	sugars 4 g
polyunsaturated fat 0.0 g	protein 2 g
monounsaturated fat 0.0 g	DIETARY EXCHANGES
cholesterol 0 mg	1 starch

SWEET POTATO–APPLE GRATIN WITH WALNUTS

SERVES 4

A sweet glaze coats this combo of sweet potato slices and tart apple pieces. Serve with Crispy Baked Chicken *(page 185).*

Cooking spray
1 medium sweet potato (about 12 ounces), peeled and cut crosswise into 3/8-inch slices
1 medium unpeeled firm tart red apple such as Braeburn or Gala, chopped into 1/2-inch pieces
1 teaspoon ground cinnamon
1/4 teaspoon ground nutmeg
1/4 teaspoon pepper
Pinch of ground cloves
1 tablespoon plus 1 teaspoon light brown sugar
2 tablespoons pure maple syrup
2 tablespoons chopped walnuts

Preheat the oven to 400°F. Lightly spray a 1- to 1 1/2-quart baking dish with cooking spray.

In a large bowl, toss together the sweet potato, apple, cinnamon, nutmeg, pepper, and cloves.

Add the brown sugar, tossing to coat.

Transfer the sweet potato mixture to the baking dish. Brush the maple syrup over the sweet potato slices and apple pieces.

Bake, covered, for 30 minutes. Increase the oven temperature to 425°F. Remove the baking dish from the oven. Uncover it and brush the slices and pieces with the juices from the dish. Sprinkle with the walnuts.

Bake for 10 to 15 minutes, or until the sweet potatoes are tender and the glaze is slightly thickened. Just before serving, brush the slices and pieces with any glaze remaining in the dish.

Cook's Tip: Use the deep-orange sweet potatoes that are often labeled as yams in the supermarket.

PER SERVING

calories 159	carbohydrates 34 g
total fat 2.5 g	fiber 4 g
saturated fat 0.5 g	sugars 21 g
trans fat 0.0 g	protein 2 g
polyunsaturated fat 2.0 g	DIETARY EXCHANGES
monounsaturated fat 0.5 g	1 starch, 1/2 fruit,
cholesterol 0 mg	1 other carbohydrate,
sodium 49 mg	1/2 fat

GLAZED SWEET POTATO CUBES

SERVES 4

This bright orange side dish adds color to any poultry, meat, or fish entrée. Serve it with a green vegetable, such as Pan-Roasted Broccoli (page 376) for a complementary contrast.

Cooking spray
2 tablespoons chopped pecans, dry-roasted
2 tablespoons fresh lemon juice
1 tablespoon light brown sugar
1 tablespoon honey
1 teaspoon olive oil
1/2 teaspoon vanilla extract
1/4 teaspoon pumpkin pie spice
1 pound sweet potatoes (about 1 large),
    peeled and cut into 1-inch cubes

Preheat the oven to 375°F. Lightly spray a shallow 1 1/2-quart baking dish with cooking spray.

In a medium bowl, whisk together all the ingredients except the sweet potato. Add the sweet potato, stirring to coat. Arrange the cubes in a single layer in the baking dish.

Bake, covered, for 40 minutes, stirring once halfway through. Stir again. Bake, uncovered, for 15 minutes, or until the sweet potato cubes are tender and the glaze has thickened.

PER SERVING

calories 136	**sodium** 64 mg
total fat 2.5 g	**carbohydrates** 28 g
saturated fat 0.0 g	fiber 4 g
trans fat 0.0 g	sugars 9 g
polyunsaturated fat 0.5 g	**protein** 2 g
monounsaturated fat 1.5 g	**DIETARY EXCHANGES**
cholesterol 0 mg	2 starch

ORANGE SWEET POTATOES

SERVES 6

No matter the season, a sweet potato casserole is a colorful dish to accompany a wide variety of entrées. Enjoy with Rosemary Chicken (page 192) or Swiss Steak (page 252).

4 medium sweet potatoes, unpeeled, or
    2 16-ounce cans sweet potatoes, packed
    without liquid or in water
Cooking spray
1/4 to 1/2 teaspoon grated orange zest
1/2 cup fresh orange juice
2 tablespoons light brown sugar
1/4 teaspoon ground cinnamon
2 dashes of bitters (optional)
1/4 cup chopped almonds

If using fresh sweet potatoes, fill a stockpot with enough water to just cover them. Bring to a boil over high heat. Boil for 30 minutes, or until tender. Discard the skins. If using canned sweet potatoes in water, drain well.

Preheat the oven to 350°F. Lightly spray a 1-quart casserole dish with cooking spray.

In a large mixing bowl, mash the sweet potatoes.

Add the remaining ingredients except the pecans. Using an electric mixer on medium speed, beat the sweet potato mixture until fluffy. Spread the mixture in the casserole dish. Sprinkle the almonds over the casserole.

Bake, covered, for 25 minutes, or until heated through.

PER SERVING

calories 156	**sodium** 64 mg
total fat 3.5 g	**carbohydrates** 30 g
saturated fat 0.5 g	fiber 4 g
trans fat 0.0 g	sugars 11 g
polyunsaturated fat 1.0 g	**protein** 2 g
monounsaturated fat 2.0 g	**DIETARY EXCHANGES**
cholesterol 0 mg	2 starch, 1/2 fat

GOLDEN LEMON-CRUMB TOMATOES

SERVES 4

Classic crumb-topped tomatoes get a makeover in this recipe. Fresh, tart lemon and Italian herbs add a sunny flavor to the luscious tomatoes, while panko adds more crunch than regular bread crumbs.

1/2 cup whole-wheat panko (Japanese-style
   bread crumbs)
2 tablespoons finely chopped fresh basil
1/2 teaspoon grated lemon zest
1 1/2 tablespoons fresh lemon juice
1/2 teaspoon dried oregano, crumbled
1 ounce goat cheese crumbles
Cooking spray
2 large tomatoes (about 8 ounces each),
   halved crosswise
1/8 teaspoon salt

Preheat the oven to 350°F.

In a small bowl, stir together the panko, basil,
lemon zest, and oregano.

Add the goat cheese, tossing gently to combine.

Lightly spray a 9-inch pie pan with cooking
spray. Place the tomato halves in the pan with
the cut sides up. Spoon the lemon juice over the
tomatoes. Sprinkle the panko mixture over the
tomatoes. Liberally spray with cooking spray.

Bake for 30 minutes, or until the tomatoes are
tender when pierced with a fork and beginning
to lightly brown.

Sprinkle with the salt. Let stand for 10 minutes
before serving.

PER SERVING

calories 86	sodium 113 mg
total fat 3.0 g	carbohydrates 11 g
saturated fat 2.0 g	fiber 2 g
trans fat 0.0 g	sugars 3 g
polyunsaturated fat 0.0 g	protein 5 g
monounsaturated fat 0.5 g	DIETARY EXCHANGES
cholesterol 7 mg	1/2 starch, 1 vegetable, 1/2 fat

"FRIED" GREEN TOMATOES

SERVES 8; 4 TOMATO SLICES PER SERVING

*This lighter version of a southern classic provides
the crunch of a cornmeal-and-flour coating, but
with fewer calories and less saturated fat and
sodium than traditional recipes.*

Cooking spray
1/3 cup white whole-wheat flour
1/2 teaspoon garlic powder
1/2 teaspoon onion powder
1/4 teaspoon salt
1/4 teaspoon pepper (freshly ground
   preferred)
1/8 teaspoon cayenne
1 large egg
2 large egg whites
1/3 cup cornmeal (yellow preferred)
1 pound green tomatoes, cored and cut into
   1/2-inch slices
1 teaspoon olive oil and 1 teaspoon olive oil,
   divided use

Preheat the oven to 400°F. Lightly spray a large
baking sheet with cooking spray.

In a medium shallow dish, stir together the
flour, garlic powder, onion powder, salt, pepper, and cayenne. In a medium shallow bowl,
whisk together the egg and egg whites. Put
the cornmeal in a separate shallow dish. Put
the dish, bowl, dish, and a large plate in a row,
assembly-line fashion. Dip the tomatoes in the
flour mixture, then in the egg mixture, and finally in the cornmeal, turning to coat at each step
and gently shaking off any excess. Place the tomatoes on the plate. Lightly spray the tops with
cooking spray.

In a large nonstick skillet, heat 1 teaspoon oil over
medium-high heat, swirling to coat the bottom.
Cook half the tomatoes with the sprayed side
down for 2 minutes, or until the bottoms are
light golden brown. Remove from the heat.

Lightly spray the tops of the tomatoes with
cooking spray. Turn over the tomatoes. Cook for
2 minutes, or until light golden brown.

Transfer the cooked tomatoes to the baking
sheet. Repeat with the remaining tomatoes and
1 teaspoon oil.

Bake for 5 minutes, or until the tomatoes are
deep golden brown.

(continued)

Cook's Tip on Coring Tomatoes: Use a paring knife to remove the tough core of a tomato. Holding the tomato in one hand, carefully cut around the core using the tip of the knife. There are also tools specially designed to make coring tomatoes easier, including the tomato shark, which resembles a melon baller, but has sharp "teeth" to dig out the core with one circular motion.

PER SERVING

calories 76	**carbohydrates** 12 g
total fat 2.0 g	fiber 2 g
saturated fat 0.5 g	sugars 2 g
trans fat 0.0 g	**protein** 4 g
polyunsaturated fat 0.5 g	**DIETARY EXCHANGES**
monounsaturated fat 1.0 g	1/2 starch, 1 vegetable,
cholesterol 23 mg	1/2 fat
sodium 103 mg	

ZUCCHINI STUFFED WITH ROASTED RED PEPPERS

SERVES 4

These baked squash shells cradle a fluffy herbed mixture of egg and vegetables. Serve with Mediterranean Fish *(page 134), which bakes at the same temperature.*

 Cooking spray
 4 medium zucchini
 2 teaspoons canola or corn oil
 1 medium garlic clove, minced
 1 medium onion, diced
 1 cup chopped roasted red bell pepper
 1/2 teaspoon dried oregano, crumbled
 1/2 teaspoon dried thyme, crumbled
 Pepper to taste (freshly ground preferred)
 1 large egg, lightly beaten using a fork, or
  2 large egg whites

Preheat the oven to 350°F. Lightly spray a shallow baking pan with cooking spray.

In a large saucepan, parboil the zucchini for 10 minutes. Drain well in a colander. Let stand to cool. Halve the zucchini lengthwise. Using a small spoon or melon baller, scoop out the pulp, leaving the shells intact. Transfer the pulp to a cutting board. Finely chop the pulp. Transfer the shells to the baking pan.

In a medium skillet, heat the oil over medium-high heat, swirling to coat the bottom. Cook the garlic for 2 minutes, or until golden brown, stirring constantly. Watch carefully so it doesn't burn.

Stir in the onion. Cook for 3 minutes, or until soft, stirring frequently.

Stir in the bell pepper, oregano, thyme, pepper, and zucchini pulp. Remove from the heat. Let stand to cool.

Stir in the egg.

Fill the cavity of each zucchini shell with the onion mixture.

Bake for 30 minutes, or until the filling is hot and bubbly.

PER SERVING

calories 89	**sodium** 65 mg
total fat 4.0 g	**carbohydrates** 11 g
saturated fat 0.5 g	fiber 3 g
trans fat 0.0 g	sugars 7 g
polyunsaturated fat 1.0 g	**protein** 4 g
monounsaturated fat 2.0 g	**DIETARY EXCHANGES**
cholesterol 47 mg	2 vegetable, 1 fat

ZUCCHINI-QUINOA PANCAKES

SERVES 4

While similar to traditional latkes or potato pancakes, this version uses a whole grain and vegetables. Serve with Lemon-Chive Sauce *(page 436) or* Sour Cream Sauce with Dill *(page 431).*

 1/4 cup uncooked quinoa, rinsed and drained
 2 small zucchini (about 8 ounces), shredded
  (about 2 cups), patted dry with paper
  towels
 1 large egg, lightly beaten using a fork
 2 tablespoons shredded or grated Parmesan
  cheese
 2 teaspoons chopped fresh dillweed
 1 medium garlic clove, minced
 1/4 teaspoon pepper
 1/2 teaspoon olive oil and 1/2 teaspoon olive
  oil, divided use

Prepare the quinoa using the package directions, omitting the salt. Transfer to a medium bowl. Fluff with a fork. Let cool completely.

Add the zucchini to the cooled quinoa. Stir in the egg, Parmesan, dillweed, garlic, and pepper until well combined.

In a large nonstick skillet, heat 1/2 teaspoon oil over medium heat, swirling to coat the bottom. Place four 1/4-cup mounds of the zucchini mixture in the skillet. Using the back of a spoon, gently press down on the mounds, spreading them to make pancakes, 3 inches in diameter. Cook for 3 minutes, or until the bottoms are browned. Turn over the pancakes. Cook for 2 minutes, or until lightly browned. Transfer to a large plate. Repeat with the remaining 1/2 teaspoon oil and zucchini mixture.

Cook's Tip: The pancakes can be made up to 8 hours in advance. To reheat them, bake them on a baking sheet in a preheated 350°F oven for 3 to 5 minutes, or until hot and lightly crisp.

PER SERVING

calories 89	carbohydrates 9 g
total fat 4.0 g	fiber 1 g
saturated fat 1.0 g	sugars 2 g
trans fat 0.0 g	protein 5 g
polyunsaturated fat 1.0 g	DIETARY EXCHANGES
monounsaturated fat 1.5 g	1/2 starch, 1/2 lean
cholesterol 48 mg	meat, 1/2 fat
sodium 66 mg	

GERMAN-STYLE WAX BEANS

SERVES 4

Reminiscent of classic German potato salad with its signature ingredients of bacon, vinegar, and a bit of sugar, the pale yellow wax beans substitute for potatoes in this side dish. Wax beans, mild in flavor, are a type of snap bean. If you prefer, you also can use the more familiar green bean.

2 ounces turkey bacon (lowest sodium available), diced
2 teaspoons canola or corn oil
1/2 cup sliced green onions
1 15.5-ounce can no-salt-added wax beans

1/4 cup white wine vinegar
1 tablespoon sugar
1 tablespoon diced pimiento, drained

In a small skillet, cook the turkey bacon over medium heat for 5 minutes, or until crisp, stirring frequently. Transfer to a plate.

Increase the heat to medium high. In the same skillet, heat the oil, swirling to coat the bottom. Cook the green onions for 3 minutes, or until soft, stirring frequently.

Stir in the remaining ingredients. Heat through.

Just before serving, sprinkle with the turkey bacon.

PER SERVING

calories 87	carbohydrates 10 g
total fat 3.5 g	fiber 3 g
saturated fat 0.5 g	sugars 5 g
trans fat 0.0 g	protein 4 g
polyunsaturated fat 1.0 g	DIETARY EXCHANGES
monounsaturated fat 1.5 g	1 vegetable, 1 other
cholesterol 10 mg	carbohydrate, 1 fat
sodium 139 mg	

BAKED VEGETABLE CASSEROLE ITALIANO

SERVES 6

Pair this casserole, which offers a variety of popular Italian vegetables, with an Italian-style entrée, such as Chicken Cacciatore (page 189).

Cooking spray
1 large eggplant, peeled and diced
1 15-ounce can crushed no-salt-added Italian plum (Roma) tomatoes, undrained
9 ounces frozen Italian green beans, thawed
1 medium zucchini, sliced into rounds
2 teaspoons dried oregano, crumbled
1 medium garlic clove, minced
Pepper to taste (freshly ground preferred)
1/4 cup shredded or grated Romano cheese

(continued)

Preheat the oven to 375°F. Lightly spray a 2-quart casserole dish with cooking spray.

In the dish, stir together the eggplant, tomatoes with liquid, green beans, and zucchini.

Stir in the oregano, garlic, and pepper. Sprinkle the Romano over the casserole.

Bake for 30 to 40 minutes, or until the casserole is bubbly and the cheese is golden brown.

PER SERVING

calories 64	**sodium** 88 mg
total fat 1.0 g	**carbohydrates** 12 g
saturated fat 0.5 g	fiber 5 g
trans fat 0.0 g	sugars 6 g
polyunsaturated fat 0.0 g	**protein** 3 g
monounsaturated fat 0.0 g	**DIETARY EXCHANGES**
cholesterol 2 mg	2 vegetable

VEGETABLE MEDLEY WITH LEMON SAUCE

SERVES 8

A peppery citrus sauce brightens this veggie trio. Serve with Crispy Baked Chicken *(page 185) or* Almond-Topped Baked Trout *(page 161).*

> 1 pound broccoli, florets separated, stems cut into 1 1/2-inch pieces
> 1 small head cauliflower, florets separated, stems cut into 1 1/2-inch pieces
> 9 ounces frozen artichoke hearts

Sauce
> 2 tablespoons light tub margarine
> 2 tablespoons finely chopped onion
> 3 tablespoons fresh lemon juice (about 1 medium lemon)
> 1/4 teaspoon paprika

■ ■ ■

> 1 pimiento, drained and diced

Keeping the vegetables in piles, steam each one separately in a large saucepan, covered, for 6 to 8 minutes, or until tender-crisp. Drain well.

To make the sauce, in a small skillet, melt the margarine over medium-high heat, swirling to coat the bottom. Cook the onion for 3 minutes, or until soft, stirring frequently. Remove from the heat.

Stir in the lemon juice and paprika.

Arrange the vegetables in groups on a serving platter. Drizzle the sauce over all. Sprinkle the pimiento over the artichoke hearts.

PER SERVING

calories 53	**sodium** 66 mg
total fat 1.5 g	**carbohydrates** 9 g
saturated fat 0.0 g	fiber 5 g
trans fat 0.0 g	sugars 1 g
polyunsaturated fat 0.5 g	**protein** 3 g
monounsaturated fat 0.5 g	**DIETARY EXCHANGES**
cholesterol 0 mg	2 vegetable, 1/2 fat

CANTONESE VEGETABLES

SERVES 8

Ginger, green onions, and garlic—the "holy trinity" of Cantonese cooking— along with chili peppers, soy sauce, and black pepper, are often used in Asian cuisine. You'll find all these ingredients flavoring this dish. Serve the vegetables on a bed of steamed brown rice. For a complementary entrée, try Fish Fillets with Kale and Garlic *(page 137).*

> 1 1/2 teaspoons finely minced peeled gingerroot
> 2 medium garlic cloves, minced
> 1/2 teaspoon curry powder
> 1/4 teaspoon salt
> 1/2 cup fat-free, low-sodium vegetable broth, such as on page 36
> 2 tablespoons sherry
> 1 tablespoon soy sauce (lowest sodium available)
> 2 teaspoons cornstarch
> 1/4 teaspoon hot chili oil and 2 teaspoons hot chili oil, divided use
> 1 1/2 cups sliced onions
> 4 medium ribs of celery, diagonally sliced

1 medium green bell pepper, cut into thin
strips
2 cups small broccoli florets
3 cups canned no-salt-added black beans,
rinsed and drained
1/2 cup chopped green onions
2 cups cherry tomatoes, quartered
1/4 cup minced fresh parsley
Pepper to taste (freshly ground preferred)

In a small bowl, stir together the gingerroot, garlic, garlic, curry powder, and salt. Set aside.

In a separate small bowl, whisk together the broth, sherry, soy sauce, cornstarch, and 1/4 teaspoon hot chili oil until the cornstarch is dissolved. Set aside.

In a wok or large skillet, heat the remaining 2 teaspoons hot chili oil over high heat, swirling to coat the bottom. Cook the gingerroot mixture for 30 seconds, or until fragrant, stirring constantly.

Stir in the onions and celery. Cook for 1 to 2 minutes, or until tender-crisp, stirring constantly. Stir in the broth mixture. Cook for 30 seconds to 1 minute, or until clear, stirring constantly.

Stir in the bell pepper, broccoli, black beans, and green onions. Cook for 1 to 2 minutes, or until the vegetables are tender-crisp, stirring constantly. Gently stir in the tomatoes. Cook for 30 seconds to 1 minute, or until heated through. Remove from the heat.

Gently stir in the parsley and pepper.

PER SERVING

calories 141	carbohydrates 25 g
total fat 1.5 g	fiber 7 g
saturated fat 0.0 g	sugars 8 g
trans fat 0.0 g	protein 7 g
polyunsaturated fat 0.5 g	DIETARY EXCHANGES
monounsaturated fat 1.0 g	1 starch, 2 vegetable,
cholesterol 0 mg	1/2 lean meat
sodium 183 mg	

ITALIAN VEGETABLE BAKE

SERVES 4

Three fresh herbs often used in Italian dishes along with garlic and balsamic vinegar accentuate the natural flavor of the fresh veggies in this side dish casserole.

Olive oil cooking spray
8 to 10 ounces mushrooms, any variety or
combination, sliced
1 small zucchini, thinly sliced
4 medium Italian plum (Roma) tomatoes,
sliced
2 small green onions, thinly sliced
1 1/2 tablespoons balsamic vinegar
1 1/2 tablespoons olive oil (extra-virgin
preferred)
2 teaspoons chopped fresh basil or
1/2 teaspoon dried basil, crumbled
2 teaspoons chopped fresh oregano or
1/2 teaspoon dried oregano, crumbled
2 teaspoons chopped fresh rosemary or
1/2 teaspoon dried rosemary, crushed
1/2 medium garlic clove, minced
Pepper to taste

Preheat the oven to 350°F. Lightly spray an 8-inch square glass baking dish with cooking spray.

Make one layer each of the mushrooms, zucchini, tomatoes, and green onions in the baking dish.

In a small bowl, stir together the remaining ingredients. Drizzle over the vegetables.

Bake, covered, for 25 minutes, or until the vegetables are tender. Using a slotted spoon, remove the vegetables from the liquid.

PER SERVING

calories 87	sodium 13 mg
total fat 5.5 g	carbohydrates 8 g
saturated fat 1.0 g	fiber 2 g
trans fat 0.0 g	sugars 5 g
polyunsaturated fat 0.5 g	protein 3 g
monounsaturated fat 3.5 g	DIETARY EXCHANGES
cholesterol 0 mg	2 vegetable, 1 fat

VEGETABLE STIR-FRY

SERVES 4

This quick side dish features the unusual seasoning combination of a sweet spice and a light, lemony herb. Try it with an equally fast entrée, such as Fish in Crazy Water *(page 134).*

> 8 ounces broccoli, florets cut to a uniform
>   size, stems trimmed, peeled, and cut
>   into 2-inch pieces
> 1 teaspoon light tub margarine
> 1 teaspoon canola or corn oil
> 8 ounces carrots, thinly sliced
> 6 ounces button mushrooms, thinly sliced
> 1 to 2 medium green onions, thinly sliced
> 1 tablespoon dry sherry
> 1 1/2 teaspoons fresh lemon juice
> 1/2 teaspoon ground nutmeg
> 1/2 teaspoon dried thyme, crumbled
> Pepper to taste

In a work or large skillet, heat the margarine and oil over medium heat, swirling to coat the bottom. Cook the broccoli, carrots, mushrooms, and green onions for 5 minutes, or until tender-crisp, stirring constantly.

Stir in the remaining ingredients.

PER SERVING

calories 74	sodium 70 mg
total fat 2.0 g	carbohydrates 12 g
saturated fat 0.0 g	fiber 4 g
trans fat 0.0 g	sugars 5 g
polyunsaturated fat 0.5 g	protein 4 g
monounsaturated fat 1.0 g	DIETARY EXCHANGES
cholesterol 0 mg	2 vegetable, 1/2 fat

RATATOUILLE

SERVES 8

When your garden's bounty comes in or it's time for a trip to the farmers' market, you'll want this recipe handy. With eggplant, tomatoes, zucchini, and bell pepper, you have the foundation for a vegetable-rich side dish. With a few changes in spices and herbs, you can use this same recipe and bring a southwestern twist to your table.

> 1 tablespoon olive oil
> 1 medium onion, finely chopped
> 1 red or green bell pepper, cut into thin strips
> 2 tablespoons minced garlic
> 4 large tomatoes, peeled, seeded, and
>   chopped
> 1 to 2 tablespoons fennel seeds (optional)
> 2 teaspoons dried oregano, crumbled
> 1/2 teaspoon dried dillweed, crumbled
> Pepper to taste (freshly ground preferred)
> 1 medium eggplant (about 1 pound), peeled
>   and diced
> 2 medium zucchini, sliced
> 1/4 cup fresh lemon juice (about 1 large
>   lemon)
> 2 tablespoons chopped fresh basil

In a large skillet, heat the oil over medium-high heat, swirling to coat the bottom. Cook the onion, bell pepper, and garlic for 3 to 4 minutes, or until the bell pepper is tender-crisp, stirring frequently. Stir in the tomatoes, fennel seeds, oregano, dillweed, and pepper. Reduce the heat and simmer for 4 to 5 minutes. Stir in the eggplant and zucchini. Simmer, covered, for 15 minutes, or until the eggplant and zucchini are tender but not mushy.

Stir in the lemon juice and basil. Serve immediately, or cover and refrigerate to serve cold.

PER SERVING

calories 70	sodium 13 mg
total fat 2.0 g	carbohydrates 13 g
saturated fat 0.5 g	fiber 4 g
trans fat 0.0 g	sugars 7 g
polyunsaturated fat 0.5 g	protein 3 g
monounsaturated fat 1.5 g	DIETARY EXCHANGES
cholesterol 0 mg	3 vegetable, 1/2 fat

SOUTHWESTERN RATATOUILLE

> 1 tablespoon olive oil
> 1 medium onion, finely chopped
> 1 red or green bell pepper, cut into thin strips
> 2 tablespoons minced garlic
> 4 large tomatoes, peeled, seeded, and
>   chopped

2 teaspoons dried oregano, crumbled

2 teaspoons chili powder

2 teaspoons ground cumin

1/4 teaspoon crushed red pepper flakes

3 sprigs of fresh thyme, leaves removed and crushed, or 1/2 teaspoon dried thyme, crumbled

1 medium eggplant (about 1 pound), peeled and diced

2 medium zucchini, sliced

2 tablespoons minced fresh parsley

1 1/2 tablespoons freshly grated Parmesan cheese

In a large skillet, heat the oil over medium-high heat, swirling to coat the bottom. Cook the onion, bell pepper, and garlic for 3 to 4 minutes, or until the bell pepper is tender-crisp, stirring frequently. Stir in the tomatoes, oregano, chili powder, cumin, red pepper flakes, and thyme. Reduce the heat and simmer for 4 to 5 minutes. Stir in the eggplant and zucchini. Simmer, covered, for 15 minutes, or until the eggplant and zucchini are tender but not mushy.

Stir in the parsley and Parmesan. Serve immediately, or cover and refrigerate to serve cold.

PER SERVING

calories 65	sodium 112 mg
total fat 1.5 g	carbohydrates 12 g
saturated fat 0.5 g	fiber 4 g
trans fat 0.0 g	sugars 7 g
polyunsaturated fat 0.5 g	protein 3 g
monounsaturated fat 0.5 g	DIETARY EXCHANGES
cholesterol 1 mg	2 vegetable, 1/2 fat

BARLEY, SQUASH, AND BELL PEPPER MEDLEY

SERVES 4

When you combine whole grains and colorful veggies, as in this dish, you can dress up even the simplest entrée.

1/2 cup uncooked quick-cooking barley

1 teaspoon olive oil and 2 teaspoons olive oil (extra-virgin preferred), divided use

1 medium yellow summer squash or zucchini, chopped

1/2 medium green or red bell pepper, thinly sliced lengthwise, then sliced crosswise into 2-inch pieces

1/2 teaspoon dried thyme, crumbled

1/8 teaspoon crushed red pepper flakes

1/8 teaspoon pepper (coarsely ground preferred)

2 tablespoons chopped fresh parsley or basil

1/4 teaspoon salt

Prepare the barley using the package directions, omitting the salt. Drain well in a colander.

Meanwhile, in a large nonstick skillet, heat 1 teaspoon oil over medium heat, swirling to coat the bottom. Add the squash, bell pepper, thyme, red pepper flakes, and pepper, stirring to combine. Cook for 5 minutes, or until the squash begins to brown on the edges, stirring frequently. Remove from the heat.

Stir the barley, parsley, salt, and the remaining 2 teaspoons oil into the squash mixture.

PER SERVING

calories 130	sodium 150 mg
total fat 4.0 g	carbohydrates 22 g
saturated fat 0.5 g	fiber 5 g
trans fat 0.0 g	sugars 2 g
polyunsaturated fat 0.5 g	protein 3 g
monounsaturated fat 2.5 g	DIETARY EXCHANGES
cholesterol 0 mg	1 1/2 starch, 1/2 fat

BRAISED BARLEY AND CORN WITH TOMATOES

SERVES 4

Chase the winter blues away with this side dish of plump kernels of corn and barley stewed with tomatoes. Because it uses ingredients found in most pantries and freezers, it's a good choice when you don't have time to go to the grocery store.

(continued)

1 teaspoon olive oil

1/4 medium onion, chopped

1 cup fat-free, low-sodium chicken broth, such as on page 36

1/2 14.5-ounce can no-salt-added diced tomatoes, undrained

1/2 teaspoon salt-free all-purpose seasoning blend

1/8 teaspoon pepper

1/8 teaspoon crushed red pepper flakes (optional)

1/4 cup uncooked pearl barley

1 cup frozen whole-kernel corn

In a medium saucepan, heat the oil over medium-high heat, swirling to coat the bottom. Cook the onion for about 3 minutes, or until soft, stirring frequently.

Stir in the broth, tomatoes with liquid, seasoning blend, pepper, and red pepper flakes. Bring to a simmer, stirring occasionally.

Stir in the barley. Reduce the heat and simmer, covered, for 30 minutes.

Stir in the corn. Simmer, covered, for 15 to 20 minutes, or until the barley is tender and the corn is heated through.

PER SERVING

calories 112	**sodium** 16 mg
total fat 1.5 g	**carbohydrates** 23 g
saturated fat 0.0 g	fiber 4 g
trans fat 0.0 g	sugars 4 g
polyunsaturated fat 0.5 g	**protein** 4 g
monounsaturated fat 1.0 g	**DIETARY EXCHANGES**
cholesterol 0 mg	1 1/2 starch

APRICOT BULGUR WITH PINE NUTS

SERVES 4

The combination of a small amount of dry-roasted pine nuts and richly browned onion gives this dish an intensely nutty flavor. Try it with Saffron-Scented Grilled Chicken *(page 201) or* Chicken with Peach Glaze *(page 190).*

1/2 cup uncooked instant, or fine-grain, bulgur

1 teaspoon canola or corn oil

1/2 medium onion, diced

5 or 6 dried apricot halves, thinly sliced

1/4 cup pine nuts, dry-roasted

1/4 teaspoon salt

Prepare the bulgur using the package directions, omitting the salt.

Meanwhile, in a large nonstick skillet, heat the oil over medium heat, swirling to coat the bottom. Cook the onion for 6 minutes, or until very richly browned (this is important), stirring frequently. Remove from the heat.

Stir the bulgur, apricots, pine nuts, and salt together with the onion. Cook, still over medium heat, for 1 to 2 minutes, or until heated through, stirring occasionally.

PER SERVING

calories 126	**carbohydrates** 19 g
total fat 5.0 g	fiber 4 g
saturated fat 0.5 g	sugars 5 g
trans fat 0.0 g	**protein** 4 g
polyunsaturated fat 2.0 g	**DIETARY EXCHANGES**
monounsaturated fat 2.0 g	1 starch, 1/2 other
cholesterol 0 mg	carbohydrate, 1 fat
sodium 150 mg	

BULGUR PILAF WITH LEMON AND SPINACH

SERVES 4

The nutty flavor of bulgur pairs well with Mediterranean entrées, such as Yemeni Lemon Chicken *(page 181) or* Mediterranean Beef and Vegetable Stir-Fry *(page 266).*

1 teaspoon canola or corn oil

1/2 cup chopped onion

1 small garlic clove, minced

1/2 teaspoon ground cumin

1/8 teaspoon ground cinnamon

1 1/2 cups water

1 cup uncooked medium-grain bulgur

1 cup chopped baby spinach

2 tablespoons chopped fresh mint

1 tablespoon fresh lemon juice

3 tablespoons pomegranate arils (seeds)

1 tablespoon slivered almonds, dry-roasted

In a medium saucepan, heat the oil over medium heat, swirling to coat the bottom. Cook the onion for 3 to 4 minutes, or until lightly browned, stirring frequently. Stir in the garlic. Cook for 30 seconds, stirring constantly. Stir in the cumin and cinnamon. Pour in the water and bulgur. Increase the heat to medium high. Bring the mixture to a boil. Reduce the heat and simmer for 12 minutes, or until the lentils are tender and the water is absorbed.

Gently stir in the spinach, mint, and lemon juice.

Just before serving, garnish with the pomegranate arils and almonds.

PER SERVING

calories 161	**sodium** 18 mg
total fat 2.5 g	**carbohydrates** 32 g
saturated fat 0.5 g	fiber 8 g
trans fat 0.0 g	sugars 2 g
polyunsaturated fat 0.5 g	**protein** 5 g
monounsaturated fat 1.5 g	**DIETARY EXCHANGES**
cholesterol 0 mg	2 starch

COUSCOUS WITH DATES AND WALNUTS

SERVES 4

This Middle Eastern side dish goes nicely with beef or chicken skewers, such as Steak and Vegetable Kebabs (page 267) or Chicken Gyros with Tzatziki Sauce (page 223).

1 cup fat-free, low-sodium chicken broth, such as on page 36

1/4 cup chopped dried dates

1/4 teaspoon ground cumin

1/8 teaspoon ground cinnamon

3/4 cup uncooked whole-wheat couscous

2 tablespoons chopped Italian (flat-leaf) parsley

2 tablespoons chopped walnuts, dry-roasted

In a medium saucepan, stir together the broth, dates, cumin, and cinnamon. Bring to a boil over medium-high heat.

Stir in the couscous. Remove from the heat. Let stand, covered, for 5 minutes. Fluff with a fork.

Gently stir in the parsley and walnuts.

Cook's Tip on Couscous: If your supermarket doesn't have whole-wheat couscous, look in the ethnic food sections or bulk food bins of natural food supermarkets. Almost all couscous takes only about 5 minutes to prepare; avoid any brand that calls for long steaming.

PER SERVING

calories 215	**carbohydrates** 43 g
total fat 3.0 g	fiber 6 g
saturated fat 0.5 g	sugars 7 g
trans fat 0.0 g	**protein** 7 g
polyunsaturated fat 2.0 g	**DIETARY EXCHANGES**
monounsaturated fat 0.5 g	2 1/2 starch, 1/2 fruit,
cholesterol 0 mg	1/2 fat
sodium 8 mg	

COUSCOUS WITH VEGETABLES

SERVES 4

The tender peas, velvety mushrooms, and fresh parsley combine with a whole grain to create a quick any-night-of-the-week side dish.

1/2 cup uncooked whole-wheat couscous

1 cup frozen green peas or any other quick-cooking vegetable, thawed and drained

1/2 cup minced onion

2 medium button mushrooms, thinly sliced

2 tablespoons dry white wine (regular or nonalcoholic)

1/2 teaspoon crushed garlic or 1/4 teaspoon garlic powder

2 tablespoons finely chopped fresh parsley

1/2 teaspoon dried basil, crumbled

1/8 teaspoon pepper

Prepare the couscous using the package directions, omitting the salt. Remove from the heat. Fluff with a fork.

(continued)

Meanwhile, in a medium nonstick saucepan, cook the green peas, onion, mushrooms, wine, and garlic over medium-high heat for 3 to 5 minutes, stirring frequently.

Stir in the parsley, basil, and pepper. Transfer to a medium bowl.

Stir in the couscous.

PER SERVING

calories 148	sodium 39 mg
total fat 0.5 g	carbohydrates 30 g
saturated fat 0.0 g	fiber 6 g
trans fat 0.0 g	sugars 3 g
polyunsaturated fat 0.5 g	protein 6 g
monounsaturated fat 0.0 g	DIETARY EXCHANGES
cholesterol 0 mg	2 starch

GRITS CASSEROLE WITH CHEESE AND CHILES

SERVES 8

Grits are a southern favorite. Here they're pumped up with two cheeses and green chiles. Partner the casserole with Salmon Cakes with Creole Aïoli *(page 151), which bakes at the same temperature.*

Cooking spray
2 cups fat-free, low-sodium chicken broth, such as on page 36
2 cups water
1 cup uncooked instant grits
1/2 cup fat-free milk
1/4 cup shredded or grated Parmesan cheese
2 3/4-ounce slices fat-free Swiss cheese, diced
2 ounces canned chopped green chiles, drained
1 tablespoon light tub margarine
2 medium garlic cloves, minced
1/4 teaspoon salt
1/8 teaspoon pepper
1/2 cup egg substitute
1/2 teaspoon chili powder

Preheat the oven to 375°F. Lightly spray a 13 x 9 x 2-inch baking pan with cooking spray. Set aside.

In a large saucepan, bring the broth and water to a boil over medium-high heat. Gradually whisk in the grits. Reduce the heat to low. Cook, covered, for 5 minutes, whisking occasionally. Remove from the heat.

Stir the milk, both cheeses, green chiles, margarine, garlic, salt, and pepper into the grits.

Stir in the egg substitute. Pour into the baking pan, smoothing the top.

Sprinkle the chili powder over the casserole.

Bake for 45 minutes. Remove from the oven. Let cool for 5 to 10 minutes.

PER SERVING

calories 113	sodium 242 mg
total fat 1.5 g	carbohydrates 18 g
saturated fat 0.5 g	fiber 1 g
trans fat 0.0 g	sugars 1 g
polyunsaturated fat 0.5 g	protein 7 g
monounsaturated fat 0.5 g	DIETARY EXCHANGES
cholesterol 3 mg	1 starch, 1/2 lean meat

ASIAN LINGUINE

SERVES 4

Serve this sassy side dish to dress up the simplest cuts of meats or poultry. Try it as a bed for Asian Beef Stir-Fry *(page 264) or* Sweet-and-Sour Pork *(page 292).*

1 3/4 cups fat-free, low-sodium chicken broth, such as on page 36
2 ounces dried whole-grain linguine, broken in half
1 large onion, thinly sliced
2 medium carrots, cut into matchstick-size strips
2 tablespoons soy sauce (lowest sodium available)
2 tablespoons cider vinegar
1 1/2 tablespoons sugar
1/8 teaspoon garlic powder
3 tablespoons slivered almonds, dry-roasted

In a medium saucepan, bring the broth to a boil over high heat. Stir in the pasta. Return to a boil. Reduce the heat to medium. Cook for 5 minutes, or until the pasta is tender. Don't drain.

Meanwhile, in a large nonstick skillet, cook the onion and carrots over medium-high heat for 6 minutes, or until the carrots are tender-crisp, stirring frequently.

In a small bowl, stir together the remaining ingredients except the almonds.

Add the pasta and any remaining liquid to the onion mixture. Pour in the soy sauce mixture. Toss gently to blend. Serve sprinkled with the almonds.

PER SERVING

calories 144	carbohydrates 26 g
total fat 3.0 g	fiber 4 g
saturated fat 0.0 g	sugars 11 g
trans fat 0.0 g	**protein** 5 g
polyunsaturated fat 1.0 g	**DIETARY EXCHANGES**
monounsaturated fat 1.5 g	1 starch, 2 vegetable,
cholesterol 0 mg	1/2 fat
sodium 233 mg	

SPINACH AND FARRO CASSEROLE

SERVES 8

Hearty and filling, you'll probably want to serve this casserole with a light entrée, such as Fillets in Lemon Dressing *(page 127), which bakes at the same temperature, or* Grilled Lemon-Sage Chicken *(page 202).*

1/2 cup uncooked farro, rinsed and drained
Cooking spray
1 cup fat-free ricotta cheese
2 tablespoons egg substitute
1 1/2 teaspoons all-purpose flour
1 1/2 teaspoons shredded or grated Parmesan cheese and 1 1/2 tablespoons shredded or grated Parmesan cheese, divided use
1/4 teaspoon dried thyme, crumbled
Pepper to taste
1 teaspoon light tub margarine

1 medium onion, chopped
1 or 2 medium garlic cloves, minced
5 ounces baby spinach, torn into bite-size pieces, or 5 ounces frozen chopped spinach, thawed and squeezed dry
4 ounces brown (cremini) mushrooms, sliced
1 tablespoon hulled unsalted sunflower seeds

Prepare the farro using the package directions, omitting the salt. Drain well in a colander.

Preheat the oven to 375°F. Lightly spray an 8-inch-square baking dish with cooking spray.

In a medium bowl, stir together the farro, ricotta cheese, egg substitute, flour, 1 1/2 teaspoons Parmesan, the thyme, and pepper.

In a large saucepan, melt the margarine over medium-high heat, swirling to coat the bottom. Cook the onion and garlic for about 3 minutes, or until the onion is soft, stirring frequently.

Reduce the heat to low. Stir in the spinach and mushrooms. Cook, covered, for 3 minutes.

Stir in the farro mixture. Spoon into the baking dish. Sprinkle the remaining 1 1/2 tablespoons Parmesan and the sunflower seeds over the farro mixture.

Bake for 25 to 30 minutes.

PER SERVING

calories 94	sodium 110 mg
total fat 1.0 g	**carbohydrates** 13 g
saturated fat 0.0 g	fiber 2 g
trans fat 0.0 g	sugars 3 g
polyunsaturated fat 0.5 g	**protein** 8 g
monounsaturated fat 0.5 g	**DIETARY EXCHANGES**
cholesterol 3 mg	1 starch, 1/2 lean meat

TOASTED FARRO WITH CARAMELIZED CARROTS AND SWEET POTATOES

SERVES 6

Farro, an ancient whole grain, pairs up with root vegetables bathed in a sweet and tart cooking liquid. Serve with Falafel with Quick-Pickled Garlic Cucumbers *(page 337) or* Slow-Cooker Brisket Stew *(page 114).*

1/2 cup uncooked pearled or semi-pearled farro
2 teaspoons grated orange zest
1/2 cup fresh orange juice
1/4 cup warm water
1 tablespoon honey
1 teaspoon cider vinegar
1/4 teaspoon nutmeg (freshly grated preferred)
2 teaspoons canola or corn oil
3 medium carrots, peeled, and sliced diagonally into 1/2-inch pieces
1 small sweet potato, peeled and cut into 1/4-inch pieces
1/2 cup finely chopped sweet onion, such as Vidalia, Maui, or Oso Sweet
1 teaspoon salt-free all-purpose seasoning blend
1 teaspoon brown sugar (light or dark)
2 tablespoons minced fresh parsley

Heat a large nonstick skillet over medium-high heat. Cook the farro for 4 to 6 minutes, or until browned, stirring constantly. Watch carefully so it doesn't burn. Transfer the farro to a medium saucepan. Set the skillet aside to cool.

Pour in water to cover the farro in the pan (water should be about 2 inches above the farro). Bring to a boil over medium-high heat. Boil for 15 minutes, or until the farro is tender, stirring frequently. Drain well in a colander. Set aside.

Meanwhile, in a small bowl, whisk together the orange zest, orange juice, water, honey, vinegar, and nutmeg.

Wipe the cooled skillet with paper towels. Heat the oil over medium-high heat, swirling to coat the bottom. Cook the carrots, sweet potatoes, onion, and seasoning blend for 5 to 8 minutes, or until the onion is very soft and the vegetables are browned, stirring frequently.

Pour the orange juice mixture over the vegetables. Bring just to a simmer. Reduce the heat to low. Cook, covered, for 5 to 8 minutes, or until the vegetables are fork-tender, stirring occasionally.

Increase the heat to medium high. Cook, uncovered, for about 2 to 3 minutes, or until the liquid has evaporated, stirring frequently.

Sprinkle the brown sugar over the vegetables. Cook for 3 to 5 minutes, or until the vegetables are glazed and beginning to caramelize, stirring constantly. Stir in the cooked farro. Cook for 1 to 2 minutes, or until heated through. Stir the parsley together with the farro mixture. Serve warm or at room temperature.

PER SERVING

calories 128	**carbohydrates** 25 g
total fat 1.5 g	fiber 3 g
saturated fat 0.0 g	sugars 8 g
trans fat 0.0 g	**protein** 3 g
polyunsaturated fat 0.5 g	**DIETARY EXCHANGES**
monounsaturated fat 1.0 g	1 1/2 starch,
cholesterol 0 mg	1 vegetable
sodium 38 mg	

LEMON-BASIL RICE

SERVES 4

This fragrant dish is mild enough to pair with nearly any entrée, and the ingredients can be found in any well-stocked kitchen.

3/4 cup uncooked instant brown rice
1 1/2 cups fat-free, low-sodium chicken broth, such as on page 36
2 teaspoons finely grated lemon zest
1 tablespoon plus 2 teaspoons fresh lemon juice
2 teaspoons olive oil (extra-virgin preferred)
1/4 teaspoon pepper
1/4 cup chopped fresh basil (about 1/2 ounce)

In a 2-quart saucepan, prepare the rice using the package directions, substituting the broth for water and omitting the salt and margarine. Remove from the heat.

Stir in the lemon zest and lemon juice. Fluff with a fork.

Stir in the oil and pepper. Fluff again. Let cool slightly, about 5 minutes (this will help keep the basil greener when added).

Sprinkle with the basil. Fluff again.

Cook's Tip on Basil: Basil can easily turn brown when washed and chopped. To help keep it green, store it carefully so it doesn't bruise. Fill a bowl with cool water to wash it. Remove the leaves from the stems. Swish the leaves in the water. Gently pat them dry with paper towels (a salad spinner can bruise the delicate leaves). Finally, chop them using a very sharp knife.

PER SERVING

calories 90	sodium 13 mg
total fat 3.0 g	carbohydrates 14 g
saturated fat 0.5 g	fiber 1 g
trans fat 0.0 g	sugars 0 g
polyunsaturated fat 0.5 g	protein 2 g
monounsaturated fat 2.0 g	DIETARY EXCHANGES
cholesterol 0 mg	1 starch, 1/2 fat

CALYPSO RICE

SERVES 4

The origin of calypso music lies deep in Trinidad. This rice hits a perfect note, providing not only color but also a taste of the Caribbean to otherwise basic rice. Serve with Jerk Chicken (page 196).

    3/4 cup fat-free, low-sodium chicken broth,
        such as on page 36
    1/4 cup 100% pineapple juice
    1/2 cup uncooked brown rice
    1/4 cup chopped onion
    1/4 cup chopped red bell pepper
    1/4 cup chopped green bell pepper
    1/4 teaspoon ground turmeric
    1/8 teaspoon salt
    1/8 teaspoon pepper
    2 tablespoons chopped fresh parsley

In a medium saucepan, bring the broth and pineapple juice to a boil over high heat. Stir in the remaining ingredients except the parsley. Reduce the heat and simmer, covered, for 40 to 50 minutes, or until the rice is tender and the liquid is absorbed. Fluff with a fork.

Just before serving, sprinkle with the parsley.

PER SERVING

calories 106	sodium 84 mg
total fat 1.0 g	carbohydrates 22 g
saturated fat 0.0 g	fiber 2 g
trans fat 0.0 g	sugars 3 g
polyunsaturated fat 0.5 g	protein 3 g
monounsaturated fat 0.5 g	DIETARY EXCHANGES
cholesterol 0 mg	1 1/2 starch

MEXICAN FRIED RICE

SERVES 6

Slightly browning the rice before cooking it imparts a mildly toasted flavor. Serve this traditional dish with Refried Beans (page 374) and Chicken Enchiladas (page 230) for a Tex-Mex feast.

    1 teaspoon canola or corn oil
    1 cup uncooked long-grain rice
    2 cups fat-free, low-sodium chicken broth,
        such as on page 36
    2/3 cup canned chopped green chiles, drained
    4 to 5 medium green onions, thinly sliced
    1/2 cup diced tomatoes
    1 medium garlic clove, minced

In a large, heavy nonstick skillet, heat the oil over medium-high heat, swirling to coat the bottom. Cook the rice for 2 to 3 minutes, or until golden brown, stirring constantly.

Stir in the remaining ingredients. Reduce the heat and simmer, covered, for 30 minutes, or until the rice is tender and the liquid is absorbed. Fluff with a fork.

PER SERVING

calories 149	sodium 112 mg
total fat 1.0 g	carbohydrates 30 g
saturated fat 0.0 g	fiber 2 g
trans fat 0.0 g	sugars 1 g
polyunsaturated fat 0.5 g	protein 3 g
monounsaturated fat 0.5 g	DIETARY EXCHANGES
cholesterol 0 mg	2 starch

MIDDLE EASTERN RICE

SERVES 8

Crunchy pine nuts and sweet raisins provide a pleasing contrast of textures in this dish, which is delicately flavored with colorful saffron and citrus. If you prefer, you can substitute ground turmeric for the saffron.

PER SERVING

calories 135	sodium 19 mg
total fat 3.0 g	carbohydrates 25 g
saturated fat 0.5 g	fiber 2 g
trans fat 0.0 g	sugars 5 g
polyunsaturated fat 1.0 g	protein 4 g
monounsaturated fat 1.0 g	DIETARY EXCHANGES
cholesterol 0 mg	1 1/2 starch, 1/2 fat

1 1/2 teaspoons light tub margarine
1/2 medium onion, minced
1 medium rib of celery, minced
1 cup uncooked brown rice
1 1/2 cups water
1 cup fat-free, low-sodium chicken broth, such as on page 36, or fat-free, low-sodium vegetable broth, such as on page 36
1/3 cup golden raisins
1 tablespoon grated orange zest
1/2 teaspoon saffron, crushed
1/4 cup pine nuts, dry-roasted
Sprigs of fresh mint (optional)

In a large saucepan, melt the margarine over medium-high heat, swirling to coat the bottom. Cook the onion and celery for 3 minutes, stirring occasionally.

Stir in the rice. Cook for 2 minutes.

Stir in the water, broth, raisins, orange zest, and saffron. Bring to a boil. Reduce the heat and simmer, covered, for 40 to 45 minutes, or until the liquid is absorbed.

Stir in the pine nuts. Just before serving, garnish with the sprigs of mint.

Cook's Tip on Raisins: Seedless raisins are made from seedless grapes. Golden raisins and dark raisins are made from the same grape but are dried differently. The golden ones are dried by artificial heat, and dark raisins are left in the sun for several weeks to achieve their deep color. This means that golden raisins are moister. Freezing raisins makes them easier to cut. If you're baking with raisins, coat them with some of the flour before adding to the batter. This will keep them from sinking to the bottom.

WILD RICE WITH MUSHROOMS

SERVES 6

The nutty flavor of wild rice pairs nicely with earthy mushrooms. Serve this dish with Turkey Cutlets with Fresh Herbs *(page 236) or* Pepper-Coated Steak *(page 258).*

1 1/4 cups uncooked wild rice (4 ounces)
1/8 teaspoon salt and 1/8 teaspoon salt, divided use
2 tablespoons light tub margarine
8 ounces button mushrooms, quartered
1/4 cup dry white wine (regular or nonalcoholic)
5 to 6 medium green onions, sliced
2 tablespoons white wine Worcestershire sauce (lowest sodium available)
1 tablespoon finely chopped fresh sage

Prepare the rice using the package directions, decreasing the salt to 1/8 teaspoon and omitting the margarine.

In a large nonstick skillet, melt the margarine over medium heat, swirling to coat the bottom. Cook the mushrooms, wine, and the remaining 1/8 teaspoon salt, covered, for 5 minutes. Increase the heat to high. Cook, uncovered, for 2 to 3 minutes, or until the juices evaporate.

Reduce the heat to medium. Stir in the green onions. Cook for 2 minutes, stirring occasionally.

Stir in the rice, Worcestershire sauce, and sage.

calories 105
total fat 2.0 g
  saturated fat 0.0 g
  trans fat 0.0 g
  polyunsaturated fat 0.5 g
  monounsaturated fat 1.0 g
cholesterol 0 mg

sodium 185 mg
carbohydrates 18 g
  fiber 3 g
  sugars 3 g
protein 4 g
DIETARY EXCHANGES
  1 starch

RISOTTO MILANESE

SERVES 8

Unlike most other risotto recipes, this one doesn't require constant stirring—all the creamy goodness without all the work! Try it with Rosemary Chicken *(page 192) or* Scallops in White Wine *(page 173).*

2 tablespoons light tub margarine

1 1/2 cups uncooked Arborio rice

3 medium green onions, finely chopped

1/4 cup dry white wine (regular or nonalcoholic)

4 cups fat-free, low-sodium chicken broth, such as on page 36

2 medium button mushrooms, chopped

1/8 teaspoon saffron or 1/2 teaspoon ground turmeric

2 tablespoons shredded or grated Parmesan cheese

In a large, heavy saucepan, melt the margarine over medium heat, swirling to coat the bottom. Stir in the rice and green onions. Cook for 2 to 3 minutes, or until the rice is milky, stirring constantly.

Stir in the wine. Cook for 2 to 3 minutes, or until the wine is absorbed, stirring constantly.

Stir in the broth, mushrooms, and saffron. Increase the heat to medium high and bring to a boil, stirring occasionally. Reduce the heat to low. Cook, covered, for 20 minutes, or until the liquid is absorbed. Just before serving, sprinkle with the Parmesan.

Cook's Tip on Arborio Rice: While there are several types of rice particularly suited for use in risotto, Arborio is perhaps the most popular due to its high starch content, giving risotto and other dishes a creaminess that no other rice provides.

Cook's Tip on Saffron: Saffron comes from the pistil of a certain crocus. Each flower has three threads called stigmas, and it takes more than 14,000 stigmas to make one ounce of saffron, which accounts for its very high cost. You can buy saffron in powder form or in threads; the threads are fresher and more flavorful. Crush them just before you use them.

calories 158
total fat 2.0 g
  saturated fat 0.0 g
  trans fat 0.0 g
  polyunsaturated fat 0.5 g
  monounsaturated fat 0.5 g
cholesterol 1 mg

sodium 59 mg
carbohydrates 30 g
  fiber 2 g
  sugars 1 g
protein 5 g
DIETARY EXCHANGES
  2 starch

RISOTTO WITH BROCCOLI AND LEEKS

SERVES 8

The key to making risotto delectably creamy is using Arborio rice. This version gets its flavor from thyme, wine, and garlic.

2 medium leeks

3 1/2 cups fat-free, low-sodium chicken broth, such as on page 36

1/2 cup dry white wine (regular or nonalcoholic) or fat-free, low-sodium chicken broth, such as on page 36

2 teaspoons chopped fresh thyme or 1/2 teaspoon dried thyme, crumbled

1/4 teaspoon salt

1/8 teaspoon pepper

1 teaspoon olive oil

3 medium garlic cloves, minced

1 cup uncooked Arborio rice

1 pound fresh or frozen broccoli florets, cut into bite-size pieces, cooked, and drained

1/4 cup shredded or grated Parmesan or Romano cheese

(continued)

Trim and discard the root ends from the leeks. Cut a 2- to 3-inch section of the white part from each leek. Cut the sections in half lengthwise, then cut crosswise into thin slices. Put the leeks in a small colander. Rinse well with cold water. Drain well.

In a large liquid measuring cup or other container with a handle and pouring spout, stir together the broth, wine, thyme, salt, and pepper. Set aside.

In a deep skillet, heat the oil over medium-high heat, swirling to coat the bottom. Cook the leeks and garlic for 2 to 3 minutes, or until the leeks are tender, stirring frequently.

Stir in the rice. Cook for 1 to 2 minutes, or until lightly toasted, stirring constantly.

Pour about 1/2 cup broth mixture into the skillet. Cook until the liquid is absorbed, stirring occasionally. Repeat the procedure until you've used all the broth mixture (the process takes 20 to 30 minutes). Reduce the heat to medium if the rice begins to stick excessively to the skillet.

Stir in the broccoli and Parmesan. Cook over medium heat for 2 to 3 minutes, or until the broccoli is heated through, stirring occasionally.

PER SERVING

calories 150	carbohydrates 27 g
total fat 2.0 g	fiber 3 g
saturated fat 0.5 g	sugars 2 g
trans fat 0.0 g	**protein** 6 g
polyunsaturated fat 0.0 g	**DIETARY EXCHANGES**
monounsaturated fat 0.5 g	1 1/2 starch,
cholesterol 2 mg	1 vegetable
sodium 150 mg	

CRANBERRY CHUTNEY

SERVES 16

Especially good with curried meat dishes, this chutney also pairs well with turkey and chicken.

- 1 pound whole fresh cranberries
- 8 ounces chopped apple (about 2 heaping cups), peeled

- 1 1/4 cups water
- 1 cup golden raisins
- 3/4 cup cider vinegar
- 2/3 cup pure maple syrup
- 1/4 cup fresh orange juice
- 1 tablespoon grated lemon zest
- 1/2 teaspoon salt
- 1/2 teaspoon ground cinnamon
- 1/2 teaspoon ground ginger
- 1/4 to 1 teaspoon crushed red pepper flakes
- 1/4 teaspoon ground allspice
- 1/8 teaspoon ground cloves

In a large saucepan, stir together all the ingredients. Bring to a boil over medium-high heat. Reduce the heat and simmer, covered, for 15 minutes, stirring occasionally.

Transfer to a glass jar with a tight-fitting lid and refrigerate. Use within two weeks.

Cook's Tip: For a longer shelf life, spoon the mixture into hot sterilized jars. Follow the jar manufacturer's directions for sealing the jars. Process for 10 minutes in a boiling water bath (the water should cover the jars by 1 to 2 inches). Remove the jars from the water. Let cool for at least 12 hours at room temperature. Then check to be sure the seal is tight. To do this, use your finger or thumb to push on the center of the lid; it should be tightly depressed when you push on it. If the center pops up when depressed, it hasn't sealed properly. If this occurs reprocess it in a new jar or store the original jar in the refrigerator.

PER SERVING

calories 92	sodium 78 mg
total fat 0.0 g	**carbohydrates** 24 g
saturated fat 0.0 g	fiber 2 g
trans fat 0.0 g	sugars 18 g
polyunsaturated fat 0.0 g	**protein** 1 g
monounsaturated fat 0.0 g	**DIETARY EXCHANGES**
cholesterol 0 mg	1 fruit, 1/2 other carbohydrate

BAKED CURRIED FRUIT

SERVES 8

When the weather turns cold, serve this spicy fruit for brunch or instead of salad at dinner.

Cooking spray
1 15.25-ounce can pineapple chunks in their
    own juice, well drained
1 15-ounce can pears in juice, well drained
1 15-ounce can apricot halves in juice,
    well drained
1 15-ounce can black cherries in juice,
    well drained
1/3 cup firmly packed light brown sugar
1 1/2 teaspoons curry powder
2 tablespoons fresh lemon juice
1 tablespoon plus 1 teaspoon light tub
    margarine

Preheat the oven to 300°F. Lightly spray an 11 x 7 x 2-inch casserole dish with cooking spray.

Spoon the pineapple, pears, apricots, and cherries into the dish, stirring to combine.

In a small bowl, stir together the brown sugar and curry powder. Sprinkle over the fruit.

Sprinkle the lemon juice over the fruit. Dot with the margarine.

Bake, covered, for 45 minutes.

PER SERVING

calories 132	**carbohydrates** 32 g
total fat 1.0 g	fiber 2 g
saturated fat 0.0 g	sugars 28 g
trans fat 0.0 g	**protein** 1 g
polyunsaturated fat 0.0 g	**DIETARY EXCHANGES**
monounsaturated fat 0.5 g	1 1/2 fruit, 1/2 other
cholesterol 0 mg	carbohyrdrate
sodium 26 mg	

Sauces and Gravies

BASIC GRAVY

SERVES 4; 1/4 CUP PER SERVING

Simple to make, but rich-tasting, serve this easy-to-make gravy with Roasted Garlic–Lemon Turkey Breast *(page 233) or* Mashed Potatoes with Parmesan and Green Onions *(page 399).*

2 to 4 tablespoons all-purpose flour
1/2 cup fat-free, low-sodium chicken or beef broth and 1/2 cup fat-free, low-sodium chicken or beef broth, such as on pages 35 and 36, divided use
1/4 teaspoon salt

In a medium skillet, cook the flour over medium-high heat for 5 to 6 minutes, or until lightly colored, stirring occasionally. Transfer to a small bowl.

Pour 1/2 cup broth into the flour, whisking until smooth. Pour into the skillet.

Whisk in the salt and the remaining 1/2 cup broth. Bring to a simmer over medium heat. Cook until the desired consistency, whisking constantly.

PER SERVING

calories 24	sodium 152 mg
total fat 29.0 g	carbohydrates 5 g
saturated fat 0.0 g	fiber 0 g
trans fat 0.0 g	sugars 0 g
polyunsaturated fat 0.0 g	protein 1 g
monounsaturated fat 0.0 g	DIETARY EXCHANGES
cholesterol 0.0 mg	1/2 starch

MUSHROOM GRAVY

In a small skillet over medium heat, cook 1/4 cup sliced button mushrooms in 2 tablespoons of the same broth as used in the gravy. Stir into the cooked gravy.

Cook's Tip: Adjust the amount of flour according to whether you want thin, medium, or thick gravy. This recipe doubles or triples well.

CREAMY CHICKEN GRAVY

SERVES 4; 1/4 CUP PER SERVING

This thick gravy pairs nicely with Baked Chicken and Vegetables *(page 187). Or pay homage to southern specialties and serve it with* Chicken-"Fried" Steak *(page 247).*

1 cup fat-free, low-sodium chicken broth, such as on page 36
1/4 cup fat-free milk
2 tablespoons all-purpose flour
1/2 teaspoon pepper, or to taste
1/8 teaspoon salt

In a medium saucepan, warm the broth over medium heat.

In a small bowl, whisk together the remaining ingredients until smooth. Gradually whisk into the broth. Cook for 3 to 5 minutes, or until thickened, whisking constantly.

PER SERVING

calories 23	sodium 86 mg
total fat 0.0 g	carbohydrates 4 g
saturated fat 0.0 g	fiber 0 g
trans fat 0.0 g	sugars 1 g
polyunsaturated fat 0.0 g	protein 1 g
monounsaturated fat 0.0 g	DIETARY EXCHANGES
cholesterol 0 mg	1/2 starch

TARTAR SAUCE

SERVES 16; 1 TABLESPOON PER SERVING

A classic pairing with seafood, this sauce is an ideal complement to Almond-Topped Baked Trout *(page 161) or* Little Shrimp Cakes *(page 177).*

1/2 cup fat-free plain Greek yogurt
2 tablespoons light mayonnaise
2 tablespoons pickle relish (lowest sodium available), drained
2 tablespoons fresh lemon juice
1 tablespoon minced onion
1 tablespoon finely chopped parsley
1 tablespoon Dijon mustard (lowest sodium available)

In a medium bowl, whisk together all the ingredients. Cover and refrigerate.

PER SERVING

calories 13	sodium 54 mg
total fat 0.5 g	carbohydrates 1 g
saturated fat 0.0 g	fiber 0 g
trans fat 0.0 g	sugars 1 g
polyunsaturated fat 0.5 g	protein 1 g
monounsaturated fat 0.0 g	DIETARY EXCHANGES
cholesterol 1 mg	free

COCKTAIL SAUCE

SERVES 4; 2 TABLESPOONS PER SERVING

This zesty dip is the perfect classic partner for shrimp cocktail. Try it with Oven-Fried Scallops with Cilantro and Lime *(page 170) or* Catfish with Zesty Slaw Topping *(page 141).*

   1/2 cup no-salt-added ketchup
   1 tablespoon fresh lemon juice
   1 tablespoon bottled white horseradish, drained
   2 teaspoons brown sugar

In a small bowl, whisk together all the ingredients. Cover and refrigerate.

PER SERVING

calories 61	sodium 16 mg
total fat 0.0 g	carbohydrates 15 g
saturated fat 0.0 g	fiber 0 g
trans fat 0.0 g	sugars 11 g
polyunsaturated fat 0.0 g	protein 0 g
monounsaturated fat 0.0 g	DIETARY EXCHANGES
cholesterol 0 mg	1 other carbohydrate

WALNUT CREAM SAUCE

SERVES 4; 1/4 CUP PER SERVING

A delicious toasted walnut flavor permeates this rich-tasting sauce. It's especially good over poached chicken or grilled fish.

   1 medium shallot, finely chopped
   2 tablespoons chopped walnuts, dry-roasted

   1 cup fat-free milk
   1 1/2 tablespoons all-purpose flour
   1 teaspoon Creole mustard or coarse-grain mustard (lowest sodium available)
   1/2 teaspoon dried marjoram, crumbled
   1/8 teaspoon salt
   2 tablespoons shredded or grated Romano or Parmesan cheese

In a medium saucepan, stir together the shallot and walnuts. Cook over medium heat for 2 minutes, or until the shallot is tender-crisp, stirring occasionally.

Whisk in the remaining ingredients except the Romano until the flour is dissolved (there may be a few lumps). Increase the heat to medium high and bring to a simmer, whisking occasionally. Reduce the heat and simmer for 2 to 3 minutes, or until thickened, whisking occasionally. Remove from the heat.

Add the Romano, whisking constantly until melted.

PER SERVING

calories 63	sodium 138 mg
total fat 3.0 g	carbohydrates 6 g
saturated fat 0.5 g	fiber 0 g
trans fat 0.0 g	sugars 3 g
polyunsaturated fat 1.5 g	protein 4 g
monounsaturated fat 0.5 g	DIETARY EXCHANGES
cholesterol 3 mg	1/2 starch, 1/2 fat

YOGURT-TAHINI SAUCE

SERVES 8; 2 TABLESPOONS PER SERVING

Serve this sauce with grilled salmon or tuna, over steamed or grilled vegetables, or even on a burger.

   3/4 cup fat-free plain Greek yogurt
   2 tablespoons chopped fresh cilantro
   2 tablespoons tahini
   1 tablespoon fresh lemon juice
   1/4 teaspoon ground cumin
   1/8 teaspoon salt
   Pinch of cayenne

(continued)

In a medium bowl, whisk together all the ingredients. Serve immediately or cover and refrigerate for up to two days.

Cook's Tip on Tahini: Tahini is made from ground sesame seeds. Depending on the amount of oil added to it, it can take the form of a slightly chunky paste or a very creamy sauce. It's a staple of Middle Eastern and Mediterranean cooking and is typically used in preparing hummus and baba ganoush. Look for it in the ethnic aisles at the supermarket.

PER SERVING

calories 34	**sodium** 46 mg
total fat 2.0 g	**carbohydrates** 2 g
saturated fat 0.5 g	fiber 0 g
trans fat 0.0 g	sugars 1 g
polyunsaturated fat 1.0 g	**protein** 3 g
monounsaturated fat 1.0 g	**DIETARY EXCHANGES**
cholesterol 0 mg	1/2 lean meat

TOMATO-MINT RAITA

SERVES 7; 1/4 CUP PER SERVING

Making delicious use of two of summer's trademark ingredients, tomatoes and mint, this sauce—like its cousin, Raita *(page 430)—complements the fiery flavors of many Indian dishes.*

> 8 ounces fat-free plain yogurt
> 2 medium tomatoes, finely chopped
> 4 medium green onions, finely chopped
> 1 medium red chile, seeds and ribs discarded, finely chopped (optional; see Cook's Tip on Handling Hot Chiles, page 24)
> 1/4 cup finely chopped fresh mint and sprigs of fresh mint, divided use
> 1/4 teaspoon cumin seeds or ground cumin
> 1/4 teaspoon salt
> Paprika to taste

In a medium bowl, whisk the yogurt until smooth.

Add the tomatoes, green onions, chile, chopped mint, cumin seeds, and salt. Stir well.

Cover and refrigerate. Just before serving, sprinkle with the paprika and garnish with the remaining sprigs of mint.

PER SERVING

calories 32	**carbohydrates** 5 g
total fat 0.0 g	fiber 1 g
saturated fat 0.0 g	sugars 4 g
trans fat 0.0 g	**protein** 2 g
polyunsaturated fat 0.0 g	**DIETARY EXCHANGES**
monounsaturated fat 0.0 g	1/2 other
cholesterol 1 mg	carbohydrate
sodium 114 mg	

RAITA

SERVES 4; 1/4 CUP PER SERVING

Cool your palate with the freshness of this Indian condiment that's made from yogurt and grated cucumber. Offer it as a side with Chana Masala *(page 338). Prepare* Indian-Spiced Rice Pudding *(page 498) for a sweet finish to your meal.*

> 1 large cucumber, peeled, seeded, and finely grated
> 1/16 teaspoon salt and 1/8 teaspoon salt, divided use
> 1 cup fat-free plain Greek yogurt
> 1/4 cup finely chopped fresh mint leaves
> 1 medium garlic clove, finely chopped
> 1/4 teaspoon ground cumin
> 1/4 teaspoon ground coriander

Put the cucumber in a colander. Sprinkle with 1/16 teaspoon salt. Let drain for 30 minutes. Using the back of a spoon, gently press the cucumber to release more of its juice. Pat the cucumber dry with paper towels.

In a medium bowl, stir together the yogurt, mint, garlic, cumin, coriander, and the remaining 1/8 teaspoon salt. Stir in the cucumber. Cover and refrigerate for at least 30 minutes before serving.

PER SERVING

calories 43	**sodium** 134 mg
total fat 0.0 g	**carbohydrates** 5 g
saturated fat 0.0 g	fiber 1 g
trans fat 0.0 g	sugars 3 g
polyunsaturated fat 0.0 g	**protein** 6 g
monounsaturated fat 0.0 g	**DIETARY EXCHANGES**
cholesterol 0 mg	1/2 fat-free milk

CREAMY DIJON-LIME SAUCE

SERVES 6; 2 TABLESPOONS PER SERVING

Serve this sauce at room temperature over chilled vegetables, such as fresh tomato slices or slightly steamed and chilled asparagus, or heat it to serve over steamed vegetables such as broccoli, cauliflower, lima beans, green beans, or carrots.

1/3 cup fat-free plain yogurt
1 tablespoon plus 1 teaspoon Dijon mustard
    (lowest sodium available)
1 teaspoon fresh lime juice
1/8 teaspoon salt
1 tablespoon olive oil (extra-virgin preferred)

In a small bowl, whisk together all the ingredients except the oil until smooth.

If using over chilled vegetables, stir in the oil. If using over hot vegetables, heat the sauce in a small saucepan over medium-low heat. Don't allow to boil. Remove from the heat. Stir in the oil.

Cook's Tip: The olive oil will have a more pronounced flavor if you add it after you take the sauce off the heat.

PER SERVING

calories 32	sodium 128 mg
total fat 2.5 g	carbohydrates 2 g
saturated fat 0.5 g	fiber 0 g
trans fat 0.0 g	sugars 1 g
polyunsaturated fat 0.0 g	protein 1 g
monounsaturated fat 2.0 g	DIETARY EXCHANGES
cholesterol 0 mg	1/2 fat

BOURBON BARBECUE SAUCE

SERVES 6; 1/4 CUP PER SERVING

Ancho powder adds deep color and a slight bite to this barbecue sauce. Use it to baste grilled chicken or beef.

1/3 cup bourbon or 100% apple juice
1/4 cup finely chopped sweet onion, such as
    Vidalia, Maui, or Oso Sweet
2 medium garlic cloves, minced
1 8-ounce can no-salt-added tomato sauce
3 tablespoons cider vinegar
2 tablespoons light or dark molasses
2 tablespoons light or dark brown sugar
1 tablespoon no-salt-added tomato paste
1 tablespoon Worcestershire sauce (lowest
    sodium available)
1 teaspoon ancho powder
1 teaspoon dry mustard
1/2 teaspoon ground cumin
1/4 teaspoon pepper
1/4 teaspoon liquid smoke (optional)

In a medium saucepan, stir together the bourbon, onion, and garlic. Bring to a boil over high heat. Reduce the heat and simmer for 4 to 6 minutes, or until the onion is soft and the liquid has nearly evaporated.

Stir in the remaining ingredients. Increase the heat to medium high and return to a boil. Reduce the heat and simmer for 6 to 8 minutes, or until the desired thickness, stirring occasionally. Refrigerate any leftover sauce in an airtight container for up to one week.

PER SERVING

calories 90	sodium 30 mg
total fat 0.5 g	carbohydrates 14 g
saturated fat 0.0 g	fiber 1 g
trans fat 0.0 g	sugars 12 g
polyunsaturated fat 0.0 g	protein 1 g
monounsaturated fat 0.0 g	DIETARY EXCHANGES
cholesterol 0 mg	1 other carbohydrate

SOUR CREAM SAUCE WITH DILL

SERVES 4; 1/4 CUP PER SERVING

Enjoy this sauce three ways. Try the dill sauce over grilled or poached salmon, the garlic variation over boiled red potatoes, and the blue cheese version over steamed broccoli.

8 ounces fat-free sour cream
1 tablespoon chopped fresh dillweed
1 tablespoon minced green onion (green
    part only)
1/2 teaspoon pepper
2 to 3 tablespoons fat-free milk (optional)

(continued)

In a medium bowl, whisk together all the ingredients except the milk. Thin the mixture with the milk, if desired. Cover and refrigerate.

For each variation, omit the dill and stir the listed ingredients into the sauce before refrigerating.

PER SERVING

calories 55	**sodium** 45 mg
total fat 0.0 g	**carbohydrates** 9 g
saturated fat 0.0 g	fiber 0 g
trans fat 0.0 g	sugars 4 g
polyunsaturated fat 0.0 g	**protein** 4 g
monounsaturated fat 0.0 g	**DIETARY EXCHANGES**
cholesterol 9 mg	1/2 starch

SOUR CREAM SAUCE WITH GARLIC

SERVES 4; 1/4 CUP PER SERVING

    1 tablespoon finely chopped fresh parsley
    1/4 teaspoon garlic powder
    Dash of red hot-pepper sauce

PER SERVING

calories 56	**sodium** 46 mg
total fat 0.0 g	**carbohydrates** 9 g
saturated fat 0.0 g	fiber 0 g
trans fat 0.0 g	sugars 4 g
polyunsaturated fat 0.0 g	**protein** 4 g
monounsaturated fat 0.0 g	**DIETARY EXCHANGES**
cholesterol 9 mg	1/2 starch

SOUR CREAM SAUCE WITH BLUE CHEESE

SERVES 5; 1/4 CUP PER SERVING

    3 tablespoons crumbled low-fat blue cheese
    1/4 teaspoon Worcestershire sauce (lowest sodium available)

Cook's Tip on Chopping Fresh Herbs: Put pieces of a fresh herb in a measuring cup or coffee mug. Using kitchen scissors, snip the herb until the pieces are the desired fineness.

PER SERVING

calories 62	**sodium** 108 mg
total fat 1.5 g	**carbohydrates** 8 g
saturated fat 1.0 g	fiber 0 g
trans fat 0.0 g	sugars 3 g
polyunsaturated fat 0.0 g	**protein** 4 g
monounsaturated fat 0.5 g	**DIETARY EXCHANGES**
cholesterol 11 mg	1/2 starch

QUICK MADEIRA SAUCE

SERVES 8; 2 TABLESPOONS PER SERVING

Madeira is a fortified wine made on the Portuguese island of Madeira. Its unique taste, which first became popular more than 200 years ago, comes from repeatedly heating the wine. Serve this flavorful sauce with roast beef, chicken, or Cornish game hens.

    1 1/4 cups fat-free, low-sodium chicken broth, such as on page 36
    1/3 cup Madeira or port and 1 tablespoon Madeira or port, divided use
    2 teaspoons cornstarch

In a small saucepan, stir together the broth and 1/3 cup Madeira. Bring to a boil over high heat. Boil for 3 to 4 minutes, or until reduced by one-third (to about 1 cup) (no stirring needed).

Put the cornstarch in a small bowl. Add the remaining 1 tablespoon Madeira, whisking until the cornstarch is dissolved. Whisk the mixture into the sauce. Cook over medium heat for 1 to 2 minutes, or until thickened, whisking constantly.

PER SERVING

calories 20	**sodium** 5 mg
total fat 0.0 g	**carbohydrates** 2 g
saturated fat 0.0 g	fiber 0 g
trans fat 0.0 g	sugars 1 g
polyunsaturated fat 0.0 g	**protein** 0 g
monounsaturated fat 0.0 g	**DIETARY EXCHANGES**
cholesterol 0 mg	free

MUSTARD AND GREEN ONION SAUCE

SERVES 20; 1 TABLESPOON PER SERVING

Serve over Crunchy Herb-Crusted Pork Chops *(page 288) or* Crispy Baked Chicken *(page 185).*

- 1/2 cup light mayonnaise
- 1/2 cup fat-free plain Greek yogurt
- 2 tablespoons Dijon mustard (lowest sodium available)
- 3 tablespoons minced green onion
- 1/8 teaspoon garlic powder

In a medium bowl, whisk together all the ingredients. Cover and refrigerate.

PER SERVING

calories 20	sodium 85 mg
total fat 1.5 g	carbohydrates 1 g
saturated fat 0.0 g	fiber 0 g
trans fat 0.0 g	sugars 0 g
polyunsaturated fat 1.0 g	protein 1 g
monounsaturated fat 0.5 g	DIETARY EXCHANGES
cholesterol 2 mg	free

MOCK HOLLANDAISE SAUCE

SERVES 4; 1/4 CUP PER SERVING

By using chicken broth and a small amount of oil instead of lots of butter, you can prepare a heart-healthy hollandaise sauce that will dress up many dishes. It's especially good over steamed or roasted asparagus.

- 1 tablespoon cornstarch
- 1 tablespoon canola or corn oil
- 3/4 cup fat-free, low-sodium chicken broth, such as on page 36
- 2 tablespoons egg substitute
- 1 to 2 tablespoons fresh lemon juice

In a small saucepan, whisk together the cornstarch and oil. Cook over low heat for 1 minute, or until smooth, whisking constantly.

Whisk in the broth. Increase the heat to medium high. Cook for 3 to 4 minutes, or until thickened, whisking constantly. Remove from the heat.

Slowly whisk the egg substitute into the sauce. Reduce the heat to low. Cook for 1 minute, whisking constantly. Remove from the heat.

Whisk in the lemon juice.

Cook's Tip on Juicing Lemons: Before you cut a lemon that has been refrigerated, let it reach room temperature. Then roll it back and forth on the counter, pressing down hard on the lemon with your hand. This will cause it to release more of its juice.

PER SERVING

calories 45	sodium 21 mg
total fat 3.5 g	carbohydrates 2 g
saturated fat 0.5 g	fiber 0 g
trans fat 0.0 g	sugars 0 g
polyunsaturated fat 1.0 g	protein 1 g
monounsaturated fat 2.0 g	DIETARY EXCHANGES
cholesterol 0 mg	1 fat

MOCK BÉARNAISE SAUCE

SERVES 4; 1/4 CUP PER SERVING

Turn poached fish or steamed vegetables into something special with this fresh herb-wine sauce.

- 1/4 cup white wine vinegar
- 1/4 cup dry white wine (regular or nonalcoholic) or dry vermouth
- 1 tablespoon minced shallot or green onion (green part only)
- 1 tablespoon minced fresh tarragon or 1 teaspoon dried tarragon, crumbled
- 1/8 teaspoon pepper (white preferred)
- 1 tablespoon cornstarch
- 1 tablespoon canola or corn oil
- 3/4 cup fat-free, low-sodium chicken broth, such as on page 36
- 2 tablespoons egg substitute

In a small saucepan, whisk together the vinegar, wine, shallot, tarragon, and pepper. Bring to a boil over medium-high heat, whisking constantly. Cook for 4 to 5 minutes, or until reduced by three-fourths (to about 2 tablespoons). Set aside.

(continued)

In a separate small saucepan, whisk together the cornstarch and oil. Reduce the heat to low. Cook for 1 minute, or until smooth, whisking constantly.

Whisk the broth into the cornstarch mixture. Increase the heat to medium high. Cook for 3 to 4 minutes, or until thickened, whisking constantly. Remove from the heat.

Slowly whisk the egg substitute into the broth mixture. Reduce the heat to low. Cook for 1 minute, whisking constantly. Remove from the heat.

Whisk in the vinegar mixture.

PER SERVING

calories 62	sodium 22 mg
total fat 3.5 g	carbohydrates 4 g
saturated fat 0.5 g	fiber 0 g
trans fat 0.0 g	sugars 0 g
polyunsaturated fat 1.0 g	protein 1 g
monounsaturated fat 2.0 g	**DIETARY EXCHANGES**
cholesterol 0 mg	1 fat

ALFREDO SAUCE

SERVES 4; 1/2 CUP PER SERVING

Versatile Alfredo sauce can go from blanketing pasta and layering lasagna to being ladled over savory crepes. You can also mix it with steamed or grilled veggies to top baked potatoes, or make a white pizza by using Alfredo sauce in place of the tomato sauce.

1 cup fat-free, low-sodium chicken broth, such as on page 36
1 cup fat-free half-and-half
2 1/2 tablespoons all-purpose flour
1 medium garlic clove, minced
1/8 teaspoon pepper
1/4 cup shredded or grated Parmesan cheese

In a medium saucepan, whisk together all the ingredients except the Parmesan. Bring to a simmer over medium-high heat, stirring occasionally. Reduce the heat and simmer for 2 to 3 minutes, or until thickened. Remove from the heat.

Add the Parmesan, stirring constantly until melted.

PER SERVING

calories 82	sodium 151 mg
total fat 1.5 g	carbohydrates 12 g
saturated fat 1.0 g	fiber 0 g
trans fat 0.0 g	sugars 4 g
polyunsaturated fat 0.0 g	protein 7 g
monounsaturated fat 0.5 g	**DIETARY EXCHANGES**
cholesterol 4 mg	1 starch, 1/2 lean meat

FRESH TOMATO AND ROASTED RED BELL PEPPER SAUCE

SERVES 8; 1/4 CUP PER SERVING

If you need a side dish for tonight's meal, serve this Italian sauce over whole-grain pasta. For an entrée instead, try it over chicken, fish, or pork.

1 tablespoon olive oil and 1 tablespoon olive oil (extra-virgin preferred), divided use
1 medium onion, finely chopped
4 medium garlic cloves, minced
1 pound Italian plum (Roma) tomatoes, coarsely chopped
3 ounces canned no-salt-added tomato paste
1 cup roasted red bell peppers, drained if bottled, chopped
1/4 cup chopped fresh basil or 1 tablespoon plus 1 teaspoon dried basil, crumbled

In a large saucepan, heat 1 tablespoon oil over medium-high heat until hot, swirling to coat the bottom. Cook the onion for about 3 minutes, or until soft, stirring frequently.

Stir in the garlic. Cook for 10 seconds, stirring constantly.

Stir in the tomatoes and tomato paste. Bring to a boil. Reduce the heat and simmer, covered, for 25 minutes, or until the tomatoes are soft. Remove from the heat.

Stir in the roasted peppers, basil, and the remaining 1 tablespoon oil. Let stand, covered, for 10 minutes so the flavors blend.

Cook's Tip: The variety of tomato makes a difference, especially when using a large amount, as in this sauce. If you substitute grape tomatoes, the sauce will be sweeter; if you use a regular tomato, the sauce will be thinner.

calories 59	sodium 25 mg
total fat 3.5 g	carbohydrates 7 g
saturated fat 0.5 g	fiber 2 g
trans fat 0.0 g	sugars 4 g
polyunsaturated fat 0.5 g	protein 1 g
monounsaturated fat 2.5 g	DIETARY EXCHANGES
cholesterol 0 mg	1 vegetable, 1 fat

SPEEDY MARINARA SAUCE

SERVES 4; 1/2 CUP PER SERVING

A combination of fresh and canned tomatoes gives this caper-spiked marinara sauce slow-cooked flavor in a short amount of time.

2 medium tomatoes
1 teaspoon olive oil
2 medium shallots, finely chopped
2 medium garlic cloves, minced
1 14.5-ounce can no-salt-added diced
    tomatoes, undrained
2 tablespoons no-salt-added tomato paste
2 teaspoons capers, drained
1 teaspoon dried oregano, crumbled
1/2 teaspoon dried basil, crumbled
1/4 to 1/2 teaspoon crushed red pepper flakes
1/8 teaspoon salt

Fill a medium saucepan three-quarters full of water. Bring to a boil over high heat.

Cut a small x in the bottom of the fresh tomatoes. Carefully put the tomatoes into the water one at a time. Reduce the heat to medium high. Cook for 1 minute, or until the tomato skins start to loosen. Using a slotted spoon, transfer the tomatoes to a cutting board. Let cool for 5 minutes.

Meanwhile, in a separate medium saucepan, heat the oil over medium heat, swirling to coat the bottom. Cook the shallots and garlic for 2 to 3 minutes, or until soft, stirring occasionally.

Stir in the remaining ingredients. Increase the heat to medium high and bring to a simmer, stirring occasionally.

Meanwhile, peel and dice the fresh tomatoes. Stir into the sauce. Reduce the heat and simmer for 15 to 20 minutes, stirring occasionally.

calories 62	sodium 137 mg
total fat 1.5 g	carbohydrates 11 g
saturated fat 0.0 g	fiber 2 g
trans fat 0.0 g	sugars 6 g
polyunsaturated fat 0.0 g	protein 2 g
monounsaturated fat 1.0 g	DIETARY EXCHANGES
cholesterol 0 mg	2 vegetable

CREOLE SAUCE

SERVES 16; HEAPING 1/4 CUP PER SERVING

This easy sauce with its traditional onion, celery, and bell pepper is delicious over chicken, shrimp, meat loaf, or stuffed bell peppers. Since it makes enough for several meals, freeze what you don't use and try it with a different entrée another time.

1 28-ounce can no-salt-added Italian plum
    (Roma) tomatoes, undrained
1 large onion, diced
1 medium green bell pepper, diced
1 medium rib of celery, chopped
2 ounces sliced button mushrooms
3 tablespoons no-salt-added tomato paste
2 medium garlic cloves, minced
1/2 teaspoon salt
1/2 teaspoon pepper, or to taste
1/2 teaspoon dried oregano, crumbled
1/2 teaspoon dried basil, crumbled

In a medium saucepan, stir together all the ingredients. Bring to a boil over medium-high heat. Reduce the heat and simmer, covered, for 20 minutes.

calories 20	sodium 156 mg
total fat 0.0 g	carbohydrates 5 g
saturated fat 0.0 g	fiber 1 g
trans fat 0.0 g	sugars 3 g
polyunsaturated fat 0.0 g	protein 1 g
monounsaturated fat 0.0 g	DIETARY EXCHANGES
cholesterol 0 mg	free

LEMON-CHIVE SAUCE

SERVES 8; 1 TABLESPOON PER SERVING

This simple no-cook sauce can be completed in 5 minutes. Its tart lemony flavor adds a bright note to a variety of dishes. Serve it over chicken, fish, broccoli, or green beans. Or, use it as a piquant vegetable dip.

1/4 cup fat-free plain yogurt

3 tablespoons low-fat mayonnaise

2 tablespoons fat-free milk

1 teaspoon grated lemon zest

2 teaspoons fresh lemon juice

2 tablespoons chopped fresh chives

1 teaspoon minced shallots

In a small bowl, whisk together the yogurt, mayonnaise, milk, lemon zest, and lemon juice until smooth. Stir in the chives and shallots.

Cook's Tip: For a slightly thinner sauce, whisk in 1 to 2 additional tablespoons of fat-free milk.

PER SERVING

calories 16	sodium 60 mg
total fat 0.5 g	**carbohydrates** 3 g
saturated fat 0.0 g	fiber 0 g
trans fat 0.0 g	sugars 2 g
polyunsaturated fat 0.0 g	**protein** 1 g
monounsaturated fat 0.0 g	**DIETARY EXCHANGES**
cholesterol 0 mg	free

MOJITO SAUCE

SERVES 6; 2 TABLESPOONS PER SERVING

The classic flavors of a mojito are all included in this dessert sauce. Serve it over Grilled Pineapple *(page 502) or other grilled fruits, such as peaches or mangoes. Try it over fresh fruit, such as berries, or baked peaches, apples, or plums.*

1/2 cup fat-free plain Greek yogurt

1/4 cup sugar

2 tablespoons fresh orange juice

2 teaspoons fresh lime juice

1/2 teaspoon spiced or white rum or

    1/8 teaspoon rum extract

3 sprigs of fresh mint

In a small bowl, whisk together the yogurt and sugar until the sugar is well blended. Whisk in the orange juice, lime juice, and rum. Add the 3 sprigs of mint. Using a muddler or the back of a spoon, crush the mint to release its flavor.

Cover and refrigerate for 30 minutes to 1 hour so the flavors blend. Discard the mint sprigs.

Stir just before serving.

PER SERVING

calories 46	carbohydrates 10 g
total fat 0.0 g	fiber 0 g
saturated fat 0.0 g	sugars 10 g
trans fat 0.0 g	**protein** 2 g
polyunsaturated fat 0.0 g	**DIETARY EXCHANGES**
monounsaturated fat 0.0 g	1/2 other
cholesterol 0 mg	carbohydrate
sodium 7 mg	

CUBAN-STYLE GARLIC AND CITRUS MOJO

SERVES 10; 2 TABLESPOONS PER SERVING

Originating in Cuba and the Caribbean, a mojo (MOH-hoh) is generally served as a condiment or used as a marinade. Try this mojo drizzled over vegetables to brighten their flavor. What sets it apart is the addition of juice from a sour orange. The juice helps tenderize meat or poultry.

1/2 cup olive oil (extra-virgin preferred)

8 medium garlic cloves, minced

3 medium shallots, minced

1/2 teaspoon dried oregano, crumbled

1/3 teaspoon ground cumin

3/4 cup fresh sour orange juice

1/4 teaspoon pepper (freshly ground preferred)

In a deep medium saucepan, gently heat the oil over medium heat. Stir in the garlic, shallots, oregano, and cumin. Cook for 1 to 2 minutes, or until fragrant, stirring constantly.

Gradually and carefully (as the sauce may sizzle), stir in the sour orange juice and pepper. Bring just to a boil. Reduce the heat to low. Cook for 3 to 5 minutes, stirring frequently.

Serve the mojo warm or at room temperature. For peak flavor, serve within a few hours of preparation.

Cook's Tip: Sour orange juice is available at Hispanic markets, in the ethnic aisle of your grocery store, or online. If you can't find it, substitute 1 teaspoon of grated orange zest, 1/2 cup fresh orange juice, and 1/4 cup fresh lime or grapefruit juice. Stir all the ingredients together until well blended.

PER SERVING

calories 111	**sodium** 2 mg
total fat 11.0 g	**carbohydrates** 4 g
saturated fat 1.5 g	fiber 0 g
trans fat 0.0 g	sugars 2 g
polyunsaturated fat 1.0 g	**protein** 0 g
monounsaturated fat 8.0 g	**DIETARY EXCHANGES**
cholesterol 0 mg	2 fat

FRESH HERB CHIMICHURRI SAUCE

SERVES 8; 2 TABLESPOONS PER SERVING

This popular sauce from Argentina is easy to keep on hand and instantly adds flavor to grilled meats or seafood. The assertive combination of parsley, cilantro, and mint is enhanced by the tartness of vinegar and lemon juice.

2 cups loosely packed fresh Italian (flat-leaf) parsley
1/2 cup loosely packed fresh cilantro
1/2 cup fat-free, low-sodium chicken broth, such as on page 36
2 tablespoons fresh mint
3 tablespoons white wine, red wine, or plain rice vinegar
1 tablespoon olive oil (extra-virgin preferred)
2 teaspoons fresh lemon juice
2 teaspoons honey
1 medium garlic clove
1/4 teaspoon salt
1/8 teaspoon pepper (freshly ground preferred)

Put all the ingredients in the order listed in a food processor or blender. Pulse five times to chop the herbs. Process for 1 to 2 minutes, or until the mixture is just smooth. Serve immediately or cover and refrigerate for up to six days.

PER SERVING

calories 30	**sodium** 84 mg
total fat 2.0 g	**carbohydrates** 3 g
saturated fat 0.5 g	fiber 1 g
trans fat 0.0 g	sugars 2 g
polyunsaturated fat 0.0 g	**protein** 1 g
monounsaturated fat 1.5 g	**DIETARY EXCHANGES**
cholesterol 0 mg	1/2 fat

SALSA CRUDA

SERVES 6; 1/4 CUP PER SERVING

Serve this zippy salsa as a dip or as a tasty topping for many Mexican dishes, such as Beef Tostadas (page 281).

2 large tomatoes, diced
1/4 cup finely chopped onion
2 to 4 teaspoons fresh lime juice
2 teaspoons chopped fresh Jalapeño, seeds and ribs discarded (see Cook's Tip on Handling Hot Chiles, page 24)
2 teaspoons finely chopped fresh cilantro, or to taste
1/4 teaspoon salt

In a medium bowl, stir together all the ingredients. Cover and refrigerate.

Cook's Tip: For a different texture, combine the ingredients in a food processor or blender and process until fairly smooth.

PER SERVING

calories 15	**sodium** 100 mg
total fat 0.0 g	**carbohydrates** 3 g
saturated fat 0.0 g	fiber 1 g
trans fat 0.0 g	sugars 2 g
polyunsaturated fat 0.0 g	**protein** 1 g
monounsaturated fat 0.0 g	**DIETARY EXCHANGES**
cholesterol 0 mg	free

TOMATILLO-CILANTRO SALSA WITH LIME

SERVES 4; 1/4 CUP PER SERVING

Tart tomatillos (tohm-ah-TEE-ohs) *join fresh cilantro, lime juice, and a bit of jalapeño for this winning salsa. Serve it as a dip for baked tortillas or to give any grilled food a Mexican flair.*

8 ounces tomatillos, papery husks discarded
1/2 cup chopped fresh cilantro
2 tablespoons chopped green onions
1 tablespoon fresh lime juice
1 medium fresh jalapeño, seeds and ribs
    discarded, quartered (see Cook's Tip on
    Handling Hot Chiles, page 24)
1/8 teaspoon salt
1 tablespoon olive oil (extra-virgin preferred)

In a food processor or blender, process all the ingredients except the oil until smooth. Pour into a small bowl.

Stir in the oil. For a stronger flavor, cover and refrigerate for up to two days.

Cook's Tip on Tomatillos: Choose firm tomatillos with close-fitting papery husks. Remove the husks and thoroughly rinse the tomatillos before cooking. To store them, leave the husks on and refrigerate the tomatillos in a paper bag for up to one month.

PER SERVING

calories 52	sodium 76 mg
total fat 4.0 g	carbohydrates 4 g
saturated fat 0.5 g	fiber 1 g
trans fat 0.0 g	sugars 3 g
polyunsaturated fat 0.5 g	protein 1 g
monounsaturated fat 2.5 g	DIETARY EXCHANGES
cholesterol 0 mg	1 fat

TOMATO-CILANTRO SALSA

Replace the tomatillos with 1 cup finely chopped tomatoes and replace the lime juice with 2 tablespoons cider vinegar. Don't use a food processor or blender with this variation; the color will be less brilliant if you do. Just chop the jalapeño and stir all the ingredients together.

PER SERVING

calories 44	sodium 78 mg
total fat 3.5 g	carbohydrates 3 g
saturated fat 0.5 g	fiber 1 g
trans fat 0.0 g	sugars 2 g
polyunsaturated fat 0.5 g	protein 1 g
monounsaturated fat 2.5 g	DIETARY EXCHANGES
cholesterol 0 mg	1 fat

CHOCOLATE SAUCE

SERVES 8; 2 TABLESPOONS PER SERVING

Need a chocolate fix? Serve this sauce warm or cold over fresh berries, grilled or broiled bananas, or fat-free, sugar-free vanilla or strawberry frozen yogurt.

2 tablespoons light tub margarine
3 tablespoons sugar
2 tablespoons unsweetened cocoa powder
2 tablespoons white corn syrup
1/4 cup fat-free evaporated milk
1 teaspoon vanilla extract

In a small saucepan, melt the margarine over medium-high heat, swirling to coat the bottom.

Whisk in the sugar, cocoa powder, and corn syrup.

Pour in the milk and bring to a boil, whisking constantly until smooth. Remove from the heat.

Whisk in the vanilla.

Cook's Tip on Cocoa Powder: Cocoa powder has much less fat than chocolate, which contains mostly saturated fat. To substitute cocoa for chocolate in baking, use 3 tablespoons of cocoa powder plus 1 tablespoon canola oil for 1 ounce of unsweetened baking chocolate.

PER SERVING

calories 57	carbohydrates 11 g
total fat 1.5 g	fiber 0 g
saturated fat 0.0 g	sugars 10 g
trans fat 0.0 g	protein 1 g
polyunsaturated fat 0.5 g	DIETARY EXCHANGES
monounsaturated fat 0.5 g	1/2 other
cholesterol 0 mg	carbohydrate
sodium 35 mg	

RASPBERRY PORT SAUCE

SERVES 4; 2 TABLESPOONS PER SERVING

For a simple yet sophisticated dessert, serve this sauce over poached or grilled fruit or fat-free, sugar-free frozen yogurt.

> 3/4 cup frozen unsweetened raspberries, blueberries, or a combination
> 2 tablespoons port
> 1 1/2 tablespoons sugar
> 1 1/2 teaspoons cornstarch
> 1/4 teaspoon vanilla extract

In a small saucepan, stir together all the ingredients except the vanilla until the cornstarch is dissolved. Bring to a boil over medium-high heat. Cook for 30 to 45 seconds, or until slightly thickened. Remove from the heat.

Stir in the vanilla. Let stand for 15 minutes. Serve at room temperature or refrigerate in an airtight container and serve cold.

PER SERVING

calories 50	carbohydrates 10 g
total fat 0.0 g	fiber 1 g
saturated fat 0.0 g	sugars 7 g
trans fat 0.0 g	**protein** 0 g
polyunsaturated fat 0.0 g	**DIETARY EXCHANGES**
monounsaturated fat 0.0 g	1/2 other
cholesterol 0 mg	carbohydrate
sodium 1 mg	

BLUEBERRY SAUCE

SERVES 6; 1/3 CUP PER SERVING

Try this fruity sauce over pancakes or waffles, such as Red, White, and Blueberry Waffles *(page 469).*

> 1 pint blueberries or 2 cups frozen unsweetened blueberries
> 1/2 cup water
> 1/4 cup sugar
> 1 tablespoon fresh lemon juice
> 1 tablespoon cornstarch
> 2 tablespoons cold water

In a medium saucepan over medium-high heat, bring the blueberries, water, sugar, and lemon juice to a boil. If using fresh blueberries, reduce the heat and simmer for 1 to 2 minutes, or until softened. If using frozen berries, there's no need to simmer.

In a small bowl, stir together the cornstarch and water until the cornstarch is dissolved. Stir into the blueberry mixture. Reduce the heat to low. Cook for 1 to 2 minutes, stirring until thick and smooth. Serve hot or cold.

PER SERVING

calories 66	carbohydrates 17 g
total fat 0.0 g	fiber 1 g
saturated fat 0.0 g	sugars 13 g
trans fat 0.0 g	**protein** 0 g
polyunsaturated fat 0.0 g	**DIETARY EXCHANGES**
monounsaturated fat 0.0 g	1/2 fruit, 1/2 other
cholesterol 0 mg	carbohydrate
sodium 2 mg	

ORANGE SAUCE

SERVES 4; 1/4 CUP PER SERVING

This sauce adds a scrumptious citrusy taste when it's drizzled over grilled pineapple, pancakes, or plain Greek yogurt.

> 1/2 teaspoon grated orange zest
> 2 cups fresh orange juice
> 1 tablespoon cornstarch
> 1 tablespoon water
> 1 tablespoon sugar
> 1 tablespoon fresh lemon juice
> 2 teaspoons light tub margarine

In a small saucepan, cook the orange juice over medium heat until reduced by half (to about 1 cup).

Put the cornstarch in a small bowl. Add the water, whisking until the cornstarch is dissolved.

Whisk in a small amount of orange juice. Whisk the cornstarch mixture into the juice remaining in the pan.

Whisk in the sugar. Cook for 1 to 2 minutes, or until thickened. Remove from the heat.

(continued)

Whisk in the lemon juice, margarine, and orange zest.

PER SERVING

calories 83	**sodium** 17 mg
total fat 1.0 g	**carbohydrates** 18 g
saturated fat 0.0 g	fiber 0 g
trans fat 0.0 g	sugars 14 g
polyunsaturated fat 0.0 g	**protein** 1 g
monounsaturated fat 0.5 g	**DIETARY EXCHANGES**
cholesterol 0 mg	1 fruit

Breads and Breakfast Dishes

WHOLE-WHEAT FRENCH BREAD

1 SLICE PER SERVING

You'll love the versatility of this nutty-flavored bread. Make a standard loaf in your bread machine, or use the dough cycle and shape the dough into baguettes to finish.

	1-pound machine (12 servings)	1 1/2-pound machine (18 servings)	2-pound machine (24 servings)
Whole-wheat flour	1 1/4 cups	2 cups	2 1/2 cups
Bread flour	1 cup	1 1/2 cups	2 cups
Fat-free dry milk	1 tablespoon	1 1/2 tablespoons	2 tablespoons
Salt	1/2 teaspoon	3/4 teaspoon	1 teaspoon
Canola or corn oil	1 tablespoon	1 1/2 tablespoons	2 tablespoons
Honey	1 tablespoon	1 1/2 tablespoons	2 tablespoons
Water	1 cup less 1 tablespoon	1 1/3 cups	1 7/8 cups
Active dry yeast	1 teaspoon	1 1/2 teaspoons	2 teaspoons

Put the ingredients in the bread machine container in the order recommended by the manufacturer. Select the basic/white bread cycle. Proceed as directed.

PER SERVING

calories 102	sodium 100 mg
total fat 1.5 g	**carbohydrates** 19 g
saturated fat 0.0 g	fiber 2 g
trans fat 0.0 g	sugars 2 g
polyunsaturated fat 0.5 g	**protein** 3 g
monounsaturated fat 1.0 g	**DIETARY EXCHANGES**
cholesterol 0 mg	1 1/2 starch

FOCACCIA

MAKES 1 LOAF; SERVES 16

Delicious on its own, useful for getting that last bite of spaghetti sauce, and even a replacement for pizza crust, this popular flatbread from Italy serves many purposes. You can either hand knead this bread or use your bread machine.

1 1/2 cups bread flour or all-purpose flour, 1 cup bread flour or all-purpose flour, plus up to 1/2 cup more as needed, divided use

1/4 cup semolina flour or all-purpose flour
1/4 cup all-purpose flour for flouring the surface, kneading, and rolling out the dough, plus more as needed
1 1/4-ounce package fast-rising yeast
1 tablespoon olive oil
2 teaspoons dried Italian seasoning, crumbled
1 teaspoon garlic powder
1/4 teaspoon salt
1 1/4 cups warm water (120°F to 130°F)
Olive oil cooking spray
1 tablespoon pine nuts
1 teaspoon dried rosemary, crushed

In a large bowl, stir together 1 1/2 cups bread flour, the semolina flour, 1/4 cup all purpose flour, the yeast, oil, Italian seasoning, garlic powder, and salt.

Pour the water into the flour mixture. Using a sturdy spoon, beat for 30 seconds.

Gradually add some of the remaining 1 cup bread flour, beating with the spoon after each addition, until the dough starts to pull away from the side of the bowl. Add more bread flour if necessary to make the dough stiff enough to handle.

Lightly flour a flat surface using the remaining all-purpose flour. Turn out the dough. Knead for 6 to 8 minutes, gradually adding enough all-purpose flour to make the dough smooth and elastic. (The dough shouldn't be dry or stick to the surface. You may not need the additional flour, or you may need up to 1/2 cup more if the dough is too sticky. See Cook's Tip on Breadmaking, page 445.) Cover the dough with a slightly damp dish towel. Let rest for 10 minutes.

Lightly spray a 14-inch pizza pan with cooking spray. Using your fingers, press the dough to the edge of the pan. Lightly spray with cooking spray. Press in the pine nuts. Sprinkle the rosemary over all. Cover with a slightly damp dish towel. Let the dough rise in a warm, draft-free place (about 85°F) for about 30 minutes.

While the dough is rising, preheat the oven to 375°F.

(continued)

Bake for 20 to 25 minutes, or until golden brown. Transfer the bread to a cooling rack. Let cool for at least 10 minutes before slicing.

BREAD MACHINE INSTRUCTIONS

Follow the manufacturer's instructions for the basic/white bread cycle.

For a flat loaf, use the bread machine only to mix the dough, following the manufacturer's directions for the dough cycle. Remove the dough when it's ready. Shape it. Press the pine nuts into the dough and sprinkle the rosemary over all. Bake as directed above. For a regular loaf, add the pine nuts and rosemary with the other ingredients.

	1-pound machine (12 servings)	1 1/2-pound machine (18 servings)	2-pound machine (24 servings)
Water	3/4 cup	1 1/4 cups	1 1/2 cups
Bread flour or all-purpose flour	1 2/3 cups	2 1/2 cups	3 1/3 cups
Semolina flour or all-purpose flour	3 tablespoons	1/4 cup	1/3 cup
All-purpose flour	3 tablespoons	1/4 cup	1/3 cup
Active dry yeast	2 teaspoons	2 1/2 teaspoons	1 tablespoon
Olive oil	2 1/4 teaspoons	1 tablespoon	1 1/2 tablespoons
Dried Italian seasoning, crumbled	1 1/2 teaspoons	2 teaspoons	1 tablespoon
Garlic powder	3/4 teaspoon	1 teaspoon	1 1/2 teaspoons
Salt	1/8 teaspoon	1/4 teaspoon	1/2 teaspoon

PER SERVING

calories 106	sodium 38 mg
total fat 1.5 g	carbohydrates 19 g
saturated fat 0.0 g	fiber 1 g
trans fat 0.0 g	sugars 0 g
polyunsaturated fat 0.5 g	protein 3 g
monounsaturated fat 1.0 g	DIETARY EXCHANGES
cholesterol 0 mg	1 1/2 starch

FOCACCIA SANDWICH LOAVES

MAKES 8 LOAVES; EACH SERVES 1

Lightly spray two baking sheets with cooking spray. After kneading, let the dough rest for 10 minutes. Divide into 8 pieces. Shape into disks. Put on the baking sheets. Cover each baking sheet with a slightly damp dish towel. Let the dough rise for 30 minutes in a warm, draft-free place (about 85°F). Press the pine nuts into the dough and sprinkle the rosemary over all. Bake as directed for 15 to 20 minutes, or until golden brown. Transfer the loaves to a cooling rack. Let cool completely before slicing in half horizontally.

PER SERVING

calories 212	sodium 76 mg
total fat 3.0 g	carbohydrates 39 g
saturated fat 0.5 g	fiber 2 g
trans fat 0.0 g	sugars 0 g
polyunsaturated fat 0.5 g	protein 7 g
monounsaturated fat 1.5 g	DIETARY EXCHANGES
cholesterol 0 mg	2 1/2 starch

HERB BREAD

MAKES 2 LOAVES; EACH SERVES 16

Sharpen your culinary skills with this step-by-step bread recipe. You'll even get a bit of exercise from lively kneading. This bread is swirled with a variety of herbs and it fills your kitchen with a divine smell while it's baking.

1/4 cup lukewarm water (105°F to 115°F)
2 1/4-ounce packages active dry yeast
1 3/4 cups fat-free milk
2 1/2 tablespoons sugar
2 tablespoons canola or corn oil
4 cups all-purpose flour, 2 cups all-purpose flour, and up to 1/2 cup all-purpose flour for flouring the surface and kneading, divided use
1 teaspoon salt
2 teaspoons caraway seeds
1/2 teaspoon ground nutmeg
1/2 teaspoon dried rosemary, crushed
1/4 teaspoon dried thyme, crumbled
Cooking spray

Pour the water into a large bowl. Add the yeast, stirring to dissolve. Let stand for 5 minutes, or until the mixture bubbles.

Stir in the milk, sugar, and oil.

Gradually stir in 4 cups flour and the salt. Using a sturdy spoon, beat for about 30 seconds, or until smooth.

Gradually add some of the remaining 2 cups flour, beating with the spoon after each addition, until the dough starts to pull away from the side of the bowl. Add more flour if necessary to make the dough stiff enough to handle.

Lightly flour a flat surface. Add the caraway seeds, nutmeg, rosemary, and thyme to the dough. Turn out the dough. Knead for 6 to 8 minutes, gradually adding enough of the remaining flour to make the dough smooth and elastic. (The dough shouldn't be dry or stick to the surface. You may not need all the flour, or you may need up to 1/2 cup more if the dough is too sticky.)

Lightly spray a large bowl with cooking spray. Put the dough in the bowl, turning to coat. Cover with a slightly damp dish towel. Let the dough rise in a warm, draft-free place (about 85°F) for about 1 hour, or until doubled in bulk.

Punch down the dough. Divide in half. Shape into loaves. Lightly spray two 9 x 5 x 3-inch loaf pans with cooking spray. Put the dough in the loaf pans. Cover each with a slightly damp dish towel. Let the dough rise in a warm, draft-free place (about 85°F) for about 30 minutes, or until doubled in bulk.

While the dough is rising, preheat the oven to 425°F.

Bake the loaves for 15 minutes. Reduce the heat to 375°F. Bake for 30 minutes, or until the bread registers 190°F on an instant-read thermometer or sounds hollow when rapped with your knuckles. Remove the bread from the pans and let cool on cooling racks for 15 to 20 minutes before cutting.

Cook's Tip on Breadmaking: The more you practice, the easier it will be to develop a feel for when the dough has the proper consistency. If you knead in too much flour or overknead the dough, it will feel dry and stiff, and the resulting loaf can be heavy. If you use too little flour or don't knead the dough enough, your loaf won't retain its shape during baking.

Resist the urge to knead the dough completely flat against your counter or board. This can cause your dough to become sticky.

For basic kneading, fold the dough toward you. Using the heels of one or both hands, push the dough forward and slightly down in an almost rocking motion. Rotate the dough a quarter turn and repeat. Follow this procedure until the dough is smooth and elastic. Add small amounts of flour when the dough starts to stick to the counter. Make note of the time you start, and knead for the amount of time called for in your recipe.

PER SERVING

calories 104	sodium 79 mg
total fat 1.0 g	**carbohydrates** 20 g
saturated fat 0.0 g	fiber 1 g
trans fat 0.0 g	sugars 2 g
polyunsaturated fat 0.5 g	**protein** 3 g
monounsaturated fat 0.5 g	**DIETARY EXCHANGES**
cholesterol 0 mg	1 1/2 starch

RYE BREAD

MAKES 2 LOAVES; EACH SERVES 18

Enjoy this whole-grain, low-sodium bread with a cup of soup such as Slow-Cooker Chicken Soup with Matzo Balls *(page 108) or use it to make a sandwich with a slice of* Thanksgiving Meat Loaf with Cranberry Glaze *(page 237).*

(continued)

Cooking spray

1/4 cup lukewarm water (105°F to 115°F)

2 1/4-ounce packages active dry yeast

1 3/4 cups fat-free milk, scalded and cooled to lukewarm

1/4 cup dark molasses

2 tablespoons canola or corn oil

2 1/2 cups rye flour

2 1/2 to 3 cups all-purpose flour, plus more as needed to dust the surface

1 tablespoon caraway seeds (optional)

Lightly spray a large bowl and a large baking sheet with cooking spray. Set aside.

Pour the water into a separate large bowl. Add the yeast, stirring to dissolve. Let stand for 5 minutes, or until the mixture bubbles.

Stir in the milk, molasses, and oil.

Gradually stir in the rye flour. Using a sturdy spoon, beat for about 30 seconds, or until smooth.

Gradually add some of the 2 1/2 cups all-purpose flour until the mixture becomes stiff enough to handle. Stir in the caraway seeds.

With some of the remaining all-purpose flour, lightly dust a flat surface. Turn out the dough. Knead for 6 to 8 minutes, gradually adding enough of the remaining flour to make the dough smooth and elastic. (The dough shouldn't be dry or stick to the surface.)

Put the dough in the prepared bowl, turning to coat the entire surface with cooking spray. Cover with a slightly damp dish towel. Let the dough rise in a warm, draft-free place (about 85°F) for about 1 hour, or until almost doubled in bulk, or when, if pressed with two fingers, an indentation remains in the dough.

Punch the dough down. Divide in half. Shape into round loaves. Let rest for 3 to 5 minutes. Transfer the loaves to the baking sheet.

Cover the dough with a slightly damp dish towel. Let the dough rise in a warm, draft-free place (about 85°F) for about 30 to 45 minutes, or until almost doubled in bulk.

While the dough is rising, preheat the oven to 425°F.

Bake the loaves for 25 to 30 minutes, or until the bread registers 190°F on an instant-read thermometer or sounds hollow when rapped with your knuckles. Transfer the baking sheet onto a cooling rack. Let the bread cool for 15 to 20 minutes before slicing.

PER SERVING

calories 77	sodium 7 mg
total fat 1.0 g	carbohydrates 15 g
saturated fat 0.0 g	fiber 1 g
trans fat 0.0 g	sugars 2 g
polyunsaturated fat 0.5 g	protein 2 g
monounsaturated fat 0.5 g	DIETARY EXCHANGES
cholesterol 0 mg	1 starch

PLUM-PECAN BREAD

MAKES 1 LOAF; SERVES 16

A slice of this fruit-and-nut-studded bread is perfect for breakfast along with a yogurt parfait, such as Blackberry-Pomegranate Yogurt Parfaits (page 479).

1 cup lukewarm water (105°F to 115°F)

1 1/4-ounce package active dry yeast

1/4 teaspoon sugar

1 1/2 cups whole-wheat flour

1 1/2 cups all-purpose flour and all-purpose flour for flouring surface, kneading, and rolling out dough, divided use

1/2 cup chopped dried plums

1/4 cup coarsely chopped pecans

2 tablespoons olive oil

1 tablespoon honey

1/4 teaspoon ground cinnamon

1/4 teaspoon salt

Cooking spray

Pour the water into a small bowl. Add the yeast and sugar, stirring to dissolve. Let stand for 5 minutes, or until the mixture bubbles.

Meanwhile, in a large bowl, stir together the whole-wheat flour and 1 1/2 cups all-purpose flour. Remove 1 cup of the mixture and set aside.

Stir the plums, pecans, oil, honey, cinnamon, and salt into the flour mixture in the large bowl.

Pour the yeast mixture into the flour mixture, stirring for about 30 seconds.

Stir in small amounts of the reserved 1 cup flour mixture until the dough starts to pull away from the side of the bowl.

Lightly flour a flat surface using the remaining all-purpose flour. Turn out the dough. Knead for 7 to 8 minutes, gradually adding enough all-purpose flour to make the dough smooth and elastic. You may not need all the flour. Shape into a ball.

Wipe the mixing bowl with a paper towel. Lightly spray the bowl with cooking spray. Put the dough in the bowl, turning to coat all sides. Cover the bowl with a slightly damp dish towel and put in a warm, draft-free place (about 85°F). Let the dough rise for 1 hour, or until doubled in bulk.

Lightly spray an 8 1/2 x 4 1/2 x 2 1/2-inch loaf pan and a cutting board with cooking spray.

Punch down the dough. Transfer to the cutting board. Press or roll the dough into a 10-inch square. Roll the dough into a cylinder and press the ends to seal. Fold the ends under the dough to form a loaf. Place the bread with the folded ends down in the loaf pan. Cover with a slightly damp dish towel and let rise in a warm, draft-free place (about 85°F) for 30 minutes, or until doubled in bulk.

While the dough is rising, preheat the oven to 375°F.

Bake the bread for 30 minutes, or until it registers 190°F on an instant-read thermometer or sounds hollow when rapped with your knuckles. Turn out onto a cooling rack. Let cool for 15 to 20 minutes before slicing.

PER SERVING

calories 122	sodium 38 mg
total fat 3.5 g	carbohydrates 21 g
saturated fat 0.5 g	fiber 2 g
trans fat 0.0 g	sugars 3 g
polyunsaturated fat 0.5 g	protein 3 g
monounsaturated fat 2.0 g	DIETARY EXCHANGES
cholesterol 0 mg	1 1/2 starch, 1/2 fat

CINNAMON BREAD

MAKES 2 LOAVES; EACH SERVES 18

While you're waiting for Quinoa Breakfast Bites *(page 477) to bake, toast this bread and melt a bit of light tub margarine on it while it's warm. Or pair it with* Stacked Sausage and Eggs *(page 476).*

> Cooking spray
> 1/4 cup lukewarm water (105°F to 115°F)
> 2 1/4-ounce packages active dry yeast
> 1 3/4 cups fat-free milk, scalded and cooled to lukewarm
> 3 tablespoons sugar
> 2 tablespoons canola or corn oil and 2 teaspoons canola or corn oil, divided use
> 3 cups all-purpose flour, 2 1/2 cups all-purpose flour, plus more as needed for flouring the surface, divided use
> 1/4 cup sugar
> 1 teaspoon ground cinnamon

Lightly spray a large bowl and two 9 x 5 x 3-inch loaf pans lightly with cooking spray. Set aside.

Pour the water into a separate large bowl. Add the yeast, stirring to dissolve. Let stand for 5 minutes, or until the mixture bubbles.

Stir in the milk, sugar, and 2 tablespoons oil.

Stir in 3 cups of flour. Using a sturdy spoon, beat for about 30 seconds, or until smooth.

Gradually add some of the remaining 2 1/2 cups flour until the mixture becomes stiff enough to handle.

With some of the remaining flour, lightly dust a flat surface. Turn out the dough. Knead for 6 to 8 minutes, gradually adding enough of the remaining flour to make the dough smooth and elastic. (The dough shouldn't be dry or stick to the surface.) Put the dough in the prepared bowl, turning to coat the entire surface with cooking spray. Cover with a slightly damp dish towel. Let the dough rise in a warm, draft-free place (about 85°F) until doubled in bulk, or when, if pressed

(continued)

with two fingers, an indentation remains in the dough. Punch the dough down. Divide in half. Shape into rectangular loaves. Let the loaves stand for 3 to 5 minutes.

Put the dough in the loaf pans. Cover each pan with a slightly damp dish towel. Let the dough rise in a warm, draft-free place (about 85°F) for about 30 to 45 minutes, or until doubled in bulk.

While the dough is rising, preheat the oven to 425°F.

In a small bowl, stir together the sugar and cinnamon. Using a pastry brush, brush the loaves with the remaining 2 teaspoons of oil. Sprinkle half the sugar mixture on top of each loaf.

Bake the loaves for 25 to 30 minutes, or until the bread registers 190°F on an instant-read thermometer or sounds hollow when rapped with your knuckles. Transfer the pans to a cooling rack. Using a metal spatula, loosen the bread from the sides of the pan. Let cool for 15 to 20 minutes before slicing.

PER SERVING

calories 94	sodium 6 mg
total fat 1.5 g	**carbohydrates** 18 g
saturated fat 0.0 g	fiber 1 g
trans fat 0.0 g	sugars 3 g
polyunsaturated fat 0.5 g	**protein** 3 g
monounsaturated fat 0.5 g	**DIETARY EXCHANGES**
cholesterol 0 mg	1 starch

RAISIN NUT BREAD

MAKES 2 LOAVES; EACH SERVES 18

Adding dried fruit and nuts to this bread gives it just the right amount of sweetness and crunch. Fire-and-Ice Cream Cheese Spread (page 14), which has a smidge of sweet of its own plus a kick of heat, is the perfect topper for this bread, especially when it's toasted.

Cooking spray
1/4 cup lukewarm water (105°F to 115°F)
2 1/4-ounce packages active dry yeast
1 3/4 cups fat-free milk, scalded and cooled to lukewarm

1/4 cup light molasses
2 tablespoons canola or corn oil
4 cups whole-wheat flour
1 to 1 1/2 cups all-purpose flour, plus more as needed for flouring the surface
1/2 cup raisins
1/2 cup coarsely chopped walnuts

Lightly spray a large bowl and two 9 x 5 x 3-inch loaf pans with cooking spray. Set aside.

Pour the water into a separate large bowl. Add the yeast, stirring to dissolve. Let stand for 5 minutes, or until the mixture bubbles.

Stir in the milk, molasses, and oil.

Gradually stir in the whole-wheat flour. Using a sturdy spoon, beat for about 30 seconds, or until smooth.

Gradually add some of the 1 cup all-purpose flour until the mixture becomes stiff enough to handle. Stir in the raisins and walnuts. With some of the remaining flour, lightly dust a flat surface. Turn out the dough. Knead for 6 to 8 minutes, gradually adding enough of the remaining flour to make the dough smooth and elastic. (The dough shouldn't be dry or stick to the surface.)

Put the dough in the prepared bowl, turning to coat the entire surface with cooking spray. Cover with a slightly damp dish towel. Let the dough rise in a warm, draft-free place (about 85°F) until doubled in bulk, or when, if pressed with two fingers, an indentation remains in the dough. Punch the dough down. Divide in half. Shape into rectangular loaves. Let the loaves stand for 3 to 5 minutes.

Put the dough in the loaf pans. Cover each pan with a slightly damp dish towel. Let the dough rise in a warm, draft-free place (about 85°F) for about 30 to 45 minutes, or until doubled in bulk.

While the dough is rising, preheat the oven to 425°F.

Bake the loaves for 25 to 30 minutes, or until the bread registers 190°F on an instant-read thermometer or sounds hollow when rapped with your knuckles. Transfer the pans to a cooling rack. Let the bread cool for 15 to 20 minutes before slicing.

PER SERVING

calories 97	**sodium** 7 mg
total fat 2.5 g	**carbohydrates** 17 g
saturated fat 0.0 g	fiber 2 g
trans fat 0.0 g	sugars 4 g
polyunsaturated fat 1.0 g	**protein** 3 g
monounsaturated fat 0.5 g	**DIETARY EXCHANGES**
cholesterol 0 mg	1 starch, 1/2 fat

CHAPATIS

MAKES 12; 1 PER SERVING

Chapati, a traditional Indian flatbread, is ideal for any meal. Serve it with all-fruit spread for breakfast or with an Indian curry, such as Chana Masala *(page 338), for dinner.*

> 2 cups whole-wheat flour, plus more as
>   needed for rolling out the dough
> 1/4 teaspoon salt
> 1 cup water
> 2 teaspoons canola or corn oil
> Cooking spray

In a large bowl, stir together the flour and salt. Slowly pour in the water while mixing with your other hand. Knead the dough for about 10 minutes, or until soft and pliable. Gently rub the oil onto the surface of the dough to prevent it from drying out. Cover the bowl with plastic wrap. Let stand for 30 minutes.

Divide the dough into 12 small balls. On a lightly floured surface, roll each ball into a very thin pancake about 4 to 6 inches in diameter, or use a tortilla press.

Lightly spray a griddle with cooking spray. Heat over high heat until very hot. Working in batches, cook the chapatis until half-done on the bottom. Turn over the chapatis. Cook until brown spots appear on the bottom. Turn over the chapatis again. Press the edges with a clean cloth until the chapatis puff up.

PER SERVING

calories 75	**sodium** 49 mg
total fat 1.5 g	**carbohydrates** 14 g
saturated fat 0.0 g	fiber 2 g
trans fat 0.0 g	sugars 0 g
polyunsaturated fat 0.5 g	**protein** 3 g
monounsaturated fat 0.5 g	**DIETARY EXCHANGES**
cholesterol 0 mg	1 starch

PEPPERCORN-DILL FLATBREAD

MAKES 60; 4 PER SERVING

Enjoy flatbread as a snack by itself or with a heart-healthy dip or spread, such as Roasted-Pepper Hummus *(page 13) or* Yellow Split Pea Dip *(page 12).*

> 2 cups all-purpose flour for flouring the
>   surface, kneading, and rolling out the
>   dough, plus more as needed
> 1 cup whole-wheat flour
> 1 tablespoon olive oil
> 2 teaspoons baking powder
> 2 teaspoons celery seeds
> 2 teaspoons dried dillweed, crumbled
> 1 teaspoon sugar
> 1 teaspoon pepper (coarsely ground
>   preferred)
> 1/2 teaspoon baking soda
> 1/4 teaspoon salt
> 1 1/4 cups low-fat buttermilk
> Cooking spray

In a large bowl, stir together 2 cups all-purpose flour, the whole wheat flour, oil, baking powder, celery seeds, dillweed, sugar, pepper, baking soda, and salt. Make a well in the center.

Pour the buttermilk into the well. Stir until the mixture forms a ball.

Lightly flour a flat surface using the remaining all-purpose flour. Turn out the dough. Knead for 2 minutes. Return the dough to the bowl. Cover with a slightly damp dish towel. Let the dough rest for 10 to 15 minutes.

Preheat the oven to 400°F. Lightly spray two large baking sheets with cooking spray.

(continued)

Lightly flour the flat surface again if more flour is needed. Roll out the dough to 1/8-inch thickness. Using a pizza cutter or sharp knife, cut the dough into strips about 1 1/2 inches wide by 4 inches long (you should have about 60). Transfer to the baking sheets. Prick each strip with a fork.

Bake for 15 minutes, or until crisp. Transfer the baking sheets to cooling racks. Let the flatbread cool for 15 to 20 minutes. Store in an airtight container for up to seven days.

PER SERVING

calories 107	**sodium** 157 mg
total fat 1.5 g	**carbohydrates** 20 g
saturated fat 0.5 g	fiber 1 g
trans fat 0.0 g	sugars 1 g
polyunsaturated fat 0.5 g	**protein** 4 g
monounsaturated fat 1.0 g	**DIETARY EXCHANGES**
cholesterol 1 mg	1 1/2 starch

DUTCH HONEY BREAD

MAKES 1 LOAF; SERVES 16

This Dutch quick bread is traditionally eaten for breakfast because it's more sweet than savory. Try it with all-fruit spread and enjoy it as a side to your favorite style of eggs.

Cooking spray
2 cups unsifted all-purpose flour
1/4 cup brown sugar
1 tablespoon baking powder
2 teaspoons ground cinnamon
1 teaspoon baking soda
1/4 teaspoon ground cloves
1/4 teaspoon ground nutmeg
1/4 teaspoon salt
1 cup low-fat buttermilk
1 large egg, beaten well using a fork
1/4 cup honey

Preheat the oven to 350°F. Lightly spray a 9 x 5 x 3-inch loaf pan with cooking spray.

In a large mixing bowl, stir together the flour, brown sugar, baking powder, cinnamon, baking soda, cloves, nutmeg, and salt.

Pour in the buttermilk, egg, and honey, stirring until the flour mixture is just moistened, but no flour is visible. Don't overmix. Pour the batter into the pan, gently smoothing the top.

Bake for 45 minutes to 1 hour, or until a wooden toothpick inserted in the center comes out clean. The finished bread will have a very firm crust.

PER SERVING

calories 98	**sodium** 212 mg
total fat 0.5 g	**carbohydrates** 21 g
saturated fat 0.0 g	fiber 1 g
trans fat 0.0 g	sugars 9 g
polyunsaturated fat 0.0 g	**protein** 3 g
monounsaturated fat 0.0 g	**DIETARY EXCHANGES**
cholesterol 12 mg	1 1/2 starch

JALAPEÑO CHEESE BREAD

MAKES 1 LOAF; SERVES 20

Smoked paprika and beer add tempting flavors to this easy-to-prepare quick bread that's the perfect complement to a bowl of Turkey Chili *(page 238).*

Cooking spray
3 cups white whole-wheat flour, plus more as needed for dusting hands
1 teaspoon baking soda
1/2 teaspoon baking powder
1 cup shredded low-fat Cheddar cheese
2 tablespoons drained and chopped pickled jalapeño
1 1/2 cups beer (light or nonalcoholic)
1 tablespoon olive oil
1/2 teaspoon smoked or regular paprika

Preheat the oven to 350°F. Lightly spray a large baking sheet with cooking spray.

In a large bowl, sift together the flour, baking soda, and baking powder.

Stir in the Cheddar and jalapeño. Make a well in the center.

Pour the beer and oil into the well. Stir until the flour absorbs the liquids (the mixture will be slightly sticky). Spoon the dough onto the center of the baking sheet.

Using lightly floured hands, shape the dough into a 9 x 6-inch oval loaf. Sprinkle the paprika over the loaf.

Bake for 40 to 45 minutes, or until the bread is golden brown and sounds hollow when rapped with your knuckles. Transfer the bread to a cooling rack. Let cool for at least 15 minutes before slicing.

Cook's Tip on Smoked Paprika: Smoked paprika, which comes from Spain, is like chipotle peppers without the heat. Use it to enhance refried beans, salsa, dips, rice dishes, marinades, and many other foods that would work well with a smoky flavor.

PER SERVING

calories 82	**sodium** 128 mg
total fat 1.5 g	**carbohydrates** 11 g
saturated fat 0.5 g	fiber 2 g
trans fat 0.0 g	sugars 1 g
polyunsaturated fat 0.0 g	**protein** 4 g
monounsaturated fat 0.5 g	**DIETARY EXCHANGES**
cholesterol 1 mg	1 starch

PARMESAN-HERB BREADSTICKS

MAKES 18; 1 PER SERVING

Nothing soaks up the last spoonful of spaghetti sauce, such as Fresh Tomato and Roasted Red Bell Pepper Sauce (page 434), or gravy, such as Mushroom Gravy (page 428), quite like these soft homemade breadsticks.

 Cooking spray
 2 cups all-purpose flour, plus more as needed for shaping breadsticks and dusting hands
 1 cup whole-wheat flour
 2 tablespoons minced green onions (green part only)
 1 tablespoon chopped fresh dillweed or 1 teaspoon dried dillweed, crumbled
 1 teaspoon baking soda
 1/2 teaspoon baking powder
 1/4 teaspoon pepper
 1/8 teaspoon salt
 1 1/2 cups low-fat buttermilk

 2 tablespoons olive oil
 2 tablespoons shredded or grated Parmesan cheese

Preheat the oven to 350°F. Lightly spray a large baking sheet with cooking spray.

In a large bowl, stir together the flours, green onions, dillweed, baking soda, baking powder, pepper, and salt. Make a well in the center.

Pour the buttermilk and oil into the well. Stir just until moistened. Don't overmix.

With lightly floured hands, divide the dough into 18 pieces. Shape each piece into a 4-inch-long cylinder (slightly wetting your hands with cold water will help keep the dough from sticking). Place the cylinders about 1 inch apart on the baking sheet. Sprinkle the Parmesan over the cylinders.

Bake for 20 to 22 minutes, or until golden brown. For a slightly crisp outside, transfer the sticks to a cooling rack. Let cool for 5 minutes before serving. For slightly warmer and less crisp sticks, put them in a bread basket lined with a dish towel. Cover and let stand for 5 minutes.

PER SERVING

calories 97	**sodium** 129 mg
total fat 2.0 g	**carbohydrates** 17 g
saturated fat 0.5 g	fiber 1 g
trans fat 0.0 g	sugars 1 g
polyunsaturated fat 0.5 g	**protein** 3 g
monounsaturated fat 1.0 g	**DIETARY EXCHANGES**
cholesterol 1 mg	1 starch

RAISIN BRAN BREAD

MAKES 1 LOAF; SERVES 16

Eat your cereal and your toast all in one with this delicious breakfast bread. Try pairing it with Cantaloupe and Honeydew Parfaits (page 480), Chèvre Omelet with Herbs (page 474), or Stacked Sausage and Eggs (page 476).

(continued)

Cooking spray
1 cup white whole-wheat flour
1 teaspoon baking soda
1/2 teaspoon salt
1/4 teaspoon ground cinnamon
1/4 teaspoon ground nutmeg
3/4 cup low-fat buttermilk
1/2 cup bran-type cereal
2 tablespoons light tub margarine, melted
1 large egg
1 teaspoon vanilla extract
1/2 cup raisins

Preheat the oven to 350°F. Lightly spray a 9 x 5 x 3-inch loaf pan with cooking spray.

In a large bowl, sift together the flour, baking soda, salt, cinnamon, and nutmeg.

In a medium bowl, stir together the buttermilk, cereal, margarine, egg, and vanilla. Pour into the flour mixture, stirring just until moistened but no flour is visible. Don't overmix; the batter should be lumpy. Stir in the raisins. Pour the batter into the pan, smoothing the top.

Bake for 40 to 45 minutes, or until a wooden toothpick inserted into the center comes out clean.

Transfer the pan to a cooling rack. Let stand for 5 minutes. Using a spatula, loosen the bread from the side of the pan. Turn out onto the cooling rack. Let cool completely before slicing.

PER SERVING

calories 61	sodium 185 mg
total fat 1.0 g	carbohydrates 11 g
saturated fat 0.0 g	fiber 2 g
trans fat 0.0 g	sugars 4 g
polyunsaturated fat 0.5 g	protein 2 g
monounsaturated fat 0.5 g	DIETARY EXCHANGES
cholesterol 12 mg	1 starch

HONEY-WHEAT OATMEAL BREAD

MAKES 1 LOAF; SERVES 16

Just stirring and baking is all this bread needs—no proofing of the yeast, kneading, or rising time. There's nothing like a slice of fresh bread to soak up soups or sauces—or just enjoy by itself.

Cooking spray
1 1/2 cups all-purpose flour
1/2 cup whole-wheat flour
1/2 cup uncooked quick-cooking oatmeal and 2 tablespoons uncooked quick-cooking oatmeal, divided use
1/4 cup toasted wheat germ
2 teaspoons baking powder
1 teaspoon baking soda
1/4 teaspoon salt
1 1/2 cups low-fat buttermilk
1/4 cup egg substitute
2 tablespoons honey
1 tablespoon olive oil

Preheat the oven to 375°F. Lightly spray an 8 1/2 x 4 1/2 x 2 1/2-inch loaf pan with cooking spray.

In a large bowl, stir together the flours, 1/2 cup oatmeal, the wheat germ, baking powder, baking soda, and salt. Make a well in the center.

Pour the buttermilk, egg substitute, honey, and oil into the well. Stir until the flour mixture is just moistened but no flour is visible. Don't overmix; the batter may have a few lumps. Spoon into the pan, gently smoothing the top. Sprinkle the remaining 2 tablespoons oatmeal over the loaf.

Bake for 40 to 45 minutes, or until a wooden toothpick inserted in the center comes out clean. Transfer the pan to a cooling rack. Let cool for 5 minutes. Turn the bread out onto the rack. Let cool for 10 minutes before slicing.

PER SERVING

calories 101	sodium 198 mg
total fat 1.5 g	carbohydrates 18 g
saturated fat 0.5 g	fiber 1 g
trans fat 0.0 g	sugars 4 g
polyunsaturated fat 0.5 g	protein 4 g
monounsaturated fat 1.0 g	DIETARY EXCHANGES
cholesterol 1 mg	1 starch

CURRANT WALNUT BREAD

MAKES 1 LOAF; SERVES 16

This fruit-nut bread makes a good complement to an egg dish, such as Country-Style Breakfast Casserole (page 473). While the bread is in the oven, prepare the casserole and let them bake together.

Cooking spray
1 1/2 cups currants or raisins
2 tablespoons canola or corn oil
2 teaspoons baking soda
1 cup boiling water
2 cups whole-wheat flour
3/4 cup chopped walnuts, dry-roasted
2/3 cup brown sugar
1 large egg or 2 large egg whites, well beaten using a fork

Preheat the oven to 350°F. Lightly spray an 8 1/2 x 4 1/2 x 2 1/2-inch loaf pan with cooking spray.

In a large bowl, stir together the currants, oil, and baking soda with the boiling water. Let stand until cool. Add the remaining ingredients. Stir together just until moistened but no flour is visible. Don't overmix; the batter will be lumpy.

Spoon the batter into the pan, smoothing the top. Bake for 40 to 45 minutes, or until a wooden toothpick inserted in the center comes out clean.

Transfer the pan to a cooling rack. Let stand for 10 minutes. Using a spatula, loosen the bread from the side of the pan. Turn the bread out onto the rack. Let cool for 10 minutes before slicing.

Cook's Tip: Soaking the dried fruit before baking first will keep it plump and moist.

PER SERVING

calories 180	**sodium** 166 mg
total fat 6.0 g	**carbohydrates** 31 g
saturated fat 1.0 g	fiber 3 g
trans fat 0.0 g	sugars 18 g
polyunsaturated fat 3.5 g	**protein** 4 g
monounsaturated fat 2.0 g	**DIETARY EXCHANGES**
cholesterol 12 mg	1 starch, 1 fruit, 1 fat

IRISH BROWN SODA BREAD

MAKES 1 LOAF; SERVES 20

The classic recipe for traditional soda bread was popular in Ireland in the mid-1800s; it didn't keep long so fresh loaves were baked every few days. This version keeps for about four days; leftovers can be frozen. Enjoy a slice for breakfast spread with all-fruit preserves or with stew or soup for dinner.

Cooking spray
3 cups whole-wheat flour
1 1/2 cups sifted all-purpose flour
1 tablespoon canola or corn oil
1 tablespoon sugar
1 teaspoon salt
1 teaspoon baking soda
1 1/2 cups raisins (optional)
3 tablespoons caraway seeds (optional)
1 1/2 cups low-fat buttermilk and 1/4 cup low-fat buttermilk, as needed, divided use

Preheat the oven to 425°F. Lightly spray a large baking sheet with cooking spray.

In a large bowl, stir together the flours, oil, sugar, salt, and baking soda. Gently stir in the raisins and caraway seeds. Make a well in the center.

Pour 1 1/2 cups buttermilk into the well. Stir until the flour mixture is just moistened but no flour is visible. Gradually add the remaining 1/4 cup buttermilk if necessary to make the dough soft but not sticky.

Lightly flour a flat surface. Turn out the dough. Knead for 15 to 20 seconds. Form the dough into a ball. With the palm of your hand, flatten the dough into a circle about 1 1/2 inches thick. With a knife, cut a cross on the top to prevent cracking during baking.

Bake for 25 minutes. Reduce the heat to 350°F. Bake for 15 minutes, or until a wooden toothpick inserted in the center comes out clean.

Transfer the baking sheet to a cooling rack. Let cool completely.

(continued)

Cook's Tip: For best results, slice 24 hours after baking.

PER SERVING

calories 113	sodium 202 mg
total fat 1.5 g	carbohydrates 22 g
saturated fat 0.5 g	fiber 2 g
trans fat 0.0 g	sugars 2 g
polyunsaturated fat 0.5 g	protein 4 g
monounsaturated fat 0.5 g	DIETARY EXCHANGES
cholesterol 1 mg	1 1/2 starch

CINNAMON-NUTMEG BREAD

MAKES 1 LOAF; SERVES 16

This sweet bread is a healthy alternative to sugary, fat-laden cinnamon rolls. Have a slice with a cup of tea for breakfast.

Cooking spray
2/3 cup sugar
1/4 cup light tub margarine
1 large egg, well beaten
1/4 cup unsweetened applesauce
2 cups sifted white whole-wheat flour
1 teaspoon ground cinnamon
1 teaspoon ground nutmeg
1/2 teaspoon baking powder
1/2 teaspoon baking soda
1 cup low-fat buttermilk

Preheat the oven to 350°F. Lightly spray a 9 x 5 x 3-inch loaf pan with cooking spray.

In a large mixing bowl, using an electric mixer on medium speed, beat the sugar and margarine for 2 to 3 minutes, or until creamed. Add the egg and applesauce. Beat until the mixture is well blended.

Put the remaining ingredients except the buttermilk in a medium bowl. Sift together twice.

Alternately add the flour mixture and buttermilk to the sugar mixture, beginning and ending with the flour and stirring after each addition until the mixture is moistened, but no flour is visible. Pour the batter into the loaf pan, gently smoothing the top.

Bake for 45 minutes to 1 hour, or until a wooden toothpick inserted in the center comes out clean. Let cool in the pan for 10 minutes. Using a metal spatula, loosen the bread from the sides of the pan. Turn out onto a cooling rack. Let cool completely.

PER SERVING

calories 106	sodium 95 mg
total fat 2.0 g	carbohydrates 19 g
saturated fat 0.0 g	fiber 2 g
trans fat 0.0 g	sugars 10 g
polyunsaturated fat 0.5 g	protein 3 g
monounsaturated fat 1.0 g	DIETARY EXCHANGES
cholesterol 12 mg	1 1/2 starch

WHOLE-WHEAT APRICOT BREAD

MAKES 1 LOAF; SERVES 16

Bits of dried apricot and walnut flavor each bite of this quick bread that's a natural with your morning coffee or a cold glass of fat-free milk.

Cooking spray
1 cup chopped dried apricots
1 cup whole-wheat flour
1 cup all-purpose flour
1/2 cup sugar
1/2 cup finely chopped walnuts, dry-roasted
2 teaspoons baking powder
1/4 teaspoon baking soda
1/2 cup unsweetened applesauce
1/2 cup fat-free evaporated milk
1/4 cup egg substitute
1 tablespoon canola or corn oil

Preheat the oven to 350°F. Lightly spray a 9 x 5 x 3-inch loaf pan with cooking spray.

In a large bowl, stir together the apricots, flours, sugar, nuts, baking powder, and baking soda.

In a small bowl, whisk together the remaining ingredients. Add to the apricot mixture. Stir just until the dry ingredients are moistened but no flour is visible. Don't overmix; the batter should be slightly lumpy. Pour into the loaf pan, gently smoothing the top.

Bake for 40 to 50 minutes, or until a wooden toothpick inserted in the center comes out clean. Transfer the pan to a cooling rack. Using a metal spatula, loosen the bread from the sides of the pan. Turn out onto the rack. Let cool for 1 hour before slicing.

BANANA PECAN BREAD

MAKES 1 LOAF; SERVES 16

A classic quick bread gets a healthy makeover with more fiber and less saturated fat and added sugar. Tuck a slice into your brown-bag lunch or even serve it as dessert, garnished with sliced bananas or fresh berries.

Cooking spray
3/4 cup whole-wheat flour
3/4 cup all-purpose flour
1/2 cup firmly packed light brown sugar
1 1/2 teaspoons baking powder
1 teaspoon ground cinnamon
1/2 teaspoon baking soda
1/8 teaspoon salt
3 very ripe medium bananas, mashed (about 1 cup)
1/2 cup chopped pecans, dry-roasted
1/2 cup egg whites (3 to 4 large) or egg substitute
3 tablespoons canola or corn oil
1 teaspoon vanilla extract

Preheat the oven to 350°F. Lightly spray a 9 x 5 x 3-inch loaf pan with cooking spray.

In a large bowl, stir together the flours, brown sugar, baking powder, cinnamon, baking soda, and salt.

Stir the remaining ingredients into the flour mixture until just moistened but no flour is visible. Don't overmix; the batter will be slightly lumpy. Spoon the batter into the pan, gently smoothing the top.

Bake for 45 to 50 minutes, or until a wooden toothpick inserted in the center comes out clean. Transfer the pan to a cooling rack. Let the bread cool for 10 minutes. Using a metal spatula, loosen the bread from the sides of the pan. Turn out onto the cooling rack. Let cool completely, about 1 hour, before slicing (a serrated knife works best).

CRANBERRY BREAD

MAKES 1 LOAF; SERVES 16

Freeze some extra cranberries when they're plentiful to enjoy this bread all year long.

Cooking spray
2 cups white whole-wheat flour
2/3 cup firmly packed light brown sugar
2 teaspoons baking powder
1/2 teaspoon baking soda
1/4 teaspoon ground allspice or ground nutmeg
1/8 teaspoon salt
1 cup fresh or frozen cranberries, chopped (don't thaw if frozen)
2 teaspoons grated orange zest
3/4 cup fresh orange juice
1/4 cup egg substitute
1 tablespoon canola or corn oil
2 teaspoons vanilla extract

(continued)

Preheat the oven to 350°F. Lightly spray an 8 1/2 x 4 1/2 x 2 1/2-inch loaf pan with cooking spray.

In a large bowl, sift together the flour, brown sugar, baking powder, baking soda, allspice, and salt. Make a well in the center.

In a medium bowl, stir together the remaining ingredients. Pour into the well. Stir just until the dry ingredients are moistened but no flour is visible. Don't overmix; the batter should be slightly lumpy. Pour into the loaf pan, gently smoothing the top.

Bake for 50 minutes to 1 hour, or until a wooden toothpick inserted in the center comes out clean. Using a metal spatula, loosen the bread from the sides of the pan. Turn out onto a cooling rack. Let cool before slicing.

PER SERVING

calories 105	sodium 118 mg
total fat 1.0 g	carbohydrates 20 g
saturated fat 0.0 g	fiber 2 g
trans fat 0.0 g	sugars 11 g
polyunsaturated fat 0.5 g	protein 3 g
monounsaturated fat 0.5 g	DIETARY EXCHANGES
cholesterol 0 mg	1 1/2 starch

Preheat the oven to 350°F. Lightly spray a 9 x 5 x 3-inch loaf pan with cooking spray.

In a large bowl, stir together the flours, wheat germ, sugar, walnuts, baking powder, and baking soda.

Add the remaining ingredients. Stir just until the dry ingredients are moistened but no flour is visible. Don't overmix; the batter should be slightly lumpy. Pour into the loaf pan, gently smoothing the top.

Bake for 55 minutes, or until a wooden toothpick inserted in the center comes out clean. Using a metal spatula, loosen the bread from the sides of the pan. Turn out onto a cooling rack. Let cool before slicing.

PER SERVING

calories 141	sodium 125 mg
total fat 2.5 g	carbohydrates 26 g
saturated fat 0.5 g	fiber 2 g
trans fat 0.0 g	sugars 9 g
polyunsaturated fat 1.5 g	protein 4 g
monounsaturated fat 1.0 g	DIETARY EXCHANGES
cholesterol 0 mg	1 1/2 starch, 1/2 fat

ORANGE WHEAT BREAD

MAKES 1 LOAF; SERVES 16

This nutty, citrusy bread is an ideal complement to Potato and Egg Scramble (page 474).

Cooking spray
2 cups all-purpose flour
1/2 cup whole-wheat flour
1/2 cup toasted wheat germ
1/2 cup sugar
1/4 cup chopped walnuts, dry-roasted
1 tablespoon baking powder
1/2 teaspoon baking soda
2 tablespoons grated orange zest
1 cup fresh orange juice
1/3 cup unsweetened applesauce
1/4 cup egg substitute
1 tablespoon canola or corn oil

VELVET PUMPKIN BREAD

MAKES 1 LOAF; SERVES 16

It's sweet and spicy and has a wonderful texture. In fact, this bread is so delicious you're not going to want to wait until the fall to make it. Try it toasted and spread with light tub margarine.

Cooking spray
1 cup canned solid-pack pumpkin (not pie filling)
1/2 cup egg substitute
1/3 cup fat-free milk
2 tablespoons light tub margarine, melted
1 tablespoon canola or corn oil
2 cups white whole-wheat flour
2 teaspoons baking powder
1 teaspoon ground cinnamon
1/2 teaspoon ground ginger
1/4 teaspoon ground nutmeg
1/8 teaspoon salt

1/2 cup chopped pecans, dry-roasted
1/3 cup sugar
1/3 cup firmly packed light brown sugar

Preheat the oven to 350°F. Lightly spray a 9 x 5 x 3-inch loaf pan with cooking spray.

In a medium bowl, whisk together the pumpkin, egg substitute, milk, margarine, and oil.

In a large bowl, sift together the flour, baking powder, cinnamon, ginger, nutmeg, and salt.

Stir the pecans and sugars into the flour mixture. Make a well in the center.

Pour the pumpkin mixture into the well. Stir just until the flour mixture is moistened but no flour is visible. Don't overmix; the batter should be slightly lumpy. Pour into the loaf pan, gently smoothing the top.

Bake for 1 hour, or until a wooden toothpick inserted in the center comes out clean. Using a metal spatula, loosen the bread from the side of the pan. Turn out onto a cooling rack. Let cool before slicing.

Cook's Tip on Leftover Canned Pumpkin: Store the leftover pumpkin in an airtight plastic container in the refrigerator for up to one week and use it in one of the other recipes in this book, such as Curried Pumpkin Soup (page 62) or Perfect Pumpkin Pancakes (page 468). For longer storage, put the pumpkin in ice cube trays to freeze. Transfer the frozen pumpkin cubes to a resealable plastic freezer bag. Add the cubes to soups or stews. Or freeze the remaining pumpkin in an airtight plastic container. Thaw in the refrigerator before using.

PER SERVING

calories 132	sodium 99 mg
total fat 4.0 g	carbohydrates 20 g
saturated fat 0.5 g	fiber 3 g
trans fat 0.0 g	sugars 10 g
polyunsaturated fat 1.0 g	protein 4 g
monounsaturated fat 2.5 g	DIETARY EXCHANGES
cholesterol 0 mg	1 1/2 starch, 1/2 fat

CHERRY-NUT BREAD

MAKES 1 LOAF; SERVES 16

This deliciously sweet bread celebrates the classic marriage of cherries and almonds. It makes a great snack with a glass of fat-free milk.

Cooking spray
2 cups white whole-wheat flour
1/2 cup firmly packed light brown sugar
2 teaspoons baking powder
1/4 teaspoon salt
1/4 teaspoon baking soda
1 cup fat-free milk
1/4 cup egg substitute
1 teaspoon grated orange zest
1/2 cup chopped almonds, dry-roasted
1/2 cup dried cherries

Preheat the oven to 350°F. Lightly spray an 8 1/2 x 4 1/2 x 2 1/2-inch loaf pan with cooking spray.

In a large bowl, sift together the flour, brown sugar, baking powder, salt, and baking soda.

In a separate large bowl, whisk together the milk, egg substitute, and orange zest.

Add the flour mixture, almonds, and cherries to the milk mixture. Stir just until the dry ingredients are moistened but no flour is visible. Don't overmix; the batter should be slightly lumpy. Pour into the loaf pan, gently smoothing the top.

Bake for 40 minutes, or until a wooden toothpick inserted in the center comes out clean. Using a metal spatula, loosen the bread from the sides of the pan. Turn out onto a cooling rack. Let cool before slicing.

PER SERVING

calories 117	sodium 122 mg
total fat 2.0 g	carbohydrates 21 g
saturated fat 0.0 g	fiber 2 g
trans fat 0.0 g	sugars 10 g
polyunsaturated fat 0.5 g	protein 4 g
monounsaturated fat 1.0 g	DIETARY EXCHANGES
cholesterol 0 mg	1 1/2 starch

ZUCCHINI BREAD WITH PISTACHIOS

MAKES 2 LOAVES; EACH SERVES 16

Some surprise ingredients—Fuji apple, olive oil, and pistachios—add a fruity nuance, color, and crunch that set this zucchini bread apart from traditional recipes.

Cooking spray
2 cups all-purpose flour
1 cup whole-wheat flour
1 cup sugar
1/3 cup firmly packed light brown sugar
1/4 cup chopped unsalted pistachios
1 teaspoon ground cinnamon
1 teaspoon baking powder
1 teaspoon baking soda
1/8 teaspoon salt
2 cups shredded zucchini (about 12 ounces)
1 medium Fuji or Granny Smith apple, peeled and shredded (about 1 cup)
3/4 cup egg substitute
1/2 cup 100% apple juice
2 tablespoons olive oil

Preheat the oven to 375°F. Lightly spray two 8 1/2 x 4 1/2 x 2 1/2-inch loaf pans with cooking spray.

In a medium bowl, stir together the flours, sugars, pistachios, cinnamon, baking powder, baking soda, and salt.

Add the remaining ingredients. Stir just until the dry ingredients are moistened but no flour is visible. Don't overmix; the batter should be slightly lumpy. Pour into the loaf pans, gently smoothing the tops.

Bake for 55 minutes to 1 hour, or until a wooden toothpick inserted in the center comes out clean. Using a metal spatula, loosen the bread from the sides of the pans. Turn out onto a cooling rack. Let cool for 20 minutes before slicing.

Cook's Tip: You can bake this bread in two 8-inch square baking pans (lightly sprayed with cooking spray) for 35 to 40 minutes, or until a wooden toothpick inserted in the center comes out clean. Cool as directed above.

PER SERVING

calories 96	**sodium** 74 mg
total fat 1.5 g	**carbohydrates** 19 g
saturated fat 0.0 g	fiber 1 g
trans fat 0.0 g	sugars 10 g
polyunsaturated fat 0.5 g	**protein** 2 g
monounsaturated fat 1.0 g	**DIETARY EXCHANGES**
cholesterol 0 mg	1 1/2 starch

EASY REFRIGERATOR ROLLS

MAKES 36; 1 PER SERVING

Enjoy these yeast rolls at your convenience. Mix and refrigerate the simple dough. When you want homemade rolls, shape them, let them rise, bake them, and enjoy!

1/4 cup lukewarm water and 1 cup lukewarm water (105°F to 115°F), divided use
1 1/4-ounce package active dry yeast
2 large egg whites
1/4 cup canola or corn oil
1/2 cup sugar
1 teaspoon salt
4 cups whole-wheat or white whole-wheat flour
Cooking spray

Pour 1/4 cup water into a small bowl. Add the yeast, stirring to dissolve. Let stand for 5 minutes, or until the mixture bubbles.

In a large bowl, lightly whisk the egg whites. Add the following ingredients in order, stirring after each addition: oil, sugar, yeast mixture, salt, the remaining 1 cup water, and the flour. Cover and refrigerate for 12 hours to four days.

Lightly spray a baking sheet with cooking spray. Make 36 rolls in your favorite shape. Transfer to the baking sheet. Cover with a slightly damp dish towel. Let rise in a warm, draft-free place (about 85°F) for 2 hours.

Preheat the oven to 375°F.

Bake for 10 minutes, or until lightly browned.

calories 72	**sodium** 68 mg
total fat 2.0 g	**carbohydrates** 13 g
saturated fat 0.0 g	fiber 2 g
trans fat 0.0 g	sugars 3 g
polyunsaturated fat 0.5 g	**protein** 2 g
monounsaturated fat 1.0 g	**DIETARY EXCHANGES**
cholesterol 0 mg	1 starch

YOGURT DINNER ROLLS

MAKES 18; 1 PER SERVING

Tangy yogurt and fragrant herbs flavor these rolls that are a delicious accompaniment for soup or salad.

  1/4 cup lukewarm water (105°F to 115°F)

  2 tablespoons sugar

  1 1/4-ounce package active dry yeast

  1 cup fat-free plain yogurt

  1 large egg

  2 tablespoons light tub margarine, melted

  2 tablespoons grated or minced onion

  2 teaspoons dried basil, crumbled

  1 teaspoon dried oregano, crumbled

  1 1/2 cups white whole-wheat flour,

      1 1/4 cups white whole-wheat flour, plus more as needed for dusting hands, divided use

  1/2 teaspoon salt

  Cooking spray

Pour the water, sugar, and yeast into a medium bowl, stirring to dissolve. Let stand for 5 minutes, or until the mixture bubbles. Stir in the yogurt, egg, margarine, onion, basil, and oregano.

In a large mixing bowl, stir together 1 1/2 cups flour and the salt.

Pour in the yogurt mixture. Using an electric mixer on low speed, beat for 30 seconds. Increase the speed to high and beat for 3 minutes. Stir in 1 1/4 cups flour. (The dough will be moist and sticky.)

Lightly spray a large bowl with cooking spray. Add the dough, turning to coat. Cover with a clean, damp dish towel. Let rise in a warm, draft-

free place (about 85°F) for 1 1/2 hours. Punch down the dough. Lightly spray a 13 x 9 x 2-inch baking pan with cooking spray. Lightly flour your hands. Form the dough into 18 balls. Put in the pan. Cover with a clean, dry dish towel. Let rise in a warm, draft-free place (about 85°F) for 40 minutes.

Preheat the oven to 400°F. Bake for 15 minutes.

calories 85	**sodium** 89 mg
total fat 1.0 g	**carbohydrates** 14 g
saturated fat 0.0 g	fiber 2 g
trans fat 0.0 g	sugars 3 g
polyunsaturated fat 0.5 g	**protein** 4 g
monounsaturated fat 0.5 g	**DIETARY EXCHANGES**
cholesterol 11 mg	1 starch

SOUTHERN RAISED BISCUITS

MAKES 30 BISCUITS; SERVES 15

You don't need to be from the South to love these tall, flaky biscuits. Try them with Seafood Jambalaya *(page 174) or* Louisiana Gumbo with Seitan *(page 366).*

  1 cup low-fat buttermilk, slightly warmed (105°F to 115°F)

  1 1/4-ounce package active dry yeast

  2 1/2 cups all-purpose flour, plus more as needed for flouring surface, kneading, rolling out dough, and cutting biscuits

  1/4 cup sugar

  1/2 teaspoon baking soda

  1/2 teaspoon salt

  1/4 cup canola or corn oil

  Cooking spray

Pour the buttermilk into a small bowl. Add the yeast, stirring to dissolve. Let stand for 5 minutes, or until the mixture bubbles.

In a large bowl, stir together 2 1/2 cups flour, the sugar, baking soda, and salt.

Add the buttermilk mixture and oil to the flour mixture. Stir just until the ingredients hold together. Don't overmix.

(continued)

Lightly flour a flat surface. Turn out the dough. Knead gently 20 to 30 times. Roll out or pat to 1/4-inch thickness. With a floured 1-inch biscuit cutter, cut out 60 biscuits, reflouring the biscuit cutter as needed. Lightly spray the top of each biscuit with cooking spray.

Lightly spray a baking sheet with cooking spray. Put 30 biscuits on it. Put a second biscuit on top of each. Cover with a slightly damp dish towel. Let rise in a warm, draft-free place (about 85°F) for about 2 hours.

Preheat the oven to 375°F.

Bake the biscuits for 12 to 15 minutes, or until light golden brown on top.

PER SERVING

calories 130	**sodium** 137 mg
total fat 4.0 g	**carbohydrates** 20 g
saturated fat 0.5 g	fiber 1 g
trans fat 0.0 g	sugars 4 g
polyunsaturated fat 1.0 g	**protein** 3 g
monounsaturated fat 2.5 g	**DIETARY EXCHANGES**
cholesterol 1 mg	1 1/2 starch, 1/2 fat

In a large bowl, stir together the flour and salt. Gradually pour in the egg white mixture. Using an electric mixer on medium speed, beat after each addition until well blended. Increase the speed to high and beat for 1 to 2 minutes.

Fill each popover cup half full of batter. Put the pan in a cold oven. Set the oven to 400°F. Bake the popovers for 45 minutes to 1 hour, or until light golden brown.

Cook's Tip: If you don't have a popover pan, substitute 12 large (about 9-ounce) or 18 medium (about 5-ounce) custard cups lightly sprayed with cooking spray. Muffin pans won't give you consistent results.

PER SERVING

calories 122	**sodium** 101 mg
total fat 3.0 g	**carbohydrates** 18 g
saturated fat 0.0 g	fiber 1 g
trans fat 0.0 g	sugars 2 g
polyunsaturated fat 1.0 g	**protein** 5 g
monounsaturated fat 1.5 g	**DIETARY EXCHANGES**
cholesterol 1 mg	1 starch, 1/2 lean meat

COLD-OVEN POPOVERS

MAKES 12; 1 PER SERVING

A popover is a light, hollow roll made with a batter similar to Yorkshire pudding. The high proportion of liquid in the batter creates steam that puffs up the bread, making it "pop over" the sides of the pan.

Cooking spray
6 large egg whites
2 cups fat-free milk
2 tablespoons canola or corn oil
1 tablespoon light tub margarine, melted
2 cups sifted all-purpose flour
1/4 teaspoon salt

Lightly spray a 12-cup popover pan with cooking spray.

In a medium bowl, beat the egg whites lightly with a fork. Add the milk, oil, and margarine, beating until well blended.

CURRY CROUTONS

SERVES 8; ABOUT 1/4 CUP PER SERVING

Low in sodium, light and crunchy, you'll want to scatter these tasty tidbits over a leafy green salad, Brussels Sprouts Caesar-Style *(page 75), or a steaming bowl of* Creamy Pumpkin Soup *(page 48).*

4 slices whole-wheat bread (lowest sodium available), cut into 1/2-inch cubes
Olive oil cooking spray
3/4 teaspoon curry powder

Preheat the oven to 300°F.

Arrange the bread cubes in a single layer on a rimmed baking sheet. Lightly spray the cubes with cooking spray. Sprinkle half the curry powder over the cubes. Bake for 8 to 10 minutes, or until crisp on top. Turn over the cubes. Lightly spray with cooking spray. Sprinkle the remaining curry powder over the cubes. Bake for 8 to 10 minutes, or until crisp and dry.

Transfer the baking sheet to a cooling rack. Let the croutons cool. Store in an airtight container.

Cook's Tip: For a Middle Eastern flavor, try using za'atar instead of curry powder. For a Greek flavor, substitute 1/4 teaspoon each of lemon zest, garlic powder, and dried oregano for the curry powder.

PER SERVING

calories 35	sodium 56 mg
total fat 0.5 g	carbohydrates 6 g
saturated fat 0.0 g	fiber 1 g
trans fat 0.0 g	sugars 1 g
polyunsaturated fat 0.0 g	protein 2 g
monounsaturated fat 0.0 g	DIETARY EXCHANGES
cholesterol 0 mg	1/2 starch

HOT SOFT PRETZELS WITH PEPPERCORN MUSTARD

MAKES 16; 1 PER SERVING

Preparing these pretzels is a fun party or family activity, and the results are warm, chewy, and much lower in sodium than the commercial kind.

Pretzels
    1 cup lukewarm water (105°F to 115°F)
    1 1/4-ounce package fast-rising yeast
    1/2 teaspoon sugar and 1 tablespoon sugar, divided use
    2 cups white whole-wheat flour, 1 1/4 to 1 3/4 cups white whole-wheat flour, 3 to 4 tablespoons white whole-wheat flour, and 1/2 cup white whole-wheat flour, divided use
    1 large egg or 1/4 cup egg substitute
    2 tablespoons light stick margarine (no trans fats)

■ ■ ■

    Cooking spray
    1 large egg white or 2 tablespoons egg substitute

    1 tablespoon water
    1/3 cup honey mustard (lowest sodium available)
    1/2 teaspoon pepper (freshly ground preferred)
    1 tablespoon plus 1 teaspoon no-salt-added herb seasoning

In a large bowl, combine 1 cup lukewarm water, the yeast, and 1/2 teaspoon sugar, stirring to dissolve. Let stand for 5 minutes.

Stir in 2 cups flour, the whole egg, margarine, and the remaining 1 tablespoon sugar. Stir rapidly with a sturdy spoon for about 30 seconds. Gradually add 1 1/4 cups flour about 1/4 cup at a time, beating with a spoon after each addition, until the dough starts to pull away from the side of the bowl.

Using 3 to 4 tablespoons flour, lightly flour a flat surface. Turn out the dough. Knead for 3 to 4 minutes, gradually adding, if needed, enough of the remaining 1/2 cup flour to make the dough smooth and elastic. (The dough shouldn't be dry or stick to the surface. You may not need any of the additional 1/2 cup flour, or you may need the entire amount if the dough is too sticky.)

Using cooking spray, lightly spray a large bowl and a piece of plastic wrap large enough to cover the top of the bowl. Transfer the dough to the bowl, turning to coat all sides with the cooking spray. Cover the bowl with the plastic wrap with the sprayed side down. Let the dough rise in a warm, draft-free place (about 85°F) for about 30 minutes, or until doubled in bulk.

Meanwhile, in a small bowl, stir together the egg white and 1 tablespoon water. Set aside.

In a separate small bowl, whisk together the mustard and pepper. Set aside.

Preheat the oven to 400°F. Lightly spray two large baking sheets with cooking spray. Punch the dough down. Divide it into 16 equal pieces. Using a small amount of flour, lightly flour a flat surface. Roll each piece of dough into an

(continued)

18-inch rope. Working with one rope, at a point about 4 inches from each end, cross one end of the rope over the other to form a circle with two 4-inch-long tails. Bring the tails together and twist them once. Lift the twist, folding the dough to the opposite side of the circle so the tails slightly overlap the circle, giving it the shape of a pretzel. Place the pretzel on a baking sheet. Repeat with the remaining dough ropes, placing 8 pretzels on each baking sheet.

Brush the egg white mixture over the top of the pretzels. Sprinkle with the herb seasoning.

Bake one sheet of pretzels for 15 to 20 minutes, or until golden brown. Transfer the pretzels to a cooling rack. Repeat with the second sheet of pretzels.

Serve with the mustard dip.

Cook's Tip: These pretzels will keep in an airtight container for up to four days, or freeze them in an airtight, rigid container for up to one month. If you are storing them, let them cool completely before putting them in a container. Store the mustard dip in the refrigerator for up to one week.

PER SERVING

calories 136	**sodium** 24 mg
total fat 2.0 g	**carbohydrates** 26 g
saturated fat 0.5 g	fiber 4 g
trans fat 0.0 g	sugars 1 g
polyunsaturated fat 0.5 g	**protein** 5 g
monounsaturated fat 0.5 g	**DIETARY EXCHANGES**
cholesterol 12 mg	2 starch

LEMON AND POPPY SEED SCONES

MAKES 16; 1 PER SERVING

A cross between a cookie and a biscuit, a scone is perfect for teatime or with a piece of fruit after dinner. This Scottish quick bread is great for dunking in tea, coffee, or fat-free milk.

  Cooking spray
  2 cups white whole-wheat flour, plus more as needed for dusting hands or rolling out the dough

  1/2 cup uncooked quick-cooking oatmeal
  1/2 cup sugar
  2 tablespoons grated lemon zest
  2 tablespoons fresh lemon juice
  1 tablespoon poppy seeds
  1 teaspoon baking powder
  1/2 teaspoon baking soda
  1/4 teaspoon salt
  2 tablespoons light tub margarine
  1/2 cup fat-free plain Greek yogurt
  1 large egg, lightly beaten

Preheat the oven to 375°F. Lightly spray a baking sheet with cooking spray.

In a large bowl, stir together the flour, oatmeal, sugar, lemon zest, poppy seeds, baking powder, baking soda, and salt.

Using a fork or pastry blender, cut the margarine into the flour mixture until crumbly. Make a well in the center. Put the lemon juice, yogurt, and egg in the well. Stir until the mixture is just moistened, but no flour is visible. Don't overmix.

Divide the dough in half and shape each half into a ball. Lightly dust your hands or a rolling pin. Flatten each ball into a circle 6 inches in diameter. Transfer the circles to the baking sheet. Using a pizza cutter or knife, cut the dough into 8 wedges, but don't separate the wedges.

Bake for 15 to 20 minutes, or until the edges are golden brown. Transfer the baking sheet to a cooling rack. Let cool for at least 5 minutes. Separate into wedges before serving.

PER SERVING

calories 101	**sodium** 119 mg
total fat 1.5 g	**carbohydrates** 18 g
saturated fat 0.0 g	fiber 2 g
trans fat 0.0 g	sugars 7 g
polyunsaturated fat 0.5 g	**protein** 4 g
monounsaturated fat 0.5 g	**DIETARY EXCHANGES**
cholesterol 12 mg	1 starch

EYE-OPENER BREAKFAST COOKIES

MAKES 30; 2 PER SERVING

Packed with good-for-you ingredients, these oatmeal cookies are a natural for breakfast, or try them as a healthy snack later in the day.

   Cooking spray
   1/2 cup unsweetened applesauce
   1/2 cup honey
   1/4 cup plus 2 tablespoons egg substitute
   1 teaspoon grated orange zest
   2 tablespoons fresh orange juice
   2 tablespoons firmly packed light
      brown sugar
   1 tablespoon canola or corn oil
   2 teaspoons vanilla extract
   3/4 cup all-purpose flour
   3/4 cup whole-wheat flour
   1 1/2 teaspoons baking powder
   1/2 teaspoon baking soda
   1 1/2 cups uncooked oatmeal
   1/2 cup fat-free dry milk
   1/2 cup toasted wheat germ
   1/2 cup chopped sweetened dried cranberries
   1/2 cup chopped pecans

Preheat the oven to 350°F. Lightly spray two large baking sheets with cooking spray.

In a large mixing bowl, using an electric mixer on medium speed, beat the applesauce, honey, egg substitute, orange zest, orange juice, brown sugar, oil, and vanilla for 1 to 2 minutes, or until smooth.

Meanwhile, in a small bowl, stir together the flours, baking powder, and baking soda. Add to the applesauce mixture, stirring just enough to combine. Beat on medium speed for 1 to 2 minutes, or until completely combined.

Add the remaining ingredients. Beat on low speed just until combined. (The dough will be slightly sticky.)

Using a small 1-tablespoon spring-loaded ice cream scoop or a tablespoon, drop by slightly heaping tablespoonfuls onto the baking sheets, allowing about 1 inch between cookies. You should have 30 cookies. Using your fingertips, slightly flatten the cookies.

Bake for 12 to 15 minutes, or until the cookies are lightly browned. Immediately transfer the cookies to cooling racks. Let cool for about 30 minutes. Store any leftover cookies in an airtight container, such as a cookie tin, for up to four days. If you prefer softer cookies, store in a resealable plastic bag. Once the cookies are completely cooled, you can freeze them in a plastic freezer bag.

Cook's Tip on Drop Cookies: Making drop cookies is a breeze when you use a small spring-loaded ice cream scoop, commonly available at supermarkets and gourmet cookware stores. The #50 scoop holds about one tablespoon and is an ideal size for most cookie recipes.

PER SERVING

calories 189	sodium 110 mg
total fat 4.5 g	carbohydrates 34 g
saturated fat 0.5 g	fiber 3 g
trans fat 0.0 g	sugars 16 g
polyunsaturated fat 1.5 g	protein 5 g
monounsaturated fat 2.5 g	DIETARY EXCHANGES
cholesterol 0 mg	1 starch, 1 other
	carbohydrate, 1 fat

APPLE MUFFINS

MAKES 18, 1 PER SERVING

These muffins are not only good for breakfast with eggs, whole-grain cereal, or yogurt, but also as a snack with fat-free cheese.

   Cooking spray
   1 cup whole-wheat flour
   1 cup buckwheat flour
   1/3 cup sugar
   1 tablespoon plus 1 teaspoon baking powder
   1/2 teaspoon ground cinnamon
   1/2 teaspoon salt
   1/4 teaspoon ground nutmeg
   1 1/2 cups fat-free milk
   1/4 cup plus 2 tablespoons canola or corn oil
   1 large egg or 2 large egg whites
   1 large apple, chopped

(continued)

Preheat the oven to 400°F. Lightly spray a standard 12-cup muffin pan and a 6-cup muffin pan with cooking spray.

In a medium bowl, stir together the whole-wheat flour, buckwheat flour, sugar, baking powder, cinnamon, salt, and nutmeg.

In a small bowl, whisk together the milk, oil, and egg.

Stir into the flour mixture until the mixture is moistened, but no flour is visible. Don't overmix; the batter should be slightly lumpy. Stir in the apple.

Spoon the batter into the muffin cups. Bake for 15 to 20 minutes, or until a wooden toothpick inserted in the center comes out clean.

Transfer the pans to a cooling rack. Let cool for 10 minutes.

PER SERVING

calories 119	**sodium** 168 mg
total fat 5.5 g	**carbohydrates** 16 g
saturated fat 0.5 g	fiber 2 g
trans fat 0.0 g	sugars 6 g
polyunsaturated fat 1.5 g	**protein** 3 g
monounsaturated fat 3.0 g	**DIETARY EXCHANGES**
cholesterol 11 mg	1 starch, 1 fat

BLUEBERRY-BANANA MUFFINS

MAKES 12; 1 PER SERVING

A fruit-lover's dream, these muffins include not only blueberries and banana but also orange juice and applesauce. Serve with Chèvre Omelet with Herbs *(page 474).*

  Cooking spray
1 cup all-purpose flour
1/2 cup whole-wheat flour
1/2 cup toasted wheat germ
1/3 cup firmly packed light brown sugar
1 tablespoon baking powder
1/2 teaspoon ground cinnamon
1/8 teaspoon ground nutmeg
1/8 teaspoon salt
1 medium very ripe banana, mashed
    (about 1/2 cup)

1/2 cup fresh orange juice
1/4 cup egg substitute
1/4 cup unsweetened applesauce
1 tablespoon canola or corn oil
1 cup blueberries

Preheat the oven to 400°F. Lightly spray a standard 12-cup muffin pan with cooking spray.

In a large bowl, stir together the flours, wheat germ, brown sugar, baking powder, cinnamon, nutmeg, and salt. Make a well in the center.

In a small bowl, whisk together the remaining ingredients except the blueberries. Pour into the well. Stir until the flour mixture is just moistened but no flour is visible. Don't overmix; the batter should be slightly lumpy. Using a rubber scraper, gently fold the blueberries into the batter. Spoon into the muffin cups.

Bake for 15 to 20 minutes, or until a wooden toothpick inserted in the center comes out clean. Transfer the pan to a cooling rack. Let cool for 10 minutes.

PER SERVING

calories 132	**sodium** 137 mg
total fat 2.0 g	**carbohydrates** 26 g
saturated fat 0.0 g	fiber 2 g
trans fat 0.0 g	sugars 10 g
polyunsaturated fat 1.0 g	**protein** 4 g
monounsaturated fat 1.0 g	**DIETARY EXCHANGES**
cholesterol 0 mg	1 starch, 1/2 fruit

CORN BREAD MUFFINS

MAKES 12; 1 PER SERVING

This classic corn bread bakes in a muffin pan, providing the perfect portions. Serve with Slow-Cooker Chili *(page 117) or* Seafood Jambalaya *(page 174).*

  Cooking spray
1 cup sifted all-purpose flour
1/4 cup yellow cornmeal
2 tablespoons sugar
2 1/2 teaspoons baking powder
1 cup fat-free milk

1 large egg or 2 large egg whites
1/4 cup canola or corn oil

Preheat the oven to 425°F. Lightly spray a standard 12-cup muffin pan (or use an 8-inch square baking pan) with cooking spray.

Sift together the flour, cornmeal, sugar, and baking powder. Add the milk, egg, and oil, stirring quickly and lightly until the flour mixture is moistened but no flour is visible. Don't beat.

Spoon the batter into the muffin cups, filling each cup two-thirds full.

Bake for 15 minutes, or until a wooden toothpick inserted in the center comes out clean and the tops are golden brown. Transfer the pan to a cooling rack. Let cool for 10 minutes.

PER SERVING

calories 110	**sodium** 98 mg
total fat 5.0 g	**carbohydrates** 14 g
saturated fat 0.5 g	fiber 0 g
trans fat 0.0 g	sugars 3 g
polyunsaturated fat 1.5 g	**protein** 3 g
monounsaturated fat 3.0 g	**DIETARY EXCHANGES**
cholesterol 16 mg	1 starch, 1 fat

FRUIT-NUT MUFFINS

MAKES 18; 1 PER SERVING

Do yourself a favor and start your day off right with a heart-smart muffin and a Strawberry-Banana Breakfast Shake (page 480) for extra protein.

Cooking spray
1 1/2 cups high-fiber oat-bran cereal
3/4 cup all-purpose flour
3/4 cup whole-wheat flour
1/2 cup chopped unsweetened dried cherries
1/2 cup chopped dried dates
1/2 cup chopped walnuts, dry-roasted
2 teaspoons baking powder
1 teaspoon baking soda
1 teaspoon ground cinnamon
1 cup low-fat buttermilk
1/2 cup honey
1/2 cup egg substitute

1/4 cup firmly packed dark brown sugar
3 tablespoons canola or corn oil

Preheat the oven to 400°F. Lightly spray a standard 12-cup muffin pan and a 6-cup muffin pan with cooking spray.

In a large bowl, stir together the cereal, flours, cranberries, dates, walnuts, baking powder, baking soda, and cinnamon. Make a well in the center.

In a medium bowl, whisk together the remaining ingredients. Pour into the well. Stir until the cereal mixture is just moistened but no flour is visible. Don't overmix; the batter should be slightly lumpy. Spoon into the muffin cups.

Bake for 15 to 20 minutes, or until a wooden toothpick inserted in the center comes out clean. Transfer the pan to a cooling rack. Let cool for about 10 minutes.

PER SERVING

calories 165	**carbohydrates** 29 g
total fat 5.0 g	fiber 2 g
saturated fat 0.5 g	sugars 17 g
trans fat 0.0 g	**protein** 4 g
polyunsaturated fat 2.5 g	**DIETARY EXCHANGES**
monounsaturated fat 2.0 g	1 starch, 1 other
cholesterol 1 mg	carbohydrate, 1 fat
sodium 167 mg	

WHOLE-WHEAT MUFFINS

MAKES 12; 1 PER SERVING

Serve these fragrant muffins fresh out of the oven with Curried Tuna Salad (page 94) and Roasted Carrot-Ginger Soup (page 39).

(continued)

Cooking spray
1 cup whole-wheat flour
3/4 cup all-purpose flour
1/4 cup toasted wheat germ
1/4 cup sugar
2 1/2 teaspoons baking powder
1/2 teaspoon ground cinnamon
1/8 teaspoon ground cloves or ground nutmeg
1/8 teaspoon salt
1 cup fat-free milk
1/2 cup grated zucchini
1/3 cup unsweetened applesauce
1/4 cup egg substitute
1 tablespoon canola or corn oil
1 teaspoon grated orange zest
3 tablespoons chopped walnuts, dry-roasted

Preheat the oven to 375°F. Lightly spray a standard 12-cup muffin pan with cooking spray.

In a large bowl, stir together the flours, wheat germ, sugar, baking powder, cinnamon, cloves, and salt. Make a well in the center.

In a medium bowl, whisk together the remaining ingredients except the walnuts. Pour into the well.

Add the walnuts. Stir until the flour mixture is just moistened but no flour is visible. Don't overmix; the batter should be slightly lumpy. Spoon into the muffin cups.

Bake for 20 to 25 minutes, or until a wooden toothpick inserted in the center comes out clean. Transfer the pan to a cooling rack. Let cool for 10 minutes in the pan before serving.

Time-Saver: For dry-roasted nuts ready at a moment's notice, prepare extras and store them in an airtight container in the freezer. You don't even need to thaw them.

PER SERVING

calories 124	sodium 128 mg
total fat 3.0 g	carbohydrates 21 g
saturated fat 0.5 g	fiber 2 g
trans fat 0.0 g	sugars 6 g
polyunsaturated fat 1.5 g	protein 4 g
monounsaturated fat 1.0 g	DIETARY EXCHANGES
cholesterol 0 mg	1 1/2 starch, 1/2 fat

APPLE-QUINOA PANCAKES
SERVES 4

This hearty breakfast dish hits the spot on a crisp autumn Sunday morning.

2 tablespoons brown sugar and 1 tablespoon brown sugar, divided use
1/2 teaspoon ground cinnamon and 1/2 teaspoon ground cinnamon, divided use
1 tablespoon light tub margarine
3 large Red Delicious apples (about 1 1/2 pounds), peeled, cored, and finely chopped
2/3 cup all-purpose flour
1/3 cup uncooked quick-cooking quinoa
1 cup egg substitute
1 cup fat-free milk
1/2 cup unsweetened applesauce
1 tablespoon vanilla extract
1/4 teaspoon salt
Cooking spray

In a small cup, stir together 2 tablespoons brown sugar and 1/2 teaspoon cinnamon.

In a large nonstick skillet, melt the margarine over medium heat, swirling to coat the bottom. Put the apples in the skillet. Sprinkle the brown sugar mixture over the apples, stirring gently to combine. Cook, covered, for 7 to 8 minutes, stirring occasionally. Remove from the heat. Set aside.

Meanwhile, using a food processor or blender, process the flour, quinoa, and the remaining 1 tablespoon brown sugar until smooth.

Add the egg substitute, milk, applesauce, vanilla, salt, and the remaining 1/2 teaspoon cinnamon to the flour mixture. Process until smooth. Stir in the apple mixture.

Preheat the oven to 200°F. Place a cooling rack on a baking sheet. Set aside.

Lightly spray a griddle or large skillet with cooking spray. Heat over medium heat.

For each pancake, ladle 1/4 cup batter onto the griddle. Cook for 2 to 3 minutes, or until bubbles are forming on the top of the pancakes and the edges are dry. Turn over the pancakes. Cook for 2 to 3 minutes. Transfer the pancakes to the cooling rack, placing them in a single layer and leaving space between. Put in the oven to keep warm. Repeat with the remaining batter (you should have a total of 8 pancakes).

PER SERVING

calories 316	carbohydrates 61 g
total fat 2.5 g	fiber 4 g
saturated fat 0.0 g	sugars 31 g
trans fat 0.0 g	protein 13 g
polyunsaturated fat 1.0 g	DIETARY EXCHANGES
monounsaturated fat 1.0 g	2 starch, 2 fruit, 1 lean
cholesterol 1 mg	meat
sodium 324 mg	

BAKED PEAR PANCAKE

SERVES 6

Baked as a large pancake rather than cooked on the stovetop as individual pancakes, this Dutch-style pancake takes about the same amount of time but requires a lot less work.

> 1 large ripe but firm pear, peeled and thinly sliced
> 1 tablespoon sugar and 2 tablespoons plus 1 teaspoon sugar, divided use
> 1/4 teaspoon ground cinnamon
> 1/8 teaspoon ground cloves
> 2 teaspoons canola or corn oil
> 3/4 cup fat-free milk
> 1/2 cup all-purpose flour
> 3 large egg whites
> 1/4 cup egg substitute
> 1/2 teaspoon vanilla extract
> 1/8 teaspoon salt
> 2 teaspoons confectioners' sugar

Preheat the oven to 425°F.

Put the pear slices, 1 tablespoon sugar, the cinnamon, and cloves in a medium bowl. Gently stir together to coat.

In a 10-inch ovenproof nonstick or cast iron skillet, heat the oil over medium-high heat, swirling to coat the bottom. Arrange the pear slices in a single layer in the skillet. Cook for 5 minutes, or until beginning to soften (don't stir).

Meanwhile, in a medium bowl, whisk together the milk, flour, egg whites, egg substitute, vanilla, salt, and the remaining 2 tablespoons plus 1 teaspoon sugar until smooth. Pour over the pear slices.

Bake for 15 to 18 minutes, or until the edge of the pancake is puffed and browned. Sprinkle with the confectioners' sugar while still in the skillet and before cutting into wedges.

Cook's Tip: Serve this delicate pancake from the skillet. It will break apart if you try to transfer the whole pancake to a serving plate.

PER SERVING

calories 129	sodium 110 mg
total fat 2.0 g	carbohydrates 24 g
saturated fat 0.0 g	fiber 2 g
trans fat 0.0 g	sugars 13 g
polyunsaturated fat 0.5 g	protein 5 g
monounsaturated fat 1.0 g	DIETARY EXCHANGES
cholesterol 1 mg	1 starch, 1/2 fruit

CINNAMON-ORANGE PANCAKES

SERVES 4

Start the weekend off right with these sweet, citrusy pancakes, served with Orange Sauce (page 439) or pure maple syrup and topped with sliced bananas or strawberries.

> 1 cup whole-wheat flour
> 3/4 cup all-purpose flour
> 2 tablespoons toasted wheat germ
> 1 tablespoon sugar
> 2 teaspoons baking powder
> 1 teaspoon ground cinnamon
> 1 cup fat-free milk
> 1 teaspoon grated orange zest
> 3/4 cup fresh orange juice
> 1/4 cup egg substitute
> Cooking spray

(continued)

Preheat the oven to 200°F. Place a cooling rack on a baking sheet. Set aside.

In a large bowl, stir together the flours, wheat germ, sugar, baking powder, and cinnamon.

In a small bowl, whisk together the remaining ingredients except the cooking spray. Pour into the flour mixture. Stir until the flour mixture is moistened but no flour is visible. Don't overmix.

Lightly spray a griddle or large skillet with cooking spray. Heat over medium heat. For each pancake, ladle 1/4 cup batter onto the griddle. Cook for 2 to 3 minutes, or until bubbles are forming on the top of the pancakes and the edges are dry. Turn over the pancakes. Cook for 2 to 3 minutes. Transfer the pancakes to the cooling rack, placing them in a single layer and leaving space between. Put in the oven to keep warm. Repeat with the remaining batter (you should have a total of 12 pancakes).

PER SERVING

calories 264	sodium 259 mg
total fat 1.5 g	carbohydrates 53 g
saturated fat 0.5 g	fiber 5 g
trans fat 0.0 g	sugars 11 g
polyunsaturated fat 0.5 g	protein 11 g
monounsaturated fat 0.0 g	DIETARY EXCHANGES
cholesterol 1 mg	3 1/2 starch

PERFECT PUMPKIN PANCAKES

SERVES 4

With canned pumpkin available year-round, you can serve these autumnal pancakes any time of the year.

3/4 cup plus 2 tablespoons whole-wheat pastry flour
1/3 cup all-purpose flour
1/4 cup toasted wheat germ
1 tablespoon pumpkin pie spice
1 1/4 teaspoons baking powder
3/4 cup canned solid-pack pumpkin (not pie filling)
3/4 cup fat-free milk

1/2 cup fat-free sour cream
1/3 cup egg substitute
1 tablespoon plus 2 teaspoons firmly packed light brown sugar
2 teaspoons canola or corn oil
2 teaspoons vanilla extract
Cooking spray

Preheat the oven to 200°F. Place a cooling rack on a baking sheet. Set aside.

In a large bowl, stir together the flours, wheat germ, pumpkin pie spice, and baking powder.

In a medium bowl, whisk together the pumpkin, milk, sour cream, egg substitute, brown sugar, oil, and vanilla. Pour into the flour mixture. Stir just until moistened but no flour is visible. Don't overmix.

Lightly spray a griddle or large skillet with cooking spray. Heat over medium-high heat. For each pancake, ladle a generous 1/4 cup of batter onto the griddle. Cook for 3 to 4 minutes, or just until bubbles begin to form on the top of the pancakes and the edges are a little dry. Reduce the heat to medium low. Gently turn over the pancakes. Cook for about 3 minutes, or until the second side is golden brown and the pancakes are fairly firm to the touch. Transfer the pancakes to the cooling rack, placing them in a single layer and leaving space between. Put in the oven to keep warm. Repeat with the remaining batter (you should have a total of 12 pancakes).

PER SERVING

calories 285	sodium 216 mg
total fat 4.0 g	carbohydrates 49 g
saturated fat 0.5 g	fiber 7 g
trans fat 0.0 g	sugars 13 g
polyunsaturated fat 1.0 g	protein 12 g
monounsaturated fat 1.5 g	DIETARY EXCHANGES
cholesterol 6 mg	3 1/2 starch

RED, WHITE, AND BLUEBERRY WAFFLES

SERVES 4

Prepare these waffles on any patriotic holiday or any other day of the year!

- 1 cup fat-free plain Greek yogurt
- 2 tablespoons honey
- 1/4 teaspoon ground cinnamon
- 4 low-fat whole-grain frozen waffles, toasted, or 4 waffles from Peanut Butter and Banana Waffle Sandwiches (in the next column)
- 1 cup sliced hulled strawberries
- 1 cup blueberries
- 1 medium banana, sliced
- 1 cup Blueberry Sauce (page 439) (optional)

In a small bowl, stir together the yogurt, honey, and cinnamon.

Place one toasted frozen or homemade waffle on each plate. Spoon 1/4 cup of the yogurt mixture over each waffle. Top with the strawberries, blueberries, and banana. Serve immediately for the best texture.

PER SERVING (WITHOUT BLUEBERRY SAUCE)

calories 208	**carbohydrates** 43 g
total fat 2.0 g	fiber 6 g
saturated fat 0.0 g	sugars 22 g
trans fat 0.0 g	**protein** 10 g
polyunsaturated fat 0.5 g	**DIETARY EXCHANGES**
monounsaturated fat 0.0 g	1 starch, 1 other
cholesterol 0 mg	carbohydrate, 1 lean
sodium 173 mg	meat

PER SERVING (WITH BLUEBERRY SAUCE)

calories 274	**carbohydrates** 60 g
total fat 2.0 g	fiber 7 g
saturated fat 0.0 g	sugars 36 g
trans fat 0.0 g	**protein** 10 g
polyunsaturated fat 0.5 g	**DIETARY EXCHANGES**
monounsaturated fat 0.5 g	1 starch, 1 fruit, 2 other
cholesterol 0 mg	carbohydrate, 1 lean
sodium 174 mg	meat

PEANUT BUTTER AND BANANA WAFFLE SANDWICHES

SERVES 4

These breakfast sandwiches are the perfect grab-and-go morning meal, especially when you make the waffles on the weekend and freeze them (see Cook's Tip on page 470) so they're ready to use throughout the week.

Waffles
- 1/2 cup whole-wheat flour
- 1/2 cup white whole-wheat flour or all-purpose flour
- 1/4 cup cornmeal
- 2 tablespoons ground flax seed
- 2 teaspoons ground cinnamon
- 1 1/2 teaspoons baking powder
- 1 teaspoon baking soda
- 1 cup low-fat buttermilk
- 2 large eggs, separated, and 1 large egg white, divided use
- 1 tablespoon canola or corn oil

■ ■ ■

- 1/4 cup creamy low-sodium peanut butter
- 1/4 cup fat-free plain yogurt
- 2 small bananas, sliced

Preheat a waffle iron using the manufacturer's directions.

Preheat the oven to 200°F. Line a baking sheet with aluminum foil. Set aside.

In a medium bowl, stir together both flours, the cornmeal, flax seed, cinnamon, baking powder, and baking soda.

In a large bowl, whisk together the buttermilk, 2 egg yolks, and oil until smooth.

Whisk the flour mixture into the buttermilk mixture until the batter is just moistened but no flour is visible. Don't overmix.

In a small metal or glass mixing bowl, using an electric mixer on high speed, beat the 3 egg

(continued)

whites until soft peaks form. Stir one-third of the egg whites into the batter. Gently fold in the remaining egg whites.

Meanwhile, heat the waffle iron until hot (follow the manufacturer's directions for spraying or oiling the surface). Pour 1/2 cup batter into the iron for each waffle (the exact amount may vary according to the size of the waffle iron). Following the manufacturer's directions for timing, cook until the steaming stops and the waffle is golden brown. Watch the first batch closely and adjust the time as necessary. Transfer the waffle to the baking sheet. Put in the oven to keep warm (uncovered). Repeat with the remaining batter.

Meanwhile, in a small bowl, stir together the peanut butter and yogurt.

To assemble the sandwiches, spread the peanut butter mixture over 4 of the waffles. Top with the banana slices and the remaining 4 waffles. Cut each sandwich in half diagonally.

Cook's Tip: You can make the waffles ahead of time, freeze them, and make the sandwiches at a later time. Cool the waffles on wire racks to avoid sogginess. Line a large baking sheet with parchment paper. Place the cooled waffles on the baking sheet. Place parchment paper between the layers. Freeze for 3 to 4 hours, or until frozen. Transfer the waffles to resealable plastic freezer bags. Freeze for up to three months. To reheat the waffles, place them in a toaster. Toast on the toast setting until hot and crispy. You can also reheat them in the oven. Preheat the oven to 350°F. Place the waffles on a baking sheet. Bake for 5 to 10 minutes, or until hot and crisp.

PER SERVING

calories 398	carbohydrates 48 g
total fat 17.0 g	fiber 7 g
saturated fat 3.0 g	sugars 13 g
trans fat 0.0 g	**protein** 17 g
polyunsaturated fat 5.5 g	**DIETARY EXCHANGES**
monounsaturated fat 7.5 g	2 starch, 1 fruit, 2 lean
cholesterol 96 mg	meat, 2 fat
sodium 594 mg	

CLASSIC FRENCH TOAST

SERVES 2

This quick and easy version of French toast can be made in just minutes. Gently wrap a slice in wax paper, grab a banana or apple, and you can be out the door with a complete breakfast in hand in no time at all.

- 2 large egg whites
- 2 tablespoons fat-free milk
- 1/4 teaspoon vanilla extract
- 1/8 teaspoon ground cinnamon
- 1 1/2 teaspoons canola or corn oil
- 2 slices day-old whole-wheat bread (lowest sodium available)

In a medium shallow bowl, whisk together the egg whites, milk, vanilla, and cinnamon.

Using a nonstick griddle over medium heat, heat the oil, swirling to coat the griddle.

Lightly dip one slice of bread in the milk mixture, turning to coat. Transfer to a plate. Repeat with the remaining bread.

Transfer both slices of bread to the griddle. Cook the bread for 2 to 3 minutes on each side, or until golden brown.

PER SERVING

calories 124	carbohydrates 13 g
total fat 4.5 g	fiber 2 g
saturated fat 0.5 g	sugars 3 g
trans fat 0.0 g	**protein** 8 g
polyunsaturated fat 1.0 g	**DIETARY EXCHANGES**
monounsaturated fat 2.5 g	1 starch, 1/2 lean meat,
cholesterol 0 mg	1/2 fat
sodium 173 mg	

APPLESAUCE TOAST

SERVES 4

Forgo the ordinary margarine or jam toast topping and try this warm-spiced autumnal spread instead. For variety, also try this fruit topping on pancakes and Classic French Toast *(above).*

4 slices whole-wheat bread (lowest sodium available)
1 cup unsweetened applesauce
1 1/2 tablespoons sugar
1 tablespoon light tub margarine
1/8 teaspoon ground cinnamon
1/8 teaspoon ground nutmeg

In a toaster or under a broiler, toast the bread.

Meanwhile, in a small saucepan, stir together the applesauce, sugar, margarine, cinnamon, and nutmeg. Bring to a simmer over medium heat.

Spread 1/4 cup of the applesauce mixture on each toasted slice of bread.

Serve immediately.

PER SERVING

calories 124	**sodium** 136 mg
total fat 2.0 g	**carbohydrates** 23 g
saturated fat 0.0 g	fiber 3 g
trans fat 0.0 g	sugars 12 g
polyunsaturated fat 0.5 g	**protein** 4 g
monounsaturated fat 1.0 g	**DIETARY EXCHANGES**
cholesterol 0 mg	1 starch, 1/2 fruit

MUESLI

SERVES 6

This no-cook, creamy cereal incorporates the goodness of traditional muesli (the German word for "mixture") ingredients. Prepare it the night before to save time in the morning.

1 cup uncooked quick-cooking oatmeal
1 cup fat-free vanilla yogurt
1/2 cup fat-free milk
1/4 cup dried currants or raisins
1/4 cup chopped dried apricots
2 tablespoons toasted wheat germ
1 tablespoon honey
2 cups blueberries
2 tablespoons chopped walnuts, dry-roasted

In a medium bowl, stir together the oatmeal, yogurt, milk, currants, apricots, wheat germ, and

honey. Cover and refrigerate for 2 hours (the oats should be plump and tender) to two days.

Just before serving, stir in the blueberries. Sprinkle with the walnuts.

PER SERVING

calories 191	**sodium** 42 mg
total fat 3.0 g	**carbohydrates** 37 g
saturated fat 0.5 g	fiber 4 g
trans fat 0.0 g	sugars 23 g
polyunsaturated fat 1.5 g	**protein** 7 g
monounsaturated fat 0.5 g	**DIETARY EXCHANGES**
cholesterol 1 mg	1 starch, 1 fruit, 1/2 fat-free milk

APPLE-BERRY COUSCOUS

SERVES 6

Couscous is a good whole grain to choose for breakfast because it cooks so quickly. This hot-grain combo uses fresh, dried, and bottled fruit and juice for flavor.

1 teaspoon canola or corn oil
2 medium apples, such as Fuji, McIntosh, or Rome Beauty, cut into 1/2-inch pieces (about 2 cups)
1/4 cup unsweetened dried cherries or cranberries
1/4 cup golden raisins
3 tablespoons dried currants or chopped dried dates
3 tablespoons light brown sugar
1 teaspoon ground cinnamon
2 cups 100% apple juice
1/2 cup water
1 teaspoon coarsely grated lime zest
3 tablespoons fresh lime juice (about 2 medium limes)
1 2/3 cups uncooked whole-wheat couscous

In a large saucepan, heat the oil over low heat, swirling to coat the bottom. Add the apples, cherries, raisins, currants, brown sugar, and cinnamon, stirring to combine. Cook, covered, for 10 minutes, or until the apples have released some of their juices, stirring occasionally.

(continued)

Stir in the remaining ingredients except the couscous. Increase the heat to high. Cover and bring to a boil.

Stir in the couscous. Remove from the heat. Let stand, covered, for 15 minutes. Fluff with a fork before serving.

Cook's Tip on Couscous: Couscous (*KOOS-koos*), which looks like tiny bits of pasta, is made from a coarse wheat flour called semolina. The name "couscous" also refers to a stew made of grain, lamb or chicken, and vegetables.

PER SERVING

calories 333	sodium 8 mg
total fat 2.0 g	carbohydrates 78 g
saturated fat 0.0 g	fiber 7 g
trans fat 0.0 g	sugars 32 g
polyunsaturated fat 0.5 g	protein 8 g
monounsaturated fat 0.5 g	DIETARY EXCHANGES
cholesterol 0 mg	3 starch, 2 fruit

BAKED PEANUT BUTTER AND APPLE OATMEAL

SERVES 10

This easy-to-throw-together casserole works for brunch or breakfast for the week as individual servings can easily be reheated each morning. A hearty combination of oats cooked in milk with fresh apples, peanut butter, and raisins provides the perfect kick-start to the day.

Cooking spray
2 cups chopped unpeeled sweet-tart apples, such as Braeburn or Gala (2 to 3 medium apples)
1 cup uncooked steel-cut oats
1 cup raisins
1/2 cup coarsely chopped walnuts
1 1/2 teaspoons ground cinnamon
1/4 teaspoon ground nutmeg
3 1/2 cups fat-free milk
1/3 cup low-sodium creamy peanut butter
1 teaspoon maple flavoring
1 teaspoon vanilla extract

Preheat the oven to 350°F. Lightly spray an 11 x 7 x 2-inch glass baking dish with cooking spray. In a large bowl, combine the apples, oats, raisins, walnuts, cinnamon, and nutmeg.

In a medium saucepan, whisk together the milk and peanut butter until smooth. Cook over medium heat for 3 to 4 minutes, or until bubbles form around the edges. Whisk in the maple flavoring and vanilla. Pour the milk mixture over the apple mixture, stirring until moistened. Pour into the baking dish.

Bake, covered, for 45 minutes, or until a knife inserted in the center comes out clean. Let stand for 10 minutes before serving.

Cook's Tip: This casserole can be served on plates, in bowls, or with milk. Cover and refrigerate any leftovers. To reheat, microwave individual servings for 30 to 50 seconds, or until heated through.

PER SERVING

calories 249	sodium 40 mg
total fat 9.5 g	carbohydrates 34 g
saturated fat 1.5 g	fiber 6 g
trans fat 0.0 g	sugars 18 g
polyunsaturated fat 4.5 g	protein 9 g
monounsaturated fat 3.0 g	DIETARY EXCHANGES
cholesterol 2 mg	1 1/2 starch, 1 fruit, 1 lean meat, 1 fat

COCOA-BANANA OATMEAL

SERVES 4

Comforting and packed with fiber, this oatmeal tastes like a chocolate-covered banana. Serve it hot or cold.

2 cups uncooked quick-cooking oatmeal
1 3/4 cups fat-free milk
1 cup thinly sliced bananas (about 2 medium bananas)
1/2 cup fat-free plain Greek yogurt
1 tablespoon plus 1 teaspoon unsweetened cocoa powder
2 teaspoons raisins (optional)
2 teaspoons pure maple syrup (optional)
1/2 teaspoon vanilla extract
1/4 teaspoon ground cinnamon

In a medium bowl, stir together all the ingredients until well blended.

To serve warm, pour the oatmeal mixture into a medium saucepan. Bring just to a boil over medium-high heat. Reduce the heat to low. Simmer for 10 minutes, stirring frequently. Gradually stir in small amounts of water if you prefer a thinner consistency.

To serve cold, cover and refrigerate overnight.

Cook's Tip: For extra nutty flavor, toast the oatmeal before using it to prepare this recipe. Preheat the oven to 200°F. Spread the oatmeal on a baking sheet. Bake for 10 to 12 minutes, or until lightly browned, stirring occasionally.

PER SERVING

calories 250	carbohydrates 43 g
total fat 3.0 g	fiber 6 g
saturated fat 0.5 g	sugars 12 g
trans fat 0.0 g	**protein** 13 g
polyunsaturated fat 1.0 g	**DIETARY EXCHANGES**
monounsaturated fat 1.0 g	2 starch, 1/2 fruit,
cholesterol 2 mg	1/2 fat-free milk
sodium 58 mg	

BREAKFAST MEAT PATTIES

SERVES 8

Skip the bacon and sausage to try this healthier morning meat option. Serve with Classic French Toast *(page 470), pancakes, or eggs. Add fresh fruit, such as berries and melon, for color on your plate and nutrients for your heart.*

> 1 pound extra-lean ground beef
> 1/2 cup fat-free, low-sodium beef broth
> 1/4 cup fine dry bread crumbs (lowest sodium available)
> 2 teaspoons grated lemon zest
> 1 tablespoon fresh lemon juice
> 1/4 teaspoon dried sage
> 1/4 teaspoon ground ginger
> 2 teaspoons canola or corn oil

In a large bowl, using your hands or a spoon, combine all the ingredients except the oil. Let stand for 15 minutes so the flavors blend.

Form into 8 patties about 1/4 inch thick. Transfer the patties to a large plate.

In a large, heavy skillet, heat the oil over medium heat, swirling to coat the bottom. Cook the patties for 7 or 8 minutes on each side, or until browned on the outside and no longer pink in the center.

PER SERVING

calories 100	**sodium** 70 mg
total fat 4.0 g	**carbohydrates** 3 g
saturated fat 1.5 g	fiber 0 g
trans fat 0.0 g	sugars 0 g
polyunsaturated fat 0.5 g	**protein** 13 g
monounsaturated fat 2.0 g	**DIETARY EXCHANGES**
cholesterol 31 mg	2 lean meat

COUNTRY-STYLE BREAKFAST CASSEROLE

SERVES 10

To enjoy this breakfast dish with no fuss in the morning, you can prepare it the night before (see Cook's Tip on page 474). Serve with fresh berries.

> Cooking spray
> 8 ounces low-fat smoked link sausage
> 2 tablespoons pure maple syrup
> 2 pounds frozen country-style hash brown potatoes (lowest sodium available)
> 2 cups fat-free milk
> 1 1/2 cups egg substitute
> 2 1-ounce slices low-fat American cheese, diced
> 1/4 cup shredded or grated Parmesan cheese
> 1/2 teaspoon dry mustard
> 1/4 teaspoon pepper
> 2 tablespoons finely chopped green onions (green part only) (optional)

Preheat the oven to 350°F. Lightly spray a 13 x 9 x 2-inch baking pan with cooking spray.

In a medium skillet, cook the sausage over medium-high heat for 3 to 4 minutes, or until browned, turning occasionally. Remove from the skillet and cut into bite-size pieces. Wipe the

(continued)

skillet with paper towels. Return the sausage to the skillet.

Pour in the maple syrup. Cook for 1 minute, stirring to coat. Arrange the sausage in a single layer in the baking pan.

Top with the potatoes.

In a medium bowl, whisk together the remaining ingredients except the green onions. Pour over the potatoes.

Bake for 1 hour, or until the center is set (doesn't jiggle when the pan is gently shaken).

Sprinkle with the green onions. Let cool for at least 10 minutes before cutting.

Cook's Tip: If you prepare this casserole ahead of time, cover and refrigerate it. When you're ready to bake it, put the cold casserole in a cold oven. Set the oven to 350°F and bake for 1 hour 10 minutes to 1 hour 15 minutes. Proceed as directed above.

PER SERVING

calories 161	carbohydrates 25 g
total fat 1.0 g	fiber 1 g
saturated fat 0.5 g	sugars 8 g
trans fat 0.0 g	protein 13 g
polyunsaturated fat 0.0 g	**DIETARY EXCHANGES**
monounsaturated fat 0.5 g	1 1/2 starch, 1 1/2 lean
cholesterol 14 mg	meat
sodium 498 mg	

POTATO AND EGG SCRAMBLE

SERVES 4

A topping of stewed tomatoes with a jolt of hot-pepper sauce adds zesty zip to this hearty breakfast dish.

> 1 cup egg substitute
> 1 1/2 ounces light tub cream cheese (about a heaping 2 1/2 tablespoons), cut into small pieces
> 1 teaspoon salt-free all-purpose seasoning blend
> 1 teaspoon olive oil
> 1 1/2 cups frozen diced hash brown potatoes (lowest sodium available)

> 2/3 cup chopped onion
> 1/4 cup diced red bell pepper
> 1/2 cup canned no-salt-added stewed tomatoes, undrained
> 1/8 to 1/4 teaspoon red hot-pepper sauce
> 4 sprigs of fresh cilantro (optional)

In a small bowl, whisk together the egg substitute, cream cheese, and seasoning blend until almost smooth (you'll still have some bits of cream cheese).

In a large nonstick skillet, heat the oil over medium-high heat for 1 minute, swirling to coat the bottom. Stir in the potatoes, onion, and bell pepper. Cook for 8 to 9 minutes, or until the potatoes are golden brown, stirring frequently. Reduce the heat to medium. Pour in the egg substitute mixture. Cook for 1 to 2 minutes, or until the mixture is set (doesn't jiggle when the skillet is gently shaken), stirring occasionally.

Meanwhile, cut the tomatoes into bite-size pieces. Put the tomatoes with liquid in a separate small bowl. Stir in the hot-pepper sauce.

Spoon the potato and egg mixture onto plates. Top with the tomato mixture. Garnish with the sprigs of cilantro.

PER SERVING

calories 147	carbohydrates 20 g
total fat 3.0 g	fiber 2 g
saturated fat 1.0 g	sugars 5 g
trans fat 0.0 g	protein 9 g
polyunsaturated fat 0.0 g	**DIETARY EXCHANGES**
monounsaturated fat 1.5 g	1 lean meat, 1 starch,
cholesterol 7 mg	1 vegetable
sodium 196 mg	

CHÈVRE OMELET WITH HERBS

SERVES 2

A touch of goat cheese, or chèvre *(SHEHV-ruh or SHEHV), and a sprinkling of a fresh herb of your choice add a delicate flavor twist to this egg dish. Round out your breakfast with a slice of* Raisin Bran Bread *(page 451) or* Blueberry-Banana Muffins *(page 464).*

2 teaspoons canola or corn oil

3 large egg whites

1 large egg

1 tablespoon water

1 teaspoon chopped fresh herb, such as basil, chives, thyme, or a combination, or 1/4 teaspoon dried herb

1/8 teaspoon salt

2 tablespoons crumbled soft herb or plain goat cheese (chèvre)

Pepper to taste

In a large nonstick skillet, heat the oil over medium-high heat, swirling to coat the bottom.

In a small bowl, whisk together the egg whites, egg, water, herb, and salt. Pour the egg white mixture into the skillet, swirling to coat the bottom. Cook for 30 seconds, or until beginning to set. Using a spatula, carefully lift the cooked edge of the omelet and tilt the skillet so the uncooked portion flows under the edge. Cook until no runniness remains, repeating the lift-and-tilt procedure once or twice at other places along the edge if needed. Remove from the heat.

Sprinkle or spread the goat cheese over half the omelet. Sprinkle with the pepper. Using a spatula, carefully fold the half with no filling over the other half. Gently slide the omelet onto a large plate. Cut the omelet in half. Transfer half to a separate large plate.

PER SERVING

calories 122	sodium 289 mg
total fat 8.5 g	**carbohydrates** 1 g
saturated fat 2.0 g	fiber 0 g
trans fat 0.0 g	sugars 1 g
polyunsaturated fat 2.0 g	**protein** 10 g
monounsaturated fat 4.0 g	**DIETARY EXCHANGES**
cholesterol 96 mg	1 1/2 lean meat, 1 fat

GREEK OMELET WITH TOMATO-FETA RELISH

SERVES 4

Much easier to prepare than a rolled omelet, this fluffy omelet brings the flavors of the Greek Isles to your brunch table. The relish topping, made with the elements of a Greek salad, could also serve as an accompaniment for baked, broiled, or grilled chicken.

Relish

1 cup grape tomatoes, quartered lengthwise

1/3 cup fat-free crumbled feta cheese

1/4 cup sliced kalamata olives

1 tablespoon minced red onion

1 tablespoon minced fresh oregano

1 tablespoon fresh lemon juice (optional)

1 teaspoon olive oil (extra-virgin preferred)

1/4 teaspoon pepper (freshly ground preferred)

Omelet

1 tablespoon olive oil and 2 teaspoons olive oil, divided use

2 medium garlic cloves, minced

1 tablespoon minced shallots and 1 teaspoon minced shallots, divided use

6 ounces baby spinach (about 4 cups)

2 large egg whites

2 large eggs

1 teaspoon minced fresh oregano

1/4 teaspoon pepper (freshly ground preferred)

■ ■ ■

1 teaspoon minced chives (optional)

In a medium bowl, stir together all the relish ingredients until well blended. Cover and refrigerate until serving time.

In a small ovenproof nonstick skillet, heat 1 tablespoon oil over medium-high heat, swirling to coat the bottom. Cook the garlic and 1 tablespoon of shallots for 1 to 2 minutes, or until fragrant, stirring constantly.

(continued)

Add the spinach to the skillet in three batches, adding a new batch as the prior one wilts. Cook for 3 to 5 minutes, or until just tender, stirring constantly. Remove the skillet from the heat. Transfer the spinach mixture to a fine-mesh strainer. Using the back of a large spoon or your fingertips, firmly press out all the liquid.

In a large metal or glass mixing bowl, using an electric mixer on high speed, beat the egg whites until soft peaks form.

Preheat the broiler.

Put the eggs in a medium bowl. Stir in the oregano, pepper, and the remaining 1 teaspoon shallots. Using an electric mixer on medium speed, beat the egg mixture until light and fluffy. Stir in the spinach. Using a spatula, gently fold the egg mixture into the egg whites, blending until no white streaks remain.

Wipe the skillet clean with paper towels. Pour the remaining 2 teaspoons oil into the skillet, swirling to coat the bottom. Heat over medium-high heat. Reduce the heat to medium. Pour the egg mixture into the skillet. Cook for 4 to 6 minutes, or until the bottom is golden.

Transfer the skillet to the broiler. Broil about 4 inches from the heat for 5 to 6 minutes, or until the omelet is browned and the eggs are set.

Slide the omelet onto a platter. Cut into wedges. Sprinkle with the chives. Serve with the relish on top or on the side.

Cook's Tip: To ovenproof a skillet, wrap the handle with aluminum foil.

PER SERVING

calories 172	**sodium** 451 mg
total fat 12.0 g	**carbohydrates** 8 g
saturated fat 2.0 g	fiber 2 g
trans fat 0.0 g	sugars 3 g
polyunsaturated fat 1.5 g	**protein** 10 g
monounsaturated fat 7.5 g	**DIETARY EXCHANGES**
cholesterol 93 mg	1 vegetable, 1 lean
	meat, 1 1/2 fat

STACKED SAUSAGE AND EGGS
SERVES 4

In this dish, you cook spiced-up eggs and vegetable-infused sausage in the same skillet for easy cleanup. Enjoy with whole-grain English muffins or Honey-Wheat Oatmeal Bread (page 452).

> 4 ounces low-fat bulk sausage
> 2 to 3 ounces button mushrooms, sliced
> 1/2 large onion, chopped
> 1/2 medium green bell pepper, chopped
> 1 cup egg substitute
> 3 tablespoons fat-free milk
> 1/8 teaspoon cayenne
> 2 tablespoons chopped fresh parsley
> 1/8 teaspoon salt

In a large nonstick skillet, cook the sausage over medium-high heat for 2 to 3 minutes, or until no longer pink, stirring constantly to turn and break up the sausage. Transfer to a medium bowl.

In the same skillet, stir together the mushrooms, onion, and bell pepper. Cook for about 3 minutes, or until the onion is soft, stirring occasionally. Stir into the sausage. Cover to keep warm.

Meanwhile, in a small bowl, whisk together the egg substitute, milk, and cayenne.

Wipe the skillet with paper towels. Heat the skillet over medium heat. Cook the egg mixture for 2 minutes, stirring frequently. Transfer to plates. Top with the sausage mixture. Sprinkle with the parsley and salt.

PER SERVING

calories 88	**sodium** 370 mg
total fat 1.0 g	**carbohydrates** 6 g
saturated fat 0.0 g	fiber 1 g
trans fat 0.0 g	sugars 4 g
polyunsaturated fat 0.0 g	**protein** 12 g
monounsaturated fat 0.0 g	**DIETARY EXCHANGES**
cholesterol 14 mg	1 vegetable, 1 1/2 lean
	meat

STRATA WITH CANADIAN BACON, SPINACH, AND TOMATOES

SERVES 4

This brunch dish is similar to a quiche or frittata because it's a mixture of bread, eggs, and cheese, but it also includes vegetables for additional flavor and nutrients. You can prepare it ahead of time and bake it later to best fit your schedule (see Cook's Tip below).

Cooking spray
3 slices whole-grain bread (lowest sodium available), cubed
10 ounces frozen chopped spinach, thawed and squeezed dry
2 medium Italian plum (Roma) tomatoes, diced
1/3 cup diced Canadian bacon
4 medium green onions, thinly sliced
1/4 cup shredded low-fat Swiss cheese
1/4 cup coarsely chopped fresh basil
1 1/2 cups fat-free milk
1 cup egg substitute
1/4 teaspoon pepper

Preheat the oven to 350°F. Lightly spray an 8-inch square baking pan with cooking spray.

In the baking pan, stir together the bread cubes, spinach, tomatoes, Canadian bacon, green onions, Swiss cheese, and basil.

In a medium bowl, whisk together the milk, egg substitute, and pepper. Pour over the bread mixture.

Bake for 55 minutes to 1 hour, or until the center is set (doesn't jiggle when the pan is gently shaken). Let cool for 10 minutes before cutting.

Cook's Tip: If you prepare this casserole ahead of time, cover and refrigerate it for up to 10 hours. When you're ready to bake it, put the cold casserole in a cold oven. Set the oven to 350°F and bake for 1 hour 5 minutes to 1 hour 10 minutes, or until the center is set. Let cool for 10 minutes before cutting.

PER SERVING

calories 177
total fat 2.0 g
   saturated fat 1.0 g
   trans fat 0.0 g
   polyunsaturated fat 0.0 g
   monounsaturated fat 0.5 g
cholesterol 12 mg
sodium 515 mg

carbohydrates 21 g
   fiber 5 g
   sugars 9 g
protein 19 g
DIETARY EXCHANGES
   1 starch, 1 vegetable, 2 lean meat

QUINOA BREAKFAST BITES

SERVES 6

Think of these quinoa bites as mini omelets. They make a great start to the day—complete with protein, vegetables, and a whole grain. They're baked in a muffin pan, so they're perfectly portable for those mornings when you need to quickly grab something and go.

Cooking spray
1/2 cup uncooked quinoa, rinsed and drained
1 medium onion, halved, cut into 1/4-inch-thick slices
1 teaspoon olive oil
10 ounces frozen chopped spinach, thawed and squeezed dry
1 small carrot, shredded (about 1/3 cup)
3 tablespoons chopped fresh chives or tarragon
1/4 teaspoon pepper
1/8 teaspoon ground nutmeg
8 large egg whites or 1 cup liquid egg whites
3/4 cup fat-free plain yogurt
3/4 cup shredded low-fat sharp Cheddar cheese

Preheat the oven to 375°F. Lightly spray a standard 12-cup muffin pan with cooking spray.

Prepare the quinoa using the package directions, omitting the salt. Transfer to a large bowl. Fluff with a fork.

In a small nonstick skillet, heat the oil over medium heat, swirling to coat the bottom. Cook the onion for 5 minutes, or until browned, stirring frequently.

(continued)

Stir the onion into the quinoa. Stir in the spinach, carrot, chives, pepper, and nutmeg.

In a medium bowl, whisk together the egg whites until frothy. Whisk in the yogurt. Stir into the quinoa mixture until just blended. Spoon into the muffin cups. Sprinkle with the Cheddar.

Bake for 15 minutes, or until a wooden toothpick inserted in the center comes out clean. Transfer the pan to a cooling rack. Let cool for 30 minutes.

Cook's Tip: Substitute 1 cup cooked buckwheat, barley, or brown rice for the cooked quinoa.

PER SERVING

calories 148	carbohydrates 17 g
total fat 3.0 g	fiber 3 g
saturated fat 1.0 g	sugars 6 g
trans fat 0.0 g	protein 14 g
polyunsaturated fat 0.5 g	DIETARY EXCHANGES
monounsaturated fat 1.0 g	1/2 starch, 1 vegetable,
cholesterol 4 mg	1 1/2 lean meat
sodium 224 mg	

BREAKFAST PIZZAS

SERVES 4

Toasted sandwich thins stand in as the crust for these morning pizzas, which are topped with tomato sauce, cheesy spinach, and poached eggs. For an Italian-style brunch, serve with Watermelon Sangría *(page 31).*

> 10 ounces frozen chopped spinach, cooked, well drained, and squeezed dry
> 1 cup fat-free ricotta cheese
> 4 large eggs
> 1/2 cup no-salt-added tomato sauce, at room temperature
> 1 teaspoon dried Italian seasoning, crumbled
> 1/4 teaspoon crushed red pepper flakes
> 2 whole-grain sandwich thins (lowest sodium available), split and toasted

In a medium bowl, stir together the spinach and ricotta.

Heat a large nonstick skillet over medium heat.

Crack the eggs into a bowl. Don't beat them. Slide the eggs, one at a time, into the skillet. Cook, covered, for 1 to 2 minutes, or until the whites are set. Uncover. Cook until the yolks are the desired doneness. Remove from the heat.

In a small bowl, whisk together the tomato sauce, Italian seasoning, and red pepper flakes. Put the sandwich thin halves on plates. Spoon the tomato mixture over the sandwich thin halves. Spoon the spinach mixture over the tomato mixture. Top with the eggs.

PER SERVING

calories 196	carbohydrates 18 g
total fat 5.5 g	fiber 5 g
saturated fat 1.5 g	sugars 5 g
trans fat 0.0 g	protein 19 g
polyunsaturated fat 1.0 g	DIETARY EXCHANGES
monounsaturated fat 2.0 g	1 starch, 1 vegetable,
cholesterol 191 mg	2 lean meat
sodium 332 mg	

BREAKFAST TACOS

SERVES 4

For a Mexican-style breakfast, wrap scrambled eggs, veggies, and cheese in a corn tortilla.

> 8 ounces button mushrooms, sliced
> 1 medium onion, chopped
> 1 medium green bell pepper, chopped
> 4 large eggs
> 1/4 cup fat-free milk
> 4 6-inch corn tortillas
> 1/4 cup low-fat 4-cheese Mexican blend
> 1/4 cup fat-free sour cream
> 1 tablespoon chopped fresh cilantro

In a large nonstick skillet, cook the mushrooms over medium-high heat for 4 minutes, or until soft, stirring occasionally. Stir in the onion and bell pepper. Cook for 4 to 5 minutes, stirring occasionally.

Meanwhile, in a medium bowl, whisk together the eggs and milk. Pour the egg mixture over the mushroom mixture, stirring with a rubber scraper to combine. Cook until the eggs are set, stirring occasionally with the scraper. Remove from the heat.

Warm the tortillas using the package directions.

Spoon the egg mixture onto the tortillas. Sprinkle the Mexican blend cheese over the egg mixture. Top with the sour cream. Sprinkle with the cilantro.

PER SERVING

calories 129	**carbohydrates** 17 g
total fat 3.0 g	fiber 3 g
saturated fat 1.5 g	sugars 7 g
trans fat 0.0 g	**protein** 11 g
polyunsaturated fat 1.0 g	**DIETARY EXCHANGES**
monounsaturated fat 0.5 g	1 starch, 1 vegetable,
cholesterol 9 mg	1 lean meat
sodium 185 mg	

MANGO SUNRISE BREAKFAST PARFAITS

SERVES 4

Start the day out bright with this parfait and its brilliantly colored fruit. Roast the mango and prepare the yogurt mixture ahead of time and store them, covered, in the refrigerator so they're ready to go in the morning.

1 medium mango
24 ounces fat-free plain Greek yogurt
1 tablespoon confectioners' sugar
1 teaspoon vanilla extract
1 teaspoon grated orange zest or grated peeled gingerroot
1/4 cup fresh orange juice
1 tablespoon sugar
3/4 cup low-fat granola, coarsely crumbled
1 cup blueberries, raspberries, blackberries, or quartered hulled strawberries

Preheat the oven to 350°F.

Put the mango on a rimmed baking sheet or in a shallow baking pan. Bake for about 1 hour, or until fork-tender. Remove from the oven. Let cool for at least 3 minutes. Peel the mango. Dice the

flesh. (If you're roasting the mango in advance, transfer to an airtight container and refrigerate.)

In a medium bowl, stir together the yogurt, confectioners' sugar, and vanilla.

In a separate medium bowl, gently stir together the mango, orange zest, orange juice, and sugar.

Spoon the mango mixture into parfait glasses or wine goblets. Top, in order, with the yogurt mixture, granola, and berries. Serve immediately or cover and refrigerate for up to 4 hours.

PER SERVING

calories 242	**carbohydrates** 44 g
total fat 1.0 g	fiber 4 g
saturated fat 0.0 g	sugars 31 g
trans fat 0.0 g	**protein** 18 g
polyunsaturated fat 0.0 g	**DIETARY EXCHANGES**
monounsaturated fat 0.0 g	1 starch, 1 fruit, 1 fat-
cholesterol 0 mg	free milk, 1 lean meat
sodium 91 mg	

BLACKBERRY-POMEGRANATE YOGURT PARFAITS

SERVES 4

Adding fruit, nuts, and seeds to plain yogurt elevates both the nutrition and the flavor to whole new levels. Preparing this homemade parfait also makes it easier to avoid the more sugary store-bought yogurt options.

1 cup fat-free plain Greek yogurt and 1/4 cup fat-free plain Greek yogurt, divided use
2 teaspoons honey and 2 teaspoons honey, divided use
1/2 cup uncooked oatmeal
2 tablespoons ground flax seed
1 cup fresh or frozen blackberries, thawed if frozen
1/2 cup 100% pomegranate juice
1 tablespoon plus 1 teaspoon pomegranate arils (seeds)
1 tablespoon plus 1 teaspoon slivered almonds, dry-roasted

(continued)

In each 8-ounce parfait glass, layer as follows: 1/4 cup yogurt, 1/2 teaspoon honey, the oatmeal, flax seed, blackberries, pomegranate juice, the remaining 1 tablespoon yogurt, and the remaining 1/2 teaspoon honey.

Sprinkle the parfait with the pomegranate arils and almonds.

Cook's Tip: Both the yogurt and the pomegranate juice add moisture to the uncooked oatmeal, giving it a creamy, muesli-like texture.

PER SERVING

calories 167	fiber 4 g
total fat 3.5 g	sugars 15 g
saturated fat 0.0 g	**protein** 10 g
trans fat 0.0 g	**DIETARY EXCHANGES**
polyunsaturated fat 2.0 g	1/2 starch, 1/2 fruit,
monounsaturated fat 1.0 g	1/2 other
cholesterol 0 mg	carbohydrate, 1 lean
sodium 32 mg	meat
carbohydrates 25 g	

CANTALOUPE AND HONEYDEW PARFAITS

SERVES 4

Breakfast parfaits are a classic, but this recipe takes it to a whole new level by layering mint-infused melon with lightly sweetened and spiced yogurt. Make these ahead of time for a grab-and-go meal.

> 4 fresh mint leaves
> 1 tablespoon light brown sugar
> 1/2 teaspoon grated lime zest
> 1 tablespoon lime juice
> 1/4 medium honeydew melon, scooped into medium-size balls or cut into bite-size cubes
> 1/4 medium cantaloupe, scooped into medium-size balls or cut into bite-size cubes
> 2 cups fat-free plain yogurt
> 1 tablespoon honey
> 1/8 teaspoon ground nutmeg
> 2 tablespoons sliced almonds, dry-roasted

Using a mortar and pestle (or put all the ingredients in a medium bowl and use a fork), crush the mint leaves together with the brown sugar, lime zest, and lime juice, separating the mint into smaller pieces and releasing its flavor.

Put the honeydew melon and cantaloupe in a medium bowl. Add the mint mixture, stirring gently to coat.

In a small bowl, whisk together the yogurt, honey, and nutmeg.

In each parfait glass, layer as follows: 1/4 cup yogurt mixture and 2 tablespoons honeydew melon mixture. Repeat the layers. Sprinkle the parfaits with the almonds.

PER SERVING

calories 156	**carbohydrates** 28 g
total fat 2.0 g	fiber 1 g
saturated fat 0.5 g	sugars 26 g
trans fat 0.0 g	**protein** 8 g
polyunsaturated fat 0.5 g	**DIETARY EXCHANGES**
monounsaturated fat 1.0 g	1/2 fruit, 1 fat-free
cholesterol 3 mg	milk, 1/2 other
sodium 116 mg	carbohydrate

STRAWBERRY-BANANA BREAKFAST SHAKE

SERVES 1

How can you make an energizing breakfast in a flash? Just throw some fruit, dairy, and ice into a blender and in less than a minute you have yourself a creamy, protein-rich shake.

> 1 cup fat-free milk
> 1/2 cup frozen unsweetened strawberries
> 1/2 medium banana
> 1/3 cup fat-free plain Greek yogurt
> 1 teaspoon vanilla extract
> 1 teaspoon sugar
> 2 ice cubes

Put all the ingredients in a blender. Blend on high speed for 45 seconds, or until smooth and creamy.

calories 231
total fat 0.5 g
  saturated fat 0.0 g
  trans fat 0.0 g
  polyunsaturated fat 0.0 g
  monounsaturated fat 0.0 g
cholesterol 5 mg
sodium 134 mg

carbohydrates 40 g
  fiber 3 g
  sugars 31 g
protein 16 g
DIETARY EXCHANGES
  1 1/2 fruit, 1 1/2 fat-free
  milk

RASPBERRY BREAKFAST SHAKE

SERVES 1

Substitute the strawberries and banana for 2/3 cup frozen unsweetened raspberries. Proceed as directed.

calories 206
total fat 0.0 g
  saturated fat 0.0 g
  trans fat 0.0 g
  polyunsaturated fat 0.0 g
  monounsaturated fat 0.0 g
cholesterol 5 mg
sodium 132 mg

carbohydrates 34 g
  fiber 3 g
  sugars 26 g
protein 16 g
DIETARY EXCHANGES
  1 fruit, 1 1/2 fat-free
  milk

Desserts

APPLE-CHERRY DROPS

MAKES 32; 1 PER SERVING

Keep lots of these plump, fruity delights on hand for play dates or when friends drop by for coffee.

Cooking spray
2 1/2 cups all-purpose flour
1 teaspoon baking powder
1 teaspoon baking soda
1 teaspoon ground cinnamon
1/4 teaspoon ground nutmeg
1/4 teaspoon salt
1 cup sugar
1/2 cup light tub margarine
1/4 cup firmly packed light brown sugar
1 teaspoon vanilla extract
1/2 teaspoon almond extract
1/4 cup egg substitute
1/4 cup unsweetened applesauce
1 cup shredded peeled apple (about 1 large; Granny Smith, Gala, or Fuji preferred)
1/2 cup unsweetened dried cherries, coarsely chopped

Preheat the oven to 350°F. Lightly spray two baking sheets with cooking spray.

In a medium bowl, stir together the flour, baking powder, baking soda, cinnamon, nutmeg, and salt.

In a large bowl, using an electric mixer on medium speed, beat the sugar, margarine, brown sugar, and vanilla and almond extracts for 3 minutes.

Add the egg substitute and applesauce. Beat for 20 to 30 seconds, or until combined.

Gradually add the flour mixture, beating on low speed for 1 minute, or until no flour is visible.

Stir in the apple and cherries. Using about half the dough, drop by heaping teaspoonfuls about 2 inches apart on the baking sheets to make 32 cookies.

Bake for 10 to 12 minutes, or until light brown. Transfer the baking sheets to cooling racks. Let the cookies partially cool on the baking sheets, about 10 minutes. Transfer the cookies to the cooling racks. Repeat with the remaining batter.

Store any remaining cookies in an airtight container at room temperature for three or four days or refrigerate for up to seven days. For longer storage, layer between pieces of wax paper in an airtight freezer container and freeze for up to four months.

PER SERVING

calories 88	**sodium** 97 mg
total fat 1.0 g	**carbohydrates** 18 g
saturated fat 0.0 g	fiber 1 g
trans fat 0.0 g	sugars 10 g
polyunsaturated fat 0.5 g	**protein** 1 g
monounsaturated fat 0.5 g	**DIETARY EXCHANGES**
cholesterol 0 mg	1 other carbohydrate

CRANBERRY-ALMOND BISCOTTI

MAKES 28; 1 PER SERVING

Biscotti are typically baked, sliced, and baked again, making them a little hard to bite into, but nicely crunchy. They soften up when dunked in hot tea or coffee.

Cooking spray
2 cups all-purpose flour, plus more as needed for flouring the surface and kneading
2/3 cup sugar
2 teaspoons baking powder
1/4 teaspoon salt
2 large eggs
2 tablespoons unsweetened applesauce
2 tablespoons canola or corn oil
1 teaspoon grated lemon zest
1/4 teaspoon almond extract
3/4 cup sweetened dried cranberries
1/4 cup chopped almonds, dry-roasted

Preheat the oven to 350°F. Lightly spray a baking sheet with cooking spray.

In a medium bowl, stir together 2 cups flour, the sugar, baking powder, and salt.

In a small bowl, whisk together the eggs, applesauce, oil, lemon zest, and almond extract.

Stir the cranberries and almonds into the egg mixture. Stir the egg mixture into the flour mixture.

Lightly flour a flat surface. Turn out the dough. Knead just until blended, 10 to 12 strokes. With slightly moistened hands, form into two 8-inch logs. Put the logs on the baking sheet. Slightly flatten to 2 1/2 inches wide.

Bake for 25 minutes. Reduce the oven temperature to 300°F. Transfer the biscotti to a cooling rack. Let cool for 10 minutes.

Cut the biscotti into 1/2-inch slices to make 28 biscotti. Place the biscotti with the cut side down on the baking sheet.

Bake for 20 minutes, turning once halfway through. Transfer to a cooling rack. Let cool completely.

PER SERVING

calories 81	sodium 55 mg
total fat 2.0 g	carbohydrates 15 g
saturated fat 0.0 g	fiber 0 g
trans fat 0.0 g	sugars 7 g
polyunsaturated fat 0.5 g	protein 2 g
monounsaturated fat 1.0 g	**DIETARY EXCHANGES**
cholesterol 13 mg	1 starch

CHOCOLATE-PISTACHIO BISCOTTI

MAKES 28; 1 PER SERVING

Whether you use regular unsweetened cocoa powder or try the dark variety, you're going to enjoy these crunchy cookies. Like all other biscotti, they need a quick dunk in a beverage such as fat-free milk to soften them a bit.

> Cooking spray
> 1 1/2 cups all-purpose flour, plus more as needed for flouring the surface and kneading
> 2/3 cup firmly packed light brown sugar
> 1/2 cup unsweetened cocoa powder
> 2 teaspoons baking powder
> 1/4 teaspoon salt
> 2 large eggs
> 2 tablespoons unsweetened applesauce

> 2 tablespoons canola or corn oil
> 1 teaspoon vanilla extract
> 1/2 cup finely chopped unsalted pistachios, dry-roasted

Preheat the oven to 350°F. Lightly spray a baking sheet with cooking spray.

In a medium bowl, stir together 1 1/2 cups flour, the brown sugar, cocoa powder, baking powder, and salt.

In a small bowl, whisk together the eggs, applesauce, oil, and vanilla.

Whisk the pistachios into the egg mixture. Whisk the egg substitute mixture into the flour mixture.

Lightly flour a flat surface. Turn out the dough Knead just until blended, 10 to 12 strokes. With slightly moistened hands, form into two 8-inch logs. Put the logs on the baking sheet. Slightly flatten to 2 1/2 inches wide.

Bake for 25 minutes. Reduce the oven temperature to 300°F. Transfer the biscotti to a cooling rack. Let cool for 10 minutes.

Cut the biscotti into 1/2-inch slices to make 28 biscotti. Place the biscotti with the cut side down on the baking sheet.

Bake for 20 minutes, turning once halfway through. Transfer to a cooling rack. Let cool completely.

PER SERVING

calories 78	sodium 56 mg
total fat 2.5 g	carbohydrates 12 g
saturated fat 0.5 g	fiber 1 g
trans fat 0.0 g	sugars 5 g
polyunsaturated fat 0.5 g	protein 2 g
monounsaturated fat 1.5 g	**DIETARY EXCHANGES**
cholesterol 13 mg	1 starch, 1/2 fat

PLUM TASTY BARS

MAKES 24; 1 PER SERVING

These bars make a welcome treat in lunch boxes or as an after-school snack. They're just as good made with other unsweetened dried fruits, such as apricots, raisins, or cranberries.

> 1 1/2 cups 100% apple juice and 1/4 cup 100% apple juice, divided use
> 1 cup dried unsweetened cherries
> 6 ounces dried unsweetened plums, chopped
> 3 tablespoons cornstarch
> 1 1/2 teaspoons grated lemon zest
> Cooking spray
> 1 1/2 cups all-purpose flour or 1 cup all-purpose flour and 1/2 cup almond flour
> 1 teaspoon baking powder
> 1 1/4 cups uncooked quick-cooking oatmeal
> 3/4 cup light brown sugar
> 1/4 cup sugar
> 2/3 cup light tub margarine

In a medium saucepan, stir together 1 1/2 cups apple juice, the cherries, and plums. Cook over medium-low heat for 20 minutes, or until the fruit is tender, stirring occasionally.

In a small bowl, whisk together the cornstarch, lemon zest, and the remaining 1/4 cup apple juice until the cornstarch is dissolved. Whisk into the fruit mixture. Increase the heat to medium high and cook for 2 to 3 minutes, or until the mixture thickens, stirring constantly. Remove from the heat. Let cool.

Preheat the oven to 375°F. Lightly spray a 13 x 9 x 2-inch baking pan with cooking spray.

Sift the flour and baking powder together in a large bowl.

Stir in the oatmeal and both sugars.

Using a pastry blender or fork, blend in the margarine until the mixture is crumbly. Press about two-thirds of the mixture into the pan.

Spread the fruit mixture over the crust. Top with the remaining flour mixture.

Bake for 30 minutes, or until the crust is light golden brown. Let cool before slicing into 24 pieces.

PER SERVING

calories 131	**carbohydrates** 27 g
total fat 2.5 g	fiber 2 g
saturated fat 0.0 g	sugars 13 g
trans fat 0.0 g	**protein** 2 g
polyunsaturated fat 0.5 g	**DIETARY EXCHANGES**
monounsaturated fat 1.0 g	2 other carbohydrate,
cholesterol 0 mg	1/2 fat
sodium 61 mg	

CASHEW AND CARDAMOM COOKIES

MAKES 24; 1 PER SERVING

Cashew nuts are actually seeds. Their sweet flavor and creamy texture are highlighted in these easy-to-make cookies.

> Cooking spray
> 1 1/2 cups all-purpose flour
> 2 tablespoons confectioners' sugar and 1/3 cup confectioners' sugar, divided use
> 1/2 cup light tub margarine
> 1 cup finely chopped cashews, dry-roasted
> 3 tablespoons cold water (as needed)
> 1 teaspoon ground cardamom
> 1 teaspoon vanilla extract

Preheat the oven to 350°F. Lightly spray a large baking sheet with cooking spray.

In a large bowl, sift together the flour and 2 tablespoons sugar. Using a fork or pastry blender, cut in the margarine. Stir in the cashews, up to 3 tablespoons water, the cardamom, and vanilla. Stir until the batter is just moistened but no flour is visible. Don't overmix.

Shape the batter into 24 small rolls, about 1 inch long and 1/2 inch thick. Transfer the rolls to the baking sheet, placing them 2 inches apart. Bake for 25 to 30 minutes, or until firm.

Meanwhile, spread the remaining 1/3 cup sugar on a separate large baking sheet. While the cookies are still warm, roll them in the sugar.

calories 84
total fat 4.0 g
  saturated fat 0.5 g
  trans fat 0.0 g
  polyunsaturated fat 1.0 g
  monounsaturated fat 2.5 g
cholesterol 0 mg
sodium 31 mg

carbohydrates 10 g
  fiber 0 g
  sugars 3 g
protein 2 g
DIETARY EXCHANGES
  1/2 other
  carbohydrate, 1 fat

calories 84
total fat 1.0 g
  saturated fat 0.0 g
  trans fat 0.0 g
  polyunsaturated fat 0.0 g
  monounsaturated fat 0.5 g
cholesterol 6 mg

sodium 58 mg
carbohydrates 17 g
  fiber 1 g
  sugars 10 g
protein 2 g
DIETARY EXCHANGES
  1 other carbohydrate

GINGER COOKIES

MAKES 60; 2 PER SERVING

If you like a spicy, soft cookie, you'll love these. The warm spices make them especially popular around the holidays

1 cup sugar
1/2 cup unsweetened applesauce
1/4 cup light tub margarine
1 large egg, lightly beaten
1/4 cup molasses
3 cups white whole-wheat flour
1 teaspoon baking soda
1 teaspoon ground cinnamon
1 teaspoon ground ginger
Cooking spray

In a large bowl, using a sturdy spoon, beat together the sugar, applesauce, and margarine.

Beat in the egg and molasses.

In a separate large bowl, sift together the remaining ingredients except the cooking spray. Stir into the sugar mixture. Cover and refrigerate the dough for 2 hours, or until thoroughly chilled.

Preheat the oven to 350°F. Lightly spray two large baking sheets with cooking spray.

Using a teaspoon, drop about 60 mounds of dough about 1 inch apart on the baking sheets.

Bake for 10 to 12 minutes.

DARK CHOCOLATE WALNUT COOKIES

MAKES 48; 2 PER SERVING

Soft, chewy, chocolaty, and studded with nuts—these cookies are a delightful way to satisfy your sweet tooth.

1/2 cup light brown sugar
1/4 cup sugar
1 large egg
3 tablespoons light tub margarine, softened
1 teaspoon vanilla, butter, and nut flavoring
    or vanilla extract
3/4 cup self-rising flour
1/3 cup unsweetened cocoa powder
1 cup chopped walnuts, dry-roasted
Cooking spray

Preheat the oven to 350°F.

In a medium mixing bowl, stir together both sugars, the egg, margarine, and flavoring just to blend. Using an electric mixer on low speed, beat until well blended.

Gradually add the flour to the batter, beating after each addition. Add the cocoa powder, beating on medium speed until well blended.

Using a rubber scraper, stir in the walnuts, scraping the side of the bowl as needed.

Liberally spray two large baking sheets with cooking spray. Spoon 12 slightly rounded teaspoons of dough onto one baking sheet. Bake for 9 minutes.

Meanwhile, on a second baking sheet, spoon out enough dough for 12 cookies.

(continued)

When the cookies have baked for 9 minutes (they may not appear done), put the baking sheet on a cooling rack for 1 1/2 minutes. Don't leave the cookies on the baking sheet for more than 2 minutes; they will harden and crumble. Put a large piece of wax paper on the counter. Using a flat, thin metal spatula (plastic is too thick), gently transfer the first batch of cookies to the wax paper. When the cookies have cooled, place them between layers of wax paper to keep them from sticking together.

Repeat the baking until all the dough is used.

Cook's Tip: The dough is very thick and similar to a brownie batter. Spray 2 teaspoons with cooking spray to help you easily drop the dough onto the baking sheet.

PER SERVING

calories 83	carbohydrates 11 g
total fat 4.0 g	fiber 1 g
saturated fat 0.5 g	sugars 7 g
trans fat 0.0 g	**protein** 2 g
polyunsaturated fat 2.5 g	**DIETARY EXCHANGES**
monounsaturated fat 1.0 g	1/2 other
cholesterol 8 mg	carbohydrate, 1 fat
sodium 66 mg	

PEANUT BUTTER COOKIES

MAKES 60; 2 PER SERVING

Enjoy these cookies fresh from the oven with a glass of ice-cold fat-free milk.

Cooking spray
1/4 cup light tub margarine, softened
3/4 cup light brown sugar
1/2 cup sugar
1/3 cup low-sodium peanut butter
1 large egg
1/4 cup unsweetened applesauce
1/2 teaspoon baking soda
2 1/2 cups all-purpose flour
1 teaspoon vanilla extract

Preheat the oven to 350°F. Lightly spray two large baking sheets with cooking spray.

In a large mixing bowl, using an electric mixer on medium speed, cream the margarine. Gradually add both sugars, beating after each addition, until the mixture is creamy. Add the peanut butter, egg, applesauce, and baking soda. Beat well. Gradually add the flour to the batter, beating after each addition. Stir in the vanilla.

Roll the dough into 60 balls about the size of a pecan or the bowl of a measuring teaspoon. Transfer to the baking sheets. Flatten the balls slightly using the back of a wet fork.

Bake for 12 to 15 minutes, or until the cookies are light brown.

Cook's Tip on Cookie Dough: Cookies are easier to roll if you moisten your hands first with cold water. Also, dip your fork in cold water before flattening the cookies.

PER SERVING

calories 98	carbohydrates 18 g
total fat 2.5 g	fiber 1 g
saturated fat 0.5 g	sugars 9 g
trans fat 0.0 g	**protein** 2 g
polyunsaturated fat 0.5 g	**DIETARY EXCHANGES**
monounsaturated fat 1.0 g	1 other carbohydrate,
cholesterol 6 mg	1/2 fat
sodium 43 mg	

SPICE COOKIES

MAKES 48; 2 PER SERVING

If you're a fan of gingerbread or gingersnaps, you'll love these gingery treats, too.

Cooking spray
1/2 cup molasses
1/2 cup light tub margarine
1/4 cup light brown sugar
1 1/2 cups all-purpose flour
1/2 cup toasted wheat germ
1 tablespoon brewer's yeast
1 1/2 teaspoons ground ginger
1 1/2 teaspoons baking soda
1/2 teaspoon ground cinnamon

Preheat the oven to 350°F. Lightly spray two baking sheets with cooking spray.

In a small saucepan, bring the molasses to a boil over medium-high heat. Stir in the margarine and sugar until melted. Remove from the heat.

In a medium bowl, stir together the remaining ingredients. Stir the molasses mixture into the flour mixture until the batter is just moistened but no flour is visible.

Using a teaspoon, drop the dough by teaspoonfuls about 1/2 inch apart on the baking sheets to make 48 cookies. Bake for 8 to 10 minutes, or until firm.

Transfer the baking sheets to cooling racks. Let stand for 5 minutes. Transfer the cookies to the cooling racks. Let cool completely.

PER SERVING

calories 80	carbohydrates 15 g
total fat 2.0 g	fiber 1 g
saturated fat 0.0 g	sugars 7 g
trans fat 0.0 g	protein 2 g
polyunsaturated fat 0.5 g	**DIETARY EXCHANGES**
monounsaturated fat 1.0 g	1 other carbohydrate,
cholesterol 0 mg	1/2 fat
sodium 113 mg	

OATMEAL AND CARROT BAR COOKIES

MAKES 24; 1 PER SERVING

Bursting with flavor, these cookies also boost the health benefits of oatmeal and carrots. Don't be surprised when you open the cookie jar and find only crumbs!

Cooking spray
1/2 cup raisins
1/2 cup light brown sugar
2 tablespoons light tub margarine, at room temperature
1/4 cup unsweetened applesauce
1 large egg
1 1/4 cups grated carrots
1/2 teaspoon ground cinnamon
1/2 teaspoon grated lemon or orange zest
1/2 teaspoon vanilla extract
1/4 teaspoon ground nutmeg
1 cup all-purpose flour
1/2 cup uncooked quick-cooking oatmeal
1 teaspoon baking powder
1 tablespoon sifted confectioners' sugar

Preheat the oven to 350°F. Lightly spray an 11 x 7 x 2-inch baking dish with cooking spray.

Put the raisins in a small bowl. Pour in boiling water to cover. Let soak for 15 minutes. Drain well in a colander. Set aside.

Meanwhile, in a large mixing bowl, using an electric mixer on medium speed, cream the brown sugar and margarine until fluffy. Add the applesauce and egg. Beat well. Stir in the carrots, cinnamon, lemon zest, vanilla, nutmeg, and raisins.

In a medium bowl, stir together the flour, oatmeal, and baking powder. Stir into the brown sugar mixture until moistened, but no flour is visible. Pour the batter into the baking dish.

Bake for 20 to 25 minutes, or until the top is lightly golden. Transfer to a cooling rack. Let cool completely.

Just before slicing into 24 pieces, sprinkle lightly with the confectioners' sugar.

PER SERVING

calories 64	sodium 33 mg
total fat 1.0 g	carbohydrates 14 g
saturated fat 0.0 g	fiber 1 g
trans fat 0.0 g	sugars 7 g
polyunsaturated fat 0.0 g	protein 1 g
monounsaturated fat 0.5 g	**DIETARY EXCHANGES**
cholesterol 8 mg	1 other carbohydrate

PUMPKIN-SPICED MERINGUE COOKIES

SERVES 24; 1 PER SERVING

Enjoy this year's fall season with these autumnal cookies. A perfect treat for a Halloween party or a sweet ending to Cider-Glazed Turkey Tenderloin with Harvest Vegetables *(page 233).*

4 large egg whites
1/2 teaspoon cream of tartar
1 cup sugar
1 teaspoon white vinegar
1 teaspoon vanilla extract
1 teaspoon pumpkin pie spice

Preheat the oven to 275°F. Line two large baking sheets with cooking parchment or aluminum foil.

In a large metal or glass mixing bowl, using an electric mixer on high speed, beat the egg whites and cream of tartar until stiff peaks form (the peaks don't fall when the beaters are lifted). Add the sugar, 2 tablespoons at a time, beating well after each addition. To test if the sugar is dissolved completely, rub the meringue mixture between your fingers; if the meringue is grainy, you may need to beat and test it again. Add the vinegar, vanilla, and pumpkin pie spice, beating well to blend.

Drop the mixture by 2 heaping tablespoonfuls about 2 inches apart on the baking sheets to make 24 meringues.

Bake for 45 minutes. Do not open the oven door.

Reduce the heat to 250°F. Bake for about 15 minutes, or until each meringue is firm and crisp, but not brown.

Transfer the meringues to a cooling rack. Let cool slightly or serve warm. Store any leftover meringues in an airtight container for a week to 10 days.

Cook's Tip: Even a single drop of egg yolk will prevent egg whites from whipping stiff, so separate eggs very carefully, one at a time.

PER SERVING

calories 36	**sodium** 9 mg
total fat 0.0 g	**carbohydrates** 9 g
saturated fat 0.0 g	fiber 0 g
trans fat 0.0 g	sugars 8 g
polyunsaturated fat 0.0 g	**protein** 1 g
monounsaturated fat 0.0 g	**DIETARY EXCHANGES**
cholesterol 0 mg	1/2 other
	carbohydrate

MERINGUE SHELLS

MAKES 12; 1 PER SERVING

Using half of each ingredient in the Pumpkin-Spiced Meringue Cookies (do not include the pumpkin pie spice), proceed as directed through beating the vinegar and vanilla into the egg white mixture. Drop the mixture by 2 heaping tablespoonfuls about 2 inches apart on the two baking sheets to create 12 mounds. Smooth each mound into a 2-inch circle. Using a teaspoon, press into the center of each to form a well, leaving a 1/2-inch border. Bake as directed. Transfer the shells to a cooling rack. Let cool before filling.

Cook's Tip: Fill these shells with fat-free, sugar-free vanilla ice cream or frozen yogurt drizzled with Blueberry Sauce (page 439). Also, try with your favorite fresh fruit and top with Raspberry Port Sauce (page 439) or Chocolate Sauce (page 438).

PER SERVING

calories 36	**carbohydrates** 9 g
total fat 0.0 g	fiber 0 g
saturated fat 0.0 g	sugars 8 g
trans fat 0.0 g	**protein** 1 g
polyunsaturated fat 0.0 g	**DIETARY EXCHANGES**
monounsaturated fat 0.0 g	1/2 other
cholesterol 0 mg	carbohydrate
sodium 9 mg	

RASPBERRY CRUMBLE BARS

MAKES 12; 1 PER SERVING

Serve these with plenty of napkins to catch those scrumptious crumbs. You won't want to miss a morsel.

Cooking spray
3/4 cup all-purpose flour
3 tablespoons sugar
1 tablespoon chopped walnuts
2 teaspoons grated lemon zest
1/8 teaspoon ground nutmeg
1/4 cup light tub margarine
2 ounces fat-free cream cheese
2 tablespoons confectioners' sugar
2 tablespoons fat-free milk
1/4 teaspoon vanilla extract
3 tablespoons all-fruit seedless raspberry
      spread

Preheat the oven to 350°F. Lightly spray an 8-inch square baking dish with cooking spray.

In a small bowl, stir together the flour, sugar, walnuts, lemon zest, and nutmeg. Using a knife or pastry blender, cut in the margarine until the mixture resembles coarse crumbs. Press the mixture firmly and evenly in the baking dish.

Bake for 15 minutes, or until the crust is golden. Transfer the dish to a cooling rack. Let cool completely.

Meanwhile, put the cream cheese in a small microwaveable bowl. Microwave, covered, on 50 percent power (medium) for 20 to 30 seconds, or until soft. Whisk in the confectioners' sugar, milk, and vanilla until smooth. Cover and refrigerate for 30 minutes, or until firm.

Spread the cream-cheese mixture over the crust.

Put the fruit spread in a small microwaveable bowl. Microwave on 100 percent power (high) for 10 seconds, or until slightly melted. Stir to melt completely. Drizzle over the cream-cheese mixture. Let cool for 5 minutes before slicing into 12 pieces.

Cook's Tip: If you have leftovers, refrigerate them for up to 24 hours.

PER SERVING

calories 79	carbohydrates 14 g
total fat 2.0 g	fiber 0 g
saturated fat 0.0 g	sugars 7 g
trans fat 0.0 g	protein 2 g
polyunsaturated fat 0.5 g	DIETARY EXCHANGES
monounsaturated fat 1.0 g	1 other carbohydrate,
cholesterol 1 mg	1/2 fat
sodium 65 mg	

PEACH-PLUM CRUMBLE

SERVES 8

Make this crumble when summer fruits are at their peak. The almonds toast as the crumble bakes, making the topping extra crisp.

Cooking spray
6 large peaches, peeled and sliced, or 4 cups
      frozen unsweetened sliced peaches,
      thawed and drained
4 large plums, peeled and sliced
2 tablespoons all-purpose flour and
      2 tablespoons all-purpose flour,
      divided use
2 teaspoons grated lemon zest
1/2 cup uncooked oatmeal
1/3 cup firmly packed light brown sugar
1/2 teaspoon ground cinnamon
2 tablespoons canola or corn oil
1/4 cup sliced almonds

Preheat the oven to 350°F. Lightly spray an 8-inch square glass baking dish with cooking spray.

In a large bowl, gently stir together the peaches, plums, 2 tablespoons flour, and the lemon zest. Spoon into the baking dish.

In a medium bowl, stir together the oatmeal, brown sugar, cinnamon, and the remaining 2 tablespoons flour.

Drizzle the oil over the topping mixture. Stir until crumbly.

(continued)

Stir the almonds into the topping mixture. Sprinkle over the filling.

Bake for 30 to 35 minutes, or until the topping is lightly browned. Transfer to a cooling rack. Let cool for a few minutes before serving.

Cook's Tip: You can vary the fruits and make this crumble throughout the summer. Use nectarines or apricots for the peaches, and substitute blackberries or raspberries for the plums.

PER SERVING

calories 183	sodium 3 mg
total fat 6.0 g	carbohydrates 33 g
saturated fat 0.5 g	fiber 4 g
trans fat 0.0 g	sugars 23 g
polyunsaturated fat 1.5 g	protein 3 g
monounsaturated fat 3.5 g	DIETARY EXCHANGES
cholesterol 0 mg	1 starch, 1 fruit, 1 fat

PEACH CLAFOUTI

SERVES 8

Traditionally a French clafouti is fresh fruit baked in an egg-custard batter. Here, we've sandwiched the fruit between two layers of batter instead—a double treat.

Cooking spray
1 1/2 teaspoons sugar
1/4 teaspoon ground cinnamon and
    1/2 teaspoon ground cinnamon,
    divided use
1 1/4 cups fat-free milk
1 cup all-purpose flour
3/4 cup egg substitute
1/4 cup firmly packed light brown sugar
1 tablespoon vanilla extract
1 teaspoon almond extract
1/4 teaspoon ground nutmeg
1/4 teaspoon salt
1 1/2 pounds peaches, peeled and sliced
    (about 3 1/2 cups)
3 tablespoons sliced almonds, dry-roasted

Preheat the oven to 350°F. Lightly spray a 9-inch square baking pan with cooking spray.

In a small bowl, stir together the sugar and 1/4 teaspoon cinnamon. Set aside.

In a food processor or blender, process the milk, flour, egg substitute, brown sugar, both extracts, nutmeg, salt, and the remaining 1/2 teaspoon cinnamon until smooth. Spread about 1/4 cup batter in the baking pan.

Bake for 5 to 10 minutes, or until set (the center doesn't jiggle when the pan is gently shaken). Arrange the peaches on the cooked batter. Pour the remaining batter on top. Bake for 20 minutes. Sprinkle the almonds, then the sugar mixture on top. Bake for 40 minutes, or until the center is set. Serve warm.

PER SERVING

calories 162	carbohydrates 31 g
total fat 1.5 g	fiber 2 g
saturated fat 0.0 g	sugars 17 g
trans fat 0.0 g	protein 6 g
polyunsaturated fat 0.5 g	DIETARY EXCHANGES
monounsaturated fat 0.5 g	1 starch, 1 fruit,
cholesterol 1 mg	1/2 lean meat
sodium 138 mg	

IRISH BOILED CAKE

SERVES 16

This traditional Emerald Isle cake is similar to a fruitcake, but instead of candied fruit it uses raisins and currants. Don't let the recipe name get in the way of your trying this recipe. The cake itself is actually not boiled; rather, the dried fruits are boiled in a sugar-margarine mixture, which is then added to the remaining ingredients and baked.

1/2 cup dark raisins
1/2 cup golden raisins
1/2 cup currants
Cooking spray
1 cup water
1/2 cup plus 2 tablespoons brown sugar
1/2 cup light tub margarine
1 cup whole-wheat flour
1 cup all-purpose flour
1 1/2 teaspoons baking powder

1 teaspoon ground cinnamon
1/8 teaspoon salt
1/4 cup sherry

Soak both types of raisins and the currants in hot water to cover for 30 minutes, or until they swell. Drain well in a colander.

Preheat the oven to 350°F. Lightly spray an 8 1/2 x 4 1/2 x 2 1/2-inch loaf pan with cooking spray.

In a large saucepan, stir together the water, brown sugar, margarine, and soaked fruits. Bring to a boil over high heat. Boil for 20 minutes, stirring occasionally. Remove from the heat. Let stand for 5 minutes to cool slightly.

Meanwhile, in a large bowl, stir together both flours, the baking powder, cinnamon, and salt.

Pour the sherry and brown sugar mixture into the flour mixture, stirring until moistened but no flour is visible.

Spoon the batter into the pan, gently smoothing the top. Bake for 45 minutes.

Reduce the heat to 325°F. Bake for 15 minutes, or until a wooden toothpick inserted in the center comes out clean.

PER SERVING

calories 153	carbohydrates 32 g
total fat 2.5 g	fiber 2 g
saturated fat 0.0 g	sugars 18 g
trans fat 0.0 g	protein 2 g
polyunsaturated fat 0.5 g	**DIETARY EXCHANGES**
monounsaturated fat 1.5 g	2 other carbohydrate,
cholesterol 0 mg	1/2 fat
sodium 106 mg	

NUT CRUST

SERVES 8

Homemade crusts are usually much healthier than the store-bought varieties, which can be high in saturated and trans fats and sodium. With so few ingredients, you can put this crust together in no time. Fill it with plain yogurt blended with your favorite fresh fruit.

1 cup all-purpose flour
1/3 cup light tub margarine, softened
1/4 cup finely chopped pecans, dry-roasted
1/4 cup confectioners' sugar

Preheat the oven to 400°F.

In a medium bowl, stir together all the ingredients until a soft dough forms. Press the dough firmly and evenly against the bottom and side (not the rim) of a 9-inch pie pan.

Bake for 12 to 15 minutes, or until lightly browned. Cool thoroughly before filling.

PER SERVING

calories 122	sodium 62 mg
total fat 5.5 g	carbohydrates 16 g
saturated fat 0.0 g	fiber 1 g
trans fat 0.0 g	sugars 4 g
polyunsaturated fat 1.5 g	protein 2 g
monounsaturated fat 3.0 g	**DIETARY EXCHANGES**
cholesterol 0 mg	1 starch, 1 fat

PUMPKIN PIE BITES

MAKES 24; 1 PER SERVING

These mini pumpkin pies are made without a crust and in mini muffin pans for just the perfect portion of sweetness. This recipe yields 24 mini pies so it's an ideal dessert to serve on a buffet table at Thanksgiving or at a Halloween party.

Cooking spray
1 cup canned solid-pack pumpkin (not pie filling)
1/4 cup mashed banana (about 1/2 medium banana)
2 large eggs
3 tablespoons firmly packed light brown sugar
1 tablespoon light or dark molasses
1 1/2 teaspoons ground cinnamon
1/2 teaspoon ground ginger
1/4 teaspoon maple extract
1/8 teaspoon ground nutmeg
2/3 cup lite coconut milk
1/2 cup fat-free aerosol whipped topping
1/4 cup unsweetened shredded coconut

(continued)

Preheat the oven to 350°F. Lightly spray a 24-cup mini muffin pan with cooking spray.

In a food processor or blender, process the pumpkin and banana until smooth. Add the eggs. Process until combined. Add the brown sugar, molasses, cinnamon, ginger, maple extract, and nutmeg. Process until blended. With the food processor running, slowly pour in the coconut milk and process until blended.

Spoon the pumpkin mixture into the muffin cups.

Bake for 20 minutes, or until a wooden toothpick inserted in the center comes out clean.

Transfer the pan to a cooling rack. Let stand for 10 minutes. Carefully transfer the mini pies to the rack. Let cool to room temperature. Refrigerate for 1 to 2 hours, or until chilled (the texture is firmer when they're chilled).

Meanwhile, spread the coconut on a baking sheet. Bake for 5 to 8 minutes, or until lightly browned, stirring occasionally.

Just before serving, top each mini pie with 1 teaspoon of the whipped topping. Sprinkle with the coconut.

Cook's Tip: The mini pies can be made up to one day in advance. Cover and refrigerate them until serving time.

PER SERVING

calories 33	carbohydrates 5 g
total fat 1.5 g	fiber 1 g
saturated fat 1.0 g	sugars 3 g
trans fat 0.0 g	**protein** 1 g
polyunsaturated fat 0.0 g	**DIETARY EXCHANGES**
monounsaturated fat 0.0 g	1/2 other
cholesterol 16 mg	carbohydrate
sodium 11 mg	

CREPES

MAKES ABOUT 22; 2 PER SERVING

For a simple dessert, fill the crepes with a chocolate-cheesecake or strawberry filling (see recipes on page 495) or your favorite fruit and serve topped with a light dusting of sifted confectioners' sugar, or a drizzle of Chocolate Sauce *(page 438) or* Raspberry Port Sauce *(page 439).*

Batter
    1 1/2 cups sifted all-purpose flour
    3/4 cup fat-free milk
    3/4 cup cold water
    2 large egg whites
    1/4 cup light stick margarine (no trans fats), melted
    2 tablespoons rum or orange-flavored liqueur (optional)
    1 tablespoon sugar
    2 to 3 tablespoons water, as needed

■ ■ ■

Cooking spray (butter flavor preferred)

In a large mixing bowl, using an electric mixer on high, beat together the batter ingredients except the water for about 1 minute, or until smooth. The batter will be thin. Cover tightly with plastic wrap and refrigerate for 2 hours to one day.

Line a plate with paper towels.

Lightly spray a small skillet with cooking spray. Heat over medium heat. When the skillet is hot, remove it from the heat. Spoon 2 tablespoons batter onto the skillet. Lift and tilt the skillet to spread the batter evenly. Return it to the heat. Cook the crepe for 2 to 3 minutes, or until the bottom is lightly browned. Turn the crepe over. Cook for about 30 seconds, or until lightly browned. Transfer the crepe to the paper towels. Repeat with the remaining batter, lightly spraying the skillet with cooking spray if necessary to make 21 more crepes. If the first crepe is too thick, whisk the water into the remaining batter.

Cook's Tip on Crepes: Test the crepe pan's readiness just as you test a pancake griddle's. Sprinkle a few drops of water on the hot surface; if they dance, your pan is hot enough. Properly cooked crepes taste delicate but actually are fairly sturdy. If one tears, it probably needed a few more seconds of cooking time. To store crepes, stack with wax paper between layers and place in airtight plastic bags. Refrigerate overnight or freeze. For ease in rolling when filled, crepes should be at room temperature when used.

CHOCOLATE-CHEESECAKE CREPES

MAKES 10; 1 PER SERVING

2 cups fat-free ricotta cheese
3 tablespoons unsweetened cocoa powder
2 large egg whites
1/4 cup plus 1 tablespoon and 2 teaspoons sugar
1/8 teaspoon salt
10 6-inch crepes, at room temperature
1 cup raspberries

In a food processor or blender, process the ricotta and cocoa until smooth. Transfer to a large bowl.

In a medium heatproof mixing bowl set over a pot of simmering water, heat the egg whites, sugar, and salt for 3 minutes, or until the sugar is dissolved and the mixture is heated through, whisking constantly. Remove the bowl from the heat. Using an electric mixer on high, beat the egg white mixture for 5 minutes, or until stiff peaks form.

Using a rubber spatula, gently fold the egg white mixture into the ricotta mixture until well combined. Cover and refrigerate for 3 hours to one day, or until set.

Just before serving time, spoon the ricotta mixture into the center of the crepes. Roll the crepes around the filling jelly-roll style. Garnish with the raspberries.

STRAWBERRY CREPES

MAKES 10; 1 PER SERVING

3 tablespoons dark brown sugar
2 tablespoons 100% orange juice
1/4 teaspoon ground cinnamon
2 1/2 cups sliced hulled strawberries
10 6-inch crepes, at room temperature

In a large bowl, stir together the brown sugar, orange juice, and cinnamon. Gently fold in the strawberries.

Spoon about 1/4 cup strawberry mixture into the center of each crepe. Roll the crepes around the filling jelly-roll style.

CHAI-SPICED FLANS WITH BLUEBERRIES

SERVES 6

The secret to success in making flans is to bake them in a water bath, or bain marie. This recipe uses boiling, not merely hot, water for the water bath; otherwise, the delicate custard will need about twice as much cooking time.

Cooking spray
2 1/2 cups fat-free half-and-half
1/2 cup egg substitute
3 tablespoons sugar and 1 tablespoon sugar, divided use
1 teaspoon vanilla extract
1/8 teaspoon ground cardamom
1/8 teaspoon ground cinnamon
1/8 teaspoon ground cloves
1 1/2 cups blueberries

Preheat the oven to 325°F. Lightly spray six 6-ounce ovenproof glass custard cups or porcelain ramekins with cooking spray.

In a large bowl, whisk together the half-and-half, egg substitute, 3 tablespoons sugar, and the vanilla. Pour into the custard cups.

Place a 13 x 9 x 2-inch baking pan in the oven. Carefully pour about 2 cups boiling water into the pan. Place the custard cups in the pan.

Bake for 40 minutes, or until a knife inserted near the center of a flan comes out clean. Carefully transfer the custard cups to a cooling rack. Let cool completely, about 1 hour. Cover and refrigerate until needed. (The flans don't need to be cold when you serve them.)

At serving time, run a knife around the edge of each flan. Place a dessert plate on each and invert.

In a small bowl, stir together the cardamom, cinnamon, cloves, and the remaining 1 tablespoon sugar. Sprinkle over each flan. Spoon 1/4 cup of blueberries around each. Serve immediately.

PER SERVING

calories 133	**carbohydrates** 28 g
total fat 0.0 g	fiber 1 g
saturated fat 0.0 g	sugars 19 g
trans fat 0.0 g	**protein** 9 g
polyunsaturated fat 0.0 g	**DIETARY EXCHANGES**
monounsaturated fat 0.0 g	2 other carbohydrate,
cholesterol 0 mg	1 1/2 lean meat
sodium 142 mg	

COFFEE-COCONUT CUSTARDS

SERVES 6

There's no need to serve coffee with this sophisticated dessert; the coffee's already included! You can use decaffeinated granules if you prefer.

Cooking spray
2 cups fat-free milk
2 tablespoons instant coffee granules
2 large eggs
1/4 cup sugar
2 teaspoons vanilla extract
1/4 teaspoon coconut extract
1/8 teaspoon salt

Preheat the oven to 350°F. Lightly spray six 6-ounce ovenproof glass custard cups or porcelain ramekins with cooking spray.

In a small saucepan, heat the milk and coffee over medium-high heat until very hot but not boiling, whisking constantly. Remove from the heat.

In a medium bowl, gently whisk together the remaining ingredients. Gently whisk in the milk mixture (don't create foam). Pour the mixture into the custard cups. Place the custard cups in a 13 x 9 x 2-inch baking pan. Pour hot tap water into the pan to a depth of 1 inch.

Bake for 30 to 40 minutes, or until a knife inserted halfway between the cup and the center of the custard comes out clean (the center won't quite be firm). Transfer the pan to a cooling rack. Carefully transfer the custard cups to a separate cooling rack for 20 minutes. For best results, cover and refrigerate until chilled.

MICROWAVE METHOD

Prepare the custard mixture as directed. Pour into microwaveable custard cups lightly sprayed with cooking spray. Put the cups in a microwaveable baking dish. Add the water as directed. Microwave on 100 percent power (high) for 12 to 15 minutes, or until the centers are just set (don't jiggle when the custard cups are gently shaken). Cool and chill as directed on page 496.

PER SERVING

calories 92	carbohydrates 14 g
total fat 1.5 g	fiber 0 g
saturated fat 0.5 g	sugars 13 g
trans fat 0.0 g	protein 5 g
polyunsaturated fat 0.5 g	DIETARY EXCHANGES
monounsaturated fat 0.5 g	1 other carbohydrate,
cholesterol 64 mg	1/2 lean meat
sodium 107 mg	

PUMPKIN CUSTARDS

SERVES 6

Need to get more fruit into your diet? Pumpkin, which is considered a fruit, is the star of this dish. Try this recipe as a healthy alternative to traditional pumpkin pie.

Cooking spray
12 ounces fat-free evaporated milk
1 cup egg substitute
1 15-ounce can solid pack pumpkin (not pie filling)
1/4 cup sugar
1 1/2 teaspoons vanilla extract
1/2 teaspoon ground cinnamon
1/4 teaspoon ground nutmeg
1 1/2 cups fat-free, sugar-free vanilla ice cream or frozen yogurt

Preheat the oven to 325°F. Lightly spray six 6-ounce ovenproof glass custard cups or porcelain ramekins with cooking spray. Place the custard cups in a 13 x 9 x 2-inch baking pan. Set aside.

In a small saucepan, heat the milk over medium heat for 5 minutes, or until hot, stirring occasionally. Don't let it boil. Remove from the heat.

In a medium bowl, using an electric mixer on medium speed, beat the egg substitute for 1 minute. Add the pumpkin, sugar, vanilla, cinnamon, and nutmeg. Beat for 1 minute. Stir in the milk. Beat for 1 minute. Pour into the custard cups.

Pour enough hot water into the baking pan to come up about halfway, being careful to keep the water out of the cups.

Bake for 40 minutes, or until a knife inserted in the center of a custard comes out clean. Carefully remove the pan from the oven. Transfer the cups from the pan to a cooling rack. Put plastic wrap directly on the surface of each custard. Let cool to room temperature. Refrigerate for at least 1 hour. (Can be made up to one day ahead.)

Just before serving, run a table knife around the edge of each custard. Invert them onto small plates. Top each custard with a scoop of ice cream. Serve immediately.

PER SERVING

calories 172	fiber 3 g
total fat 0.5 g	sugars 21 g
saturated fat 0.0 g	protein 12 g
trans fat 0.0 g	DIETARY EXCHANGES
polyunsaturated fat 0.0 g	1 fat-free milk,
monounsaturated fat 0.0 g	1 vegetable, 1 other
cholesterol 3 mg	carbohydrate,
sodium 185 mg	1 1/2 lean meat
carbohydrates 31 g	

CHOCOLATE-MINT PUDDING

SERVES 4

Skip the boxed pudding mixes full of added sugar and sodium and treat yourself to this creamy, chocolaty pudding with zingy notes of fresh mint.

2 cups fat-free milk
1/2 cup tightly packed sprigs of fresh mint and 4 sprigs of fresh mint, divided use
1/4 cup egg substitute
2 tablespoons plus 2 teaspoons sugar
2 tablespoons cornstarch
2 tablespoons unsweetened dark cocoa powder
1/4 teaspoon mint extract

(continued)

In a heavy, medium saucepan, bring the milk to a boil over medium-high heat. Remove from the heat. Stir in the 1/2 cup of mint sprigs. Let stand, covered, for 15 minutes.

Strain the milk through a fine-mesh sieve into a medium bowl. Pour the strained milk back into the pan.

Whisk in the egg substitute, sugar, cornstarch, and cocoa powder until the sugar and cornstarch are dissolved. Cook, still over medium-high heat, for 8 to 10 minutes, or until the mixture comes to a full boil and begins to thicken, whisking constantly. Remove from the heat. Stir in the mint extract.

Spoon the pudding into dessert dishes. Garnish with the remaining 4 sprigs of mint.

Cook's Tip: If you prefer cold pudding, cover the surface of the pudding with plastic wrap before refrigerating to prevent skin from forming. Chill at least 3 hours.

PER SERVING

calories 109	carbohydrates 20 g
total fat 0.5 g	fiber 1 g
saturated fat 0.0 g	sugars 15 g
trans fat 0.0 g	protein 6 g
polyunsaturated fat 0.0 g	DIETARY EXCHANGES
monounsaturated fat 0.0 g	1/2 fat-free milk,
cholesterol 3 mg	1 other carbohydrate
sodium 83 mg	

INDIAN-SPICED RICE PUDDING

SERVES 6

You'll have a whole new appreciation for rice pudding when it's been updated with fragrant Indian spices. Raisins and pistachios add textural contrast to the creamy pudding.

Cooking spray
1/2 cup uncooked quick-cooking brown rice
2 cups fat-free milk, heated
1/4 cup sugar
2 teaspoons coconut extract
1/4 teaspoon ground cardamom
1/4 cup egg substitute
1/4 cup golden raisins

1/4 cup chopped unsalted pistachios, dry-roasted

Lightly spray a 1-quart casserole dish with cooking spray. Set aside.

Prepare the rice using the package directions, omitting the salt and margarine. Transfer to the casserole dish.

Meanwhile, preheat the oven to 350°F.

Add to the casserole dish, in order, the milk, sugar, coconut extract, cardamom, and egg substitute. Stir well. Gently stir in the raisins and pistachios. Cover the dish and set in a 13 x 9 x 2-inch baking pan. Pour hot tap water into the pan to a depth of 1 inch.

Bake for 1 hour, or until the mixture is thick. Serve warm or cover and refrigerate to serve chilled.

Cook's Tip on Bain Marie: Using a *bain marie* (*bahn mah-REE*), or water bath, is a technique for cooking custards and some other fragile foods. The container holding the food is placed in a larger pan (also called a *bain marie*) that holds a small amount of hot water. The technique keeps the food from separating or curdling.

PER SERVING

calories 148	carbohydrates 26 g
total fat 2.5 g	fiber 1 g
saturated fat 0.5 g	sugars 17 g
trans fat 0.0 g	protein 6 g
polyunsaturated fat 1.0 g	DIETARY EXCHANGES
monounsaturated fat 1.5 g	1 1/2 other
cholesterol 2 mg	carbohydrate, 1 lean
sodium 58 mg	meat

GREEK YOGURT WITH HONEY AND WALNUTS

SERVES 4

Called Yiaourti me Mele, *this simple dish is often served for dessert in tavernas throughout Greece. A touch of honey tames the tartness of the creamy yogurt, while the nuts add a contrasting crunch.*

2 cups fat-free plain Greek yogurt
1/2 teaspoon vanilla extract (optional)

1/4 cup chopped walnuts, dry-roasted

2 tablespoons plus 2 teaspoons honey

Ground cinnamon to taste

In a medium serving bowl, stir together the yogurt and vanilla. Sprinkle with the walnuts. Drizzle with the honey. Sprinkle with the cinnamon.

PER SERVING

calories 150	carbohydrates 17 g
total fat 5.0 g	fiber 1 g
saturated fat 0.5 g	sugars 16 g
trans fat 0.0 g	**protein** 11 g
polyunsaturated fat 3.5 g	**DIETARY EXCHANGES**
monounsaturated fat 0.5 g	1 other carbohydrate,
cholesterol 0 mg	1 1/2 lean meat
sodium 43 mg	

BLUEBERRY-POMEGRANATE PARFAITS WITH A MINT RUM SAUCE

SERVES 4

Jewel-toned fruits are layered with a mint rum cream sauce in this patriotic red, white, and blue dessert. If you prefer, you can use raspberries, pitted cherries, or sliced strawberries in place of the pomegranate arils.

1 cup fat-free milk and 1/4 cup fat-free milk, divided use

2 tablespoons plus 2 teaspoons sugar

1 tablespoon plus 1 teaspoon cornstarch

1 tablespoon chopped fresh mint and 4 sprigs of fresh mint, divided use

1 tablespoon rum or rum extract

6 ounces blueberries

6 ounces pomegranate arils (seeds) and 1 tablespoon plus 1 teaspoon pomegranate arils (seeds), divided use

In a small saucepan, whisk together 1 cup milk and the sugar. Bring to a boil over medium-high heat, whisking occasionally until the sugar is dissolved.

Meanwhile, in a small bowl, whisk together the remaining 1/4 cup milk and the cornstarch until the cornstarch is dissolved. Whisk into the sugar

mixture. Cook for 2 to 3 minutes, or until thickened, whisking constantly. Remove from the heat.

Whisk the chopped mint and rum into the sauce. Let cool for 20 minutes to set slightly.

Spoon the 6 ounces pomegranate arils into the parfait glasses, dividing evenly. Spoon about 1/4 cup sauce into each glass. Spoon one-fourth of the blueberries into each glass. Top with the remaining sauce. Garnish each parfait with 1 teaspoon of the remaining pomegranate arils and the sprigs of mint. Cover and refrigerate for about 2 hours.

Cook's Tip on Pomegranate Arils: Look for pomegranate arils (seeds) in the frozen section of your grocery store. The frozen variety are not as brightly colored as fresh arils, but they still provide color and a tangy flavor to dishes.

PER SERVING

calories 140	carbohydrates 30 g
total fat 0.5 g	fiber 3 g
saturated fat 0.0 g	sugars 23 g
trans fat 0.0 g	**protein** 4 g
polyunsaturated fat 0.0 g	**DIETARY EXCHANGES**
monounsaturated fat 0.0 g	1 fruit, 1 other
cholesterol 2 mg	carbohydrate
sodium 35 mg	

PEACH MELBA PARFAITS

SERVES 4

Our lightened version of Peach Melba requires some planning to accommodate the freezing time. But because you can freeze the mixture for up to five days, this is an ideal make-ahead dessert.

1 cup raspberries and 1/2 cup raspberries, divided use

1 1/2 cups fat-free, sugar-free vanilla yogurt

1 medium peach, peeled and cut into 16 slices

In a food processor or blender, process 1 cup raspberries until smooth. Pour into a fine-mesh sieve. Holding the sieve over a small bowl, use the back of a spoon to press the raspberries

(continued)

through the sieve to remove the seeds. Discard the seeds. Pour the raspberries back into the food processor.

Add the yogurt. Process until smooth. Spoon into a freezer-proof bowl. Freeze, covered, for 6 to 8 hours, or until solid.

About 20 minutes before serving time, remove the raspberry mixture from the freezer. Let stand at room temperature to soften slightly. Spoon the mixture into the food processor and process, scraping the side once, until smooth.

Spoon about 3 tablespoons of the raspberry mixture into each parfait glass. Place 2 peach slices on the raspberry mixture. Repeat the layers. Spoon the remaining raspberry mixture onto each parfait. Garnish with the remaining 1/2 cup raspberries. Serve immediately.

Cook's Tip: If you prefer using frozen unsweetened raspberries instead of fresh, let them thaw until just icy. Using both the fruit and its juice, proceed as directed. Fresh raspberries, however, will make the most attractive garnish for topping the parfaits.

PER SERVING

calories 78	carbohydrates 16 g
total fat 0.5 g	fiber 4 g
saturated fat 0.0 g	sugars 12 g
trans fat 0.0 g	**protein** 4 g
polyunsaturated fat 0.0 g	**DIETARY EXCHANGES**
monounsaturated fat 0.0 g	1/2 fat-free milk,
cholesterol 2 mg	1/2 fruit
sodium 55 mg	

GINGER-BERRY WONTON BASKETS

MAKES 12; 2 PER SERVING

With its flavor flexibility from savory to sweet dishes, ginger is a perfect complement to the sweet tartness of the berries in this dish. Combined with the tang of lemon and the crunch of the baked wonton shell, this mini dessert makes a memorable mouthful.

Cooking spray
12 wonton wrappers

12 ounces frozen mixed berries, thawed and drained, 1/2 cup liquid reserved (squeezing from fruit as needed)
1 tablespoon plus 1 teaspoon sugar
1 1/2 teaspoons cornstarch
1 tablespoon fresh lemon juice
1/2 teaspoon ground ginger
8 sprigs of mint (optional)

Preheat the oven to 400°F. Lightly spray 12 cups of a 12-cup mini muffin pan with cooking spray.

Place the wonton wrappers in a single layer on a flat surface. Lightly spray both sides of the wrappers with cooking spray. Place a wonton wrapper in each muffin cup. Press down gently on the bottom of each so the wrappers mold to the shape of the cups and the tips point out in a decorative fashion.

Bake for 6 to 8 minutes, or until golden brown. Transfer the pan to a cooling rack. Let cool for at least 15 minutes before removing wonton baskets from the pan. Let wonton baskets cool completely.

Meanwhile, in a small saucepan, stir together the liquid from the berries, sugar, and cornstarch until the sugar and cornstarch are dissolved. Cook over medium heat for 10 to 12 minutes, or until the mixture has thickened, stirring occasionally. Stir in the thawed berries, lemon juice, and ginger. Cook for 3 to 5 minutes, or until the fruit is warm. Let cool slightly, about 5 minutes.

Spoon the berry mixture into the baskets. Garnish with the mint. Serve immediately.

PER SERVING

calories 128	sodium 15 mg
total fat 0.5 g	**carbohydrates** 30 g
saturated fat 0.0 g	fiber 3 g
trans fat 0.0 g	sugars 11 g
polyunsaturated fat 0.0 g	**protein** 3 g
monounsaturated fat 0.0 g	**DIETARY EXCHANGES**
cholesterol 2 mg	1 starch, 1 fruit

CINNAMON PECAN BAKED APPLES

SERVES 4

Fresh citrus and earthy spices stuff these warm nutty apples with a culinary treasure. Serve warm just as is or with a small scoop of fat-free, sugar-free vanilla ice cream or frozen yogurt on top.

1/4 cup uncooked oatmeal

1/4 cup chopped pecans or walnuts

1 teaspoon grated lemon zest

2 tablespoons fresh lemon Juice

2 teaspoons brown sugar

1 teaspoon ground cinnamon

1 teaspoon olive oil

1/2 teaspoon ground nutmeg

4 medium baking apples, such as Rome or Winesap, cored and seeded

1 cup fresh orange juice

Preheat the oven to 400°F.

In a small bowl, stir together the oatmeal, pecans, lemon zest, lemon juice, brown sugar, cinnamon, oil, and nutmeg.

Cut a small layer off the bottom of each apple to create a flat, stable surface. Put the apples upright in a 2-quart baking dish. Spoon the oatmeal mixture into the cavities of the apples. Pour the orange juice around the apples.

Bake for 1 hour, or until the apples are tender. Transfer the baking dish to a cooling rack. Let stand for 10 minutes. Reserve the juice.

Transfer the apples to shallow dessert bowls. Drizzle the juice over the apples.

Cook's Tip: To easily and safely check if the apples are done baking, use tongs to gently squeeze them. If they give, they are done.

PER SERVING

calories 212	**carbohydrates** 39 g
total fat 7.0 g	fiber 6 g
saturated fat 1.0 g	sugars 27 g
trans fat 0.0 g	**protein** 2 g
polyunsaturated fat 2.0 g	**DIETARY EXCHANGES**
monounsaturated fat 4.0 g	2 fruit, 1/2 other
cholesterol 0 mg	carbohydrate, 1 1/2 fat
sodium 3 mg	

ORANGE-POACHED ORANGES

SERVES 6

With its fresh, rich citrus flavors and simple, but elegant presentation, this dessert is a distinctive way to enjoy fruit.

2 1/2 cups fresh orange juice and (if needed) 1 cup fresh orange juice, divided use

1/2 cup orange liqueur, such as Grand Marnier (optional)

2 tablespoons sugar

1 cinnamon stick (about 3 inches long)

4 large seedless oranges, peeled and cut into 1/2-inch slices

In a medium saucepan, stir together 2 1/2 cups orange juice, the liqueur, sugar, and cinnamon stick. Bring to a simmer over medium heat, stirring until the sugar is dissolved.

Gently place the oranges in the orange juice mixture. If necessary, pour in enough of the remaining 1 cup orange juice to barely cover the oranges. Increase the heat to high and bring to a simmer. Reduce the heat and simmer for 5 to 7 minutes, or until the oranges are tender, stirring frequently.

Using a slotted spoon, transfer the oranges to dessert dishes.

Increase the heat to high and bring the orange juice mixture to a boil. Boil for 10 to 12 minutes, or until reduced by half (to about 1 1/2 cups), stirring constantly. Discard the cinnamon stick. Spoon the sauce over the oranges.

PER SERVING

calories 139	**sodium** 2 mg
total fat 0.5 g	**carbohydrates** 34 g
saturated fat 0.0 g	fiber 3 g
trans fat 0.0 g	sugars 28 g
polyunsaturated fat 0.0 g	**protein** 2 g
monounsaturated fat 0.0 g	**DIETARY EXCHANGES**
cholesterol 0 mg	2 fruit

BAKED GINGER PEARS

SERVES 8

These Asian-influenced pears are a perfect ending to stir-fry entrées, such as Chicken and Snow Pea Stir-Fry *(page 204) or* Asian Beef Stir-Fry *(page 264).*

8 canned pear halves in fruit juice, well
　　drained, juice reserved
1/3 cup firmly packed light brown sugar
2 tablespoons chopped pecans, dry-roasted
1 teaspoon fresh lemon juice
1/4 teaspoon ground ginger

Preheat the oven to 350°F.

Arrange the pears with the cut side up in a glass baking dish just large enough to hold them.

In a small bowl, stir together the brown sugar, pecans, lemon juice, and ginger. Spoon into the cavities of the pear halves.

Pour the reserved juice around the pears.

Bake for 15 to 20 minutes. Serve warm or cover and refrigerate to serve chilled.

MICROWAVE METHOD

Drain the juice from the pears, reserving 1 cup. Arrange the pear halves with the cut side up in a microwaveable glass pie pan. Prepare as directed. Microwave on 100 percent power (high) for 5 minutes. Let cool for at least 10 minutes before serving.

PER SERVING

calories 86	**carbohydrates** 19 g
total fat 1.5 g	fiber 1 g
saturated fat 0.0 g	sugars 17 g
trans fat 0.0 g	**protein** 0 g
polyunsaturated fat 0.5 g	**DIETARY EXCHANGES**
monounsaturated fat 0.5 g	1 fruit, 1/2 other
cholesterol 0 mg	carbohydrate
sodium 6 mg	

GRILLED PINEAPPLE

SERVES 6

When you've finished grilling your entrée, put some fruit on the grill for dessert. If you've tried pineapple, it's time to branch out to other seasonal fruits (see the Cook's Tip below). You can brush the lemon-honey mixture in this recipe on any of these alternatives.

1/4 cup honey
1/2 teaspoon grated lemon zest
1 tablespoon fresh lemon juice
1/4 teaspoon ground cinnamon
1 medium pineapple, peeled and cut into
　　12 spears

Preheat the grill on medium.

In a small bowl, stir together all the ingredients except the pineapple.

Grill the pineapple directly on the grill rack for 6 to 8 minutes, or until tender, turning once halfway through. Transfer to plates. Brush with the honey mixture. Serve immediately.

Cook's Tip for Grilled Fruit: For the best results, all fruit for grilling should be ripe but still firm. Peaches should be halved and pitted, then grilled for 8 to 10 minutes. Cut peeled mangoes lengthwise into slabs (about 4 per mango); grill for 4 to 6 minutes. Grill whole bananas or halve them lengthwise, then grill for 4 to 6 minutes. Regardless of the fruit you choose, turn it once about halfway through the grilling time.

PER SERVING

calories 119	**carbohydrates** 32 g
total fat 0.0 g	fiber 2 g
saturated fat 0.0 g	sugars 26 g
trans fat 0.0 g	**protein** 1 g
polyunsaturated fat 0.0 g	**DIETARY EXCHANGES**
monounsaturated fat 0.0 g	1 fruit, 1 other
cholesterol 0 mg	carbohydrate
sodium 2 mg	

SPICED SKILLET BANANAS

SERVES 4

Sample a taste of the Deep South with these bananas in a brown sugar glaze.

- 1 tablespoon light tub margarine
- 2 tablespoons dark brown sugar
- 1/4 teaspoon ground cinnamon
- 1/4 teaspoon ground nutmeg
- 2 cups sliced bananas (about 3 medium bananas)
- 1/4 cup chopped pecans, dry-roasted

In a large nonstick skillet over medium-high heat, melt the margarine, swirling to coat the bottom. Add the brown sugar, cinnamon, and nutmeg, stirring until the mixture is bubbly and the brown sugar is dissolved.

Add the bananas, stirring gently to coat. Cook for 3 minutes, or until just softened and beginning to glaze and turn golden. Don't overcook, or the bananas will break down. Remove from the heat.

Just before serving, sprinkle with the pecans. Serve immediately.

PER SERVING

calories 151	carbohydrates 25 g
total fat 6.5 g	fiber 3 g
saturated fat 0.5 g	sugars 16 g
trans fat 0.0 g	protein 2 g
polyunsaturated fat 2.0 g	DIETARY EXCHANGES
monounsaturated fat 3.5 g	1 fruit, 1/2 other
cholesterol 0 mg	carbohydrate, 1 fat
sodium 25 mg	

SPICED SKILLET APPLES

Replace the bananas with thinly sliced peeled apples, such as Red Delicious; the cinnamon and nutmeg with 3/4 teaspoon ground cumin; and the pecans with walnuts. Cook over medium heat for 6 to 8 minutes, or until the apples are just tender.

PER SERVING

calories 111	carbohydrates 15 g
total fat 6.0 g	fiber 1 g
saturated fat 0.5 g	sugars 13 g
trans fat 0.0 g	protein 1 g
polyunsaturated fat 3.5 g	DIETARY EXCHANGES
monounsaturated fat 1.5 g	1/2 fruit, 1/2 other
cholesterol 0 mg	carbohydrate, 1 fat
sodium 25 mg	

STRAWBERRY-RASPBERRY ICE

SERVES 8

A cool double dose of berries, this ice looks attractive in chilled wine or champagne glasses, garnished with sprigs of fresh mint.

- 6 ounces frozen 100% white grape juice concentrate
- 1 cup water
- 2 tablespoons confectioners' sugar
- 8 ounces frozen unsweetened strawberries, slightly thawed
- 6 ounces frozen unsweetened raspberries, slightly thawed
- 6 ice cubes (about 1 cup), slightly chopped
- Sprigs of fresh mint (optional)

In a food processor or blender, combine all the ingredients except the mint in the order listed. Process until smooth (except for the seeds), stirring occasionally. Pour into a large resealable plastic freezer bag and seal tightly. Place the bag on its side in the freezer and let the mixture freeze solid, at least 2 hours.

About 15 minutes before serving, remove the bag from the freezer and let the ice thaw slightly, mashing with a fork if necessary. At serving time, spoon into chilled glasses. Garnish with the mint sprigs. Serve immediately.

PER SERVING

calories 91	sodium 2 mg
total fat 0.0 g	carbohydrates 23 g
saturated fat 0.0 g	fiber 2 g
trans fat 0.0 g	sugars 19 g
polyunsaturated fat 0.0 g	protein 0 g
monounsaturated fat 0.0 g	DIETARY EXCHANGES
cholesterol 0 mg	1 1/2 fruit

FROZEN BANANA-ORANGE PUSH-UPS

MAKES 6; 1 PER SERVING

The kid-friendly flavors and the fun way to eat this treat make this an easy way to get your children to eat more fruit!

2 medium bananas, sliced
6 ounces frozen 100% orange juice
    concentrate, thawed
1/2 cup fat-free dry milk
1/2 cup water
1 cup fat-free plain Greek yogurt

In a food processor or blender, process all the in-gredients for 2 to 3 minutes, or until foamy. Pour into six small paper cups. Freeze for 2 to 3 hours, or until frozen.

To eat, squeeze the bottom of the cup.

Cook's Tip: This recipe is also delicious with pine-apple juice concentrate instead of orange.

PER SERVING

calories 135	sodium 50 mg
total fat 0.5 g	**carbohydrates** 27 g
saturated fat 0.0 g	fiber 1 g
trans fat 0.0 g	sugars 22 g
polyunsaturated fat 0.0 g	**protein** 7 g
monounsaturated fat 0.0 g	**DIETARY EXCHANGES**
cholesterol 2 mg	1 fruit, 1 lean meat

APPLE PIE POPS

MAKES 10; 1 PER SERVING

This frozen delight is so simple you'll want to keep it on hand all year round. Pop the filled frozen ice cube tray in a cooler to bring as a refreshing snack when the kids are finished with sports practice or playing in the park.

4 cups 100% apple juice
1 cup unsweetened applesauce
1 to 2 teaspoons apple pie spice, or to taste
3 tablespoons graham cracker crumbs

In a medium bowl, whisk together the apple juice, applesauce, and apple pie spice. Sprinkle the graham cracker crumbs into 10 sections of an ice cube tray. Pour the apple juice mixture over the crumbs. Freeze for 1 to 2 hours, or until partially frozen.

Insert a wood, paper, or plastic dessert stick (that's not pointed) into each pop. Freeze completely.

PER SERVING

calories 65	sodium 14 mg
total fat 0.5 g	**carbohydrates** 16 g
saturated fat 0.0 g	fiber 1 g
trans fat 0.0 g	sugars 12 g
polyunsaturated fat 0.0 g	**protein** 0 g
monounsaturated fat 0.0 g	**DIETARY EXCHANGES**
cholesterol 0 mg	1 fruit

WATERMELON-CILANTRO SORBET

SERVES 12

A scoop of chilled watermelon sorbet is a perfect way to cool down on a hot summer's day.

1/3 cup sugar
1/3 cup water
8 cups cubed seedless watermelon (about
    half of 1 20-pound watermelon)
1/2 cup fresh lime juice (about 4 large limes)
1/4 cup tequila (optional)
1/4 cup minced fresh cilantro and
    1 tablespoon minced fresh cilantro,
    divided use
1 large lime, cut into 12 thin slices, each slice
    notched with 1/4-inch cut

In a small saucepan, stir together the sugar and water. Bring to a boil over medium-high heat. Reduce the heat and simmer for 2 to 3 minutes, stirring constantly until the sugar is dissolved. Remove from the heat.

Pour the liquid into a small bowl. Cover and re-frigerate for 10 to 15 minutes, or until cool.

In a large bowl, stir together the cooled sugar mixture, watermelon, lime juice, and tequila.

Ladle half the mixture into a food processor or blender. Process until smooth. Pour the mixture into a separate large bowl. Process the remaining watermelon mixture then pour it into the large bowl to combine all the watermelon mixture. Gently stir in 1/4 cup cilantro.

Transfer the mixture to a 13 x 9 x 2-inch metal pan. Cover with plastic wrap and freeze for about 2 hours, or until the top layer of the mixture is frozen.

Remove from the freezer. Using a large spoon or fork, lightly scrape the top layer. Re-cover the pan and return to the freezer. Allow the top layer to refreeze for about 30 minutes.

Again remove from the freezer. Repeat the scraping of the frozen top layer. Again re-cover the pan and return to the freezer.

Repeat the scraping and refreezing process until the sorbet is fluffy and light pink, about 2 hours total.

At serving time, spoon 1/2 cup sorbet into sherbet or parfait glasses. Sprinkle with the remaining 1 tablespoon cilantro. Garnish the rim of each glass with a lime slice.

Cook's Tip: For a quicker result, pour the processed watermelon mixture into an ice cream/sorbet maker. Freeze according to the manufacturer's directions.

Cook's Tip: For a cool and icy summer treat, pour the processed watermelon mixture into ice pop molds. (Omit the tequila for children's pops.)

PER SERVING

calories 55	sodium 2 mg
total fat 0.0 g	carbohydrates 14 g
saturated fat 0.0 g	fiber 1 g
trans fat 0.0 g	sugars 12 g
polyunsaturated fat 0.0 g	protein 1 g
monounsaturated fat 0.0 g	**DIETARY EXCHANGES**
cholesterol 0 mg	1 fruit

COFFEE AND CREAM SORBET

SERVES 6

Here's a way of using up the extra coffee from your morning pot. Skip buying an expensive cold coffee drink from your local shop that's full of fat and sugar and instead make your own version by adding a serving of sorbet to a glass of unsweetened iced coffee.

1 1/2 cups strong dark coffee, warmed
1/4 cup light corn syrup
2 tablespoons fat-free half-and-half
1 tablespoon coffee liqueur (optional)

In a medium bowl, whisk together the coffee and corn syrup until the corn syrup is dissolved. Cover and refrigerate until cold.

Stir the half-and-half and liqueur into the coffee mixture.

Pour the coffee mixture into an ice cream maker. Freeze according to the manufacturer's directions.

At serving time, spoon 1/3 cup sorbet into sherbet or parfait glasses.

Cook's Tip: The sorbet will be soft when it comes out of the ice cream machine. Freeze it for 2 to 3 hours for a firmer texture.

PER SERVING

calories 45	sodium 15 mg
total fat 0.0 g	carbohydrates 12 g
saturated fat 0.0 g	fiber 0 g
trans fat 0.0 g	sugars 12 g
polyunsaturated fat 0.0 g	protein 0 g
monounsaturated fat 0.0 g	**DIETARY EXCHANGES**
cholesterol 0 mg	1 other carbohydrate

COFFEE AND CREAM GRANITA

Follow the directions for the sorbet, thoroughly combining the half-and-half and liqueur with the coffee mixture. Pour the coffee mixture into an 8-inch square metal pan. Freeze for 2 to 4 hours, scraping the mixture every 30 minutes with a fork, until slushy and smooth.

(continued)

Cook's Tip: The granita has larger ice crystals than the sorbet so it will have a more granular texture. For best results, serve either the sorbet or the granita the day it is made.

SUNNY MANGO SORBET

SERVES 4

Thick, creamy, rich, tart, and sweet—this super-simple sorbet is all these! Enjoy after Tandoori-Spiced Swordfish-and-Vegetable Kebabs *(page 156)* or Indonesian Chicken Curry *(page 227).*

> 4 cups coarsely chopped mangoes (about 5 medium)
> 1/2 cup fresh lime juice (about 4 large limes)
> 2 tablespoons sugar

In a food processor or blender, process the ingredients until smooth. Pour into a large resealable plastic freezer bag and seal tightly. Place the bag on its side in the freezer for about 2 hours, or until the mixture is thick. If frozen solid, remove the bag from the freezer about 30 minutes before serving time. Stir the sorbet before serving.

Cook's Tip: If you want a completely smooth sorbet, strain the processed mixture before freezing.

PER SERVING

calories 131	**sodium** 2 mg
total fat 0.5 g	**carbohydrates** 34 g
saturated fat 0.0 g	fiber 3 g
trans fat 0.0 g	sugars 29 g
polyunsaturated fat 0.0 g	**protein** 2 g
monounsaturated fat 0.0 g	**DIETARY EXCHANGES**
cholesterol 0 mg	2 fruit

CHERRY-BERRY CHILL

SERVES 8

This dessert has the texture of soft-serve ice cream, and it's a refreshing way to incorporate more fruit into your day.

> 1 pound frozen unsweetened mixed berries
> 3/4 cup 100% white grape juice
> 1/3 cup sugar
> 1/4 cup fat-free half-and-half
> 2 teaspoons vanilla extract
> 8 ounces frozen unsweetened pitted dark (sweet) cherries, partially thawed

In a food processor or blender, process all the ingredients except the cherries until smooth.

Add the cherries. Process until smooth. Serve immediately for soft serve or transfer to an airtight freezer container and freeze for at least 4 hours. If frozen, let stand at room temperature for 15 minutes before serving for peak flavor and texture.

PER SERVING

calories 98	**carbohydrates** 25 g
total fat 0.0 g	fiber 2 g
saturated fat 0.0 g	sugars 21 g
trans fat 0.0 g	**protein** 1 g
polyunsaturated fat 0.0 g	**DIETARY EXCHANGES**
monounsaturated fat 0.0 g	1 fruit, 1/2 other
cholesterol 0 mg	carbohydrate
sodium 9 mg	

Index

S

saffron, cook's tip on, 423

salad dressings
Chunky Cucumber and Garlic Dressing, 106
Lemon Dressing, 106
Poppy Seed Dressing with Kiwifruit, 105
Zesty Tomato Dressing, 105

salad greens
Arugula Salad with Roasted Beets and Pomegranate Vinaigrette, 67
Asian Beef Lettuce Wraps with Vietnamese Dipping Sauce, 270
Cajun Chicken Salad, 96
Chef's Salad, 100
Eight-Layer Salad, 101
Fattoush Salad, 70
French Peas, 396
Ginger-Infused Watermelon and Mixed Berries, 87
Hot and Spicy Arugula and Romaine Salad, 71
Layered Taco Salad with Tortilla Chips, 98
Mexican Shrimp Salad, 95
Orange Chicken Lettuce Wraps, 19
Roasted Beet Salad, 74
Salmon and Spring Greens with Tangy-Sweet Dressing, 93
Southwestern Pork Salad, 99

salads, list of recipes, 65–66

salmon
Baked Salmon with Cucumber Relish, 147
Broiled Salmon over Garden-Fresh Corn and Bell Peppers, 149
Broiled Salmon with Minty Citrus Relish, 148
Ginger-Walnut Salmon and Asparagus, 146
Grilled Pineapple-Lime Salmon, 150
Grilled Salmon with Cilantro Sauce, 150
Salmon and Orzo Salad, 93
Salmon and Spring Greens with Tangy-Sweet Dressing, 93
Salmon Cakes with Creole Aïoli, 151
Salmon Fillets with Mango-Strawberry Salsa, 148
Salmon with Cucumber-Dill Sauce, 147
Sesame-Orange Salmon, 151
Smoked Salmon Party Dip, 12

sandwiches and wraps
Chicken Gyros with Tzatziki Sauce, 223
Chipotle Chicken Wraps, 196
Creole Tuna Steak Sandwich with Caper Tartar Sauce, 165
Meatball Sliders with Beer Sauce, 20
Meatball Wrap, 282
Peanut Butter and Banana Waffle Sandwiches, 469
Philadelphia-Style Cheese Steak Wraps, 259
Southwestern Turkey Wraps, 241
Spicy Tuna Pitas, 168

Sardines, Sautéed Lemon-Garlic, and Fennel with Fettuccine, 152

saturated fats, limiting, 4–5

sauces, list of recipes, 427

sauerkraut
Cabbage Rolls with Sauerkraut, 276
Pork with Spiced Sauerkraut, 289

sausages
Baked Tilapia with Sausage-Flecked Rice, 157
bulk, cook's tip on, 158
Country-Style Breakfast Casserole, 473
Paella, 220
Stacked Sausage and Eggs, 476

scallops
Linguine with Scallops and Asparagus, 171
Oven-Fried Scallops with Cilantro and Lime, 170
Scallops in White Wine, 173

Scones, Lemon and Poppy Seed, 462

seafood. See fish; shellfish

seeds, adding to diet, 4

seitan
Louisiana Gumbo with Seitan, 366
Roasted Seitan and Vegetables with Cranberry–Red Wine Sauce, 365
Veggie Tacos with Seitan, 366

serving sizes, 6

shallots, cook's tip on, 248

shellfish
Linguine with White Clam Sauce, 168
Oven-Fried Oysters, 172
see also crabmeat; scallops; shrimp

shrimp
Curried Shrimp Risotto, 175
Fiery Shrimp Dijon, 175

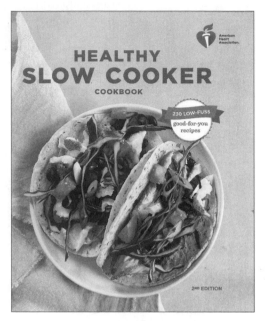
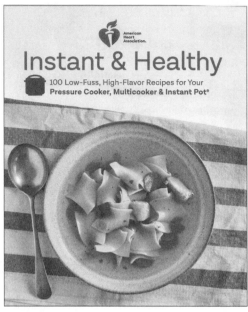
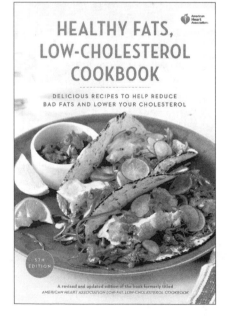
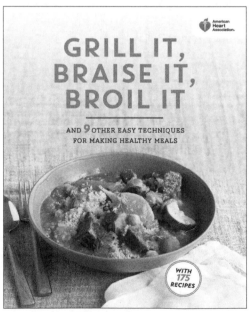